Laboratory Haematology
An Account of Laboratory Techniques

MURRAYFIELD HOSPITAL
122 CORSTORPHINE ROAD
EDINBURGH EH12 6UD
Tel: 031-334 0363

Laboratory Haematology
An Account of Laboratory Techniques

EDITED BY

I. Chanarin BSc MD FRCPath
Head of the Section of Haematology, MRC Clinical Research Centre, Harrow, Middlesex;
Consultant Haematologist, Northwick Park Hospital, Harrow, Middlesex, UK

SECTION EDITORS

J. C. Cawley MD PhD MRCPath FRCP
Professor of Haematology, University of Liverpool, Liverpool, UK

I. Chanarin BSc MD FRCPath
Head of the Section of Haematology, MRC Clinical Research Centre, Harrow, Middlesex;
Consultant Haematologist, Northwick Park Hospital, Harrow, Middlesex, UK

Marcela Contreras MD
Director, North London Blood Transfusion Centre; Honorary Senior Lecturer,
Department of Haematology, St Mary's Hospital Medical School, London, UK

Robin C. Knight FIMLS
Senior Chief MLSO, North London Blood Transfusion Centre; Visiting Lecturer (Transfusion Sciences),
Paddington College, London, UK

Samuel J. Machin MB MRCPath
Consultant Haematologist, The Middlesex Hospital, London, UK

Ian J. Mackie BSc FIMLS
Lecturer in Haematology, The Middlesex Hospital, London, UK

D.A.W. Waters FIMLS
Principal MLSO, Northwick Park Hospital, Harrow, Middlesex, UK

Colin P. Worman BA PhD
Senior Biochemist, Department of Haematology, University College Hospital,
London, UK

CHURCHILL LIVINGSTONE
EDINBURGH LONDON MELBOURNE AND NEW YORK 1989

CHURCHILL LIVINGSTONE
Medical Division of Longman Group UK Limited

Distributed in the United States of America by Churchill
Livingstone Inc., 1560 Broadway, New York, N.Y. 10036,
and by associated companies, branches and representatives
throughout the world.

ISBN 0-443-03343-9

First edition 1989

British Library Cataloguing in Publication Data
Laboratory haematology: an account of laboratory techniques
    1. Man. Blood. Diagnosis. Laboratory techniques
    I. Chanarin, I. (Israel)
    616.1′5075

Library of Congress Cataloging in Publication Data
Laboratory haematology: an account of laboratory techniques

    Includes index.
    1. Blood — Examination.   2. Hematology — Technique.
    3. Diagnosis, Laboratory.   I. Chanarin, I. (Israel)
[DNLM: 1. Hematologic Diseases — diagnosis.
2. Hematologic Diseases — therapy.   3. Hematology —
methods. WH 100 L126]
RB45.L23   1989   616.1′5   88-28490

Produced by Longman Group (FE) Ltd
Printed in Hong Kong

Preface

'It is a truth universally acknowledged that a single man in possession of a good fortune must be in want of a wife'.

Jane Austen,
Pride and Prejudice.

Another truth perhaps not as widely acknowledged is that the best account of how to carry out and interpret the wide range of investigations required in modern haematology can only be provided by the co-operation of medical and laboratory scientists. This has formed the basis of this book. Each of the four major sections, red cells, white cells, haemostasis and immunohaematology has been edited by a doctor and senior technologist.

Each method has been contributed by a doctor/technologist team which has a special interest in the method and in the related disorders. In this way it is hoped that the technical details of performance will be derived from experience at the bench and indications and interpretation of the data will carry the hallmark of clinical experience.

This text is the result of immense team work by many contributors. The editors would be grateful to receive advice of error of any kind that may have crept into the text as well as suggestions for improvements in future editions.

Harrow, Middlesex, 1989   I. C.

Contributors

ERYTHROCYTES SECTION 1

Edited by I. Chanarin, D. A. W. Waters

Susan P. Baker BSc MSc FIMLS
Senior Biochemist, Department of Chemical
Pathology, Queen Charlotte's Hospital, London, UK

Ian C. Barr FIMLS
Chief MLSO, Department of Clinical Chemistry,
Northwick Park Hospital, Harrow, Middlesex, UK

M. Bartlett
Brooklyn Veterans Administration, Downstate Medical
Centre, Brooklyn, New York, USA

C. S. Bowring BSc PhD CPhys MInstP
Principal Physicist, Exeter Health Authority;
Honorary Research Fellow, University of Exeter,
Exeter, UK

Brian S. Bull MD
Professor and Chairman, Department of Pathology,
Loma Linda University School of Medicine, Loma
Linda, California, USA

I. Chanarin BSc MD FRCPath
Head, Section of Haematology, MRC Clinical
Research Centre; Consultant Haematologist,
Northwick Park Hospital, Harrow, Middlesex, UK

Bernard A. Cooper MD FRCP(C) FACP
Professor, McGill University, Montreal; Director,
Hematology and Medical Oncology, Royal Victoria
Hospital, Montreal, Quebec, Canada

Maria da Costa MD
Chief of Hematology, City Hospital Center at
Elmhurst; Professor of Medicine, The City University
of New York, New York, USA

John H. Darley FIMLS
Department of Haematology, John Radcliffe Hospital,
Oxford, UK

Pauline M. Emerson MD FRCPath
Consultant Haematologist, John Radcliffe Hospital,
Oxford, UK

Karen Hay MS MT(ASCP)
Clinical Instructor, School of Allied Health
Professions, Loma Linda University, Loma Linda,
California, USA

Erika Jones
Royal Victoria Hospital, McGill University, Montreal,
Canada

Elizabeth A. Letsky MB BS FRCPath
Consultant Haematologist, Hammersmith and Queen
Charlotte's Special Health Royal Postgraduate Medical
School, Hammersmith Hospital, London, UK

J. H. Matthews MA MRCP MRCPath
Senior Lecturer in Haematology, St Mary's Hospital
Medical School, London, UK

M. J. Muir
MRC Clinical Research Centre, Northwick Park
Hospital, Harrow, Middlesex, UK

E. J. Parker-Williams MB BS FRCPath
Senior Lecturer in Haematology, St George's Hospital
Medical School; Honorary Consultant Haematologist,
St George's Hospital, London, UK

Martin J. Pippard BSc MB ChB MRCP (UK)
MRCPath
Consultant Haematologist, MRC Clinical Research
Centre, Northwick Park Hospital, Harrow, Middlesex,
UK

M. G. Rinsler MD FRCPath
Consultant Chemical Pathologist, Northwick Park
Hospital, Harrow, Middlesex, UK

Mary Rossi BA
Staff Research Associate, MacMillan-Cargill
Hematology Research Laboratory, Cancer Research
Institute, San Francisco, California, USA

J. A. Sharpe
MLSO, MRC Molecular Haematology Unit, John
Radcliffe Hospital, Oxford, UK

J. Sheerman-Chase FIMLS
Chief MLSO, Haematology Department, Queen
Charlotte's Maternity Hospital, London, UK

S. B. Shohet MD
Professor of Laboratory Medicine and Medicine;
Director, MacMillan-Cargill Hematology Research
Laboratory, University of California, San Francisco,
USA

A. D. Stephens MD FRCPath
Consultant Haematologist, St Bartholomew's Hospital,
London, UK

P. C. W. Stone
Senior MLSO, Department of Haematology,
University of Birmingham, Birmingham, UK

John Stuart MD FRCP FRCPath
Head of Department of Haematology, University of
Birmingham; Consultant Haematologist, Queen
Elizabeth Hospital, Birmingham, UK

Jaak Tikerpäe MSc
Senior Research Officer, Clinical Research Centre,
Harrow, Middlesex, UK

David C. Warhurst BSc PhD MRCPath
Honorary Microbiologist, PHLS Malaria Reference
Laboratory; Senior Lecturer, Department of Medical
Protozoology, London School of Hygiene and Tropical
Medicine, London, UK

D. A. W. Waters FIMLS
Principal MLSO, Northwick Park Hospital, Harrow,
Middlesex, UK

S. N. Wickramasinghe ScD MRCP FRCPath FIBiol
Professor of Haematology, St Mary's Hospital Medical
School, University of London, London, UK

Barbara J. Wild PhD
Senior Chief MLSO, Haemoglobulin Laboratory,
Department of Haematology, St Bartholomew's
Hospital, London, UK

J. E. Williams CBiol MIBiol AIMLS
Senior Chief MLSO, Department of Medical
Parasitology, London School of Hygiene and Tropical
Medicine, London, UK

W. G. Wood BSc PhD
MRC Staff Scientist, Molecular Haematology Unit,
John Radcliffe Hospital, Oxford, UK

LEUCOCYTES SECTION 2

Edited by J. C. Cawley and C. P. Worman

I. E. Addison PhD
Senior Biochemist, Department of Haematology,
University College Hospital, London, UK

Glen C. Begley MB BS FRACP
Research Fellow, Walter and Eliza Hall Institute of
Medical Research, Royal Melbourne Hospital,
Victoria, Australia

Gordon F. Burns PhD
Assistant Director of Research, Division of
Immunology, Institute of Medical and Veterinary
Science, Adelaide, Australia

Dario Campana MD
Lecturer in Immunology, Royal Free Hospital Medical
School, London, UK

J. C. Cawley MD PhD MRCPath FRCP
Professor of Haematology, University of Liverpool,
Liverpool, UK

I. Chanarin BSc MD FRCPath
Consultant Haematologist; Head, Section of
Haematology, MRC Clinical Research Centre,
Northwick Park Hospital, Harrow, Middlesex, UK

Elaine Coustan-Smith FIMLS Haematology, FIMLS
Immunology
Chief MLSO, Department of Immunology, Royal Free
Hospital, London, UK

Wendy N. Erber MB BS DPhil
Haematology Registrar, Royal North Shore Hospital,
Sydney, Australia

R. J. Flemans
Consultant Technical Adviser, Department of
Haematological Medicine, Cambridge University,
Cambridge, UK

Rodolfo C. Garcia PhD
Research Fellow, Department of Medicine, University
College and Middlesex School of Medicine, London,UK

F. G. J. Hayhoe MA MD FRCP FRCPath
Leukaemia Research Fund Professor of
Haematological Medicine, Cambridge University,
Cambridge, UK

George Janossy MD PhD MRCPath DSc
Professor of Immunology, Royal Free Hospital,
London, UK

H. M. Jones FIMLS
Senior MLSO, Department of Haematology,
University College and Middlesex School of Medicine,
London, UK

F. Lauriola Dip Appl Sci
Laboratory Technician, Walter and Eliza Hall
Institute of Medical Research, Royal Melbourne
Hospital, Victoria, Australia

D. Y. Mason DM FRCPath
Lecturer in Haematology, Medical School, University
of Oxford, Oxford, UK

Donald Metcalf MD FRACS FRCPA FAA FRS
Research Professor of Cancer Biology, Walter and
Eliza Hall Institute of Medical Research, Royal
Melbourne Hospital, Victoria, Australia

A. W. Segal MB ChB MD DSc PhD FRCP
Charles Dent Professor of Medicine, University
College and Middlesex School of Medicine,
London, UK

J. L. Smith PhD MRCPath
Head of Wessex Regional Immunology Services,
Southampton General Hospital, Southampton, UK

Freda K. Stevenson MSc DPhil
Top Grade Biochemist, Regional Immunology Service,
Southampton General Hospital; Honorary Visiting
Fellow, University of Southampton, Southampton,
UK

C. A. Strange FIMLS
Chief MLSO, Department of Haematology, Royal
Liverpool Hospital, Liverpool, UK

A. M. Timms BSc FIMLS
Chief MLSO, Department of Immunology, Royal Free
Hospital Medical School, London, UK

Colin P. Worman BA PhD
Senior Biochemist, Department of Haematology,
University College Hospital, London, UK

HAEMOSTASIS SECTION 3

Edited by S. J. Machin, I. J. Mackie

H. Bull BSc PhD
Research Fellow, Department of Haematology, The
Middlesex Hospital, London, UK

Judith Chapman FIMLS
Senior Chief MLSO, Blood Transfusion Department,
St Bartholomew's Hospital, London, UK

Hannah Cohen MB ChB MRCP MRCPath
Clinical Research Associate, Department of
Haematology, The Middlesex Hospital, London, UK

Robert G. Dalton MB MRCP MRCPath
Research Fellow, Haemophilia Centre, St Thomas'
Hospital, London, UK

Paul Harrison BSc
Research Associate, Haemophilia Centre, St Thomas'
Hospital, London, UK

Leslie Holland MSc FIMLS
Chief MLSO, Haemophilia Centre, St Thomas'
Hospital, London, UK

Samuel J. Machin MB MRCPath
Consultant Haematologist, The Middlesex Hospital,
London, UK

Ian J. Mackie BSc FIMLS
Lecturer in Haematology, The Middlesex Hospital,
London, UK

P. Metcalfe BTech (Hons)
Senior MLSO, Blood Transfusion Department,
St Bartholomew's Hospital, London, UK

Michael Murphy MRCP MRCPath
Senior Lecturer in Haematology and Honorary
Consultant, St Bartholomew's Hospital, London, UK

A. M. Peters BSc MD MRCPath MSc (Neul Med)
Senior Lecturer in Diagnostic Radiology, Royal
Postgraduate Medical School; Honorary Consultant in
Diagnostic Radiology, Hammersmith Hospital and in
Paediatric Radiology, Hospital for Sick Children,
London, UK

R. H. Saundry MSc PhD
Senior Biochemist, Division of Haematology, St
Thomas' Hospital, London, UK

G. F. Savidge BA MB BChir MA MD
Haemophilia Centre Director, St Thomas' Hospital,
London, UK

Martin J. Shearer BSc PhD
Principal Biochemist, Haematology Department, Guy's
Hospital, London, UK

Yvonne Stirling FIMLS
Senior Chief MLSO, Coagulation Laboratory, MRC
Epidemiology and Medical Care Unit, Northwick Park
Hospital, Harrow, Middlesex, UK

Dominic Wall BSc
Research Fellow, Department of Haematology, The
Middlesex Hospital, London, UK

K. Walshe FIMLS
Research Fellow, Department of Haematology, The
Middlesex Hospital, London, UK

Anne Yardumian MB MRCP
Research Fellow, Haematology Department, The
Middlesex Hospital, London, UK

IMMUNOHAEMATOLOGY SECTION 4

Edited by M. Contreras, R. C. Knight

Malcolm L. Beck FIMLS MIBiol
Technical Director, Community Blood Center of
Greater Kansas City, Kansas City, Missouri, USA

G. W. G. Bird DSc FRCPath
Director, Blood Group Reference Laboratory, Oxford;
Honorary Consultant, Blood Transfusion Service,
Birmingham, UK

Albert E. G. von dem Borne MD PhD
Senior Investigator, Department of Immunological
Haematology, Central Laboratory Department of
Haematology, Academic Medical Centre, Amsterdam,
The Netherlands

Marcela Contreras MD
Director, North London Blood Transfusion Centre;
Honorary Senior Lecturer, Department of
Haematology, St Mary's Hospital Medical School,
London, UK

C. M. van Dalen
Department of Immunohaematology, Central
Laboratory of the Netherlands Red Cross Blood
Transfusion Service, Amsterdam, The Netherlands

Hilliard Festenstein MB ChB DipBact FRCPath
MRCPath FIBiol
Professor of Immunology, London Hospital Medical
College, London, UK

Robin C. Knight FIMLS
Senior Chief MLSO, North London Blood
Transfusion Centre; Visiting Lecturer (Transfusion
Sciences) Paddington College, London, UK

Cristina Navarrete PhD
Lecturer, Department of Immunology, London
Hospital Medical College, London, UK

Willem Hendrik Ouwehand MD PhD
Department of Immunohaematology, Central
Laboratory of the Netherlands Red Cross Blood
Transfusion Service, Amsterdam, The Netherlands

Fred V. Plapp MD PhD
Director of Hematology, Immunology, and
Transfusion Service, and Clinical Pathologist, St
Luke's Hospital, Kansas City, Missouri, USA

Contents

PLATE 1

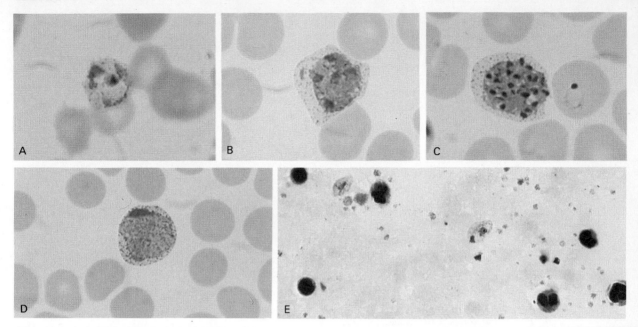

Plate 1.1 A *P. vivax* trophozoite (× 520).
B *P. vivax* developing schizont (× 520).
C *P. vivax* mature schizont and young trophozoite (× 520).
D *P. vivax* gametocyte (× 520).
E *P. vivax* thick blood film (× 160).

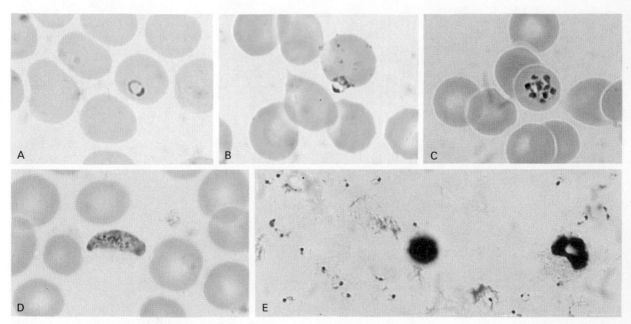

Plate 1.2 A *P. falciparum* ring form (× 520).
B *P. falciparum* young trophozoite (accole form) with clefts (× 520).
C *P. falciparum* developing schizont (× 520).
D *P. falciparum* gametocyte (× 520).
E *P. falciparum* thick blood film (× 260).

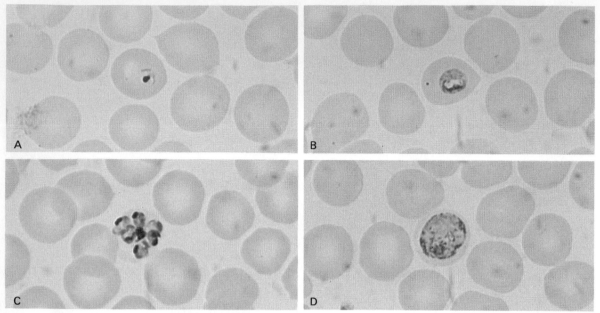

Plate 1.3 A *P. malariae* 'birds-eye' ring (× 520).
             B *P. malariae* compact trophozoite (× 520).
             C *P. malariae* schizont (× 520).
             D *P. malariae* gametocyte (× 520).

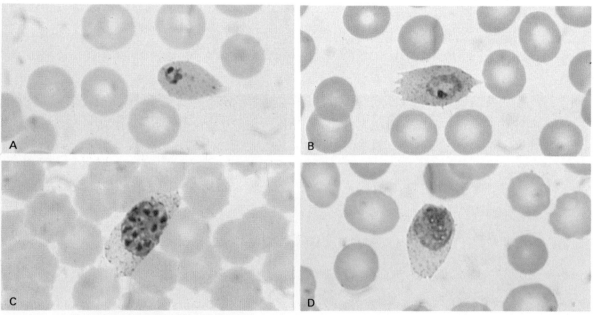

Plate 1.4 A *P. ovale* young trophozoite (× 520).
             B *P. ovale* mature trophozoite (× 520).
             C *P. ovale* mature schizont (× 520).
             D *P. ovale* gametocyte (× 520).

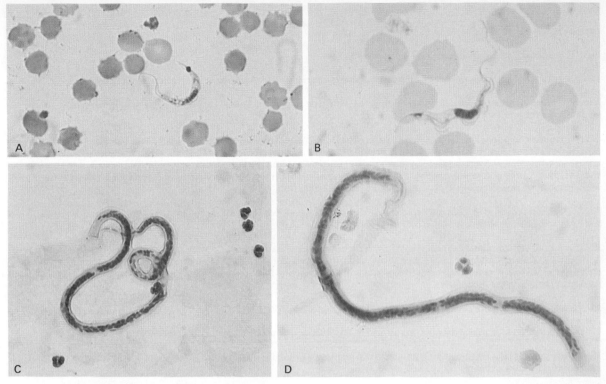

1.5 A *T. cruzi* in blood (mouse) (× 320).
B *T. b. rhodesiense* in blood (× 520).
C *L. loa* microfilaria in thick blood film (× 128).
D *L. loa* microfilaria in thick blood film (× 160).

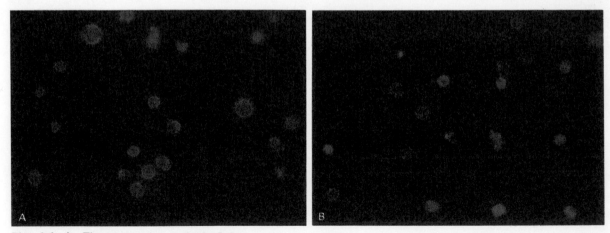

Plate 1.6 A Fluorescence due to platelet IgG.
B Fluorescence due to chloroquine damage.

PLATE 2

Figs. 1–19.

1–3. Romanowsky stains of normal bone marrow cells.

1. Leishman stain: good colours but weak granule staining especially of azurophil and neutrophil specific granules.

2 & 3. Heyl stain: strong colour characteristics shown with good staining of azurophil promyelocyte granules and most later granulocyte neutrophil specific granules.

4–7. A sequence of Sudan black (SB), benzidine peroxidase, diaminobenzidine peroxidase (DAB) and 3-amino-9-ethyl carbazole peroxidase (3AC) in normal buffy coat leucocytes. Monocyte granules are shown best in SB, the benzidine peroxidase is heavy but diffuse in neutrophils and weak diffuse in monocytes, DAB gives a crisp granular pattern, most like SB but darker in monocytes, and 3AC gives strong neutrophil reactions with local diffusion, weaker reactions in monocytes but again with some diffuse spread, and a notable reaction in lymphocytes and around a platelet clump.

8–11. A similar sequence in a strongly reacting AML (with 8;21 translocation). All reactions are strong, SB the heaviest and DAB and 3AC both show Auer rods.

12–15. A third similar sequence in an AMML with numerous monoblasts; the SB shows strong reactions with some localised positivity and scattered granules in two monoblasts and parts of two more at the edge, and heavy positivity in an early eosinophil. Of the three peroxidase reactions, each shows a similarly heavy reaction in an eosinophil precursor, but negative or only weak and localised reactions in the monoblasts.

16. Heavy overall positivity to SB in acute promyelocytic leukaemia (APL).

17. Scattered discrete granular positivity to SB in AMML with predominance of maturing promonocytes.

18. Mixed sudanophilia, with scattered granules in monoblasts and localised reaction in myeloblasts in AMML with both granulocyte and monocyte precursors, well represented.

19. Localised strong cytoplasmic sudanophilia in the myeloblasts of a mixed erythroleukaemia; erythroblasts are negative.

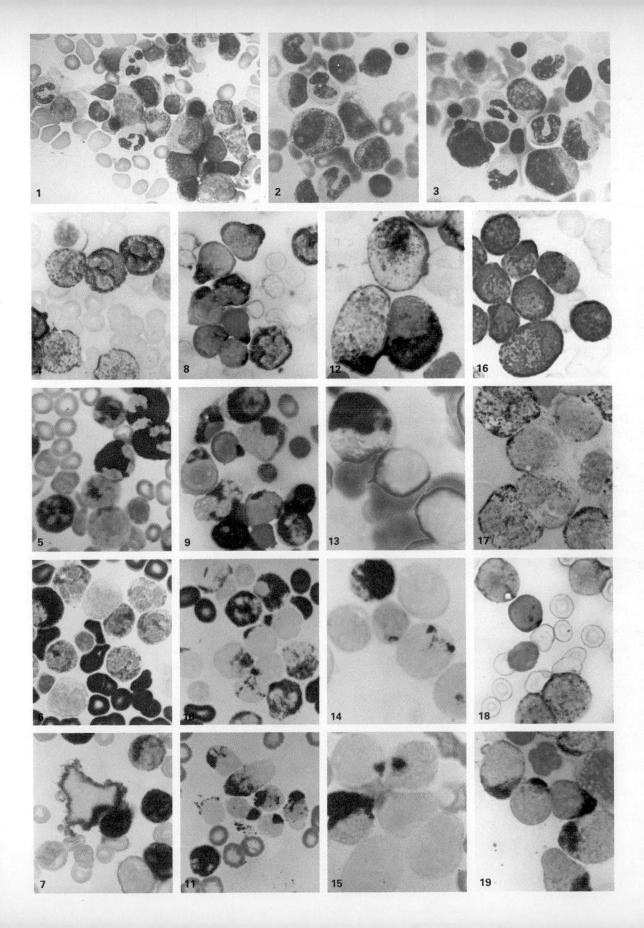

PLATE 2 (contd)

Figs. 20–37.

20. PAS reaction in normal bone marrow showing increasing diffuse and granular positivity in granulocytes with increasing maturity: the erythroblast is negative.

21–28. PAS reactions in various myeloid leukaemia states.

21. AML with minimal maturation: largely PAS negative (there is a normally reacting neutrophil polymorph present).

22. AML with some maturation: a weak diffuse tinge is found in the cytoplasm of most blast cells.

23. APL with strong diffuse and finely granular positivity.

24. AMML with some diffuse tinging of both granulocyte and monocyte precursors.

25 & 26. Extremes of PAS reactivity in predominantly monoblastic AMML: reactions may range from almost negative with possible weak diffuse tinge as in Plate 2.25, to coarse granular positivity, usually on a diffusely tinged background, as in Plate 2.26.

27. A combined SB and PAS stain in a mixed myeloid leukaemia with megakaryoblastic component. Granulocyte and monocyte precursors show mixed SB and PAS reactions; the megakaryocyte precursors show coarse granular PAS reaction with diffuse background staining.

28. PAS reaction in an erythroleukaemia; erythroid precursors from proerythroblast to late normoblast are shown, most with strong PAS positivity, ranging from coarse granularity in early and intermediate erythroblasts to a weak or moderate tinge in late normoblasts, several of which show nuclear rosette formation. The accompanying PAS-negative blast cells are myeloblasts.

29. Dual esterase reaction in normal bone marrow cells; granulocytes and their precursors show bright blue positivity to chloroacetate esterase (CE) while two monocytes show butyrate esterase (BE) positivity as a reddish brown colour. Erythroblasts are negative.

30–37. Dual esterase reactions in various myeloid leukaemic states. Plate 2.34 is from a preparation stained by the single incubation method using Fast Blue B as receptor for both esterase reactions. The remaining stains are with the double incubation procedure with Fast Blue B for CE and Fast Garnet GBC for BE.

30 & 31. APL showing CE granular positivity and both solid and hollow Auer rods, frequently multiple.

32. AMML with CE positive granulocyte precursor and BE positive promonocyte.

33. AMML with predominantly monocyte precursors; all except one cell show BE positivity.

34. AMML of similar cytology with BE positivity as brownish black granules with the single incubation staining method.

35. Two early erythroblasts from an erythroleukaemia, showing BE positivity — contrasting with the CE reaction in a granulocyte at the bottom corner.

36 & 37. Bone marrow from a case of mixed myeloid leukaemia with megakaryoblastic predominance: the blast cells show only weak BE positivity in Plate 2.36, but much stronger reactions with α-naphthyl acetate as substrate in Plate 2.37.

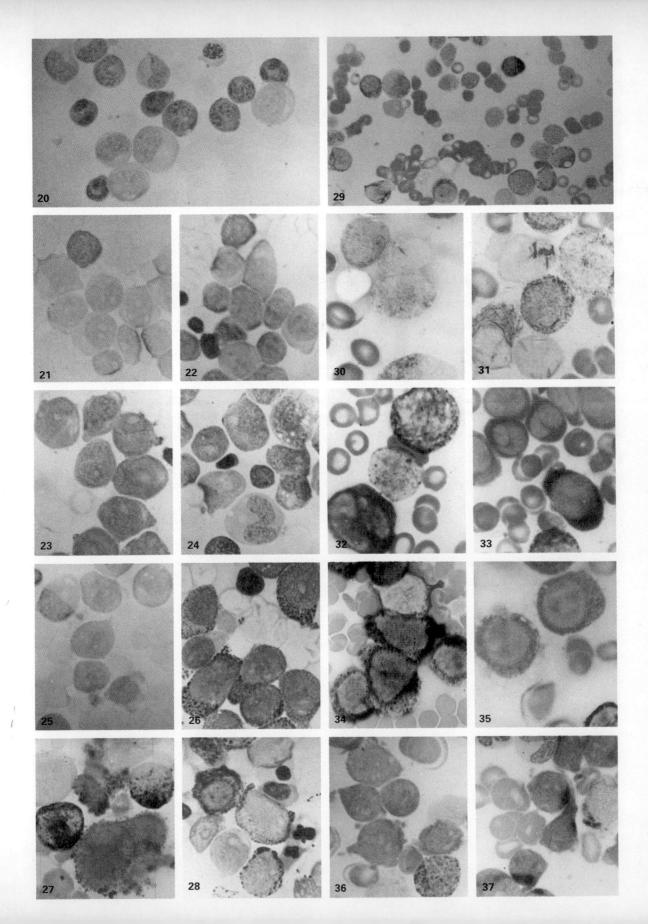

PLATE 2 (contd)

Figs. 38–57

38–41. Romanowsky (Heyl), SB, PAS and dual esterase reactions in marrow cells from a case of AMML with Inv 16. The mixture of monocyte and granulocyte precursor reactivity to PAS and dual esterase is well shown in Plates 2.40 and 2.41, as are the eosinophils, sometimes atypical in Plates 2.38 and 2.39.

42–45. A typical example of ALL, with Heyl reaction (Plate 2.42), negative SB (Plate 2.43) and with the variably coarse PAS positivity against a negative background shown in low and higher power views in Plates 2.44 and 2.45.

46–49. Hairy-cell leukaemia (HCL) — buffy coat preparations.

46. PAS reaction with characteristic diffuse and granular positivity.

47. Acid phosphatase (tartrate resistant) with coarse granular positivity and occasional rods perhaps representing ribosome lamellar bodies.

48. Dual esterase reaction, showing BE positivity in most HCs, often with a crescentic disposition.

49. Alkaline phosphatase is strongly positive in the neutrophils of HCL, though HCs themselves are negative.

50. Localised acid phosphatase blocks of positivity in a T-cell CLL.

51. Similar localised BE reaction in the same case.

52. Another example of polar acid phosphatase reaction in a T-cell prolymphocytic leukaemia.

53. A range of positivity to alkaline phosphatase in neutrophils, showing one cell with a score of 1+, two cells with 3+, and one with 4+ ratings. The negative cells present are lymphocytes.

54. Acid phosphatase positivity in a monocyte/macrophage among negative lymphoblasts from a pleural exudate in ALL.

55. PAS reaction in the lymphoblasts from the same aspirate.

56. Erythroblasts from a case of erythroleukaemia stained for acid phosphatase, showing strong positivity with a tendency to polar concentration.

57. Alkaline phosphatase reaction in a spreading macrophage from normal bone marrow; neighbouring erythroblasts are negative.

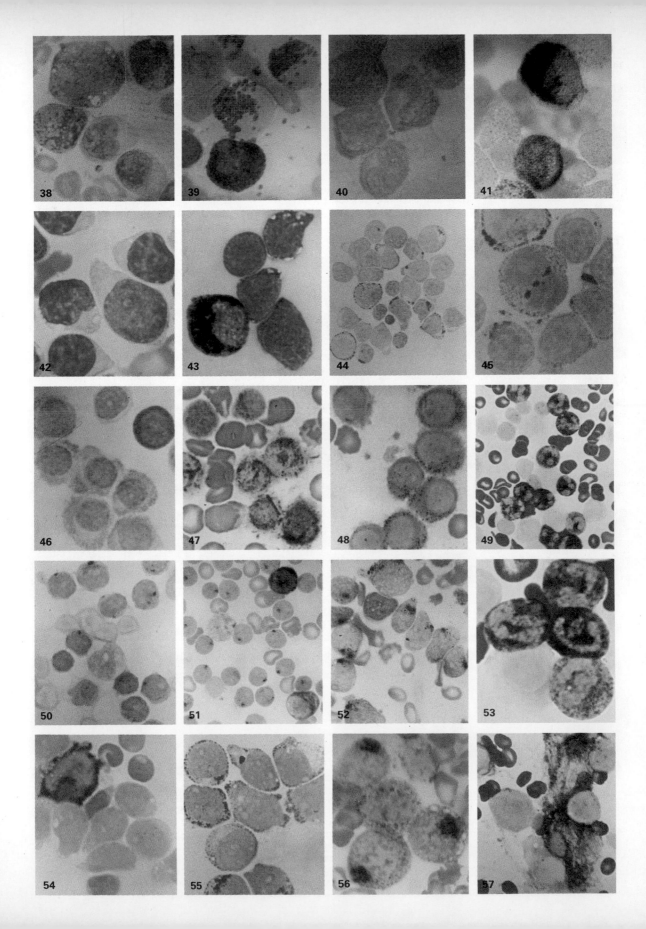

PLATE 3

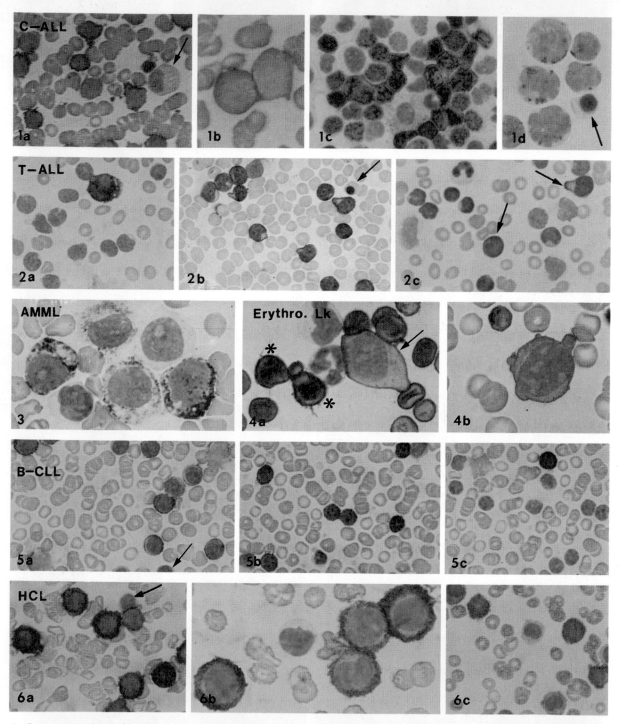

1. *Common acute lymphoblastic leukaemia*: Positive reactions for (a) HLA-DR (negative myeloid cell arrowed); (b) common acute lymphoblastic leukaemia antigen; (c) terminal transferase; and (d) intracytoplasmic mu chains (unstained normoblast arrowed).
2. *T-cell acute lymphoblastic leukaemia*: (a) HLA-DR is absent (note on HLA-DR positive normal monocyte); (b) T-cell antigen CD7 is strongly expressed (unstained normoblast arrowed); (c) cortical thymocyte antigen CD1 is expressed with variable intensity (two strongly stained blasts arrowed). 3. *Acute myelomonocytic leukaemia*: Positivity for antibody DAKO-Macrophage.
4. *Erythroleukaemia*: Labelling for (a) glycophorin A, showing positive normoblasts (asterisks) and blast cell (arrowed), and (b) transferrin receptor. 5. *B-cell chronic lymphocytic leukaemia*: Expression of (a) HLA-DR (negative normal lymphocyte arrowed) and (b) CD5 antigen (T1); and (c) absence of the pan-T antigen CD3 (T3). 6. *Hairy-cell leukaemia*: Positivity for (a) p150,95 antigen (unstained normal lymphocyte arrowed); (b) CD22 B-cell antigen; and (c) CD25 (Tac) antigen.

Erythrocytes

1

The blood count, its quality control and related methods

The routine 'blood count' is the commonest of all laboratory investigations, and there are very few patients coming into hospital who do not have one done. As a general principle, no test should be done unless there is a specific clinical need for it, and the information it provides is of material benefit to the patient and the clinician. These days no anaesthetist is likely to allow an operation to proceed without knowing the haemoglobin level of the patient. Whatever the laboratory workers feel about routine blood counts, they are going to be asked for, and it does provide some measure for population screening.

Both in the collection of the blood sample, and its subsequent handling in the laboratory, a rigid identification procedure must be followed. Any further manoeuvres in the laboratory require the same process of identification. All procedures require adequate mixing of the sample, and all tests are carried out with the sole aim of providing an accurate, repeatable result, with quality control measures rigidly adhered to.

Blood-borne pathogens make the life of the laboratory worker more difficult. It is to be hoped that the clinician requesting the test will inform the laboratory of any patient having, or suspected of having, a dangerous pathogen, and will identify the sample clearly. Conditions such as hepatitis and HIV infections constitute a handling risk for *everyone*. However, *any* sample is potentially pathogenic. Good working practices in the laboratory must always be observed; accidents will happen and all staff must know what procedure to follow should an accident occur. Mouth pipetting should not be undertaken for any specimens.

Estimation of the haemoglobin concentration, red cell, white cell and platelet count and absolute values can be made by manual methods or by automated counters. Automated counters have brought a high degree of precision and reproducibility to what was once a very tedious task in the laboratory. The speed makes it possible to handle large numbers of blood samples and the quality of the result makes it suitable for even relatively small laboratories with relatively few technicians. Indeed, the only contraindication apart from

cost, is remoteness of a laboratory from access to service engineers since breakdowns are a not infrequent occurrence. The larger machines incorporate a facility for complete or partial differential white cell counts.

In using automated counters the instructions of the manufacturer are followed and it is not appropriate to set these out here. However, the output of the machine has to be set by the operator and hence quality control procedures in monitoring the output are of considerable importance. These are dealt with in detail in this chapter.

Manual methods are still in use in many smaller centres, particularly where it would be inappropriate to use electronic equipment, and hence an account of these methods is given.

$\bar{X}_B$ CALIBRATION AND CONTROL OF THE MULTICHANNEL HAEMATOLOGY ANALYSERS

Traditionally, quality control of the various multichannel haematology analysers has utilised fixed or inhouse control material with assigned values. The operator subjects the control material to analysis, and evaluates the results for discrepancies from assigned values. After rechecking and confirming any deviant results, the operator troubleshoots and/or recalibrates the test channel in question, and proceeds with patient testing.

There are a number of significant disadvantages to this approach (Table 1.1). These should be considered when selecting a quality control method for a multichannel analyser. Some of these disadvantages can be overcome by the use of the $\bar{X}_B$ system for quality control of the red blood cell parameters. Further application of the $\bar{X}_B$ analysis also permits WBC calibration and control of instruments which utilise the impedance counting principle. Although the $\bar{X}_B$ algorithm is somewhat unwieldy for long-hand use, it is easily accessible to even small laboratories due to the availability of programmable calculators. The algorithm is also available as part of the computer package of the larger

Table 1.1 Advantages and disadvantages of the different available methods for quality control of the red cell analytical channels.

QC method	Advantages	Disadvantages
In-house controls	Inexpensive. Utilises fresh blood.	Time-consuming preparation. Parameters are unstable. Values assigned by user require reference instrumentation/methodology for determination of expected values. 'Out of limits' results frequently indicate problems with control material rather than with instrument. Requires external reference for instrument calibration. No generally accepted reference method for particle counts (WBC, RBC or platelet).
Commercial controls	Values assigned by independent analysis. Simple to use.	Expensive. Relative instability of parameters. Fixed blood behaves in different manner to fresh, so insufficiently assesses instrument function. 'Out of limits' results frequently indicate problems with control material rather than with instrument. Requires external reference for instrument calibration.
$\bar{X}_B$ analysis	Inexpensive. Simple to use. Utilises unfixed blood. $\bar{X}_B$ algorithm incorporated into current instrumentation. QC data made available every 20 samples. May be used as calibrator.	Requires general patient population. Requires workload of >60 samples/24 hours.

haematology analysers manufactured by companies such as Coulter, Ortho, Technicon and TOA.

This algorithm is based on the inherent stability of the red blood cell indices in a general hospital population. It utilises patient data, recording the MCV, MCH and MCHC of each patient sample. Smoothing and trimming functions are applied to minimise the effects of haematologically abnormal samples and stat-istical variability due to small sample size. Every 20 patient samples, quality control information is calculated and made available to the operator. Any significant shift or trend in the data infers either a non-random sampling of the patient population (e.g. a preponderance of nursery or haematology/oncology patients) or an instrument malfunction. The $\bar{X}_B$ formula and an example of its component steps are given in Table 1.2.

The algorithm's smoothing function is achieved by incorporation of the $\bar{X}_B$ mean from the previous patient batch into the calculation step involving each individual patient. Note how the previous batch $\bar{X}_B$ mean of 90 is subtracted from each individual patient sample in Table 1.2. The effect of this step is to incorporate

Table 1.2 Explanation of $\bar{X}_B$ calculations.

1. Subtract each individual patient sample from the, previous $\bar{X}_B$ mean to obtain a positive or negative 'difference' value.
2. Calculate the square root of each 'difference', but maintain the mathematical sign by multiplying the square root result by either +1 or −1, depending on the sign of the original difference. For example, the square root of −4 would become 2(−1), or −2.
3. After 20 values have been obtained, add these together and divide by 20 to obtain the mean 'difference'.
4. Square this value, maintaining the mathematical sign. For example, a difference of −0.3 would be squared to −0.09.
5. Add this value to the previous $\bar{X}_B$ mean to obtain the new mean.
6. Repeat steps 1–6 on the next batch of 20 patients.

$$\bar{X}_{B,i} = \bar{X}_{B,i-1}$$
$$+ \text{sgn}\left(\sum_{j=1}^{N} \text{sgn}(X_{ji} - \bar{X}_{B,i-1}) \sqrt{|X_{ji} - \bar{X}_{B,i-1}|} \right)^2$$
$$\times \left(\frac{\sum_{j=1}^{N} \text{sgn}(X_{ji} - \bar{X}_{B,i-1}) \sqrt{|X_{ji} - \bar{X}_{B,i-1}|}}{N} \right)^2$$

where sgn = the arithmetic sign of the number in parentheses, N is commonly taken to be 20, and $\bar{X}_{B(i-1)}$ is the average after (i − 1) batches.

Example:

Pt #	Patient value	− Previous mean	= Diff	Square root (maintain sign)
1	90	90	0	0
2	89	90	−1	−1
3	91	90	1	1
4	86	90	−4	−2
5	74	90	−16	−4
•	•	•	•	•
•	•	•	•	•
•	•	•	•	•
20	95	90	5	2.2

Mean difference	−3.8/6 = −0.6
Mean difference squared	−0.36
New $\bar{X}_B$ mean	90 − 0.36 = 89.64

information about the previous mean value into the present computation. Thus, this step makes the $\bar{X}_B$ calculation behave in some respects like a running mean or moving average. This serves to reduce the coefficient of variation (CV) of the calculation to less than one per cent, enabling the operator to obtain a quality control data point every 20 samples. Without the smoothing function, batches of 80–100 patients would be required for comparable effectiveness.

Trimming is achieved by the use of the square root function. The example in Table 1.2 demonstrates that the net effect of sample #5 (with an MCV of 74) is reduced from -16 to -4 by use of the square root function. In contrast, since samples #2 and #3, are each within one unit of the previous mean, their effect is unchanged by the square root manipulation of the data. The effect of samples close to the mean is thereby maximised, while the effect of outliers is minimised. It is evident, therefore, that an occasional haematologically abnormal sample will have relatively little effect on the quality control program, while an instrument malfunction or drift causing a consistent change of even one per cent will be clearly demonstrated by a change in the $\bar{X}_B$ quality control points. In this way, the algorithm provides an extremely sensitive mechanism for monitoring instrument function even if the $\bar{X}_B$ data has not yet exceeded acceptable limits.

Initialising the $\bar{X}_B$ quality control system

Any laboratory servicing a general patient population is a potential candidate for the $\bar{X}_B$ system. On the other hand, hospitals catering primarily for paediatric or haematologically abnormal populations would be unlikely to find the system effective since the inherent population CV would be too great. Very small laboratories would also be advised to use an alternative method of quality control, as their workload would be insufficient to provide an adequate number of quality control data points. At minimum, 60 samples/day should be processed through the instrument in question, providing at least three data points in a 24-hour period.

To initiate the $\bar{X}_B$ quality control system, the instrument's red cell channels are first calibrated to the internationally determined target values given in Table 1.3 and to reference cyanmethaemoglobin determinations.

Table 1.3 Internationally derived indices target values for $\bar{X}_B$ analysis.

Index	Target	Acceptable QC limits
MCV	= 89.5	± 3.0 fl
MCH	= 30.5	± 1.0 pg
MCHC	= 34.0	± 1.0 g/dl

The initial calibration is most easily achieved as follows:

1. Perform haemoglobin calibration procedure (Table 1.8) and calibrate haemoglobin channel accordingly.
2. Calibrate the other RBC parameters to approximate values using a fresh blood sample whose values were assigned by another instrument, or using a commercial control or calibrator.
3. Run patient samples through the system to generate $\bar{X}_B$ data.
4. Monitor the results as outlined below, and adjust the calibration as indicated by any $\bar{X}_B$ bias. All further calibration will be based on the biases derived from the $\bar{X}_B$ manipulation of the indices combined with the haemoglobin data. All bias is expressed as $100 \pm$ channel deviation i.e. 102.3% for a channel deviating $+ 2.3\%$.

Monitoring the $\bar{X}_B$ quality control system

The algorithm utilises incoming patient indices data to generate updated quality control information every 20 samples. These values are examined for any significant deviation from the target values. The basic steps for effective utilisation of this quality control method are as follows:

1. Monitor $\bar{X}_B$ data for any of the conditions listed in Table 1.4. Any Category I condition requires that patient testing be stopped until the problem is resolved. Category II conditions can be handled in a more leisurely manner. Since the index values may not yet be out of limits, Category II action may be temporarily delayed.

Table 1.4 $\bar{X}_B$ criteria for evaluation/action.

Category I: Immediate evaluation/action
  * Shift of any parameter by $\geq 3\%$
  * Any index exceeding $\pm 3\%$ limits
  * Haemoglobin calibration exceeding $\pm 2\%$ limits
  * Any index exceeding $\pm 2\%$ limits for >5 points

Cateogry II: Evaluate when convenient
  * Trend in >5 sequential data points
  * Any index exceeding $\pm 2\%$ limits for >3 points

2. Interpret $\bar{X}_B$ pattern to isolate possible cause (Table 1.6).
3. Differentiate between non-random patient-sampling and instrument malfunction/miscalibration defects (Table 1.7). If a non-random patient batch seems to be the most likely cause, proceed with testing.
4. Perform haemoglobin calibration verification (Table 1.8) to obtain haemoglobin bias.
5. Calculate bias of all primary RBC parameters (Table 1.9).

6. Troubleshoot/calibrate instrument for involved parameters as per manufacturer's instructions.

Pattern recognition

Because of the mathematical relationships between the different red cell parameters, specific instrument defects — hydraulic, pneumatic or calibration — result in specific recognizable $\bar{X}_B$ pattern changes. This greatly simplifies the troubleshooting process. The interpretation will differ depending upon the type of instrument used. Examination of the mathematical relationships outlined in Table 1.5 will aid in pattern recognition.

Table 1.5 Derivation of red blood cell parameters.

Parameter	Instrument type	
	MCV directly measured	Hct directly measured
RBC	Directly measured	Directly measured
Haemoglobin	Directly measured	Directly measured
Haematocrit	$\dfrac{MCV \times RBC}{10}$	Directly measured
MCV	Directly measured	$\dfrac{Haematocrit \times 10}{RBC}$
MCH	$\dfrac{Haemoglobin \times 10}{RBC}$	$\dfrac{Haemoglobin \times 10}{RBC}$
MCHC	$\dfrac{Haemoglobin \times 100}{MCV \times RBC}$	$\dfrac{Haemoglobin \times 100}{Haematocrit}$

Table 1.6 Possible $\bar{X}_B$ patterns and their interpretation.

Observed pattern change	Interpretation	
	Instrument type	
	MCV directly measured	Hct directly measured
Increased MCH and MCHC	Increased Hgb or decreased RBC	Increased Hgb
Decreased MCH and MCHC	Decreased Hgb or increased RBC	Decreased Hgb
Increased MCV with decreased MCHC	Increased MCV	Increased Hct
Decreased MCV with increased MCHC	Decreased MCV	Decreased Hct
Increased MCV and MCH	Non-random samples or protein buildup (↑ MCV plus ↓ RBC)	Non-random samples or decreased RBC
Decreased MCV and MCH	Non-random samples	Non-random samples or increased RBC

When instrument malfunction or miscalibration occurs in one of the directly measured parameters, it can be seen from the mathematical relationships that at least two of the indices will show a corresponding change. For example, an erroneously high haemoglobin will result in erroneously high MCH and MCHC data, with the MCV remaining unchanged. An erroneously low RBC count will result in an artificially elevated MCH and MCHC on instruments which obtain the MCV by direct measurement. On the other hand, the same error in the RBC count will result in erroneously elevated MCV and MCH on instruments which measure haematocrit directly. Miscalibration of any of the primary parameters, therefore, can be monitored by corresponding changes in the affected indices. Table 1.6 outlines the various possible patterns which may be obtained, and how they should be interpreted.

It is apparent that patterns involving a simultaneous increase or decrease in the MCV and MCH can be caused by a non-random batch of patient data as well as by analyser malfunction. This sometimes happens when a twenty-patient batch includes a preponderance of samples from one patient subpopulation — for example, several paediatric or haematology/oncology patient samples analysed back-to-back rather than intermixed with other patients. When a simultaneous MCV and MCH jump occurs, it becomes necessary for the operator to determine whether the cause is a non-random patient sampling or an instrument malfunction. Table 1.7 outlines two methods which can be used to accomplish this.

Simultaneous pattern changes in the MCH and MCHC require an added evaluation step with all instruments which measure the MCV directly. It is impossible, simply by evaluating the $\bar{X}_B$ patterns, to differentiate between problems involving the haemoglobin or red cell channels on these instruments. To resolve the question, perform a haemoglobin calibration verification procedure (Table 1.8) to first determine the haemoglobin bias. Then use this data and the $\bar{X}_B$ data to calculate the RBC bias (Table 1.9). The haemoglobin calibration verification procedure should be performed at least weekly as a check on all systems, even if there are no problems evident.

Platelet calibration

The calibration of the platelet channel through indirect utilization of the red cell $\bar{X}_B$ data turns out to be rela-

Table 1.7 Methods for differentiating non-random samples from instrument defects.

Method I:
* Obtain five fresh blood samples tested just prior to development of $\bar{X}_B$ change.
* Rerun the samples on the instrument in question, noting the MCV's.
* Look up the original MCV's.
* Express the current MCV of each sample as a percentage of the original MCV to determine percent change.
* Calculate the average percent change, and evaluate as follows:

Non-random population	≤2.2%
Instrument defect	>2.2%

Method II:
* If MCV and MCH on $\bar{X}_B$ plot are increased, look up the five patients in that batch with the highest MCV's. Look up the five lowest MCV's if the MCV and MCH are decreased.
* Evaluate patient demographic data and prior patient MCV data to differentiate between a non-random sample and an instrument defect as shown below:

Non-random samples .... 1. predominantly nursery or haematology/oncology patients (MCV and MCH spike)
2. predominantly paediatric (MCV and MCH drop)
3. prior MCV data within two units of current data

Instrument defect .... 1. no obvious patient sampling bias
2. prior MCV data differing by more than two units from current data

Table 1.8 Haemoglobin calibration verification procedure (to be performed weekly or more frequently if indicated by conditions in Table 1.4).

* Obtain four normal EDTA blood samples.
* Run each sample twice (following itself). Use the second haemoglobin value for all subsequent calculations.
* Perform duplicate manual haemoglobin determinations on each sample using reference methods and a certified cyanmethaemoglobin standard. Use the average haemoglobin value for all subsequent calculations.
* Express each instrument haemoglobin value as a percent of the reference value to obtain the average *haemoglobin bias* for the instrument.

$$\frac{\text{Haemoglobin}}{\text{bias}} = \frac{\text{Instrument haemoglobin}}{\text{Reference haemoglobin}} \times 100\%$$

Table 1.9 Determination of instrument bias.

Hgb bias	derived from haemoglobin calibration verification (Table 1.8)
MCV bias (if MCV measured directly)	$\dfrac{\text{Current } \bar{X}_B \text{ MCV value}}{89.5} \times 100\%$
Hct bias (if Hct measured directly)	$\dfrac{\text{Haemoglobin bias} \times 34.0}{\text{Current } \bar{X}_B \text{ MCHC value}}$
RBC bias	$\dfrac{\text{Haemoglobin bias} \times 30.5}{\text{Current } \bar{X}_B \text{ MCH value}}$

channels is extremely rare and can be monitored by regular performance of the daily electronic checks recommended by the manufacturer; the vast majority of changes in the X_B indices patterns reflect changes in the dilutional and flow characteristics of the instrument. Thus virtually all changes affecting the RBC count will affect the platelet count similarly.

Secondly, a constant mathematical relationship exists between the amplification factors applied to the raw RBC data and to the raw platelet data. A corresponding relationship exists between the calibration factors for the two parameters. When using the Coulter S-Plus IV, for example, the relationship can be expressed as follows:

$$\text{Cal factor}_{\text{platelet}} = \text{Cal factor}_{\text{RBC}} \times 0.875$$

Different models may have different factors, and these should be determined and/or verified initially. After initial instrument calibration, this relationship is maintained by adjusting the RBC and platelet channels identically at the time of each recalibration. If desired, platelet calibration may be periodically verified by cross-checking samples against values obtained on a primary instrument such as the ultra-Flo 100, commercial platelet calibrators or nationally referenced quality control survey specimens.

White blood cell calibration

Control of the WBC channel is considerably more difficult than control of the platelet channel, since WBCs are counted on a different dilution and in a different bath than are RBCs. There are, however, two alternative ways of applying the X_B methodology to control of the white cell channel on impedance counters. (Instruments which rely on light scatter for the WBC determination may require a more traditional method of WBC quality control.)

The first method utilises a fixed RBC suspension as a WBC control after initial calibration of the instrument to reference methodology. Table 1.10 outlines the steps necessary to initially calibrate the instrument. Tables 1.11 and 1.12 outline the reagents and procedural steps

tively simple on impedance counters. This is due to two facts.

First, these instruments analyse platelets on the same dilution, in the same suspension and through the same apertures as they do red blood cells. Any dilutional and flow changes affecting the RBC count can therefore be expected to similarly affect the platelet count. Fortunately, isolated electronic drift of individual instrument

Table 1.10 Calibration of the WBC channel to reference methodology.

* On each of three normal blood samples, obtain duplicate WBC counts on the analyser in question.
* Prepare duplicate 1 : 500 dilutions of the same three blood samples using Grade A glassware.
* Analyse these dilutions on a primary instrument such as the Coulter Model ZBI.
* Correct these counts for coincidence.
* Express the original analyser counts as a percentage of these corrected reference counts. The average value is the analyser bias.
* Calibrate the analyser to correct for any bias.

Table 1.11 Reagent list for preparation of fixed RBCS for WBC control (impedence counters only).

STOCK REAGENTS

Solution A 0.2 M/L dibasic sodium phosphate
Na_2HPO_4 30.02 g
Fill to 1000 ml with distilled water.
Store at 4°C.

Solution B 0.2 M/L monobasic sodium phosphate
$NaH_2PO_4.H_2O$ 27.6 g
Fill to 1000 ml with distilled water.
Store at 4°C.

50% Glutaraldehyde
Reagent grade stock solution available commercially.

WORKING REAGENTS

Sorensen's phosphate buffer, pH 7.2
Solution A   72 ml
Solution B   28 ml
Stable for six months at 4°C.

Glutaraldehyde (4%) in distilled water
Glutaraldehyde, 50% 8 ml
Fill to 100 ml with distilled water.
Stable for six months at 4°C.

necessary for the preparation of the fixed control. The fixed cells are resistant to lysis, and so are counted as white blood cells by the impedance counter. For effective use, the fixed material should be cycled at least daily as a check on the WBC channel. As with all fixed cell controls, however, the results should be used with caution since fixed cells are not always 'seen' by the instrument in the same way as are fresh cells. When this happens, a measurement bias is introduced which reflects the idiosyncrasies of the instrument/fixed cell combination rather than true calibration bias. If this is not recognised by the operator and the 'measurement bias' is interpreted as 'calibration bias', any resultant recalibration will introduce a consistent error of equal but opposite amount into the measurement of all later fresh cells. The user should therefore verify that each instrument will analyse fixed cells in the same manner as fresh cells before relying on this or any fixed cell methodology.

Table 1.12 Preparation of fixed red cells for WBC control of impedence counters.

* Centrifuge a normal EDTA blood sample and discard the plasma.
* Resuspend the cells approximately 50:50 in isotonic instrument diluent. Mix well.
* Obtain replicate RBC counts on the sample using a multichannel haematology analyser that is recovering the mean indices shown in Table 1.3. Use the average RBC count for further calculations.
* Dilute the blood 1:500 in a 100 ml volumetric flask as follows:

— Add 10 ml Sorensen's phosphate buffer to flask.
— Add 10 ml glutaraldehyde (4%).
— Fill almost to the 100 mark with isotonic instrument diluent.
— Add 200 μl well-mixed blood using a Grade A pipette.
— Fill to volume with isotonic instrument diluent, and mix well.
— Allow to fix overnight at room temperature.
— Dispense into aliquots for daily use.
— Stable at refrigeration temperatures for at least six months.

* Calculate the target value for the fixed cells as follows, utilizing the average RBC count obtained above, the RBC bias for the instrument (Table 1.9) and the 1:500 dilution factor.

$$\text{Target WBC} \times 10^9/l = \frac{RBC \times 10^{12}/l}{500} \times \frac{100}{RBC \text{ bias}}$$

* Before using, return an aliquot to room temperature with mixing, and cycle through the instrument as a whole blood sample. The WBC readout should fall within ±5% of the assigned target value.

The second method of WBC control (Table 1.13) avoids the pitfalls of fixed cell measurement bias by utilising fresh red blood cells as WBC surrogates. Fresh red blood cells of known concentration — minus the usual lysing reagent — are introduced into the WBC bath and analysed as white blood cells. As before, the method utilises the RBC bias as determined by the indices means and reference haemoglobin checks.

Whichever method is used, the bias of the WBC channel should be minimised (i.e. the WBC channel should be recalibrated) whenever the average bias exceeds 5%.

Conclusion

When an instrument is running smoothly, the $\bar{X}_B$ plots show little variability. When pneumatic/hydraulic problems develop, the plots may show greater than usual variability — even though the instrument is not yet out of control. And when calibration becomes necessary, the calculated biases for each parameter can be used to

Table 1.13 Fresh RBCs as WBC surrogates.

---

* Obtain a normal blood sample and cycle several times through the analyser to obtain an average RBC count. (NOTE: The instrument must be stable so far as the RBC parameters are concerned, and the RBC bias must be known.)
* Obtain the 'true' RBC count by mathematically correcting the average RBC count for any RBC analyser bias.
* Remove the lysing agent from the machine and replace with reagent diluent as follows:
  — Remove pickup lines from the lysing agent container.
  — Prime 2–3 times with air.
  — Wash down the outside of the pickup lines with reagent diluent.
  — Install the pickup lines in a container of reagent diluent.
  — Prime until all residual lyse is removed from the system. (If the instrument provides haemoglobin voltage readings for the haemoglobin blank and test, these two readings will be virtually identical if all of the lyse has been removed from the system.)
* Prepare a 1 : 500 reference dilution of the blood in instrument diluent using Grade A glassware.
* Cycle through the analyser several times to obtain an average WBC count. (Since there is no lyse in the dilution, the RBCs will be counted as WBCs.)
* Calculate the bias of the WBC channel as follows:

$$\text{WBC bias} = \frac{\text{WBC} \times 10^7/\text{l} \times \text{RBC bias} \times 500}{\text{RBC} \times 10^{12}/\text{l}}$$

* Troubleshoot/recalibrate as necessary if the bias exceeds $\pm 5\%$.

---

directly calibrate the instrument without the need for an externally analysed calibration sample. The algorithm, therefore, provides a global system for quality control of the red cell analytical channels on the multiparameter haematology instruments.

GENERAL COMMENTS ON MANUAL CELL COUNTS

Purpose
The absolute measurement of any cell or particle provides an integral component in the assessment of a haematological disorder. Even with the widespread use of electronic cell counters, the manual method is still the reference method for calibrating these counters. The pipettes and counting chambers used for the manual counting of cells can be accurately calibrated, and manufacturers of such equipment must conform to national specifications.

Principles of cell counting
This requires the enumeration of cells in a precisely measured sample of blood which has been accurately diluted; the count must be reproducible. The diluting fluid must allow selective counting of the cells.

Test samples
The anticoagulant of choice in collecting venous blood is the dipotassium salt of EDTA, 1.50 ± 0.2 mg per ml of blood. Throughout this section, it will be assumed that blood will be collected into EDTA.

Equipment
○ Glass or plastic tubes 75×12 mm with tightly fitting bung.
○ Glass capillary tubes, 75×1 mm.
○ Graduated pipettes, volume depending on test being performed.
○ Accurate Schellback 20 μl pipette or precision positive displacement pipette 25 μl (Gilson).
○ Improved Neubauer chamber for red cell, white cell and platelet counting. Fuchs Rosenthal chamber for eosinophil counting.

Comments
There are many sources of error in performing manual cell counts, one of the most important being that too few cells are counted, particularly in comparison with electronic cell counters. The more cells that can be counted, the more valid is the result likely to be. However, time frequently does not permit this approach. A scrupulous technique is vital; counting errors are due to:

1. Dilution
The potential error is large as only a small volume of blood is diluted in a large volume of diluent. This is especially true for red cells as the degree of dilution is so much greater.

2. Sampling
The blood sample must be thoroughly mixed, the aliquot obtained for dilution should be measured precisely, the diluted sample itself must be adequately mixed, and the transfer of fluid to the counting chamber should be smooth, uninterrupted and stopped at the right moment. The fluid must not be allowed to overflow into the moat. The counting chamber permits a precise volume of diluted blood to be examined.

3. Counting
The cells must be recognised and counted by the operator, and care taken to count *all* the cells in the appropriate area of the grid (see Fig. 1.1). With practice, superimposition or physical abnormalities of cells are recognised and counted correctly. Observer error in counting is quite common, particularly between indi-

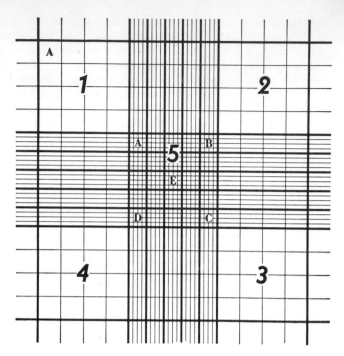

Fig. 1.1 Improved Neubauer counting chamber. The solid black lines are in fact triple lines. The white cells are counted in squares 1, 2, 3 and 4. Red cells and platelets are counted in square 5A, B, C, D, E. (Reprinted by permission from Page L B and Culver P J, Syllabus of Laboratory Examinations in Clinical Diagnosis, Harvard University Press)

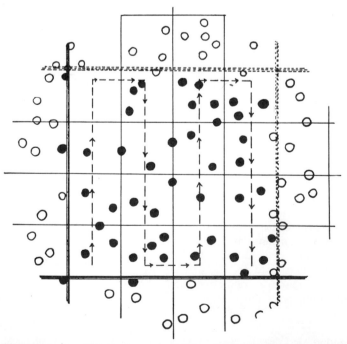

Fig. 1.2 Counting sequence. The picture is a diagramatic representation of the red cell count, showing the sequence of counting which should be followed, the square shown is 5A in Figure 1.1. The same sequence of counting would be followed for any other cell count. (Reprinted by permission from Page L B and Culver P J, Syllabus of Laboratory Examinations in Clinical Diagnosis, Harvard University Press)

vidual observers. It is most important to avoid drying of the preparation as this will affect the distribution of the cells.

There are statistical considerations as well, whatever method of counting is employed. The variation in repeated counts of randomly distributed cells follows a Poisson distribution. The standard deviation of repeated observations is equal to the square root of the mean number of cells counted; the more cells counted, the greater the precision.

General points

Red and white cell bulb pipettes should not be used as these involve mouth pipetting and are more difficult to calibrate. Glass or plastic tubes to which accurately measured volumes of blood and diluting fluid are added are preferable as these can be sealed and placed on a mechanical mixer to ensure adequate mixing. With capillary tubes, the transfer of the diluted sample is easily achieved and filling of the counting chamber carried out more smoothly. The counting chamber and coverglass should be treated as precision instruments, and when charged, hold a precise volume of fluid in the ruled area. The coverglass is specially ground to a uniform flatness. Under no circumstances should ordinary coverglasses be used. To achieve this precision, they must be absolutely free of dust, grease and protein. The coverglass must be handled by the edges, and applied firmly to the chamber, so that Newton's rings are seen where it is in contact with the chamber.

The counting of the cells should follow a specific pattern as illustrated (see Fig. 1.2). The procedure for counting must follow a sequence so that cells touching the lines on two sides of each square are counted as within the square; cells touching the other two sides are outside the square. In this way, every cell is assigned to one square and no cell is counted twice.

Cell counting is made easier if the microscope is 'set up' to reduce the amount of light by lowering the condenser a little, and partly closing the diaphragm. Examine under the low power ($\times$ 10) objective first to see if the distribution of cells is uniform; if not, recharge the chamber.

RED CELL COUNT

Reagents
Red cell diluting fluid

Method
1. Add 20 μl of blood to 4 ml diluting fluid (dilution 1 in 200), and seal the tube.
2. Mix well for at least two minutes, on a mechanical mixer.

3. The red cell suspension is taken up into a glass capillary tube, and each side of the counting chamber is filled in a single smooth action, making sure that no fluid overflows into the moat.
4. Place the chamber inside a moistened petri dish for five minutes to allow the cells to settle.
5. Using $\times$ 40 objective and $\times$ 10 eyepieces count the cells in at least 80 small squares; 500 cells is the minimum number to be recorded.

Calculation
Red cell count
$$= \frac{\text{no. of cells counted}}{\text{volume counted (0.02)}} \times \text{dilution} \times 10^6 \text{ per l.}$$

$$= N \times 10\,000 \times 10^6/l$$
Normal $3.8 - 6.0 \times 10^9/l$

Composition of reagents

Red cell diluting fluid
10 ml of 40% formalin made up to 1 litre with 32 g/l trisodium citrate.

WHITE CELL COUNT

Principle
The red cells have to be lysed, and a colouring agent can be added to aid recognition of the leucocytes.

Reagents
White cell diluting fluid

Method
1. Add 20 μl of blood to 0.38 ml diluting fluid (dilution 1 in 20), seal tube.
2. Mix well for two minutes on a mechanical mixer.
3. Smoothly fill the counting chamber as for RBC, and place chamber in a moistened petri dish for two minutes.
4. All the stained leucocytes in an area of 4 mm^2 should be counted, using a $\times$ 10 objective and $\times$ 10 eye-pieces.

Calculation
White cell count
$$= \frac{\text{no. of cells counted}}{\text{volume counted (0.4)}} \times \text{dilution} \times 10^6 \text{ per l}$$

$$= N \times 50 \times 10^6/l$$

Interpretation

Normal range
Adults $4-11 \times 10^9/l$
Infants at birth $10-24 \times 10^9/l$

| Infants 1 year | $6-18 \times 10^9/l$ |
| Children <10 yrs | $5-14 \times 10^9/l$ |

Comments (See general normal range table)
— If the count is low, greater accuracy may be obtained by counting all the white cells in the whole ruled area (= 9 mm²).
— Debris and dust may be mistaken for white cells by the inexperienced.
— Nucleated red cells will also be counted, but examination of a stained blood film will give warning of their presence.
— If the white cell count is very high, it is permissible to count the cell in the central ruled area and multiply the result by 200 to obtain the total white cell count.

Composition of reagents

White cell diluting fluid

Glacial acetic acid	2 ml
1% Methylene Blue	1–2 drops
Distilled water	98 ml

PLATELET COUNT

Purpose

In most instances, platelet numbers can be adequately assessed by examination of a blood film, only low or high numbers of platelets need to be enumerated by counting. With the increasing use of cytotoxic drugs, knowing the number of platelets is important for patient management. The red cells have to be lysed.

Reagents

1% oxalate (for the experienced)
or
Barr's fluid (for the inexperienced).

Method

1. Place the 20 μl blood into 0.38 ml diluting fluid (dilution 1 in 20), seal tube.
2. Mix for at least 10 minutes on mechanical mixer.
3. Fill a Neubauer chamber as for RBCs. Place the chamber in a moist petri dish for at least 20 minutes to allow platelets to settle.
4. Using a × 40 objective and × 10 eye-pieces, count the number of platelets in the same 80 small squares as for RBCs. The platelets appear as small, highly refractile particles.

Calculation

Platelet count
$$= \frac{\text{no. of cells counted}}{\text{volume counted (0.02)}} \times \text{dilution} \times 10^6 \text{ per l}$$

$$= N \times 1000 \times 10^6/l$$

Normal range $150 - 400 \times 10^9/l$

Comments

— Dust and other debris in the diluting fluid must be rigidly excluded. The diluting fluid should be filtered and centrifuged each day at 1200–1500 g for 15 minutes.
— Counting chamber and coverglass must be absolutely clean and dust free.
— Adequate mixing of the diluted sample is essential; platelets take longer to mix than red cells or white cells. A vortex mixer will be much quicker, although this will tend to create bubbles.
— If the numbers are reduced, count the platelets in the whole central area of small squares (0.1 μl).
— Platelets in EDTA are rounded; with directly-collected capillary samples, the platelets will be irregular in shape and show filamentous pseudopods.
— Platelets should be single; the occasional clump of two or three is acceptable, but larger aggregates invalidate the count.
— The white cells can also be counted with ammonium oxalate as the diluting fluid. Barr's fluid stains the white cells and platelets blue-black, and makes the counting easier for the less experienced.
— Phase-contrast microscopy provides better resolution for platelet counting, and platelets can be more easily differentiated from dust and cellular debris. A special thin counting chamber is required for this.

Composition of reagents

Platelet fluid

| Ammonium oxalate | 1 gm |
| Glass distilled or deionized water | 100 ml |

Filter and centrifuge at 1200–1500 g for 15 minutes prior to use.

Barr's fluid for platelet counts

Saponin	0.25 g
Trisodium citrate	3.5 g
Brilliant Cresyl Blue	0.1 g
40% formalin	1.0 ml
Distilled water	to 100 ml

Filter before use and centrifuge as above.

EOSINOPHIL COUNT

Purpose

To count the number of circulating eosinophils.

Principle

The particular property of eosinophil granules is that they take up Eosin and this allows them to be counted directly on a counting chamber. The staining solution lyses red cells and the other white cells do not take up the stain.

Reagents
Dunger's hypotonic Eosin solution.

Equipment
Fuchs-Rosenthal counting chamber 4 mm × 4 mm (or 3 mm × 3 mm).

Method
1. Add 20 μl of blood to 0.38 ml Dunger's fluid. (Dilution 1 in 20).
2. Mix for no more than 30 seconds and fill the counting chamber.
3. Place the chamber in a moistened petri dish for at least three minutes for the eosinophils to settle.
4. Use a × 10 objective and × 10 eye-pieces; the eosinophils stain deeply orange/red.
5. The light source should be as bright as can be tolerated to highlight only the eosinophils and to exclude all other cells.
6. Count all the eosinophils within the total ruled area. If the count is low, count both sides of the counting chamber.

Calculation
The ruled area of the Fuchs-Rosenthal chamber is a 4 mm square, and has a depth of 0.2 mm and volume of 3.2 μl. (1.8 μl if it is a 3 mm square).
Eosinophil count

$$= \frac{\text{no of cells counted}}{\text{volume counted}} \times \text{dilution} \times 10^6 \text{ per l}$$

$$= \frac{N \times 20}{3.2} \times 10^6/l$$

Normal range of eosinophils 0.04–0.4 × 10^9/l

Comments
The general guidelines for chamber counts apply and in addition:
— Delay in counting should not be longer than 30 minutes as the eosinophils will disintegrate if left longer.
— If the count is very low, a 1 in 10 dilution can be used.
— There is a diurnal fluctuation in the eosinophil count and it is lowest in the morning.

Interpretation
There is an inverse relation between adrenal cortical activity and the eosinophil count. In Cushing's syndrome, the number of eosinophils is low, whereas in adrenocortical insufficiency (Addison's disease) the eosinophils are at the upper limit of normal or higher. Following an injection of ACTH, normal subjects would show a fall in eosinophils whereas there would be no fall in the eosinophil count in Addison's disease.

The eosinophil count may be raised in parasitic infestations (nematodes including hookworm, ascaris, filaria, schistosomiasis, cysticercosis, toxoplasma, amoebiasis, malaria, etc.), arthropod infections (scabies), allergic disorders (asthma, hay fever, urticaria, etc.), skin disorder (psoriasis, eczema, etc.), gastrointestinal disorders (milk sensitivity, ulcerative colitis, Crohn's disease, etc.), hyperosinophilic syndromes and some tumours (Hodgkin's). An increase may be familial.

Composition of reagents

Dunger's hypotonic Eosin solution
Eosin A (200 g/l)   5 ml
Acetone   5 ml
Distilled water   90 ml
The solution is stored at 4°C, filtered prior to use and should be prepared fresh every two weeks.

HAEMOGLOBIN DETERMINATION BY THE CYANMETHAEMOGLOBIN METHOD

Measurement of haemoglobin concentration in a whole blood sample is a basic screen for anaemia or for polycythaemia.

Principle
Blood is diluted in a solution containing potassium cyanide and potassium ferricyanide (Drabkin's solution). Haemoglobin, methaemoglobin and carboxyhaemoglobin are all converted to cyanmethaemoglobin. The absorbance of the solution is measured against a reference standard solution of cyanmethaemoglobin.

Test samples
Venous or capillary blood collected into dry EDTA. Alternatively, free flowing capillary blood may be measured and added to the diluting fluid without anticoagulation.

Standard
Standard solutions of cyanmethaemoglobin are widely available commercially. They have a shelf life of 5 years and contain 700 ± 150 mg of cyanmethaemoglobin per litre. Each ampoule is labelled to the nearest mg of cyanmethaemoglobin. Accurate calibration of a blood sample which can serve as a standard can be prepared by making a dilution of blood in Drabkin's solution and measuring the extinction at 540 nm. One millimole of cyanmethaemoglobin (M.Wt. 64, 458) has an extinction coefficient of 44.0.

Reagents

Drabkin's solution

It is usual to prepare this solution by dissolving a tablet or diluting an ampoule as directed by the supplier. Alternatively the solution may be prepared (see below). Its absorbance should be zero at 540 nm against a water blank.

Method

1. Add 20 μl of blood to 4 ml of cyanmethaemoglobin reagent.

2. Mix well and leave to stand at room temperature for at least three minutes.

3. Read the absorbance on a photoelectric colorimeter at 540 nm against a reagent blank.

4. Read the absorbance of the contents of an ampoule of cyanmethaemoglobin standard at 540 nm against a reagent blank.

Calculation

$$\frac{\text{Absorption of test sample}}{\text{Absorbance of standard}}$$

$$\times \frac{\text{Concentration standard} \times \text{dilution factor}}{100}$$

= Haemoglobin (g/l)

Notes on technique

— The blood sample must be properly mixed before sampling and allowed to warm.
— The standard solution of cyanmethaemoglobin should be at room temperature when its absorbance is measured.
— When the haemoglobin level of a number of blood samples is to be measured it is convenient to prepare a table relating colorimeter readings to haemoglobin concentration.
— When blood samples contain more than 40×10^9 white cells/litre the diluted samples should be centrifuged at 3000 rpm for 10 minutes before reading to avoid a false reading due to turbidity imparted by the white cells.
— Care should be exercised when handling potassium cyanide.
— Prolonged pressure on the arm during venepuncture must be avoided as this can increase the haemoglobin concentration. The haemoglobin concentration is lower when the specimen is collected from the patient in the supine as compared to the erect posture. The variation may be as great as 15 g/l.

Comment

The cyanmethaemoglobin method is the reference method for haemoglobin estimation because all haemo-globin compounds except sulphaemoglobin are estimated. Highly reliable and stable standards are available.

Interpretation

Normal range (sea level)

Adult males	155 ± 25 g/l
Adult females	140 ± 25 g/l
Newborn infants	165 ± 30 g/l
Children aet 3 months	110 ± 15 g/l
Children aet 1 year	120 ± 10 g/l
Children aet 3–6 years	130 ± 10 g/l

The mean haemoglobin level in those normally resident at altitude is as follows:
4000 feet above sea level 169 g/l
15 000 feet above sea level 208 g/l

Composition of solutions

Drabkin's solution (pH 7.0–7.4)

Potassium ferricyanide	200 mg
Potassium cyanide	50 mg
Potassium dihydrogen orthophosphate	140 mg
Nonidet P40 (Shell Chemical Co)	1 ml
Distilled water to	1 litre

Check pH and store solution in a dark bottle at room temperature. It must not be allowed to freeze.

Care: Potassium cyanide is poisonous.

HAEMATOCRIT OR PACKED CELL VOLUME (PCV) DETERMINATION

Purpose

The haematocrit (packed cell volume — PCV) is the percentage of a volume of blood occupied by red cells. It is a screening test for anaemia, or polycythaemia, and when accurate measurements of the haemoglobin level and red cell count are available the 'absolute values' (p. 16) for red cells can be calculated.

Principle

A volume of anticoagulated (or capillary) blood is placed in a glass tube which is centrifuged so that the blood is separated into its three main components — red cells, white cells and platelets (buffy coat, p. 22) and plasma. Ideally, there should be complete separation of cells and plasma, but this is not achieved. The haematocrit is the ratio of the height of the red cell column to that of the whole blood sample in the tube.

Test samples

1. Venous blood, anticoagulated with dry K_2 — EDTA

2. Capillary blood, freely flowing, drawn up directly

into a microhaematocrit capillary tube which has been coated inside with heparin.

Equipment

Microhaematocrit method
○ Microhaematocrit centrifuge, with a pre-set speed providing a centrifugal force of 12 000 g.
○ Capillary tubes, 75 mm long and internal diameter of 1 mm :
  a. plain for anticoagulated blood
  b. heparinized for capillary blood.
○ Plasticine sealer (e.g. Cristaseal) or
○ Bunsen burner

Macro-method of Wintrobe
○ Wintrobe graduated haematocrit tubes.
○ Long-stemmed capillary pipette (the delivery tip must reach the bottom of the haematocrit tube).
○ Bench centrifuge capable of generating at least 2500 g at the bottom of the cup.

Method

With both methods, the blood sample should be as fresh as possible and well mixed

Micromethod
1. Using capillary action, allow blood to enter micro-haematocrit capillary tube, stopping at 10–15 mm from the end. Wipe the outside of the tube.
2. a. Seal the dry end by pushing into the plasticine two or three times.
  b. If heat sealing is used rotate the dry end of the capillary tube in a fine Bunsen burner flame.
3. Place the tube into one of the centrifuge plate slots, with the sealed end against the rubber gasket of the centrifuge plate. Keep a record of patient's name against centrifuge plate numbers.
4. If using a Hawksley microhaematocrit centrifuge, screw down solid plate then close lid. If using a Crist microhaematocrit centrifuge, close lid.
5. Centrifuge for five minutes.
6. Read the PCV in the Microhaematocrit Reader by placing the base of the red cell column on the '0' line, the meniscus of the plasma on the '100' line, then moving the silver line on the adjuster until it is touching the red cell/white cell-platelet interface. Avoiding parallax error read the PCV from the scale.
Units. The haematocrit is the ratio of the packed red cells to the volume of blood (1/1), e.g. 0.45.

Comments

— It is preferable to perform tests in duplicate, as the fragile microhaematocrit capillary tubes may shatter (see below), but if large numbers are being tested, it is impracticable.

— Shattering of the capillary tubes is due to the very rapid acceleration of high speed microhaematocrit centrifuges. This can be prevented to some extent by first spinning the centrifuge head by hand so that the bottom of the capillary tube is in firm contact with the shoulder of the centrifuge plate.
— It is preferable, although not essential, to balance the microhaematocrit capillary tubes in the centrifuge.
— The amount of blood added to the EDTA-tube should be as indicated on the label. An excess of EDTA leads to red cell shrinkage.
— Oxygenation of the blood produces a 2% decrease in the PCV and, therefore, the sooner the PCV is measured the better. Prolonged mixing will usually aerate the blood satisfactorily.
— With heat sealing, a rubber gasket is not required, with plasticine-sealed tubes a gasket is necessary.
— With a raised haematocrit, as in polycythaemia, there may be reduced red cell packing even with a high speed centrifuge; centrifugation for a further five minutes may be required. A further 30 minutes is required in the Wintrobe method.
— Red cell size and shape may influence the PCV reading; abnormally shaped red cells such as sphero-cytes, sickled cells, microcytic hypochromic cells and macrocytes, etc. may lead to increased plasma trapping.
— Inspection of the plasma and buffy coat will sometimes provide valuable diagnostic information, e.g. jaundice, thrombocytosis, leukaemia.

Interpretation

Normal range

Males	0.40–0.52
Females	0.37–0.47

RETICULOCYTE COUNT

Purpose

To enumerate the number of immature red cells (reticulocytes).

Principle

Residual RNA in immature red cells is precipitated and stained with a supravital dye.

Test samples

Venous or capillary blood.

Reagents

Brilliant Cresyl Blue 1% in citrate saline or New Methylene Blue 1% in citrate saline.

Equipment

○ Glass or plastic test tube 75 × 10 mm.
○ Dropper bottle containing Brilliant Cresyl Blue or New Methylene Blue solution.
○ Pasteur pipette.
○ Capillary tube.
○ Microscope slides.
○ Test tube rack.
○ Reducing eyepiece.

Method

1. Transfer two drops of blood to the test tube and add two drops of Brilliant Cresyl Blue or New Methylene Blue. Mix by flicking the bottom of the tube.
2. Leave in rack for 15–20 minutes
3. Remix contents. With the capillary tube, take up some of the mixture and place a drop near the end of a glass slide; spread in the same way as for a blood smear.
4. When dry, the film is examined using the × 100 oil-immersion objective and × 10 eyepieces. The reticular material (RNA) is stained blue-black and the mature (non-reticulated) cells pale green. For accurate counting, the red cells should not overlap.

Counting

There are several means available:

1. Insert an adjustable diaphragm into one of the eye-pieces.
2. Insert a circle of paper with a central square cut out of it into one of the eyepieces. In both 1. and 2. the number of red cells and reticulocytes are counted as they pass through the central area.
3. The field method. Count all the red cells and reticulocytes in one high power field; moving across the film, count all the reticulocytes in successive fields, and keep a tally of the number of reticulocytes and fields examined; usually 10 fields will be adequate.

Calculation

Reticulocytes

$$= \frac{\text{number of reticulocytes counted}}{\text{number of red cells and reticulocytes counted}} \times 100$$

Absolute reticulocyte count/l

$$= \frac{\% \text{ reticulocytes} \times \text{total RBC/l}}{100}$$

Comments

— If the patient is anaemic, add half the amount of staining fluid.
— Do not counterstain; methanol will dissolve Heinz bodies if present.

— Ideally 100 reticulocytes should be counted; in practice count 1000 red cells. With the field method this is quite easy, and in 10 fields an adequate number of reticulocytes and red cells will be counted.
— Whether Brilliant Cresyl Blue or New Methylene Blue is chosen is a matter of personal choice. If haemoglobin 'H' bodies are to be looked for, Brilliant Cresyl Blue is preferable.

Interpretation

Normal reticulocyle count 0.2–2.0%
Normal absolute reticulocyte count 20–100 × 10^9/l.

The reticulocyte count gives a good guide to the state of the erythroid activity of marrow. A low reticulocyte count in the presence of anaemia indicates an inappropriate response to the anaemia as may be seen in bone marrow depression (from whatever cause), or a lack of an essential haematinic. An increased reticulocyte count is expected when haemorrhage or haemolysis is present, or with the response to specific haematinic therapy.

Composition of reagents

Reticulocyte fluid
3% trisodium citrate

Trisodium citrate	1.5 g
Distilled water	50 ml

To make stain:

Brilliant Cresyl Blue	1 g
3% trisodium citrate	20 ml
0.9% sodium chloride	80 ml

Ensure dissolving of powder by mixing in a magnetic stirrer for 5–10 minutes. Filter. Stain is now ready for use.

New Methylene Blue

New Methylene Blue	1 gm
Citrate- saline solution	100 ml

(20 mls of 30 g/l sodium citrate)
(80 mls of 9.0 g/l sodium chloride)
Add some glass beads and shake at intervals over 24 hours. Filter. Ready for use.

ABSOLUTE VALUES

Besides determining the shape of a red cell, measurement of the actual haemoglobin concentration and size of the red cells will often be helpful in determining the likely cause of the anaemia. The measurements of the average haemoglobin content and size of the red cell can be calculated from knowledge of the number of red cells, the haemoglobin content, and the packed cell volume. The mean cell haemoglobin (MCH) and the mean cell volume (MCV) provide this information, and together with the mean cell haemoglobin concentration (MCHC) are referred to as the 'absolute values' for red cells. Electronic cell counters can measure and calculate these absolute values quickly and reliably. Manual methods, besides being time-consuming, are less accurate.

Mean cell haemoglobin (MCH)

$$= \frac{\text{haemoglobin content (g/l)}}{\text{red cell count } (\times 10^{12})}$$

normal range 27–32 pg/cell

Mean cell volume (MCV) $= \dfrac{\text{PCV (1/1)}}{\text{RBC } (\times 10^{12})}$

normal range 80–94 fl

Mean cell haemoglobin concentration (MCHC)

$$= \frac{\text{haemoglobin content (g/l)}}{\text{PCV (1/1)}}$$

normal range = 31.5–36.5%

In normal adults these indices of red cell size and haemoglobin content are constant, but they only represent mean values. It is essential to check the appearance of the red cells on the stained blood film against these calculated values. Examination of a blood film may be much more revealing, particularly if a dimorphic population of red cells is present. The two tests should complement each other.

NORMAL VALUES (Table 1.14)

Differential white cell count (adults)

Neutrophils	2.0–7.5 × 10^9/l	(40–75%)
Lymphocytes	1.5–4.0	(20–45%)
Monocytes	0.2–0.8	(2–10%)
Eosinophils	0.04–0.4	(1– 6%)
Basophils	<0.1	(<1%)

THE BLOOD FILM

Spreading the blood film

To evaluate the change in numbers or cytology of the red cells, white cells and platelets a well-made, well-stained blood film forms the cornerstone of haematological diagnosis; the experienced microscopist learns more from this examination than from any other single test.

Table 1.14 Normal values.

Normal values	Men	Women
White cell count × 10^9/l	4–11	4–11
Red cell count × 10^{12}/l	4.5–6.0	3.8–5.2
Haemoglobin g/l	130–180	120–160
Packed cell volume (haematocrit) 1/l	0.40–0.52	0.37–0.47
Mean cell volume* (MCV) fl/cell	80–94	80–94
Mean cell haemoglobin (MCH) pg/cell	27–32	27–32
Mean cell haemoglobin concentration (MCHC)%	31.5–36.5	31.5–35.5
Platelet count × 10^9/l	150–140	150–400
Erythrocyte sedimentation rate mm/hour	1–7	3–9
Reticulocytes % × 10^9/l	0.2–2.0 20–100	0.2–2.0 20–100
Plasma haemoglobin mg/l	<40	<40

* There is no consensus between different laboratories about the range of the normal MCV since minor variations in machine setting of automated counters produce variations; nor is there any absolute standard.

Test samples

Venous blood collected in K_2-EDTA, or capillary blood. Fresh films are best.

Equipment

○ Glass microscope slides or cover slips may be used; the techniques using glass slides will be described. The slides must be absolutely clean and dust free.

○ 'Spreader'. A microscope slide, with one corner removed at each end, provides the easiest method for making a spreader; the edges at the ends should be free of nicks and defects and preferably bevelled. A diamond pencil is used to make a cut across a corner, which is then broken off, providing a spreader which is narrower than the slide for the blood film preparation.

○ Glass capillary tubes (size 75 × 1 mm).

Method

Using a glass capillary tube, a small drop of blood, whether from EDTA-anticoagulated blood or direct from a finger puncture, is placed on the slide, 1 cm from one end in the midline. The slide is placed on a flat surface and held down firmly, with the thumb and forefinger at opposite ends. As quickly as possible, the spreader, held at an angle of 45°, is placed just in front of the drop of blood, and drawn back to touch the drop of blood and to allow the blood to spread all the way along the contact line between the two slides. The spreader is pushed forward smoothly and rapidly, maintaining contact between the two slides. The blood film formed should be 3–4 cm long, evenly spread with no ragged tails. If the patient is anaemic, the film may be too thin, in which case spread it more quickly and use a steeper angle than 45° between the two slides. Conversely, if the patient is polycythaemic, spread the film more slowly and use a less steep angle for the spreader.

Allow the film to dry before labelling with a 4B pencil at the thick end of the blood film. In humid conditions, it may be advisable to use a fan or hand-held hairdryer to dry the film more quickly. The thickness should be such as to allow the erythrocytes to be separated from each other in the last quarter of the film.

The film should be fixed and stained as soon as possible, as the results of staining become less satisfactory the longer it is delayed.

The preparation and use of thick blood films is described on page 154.

FIXATION AND STAINING OF BLOOD AND BONE MARROW FILMS (see also p. 23)

Purpose
Staining of blood and marrow films with polychrome stains allows for the identification of the various cell types.

Principle
Blood and marrow films are stained by the Romanowsky dyes which are compound dyes consisting of a mixture of Methylene Blue and Eosin, with a number of contaminating dyes which can alter the staining characteristics. Methylene Blue stains acidic cell components, such as nuclei and cytoplasmic RNA. Eosin is red and stains more basic components such as haemoglobin. In practice, a number of structures are stained with both components, and the contaminants contribute. These dyes are dissolved in methyl alcohol, which also acts as a fixative.

Reagents
A number of Romanowsky stains are available, which are used singly or in combination:
- Leishman's stain
- May-Grünwald Giemsa stain
- Jenner-Giemsa stain
- Giemsa stain (see malarial staining p. 153)
- Buffered distilled water pH 6.8.

Fixation
Good fixation is essential for good staining and presentation of cellular detail. Contamination of methyl alcohol with water leads to poor fixation and loss of cell detail, and it is most important to prevent this from happening. Methyl alcohol readily takes up water

vapour. All staining solutions must be kept stoppered, and any glass ware used in the preparation of home-made stains must be absolutely dry. In very humid conditions, fixation artefacts are common, especially in the tropics. High grade, or redistilled methanol, should be used for making up Romanowsky stains; this is particularly true of Leishman's stain. If slides are first fixed in a Coplin jar containing methanol, it is important to change the methanol frequently. This is also true if an automatic staining machine is used, as water vapour is soon taken up.

Staining

Leishman's method
1. Support film in a horizontal position on two parallel glass or metal rods 5 cm apart, over a sink.
2. Flood the slide with Leishman's stain and leave for two minutes to fix the film. In hot weather, evaporation will be rapid and the stain will precipitate on the film; this can be avoided by adding more stain.
3. Add double the volume of buffered distilled water, making sure that none of the diluted stain runs off. The stain and water can be mixed by blowing gently over the surface, or by using a Pasteur pipette with a rubber teat, making sure that the surface of the film is not touched. A metallic scum will appear on the surface.
4. Leave for eight minutes.
5. Wash the stain off with buffered water until no blue washes off; give a final rinse with running tap water. Immediately clean the back of the slide with a tissue and stand upright to dry; if it is very dirty, adding a drop of methanol to the tissue will quickly remove any stain deposit. DO NOT BLOT THEM DRY.
6. When completely dry, the thinner end of the film should be covered with a 22 × 22 mm coverglass, using a mountant.

Coplin jar method
1. Fix slides in a Coplin jar of anhydrous methanol for ten minutes.
2. Transfer slides to another jar, containing May-Grünwald (or Jenner) stain, freshly diluted 1:1 with buffered distilled water; leave for ten minutes.
3. Transfer slides without rinsing to a jar containing Giemsa stain (diluted 1 in 10 with buffered distilled water). Leave for ten minutes.
4. Transfer slides to a jar containing buffered distilled water, raising and lowering the slide a few times in the water before leaving it undisturbed for five minutes to differentiate.
5. The film should not leach out any more blue stain, and may now be rinsed in tap water and stood upright to dry.

6. When completely dry, the thinner end of the film should be covered with a 22 × 22 mm coverglass using a mountant.

Comments
— The quality of staining can be monitored by inspecting the wet film under the low power of the microscope.
— Preservation of cellular detail in stained blood films is probably best if they are left unmounted, however they will inevitably become scratched and collect dust. Mounting with a coverglass is a reasonable compromise, and a neutral mounting medium, miscible with xylol, allows good preservation.

Complications in staining
The appearance of films can be variable. A well-stained film usually appears pink, but it may be blue, and the nuclei deeply stained.

Different batches of stain, the pH of the diluting fluid, the thickness of the blood film or the glass slides themselves may contribute to this variation. If the slides appear very pink, there is usually under-staining of the cells, perhaps because differentiation has been prolonged, or the buffer is too acid. Whenever staining is unsatisfactory, the technique, simple as it is, should be reviewed, and in particular the pH of the buffer checked. Freshly collected blood films will always stain more vividly than films made from blood collected into EDTA. Vacuolation of the red cells indicates the presence of water vapour, either because the methanol used for fixation is no longer water-free, or the slides have taken too long to dry in a humid atmosphere. If films are made in an air-conditioned room, they must be fixed in methanol before leaving those conditions.

Composition of reagents

Slide cleaning solution
Absolute ethanol	3 parts
Acetone	1 part

Leave slides in the solution; remove and polish with a clean cloth. Store in dust-free boxes.

Leishman's stain
Leishman's stain powder	0.2 g
Methyl alcohol (analar or re-distilled)	100 ml

Swirl to mix, then warm in a 56° water bath for 15 minutes, with occasional stirring. Filter the solution into a clear bottle and allow to 'ripen' for two or more weeks in daylight.

May-Grünwald's stain
May-Grünwald's stain powder	0.3 g
Methyl alcohol	100 ml

Swirl to mix then warm in a 56°C water bath for 15 minutes. Allow to cool to room temperature, shaking the solution several times in 24 hours. Filter the solution, which is now ready for use.

Jenner's stain
Jenner's stain powder	0.5 g
Methyl alcohol	100 ml

Prepare as for May-Grünwald stain

Giemsa stain
Gurr's improved Giemsa stain R66	1.0 g
Glycerol	66 ml
Methyl alcohol	66 ml

Add the Giemsa stain to the glycerol then heat in a 56°C water bath for 90–120 minutes. Occasional mixing is advised. 66 ml of methyl alcohol is then added, and after thorough mixing the solution is allowed to stand at room temperature for seven days, then filtered. It is then ready for use.

Sorensen's buffer pH 6.8
M1 Sorensen's Buffer (concentrated) (Mercia-Brocades Ltd)	25 ml

Dilute the concentrate to 5 litres with distilled water to give a M/300 working solution. Check the pH and adjust.

EXAMINATION OF BLOOD FILM

Examination of a well-spread, well-stained blood film provides useful information about all the formed elements of the blood. The stained blood film should be examined with the naked eye to see if there is any unusual staining, and then with both low and higher power objectives. Rouleaux formation, red cell agglutination and background protein staining may be noted.

Red cell morphology
The erythrocytes, examined in that area of the film where they do not touch each other, should be assessed for size, shape, haemoglobin concentration and distribution, and for the presence of abnormal forms or inclusion bodies.

Erythrocyte size, particularly if there are very small or large cells, is quite easy to assess, but a slight uniform increase in size (such as occurs in alcoholism) may be much more difficult to pick up. The red cell haemoglobin content should be noted, in particular if it is decreased (hypochromia), abnormally distributed (target cells, eccentrocytes) or appears bluer (polychromasia).

Red cell shape, if abnormal (poikilocytosis), depends on recognising the dominant abnormality, and this may be diagnostic of the underlying disorder — e.g. sickled cells, spherocytes, fragmented cells, etc.

Red cell inclusions, such as nucleated red cells, Howell-Jolly bodies, basophil stippling or the presence of malarial parasites can all provide clues to the underlying haematological or disease pathology. Some of these abnormalities are set out in Table 1.15.

Table 1.15 Red cell abnormalities.

Abnormality	Description	Associated disorders
Acanthocytosis	Small cells (almost spherical) with multiple thorny projections	A-β-lipoproteinaemia
Anisochromasia	Twin population of cells	Iron deficiency being treated with iron (or transfused); sideroblastic anaemia; combined deficiency anaemia (iron and vitamin B_{12} or folic acid)
Anisocytosis	Unequal variation in size	A non-specific feature but more pronounced in severe anaemia
Crenated cells	Cell with multiple evenly-spaced blunt projections	Artefact, old people, thyroid deficiency, delay in making film
Elliptocytosis	Thin, elongated cells, or oval cells if less pronounced	Iron deficiency, megaloblastic anaemia, hereditary elliptocytosis
Howell-Jolly Bodies	Spherical, darkly-staining bodies within the red cell (nuclear debris)	Hyposplenism
Hypochromia	Pale cells (MCH < 27 pg)	See microcytosis
Macrocytosis	Large cells (MCV > 94 fl)	Megaloblastic anaemias, liver disease, reticulocytosis, newborn, alcoholism
Microcytosis	Small cells (MCV < 80 fl)	Iron deficiency, thalassaemia, anaemia of chronic disorders, hyperthyroidism, childhood.
Nucleated red cells	Erythrocytes with nuclei	Any severe anaemia (except aplastic) myelofibrosis, carcinomatosis, leukaemia, severe heart failure, haemolytic disease of the newborn
Poikilocytosis	Abnormal shape	Any anaemia; more prominent if severe. The abnormal shape may be diagnostic e.g. sickle cells
Polychromasia	Cells stain bluish grey; slightly larger cells than normal (reticulocytosis)	Response to blood loss, haemolysis or haematinic therapy
Rouleaux	'Aggregated' red cells, arranged side by side into columns like stacks of coins	Chronic inflammatory, and malignant disease, myeloma, macroglobulinaemia
Schistocytes	Fragmented; irregularly-contracted cells	Carcinoma, uraemia, disseminated intravascular coagulation, mechanical damage to cells; drugs and toxins
Sickle cells	Crescent shape	Sickle cell anaemia
Spherocytosis	A spherical cell with no central pallor	Hereditary spherocytosis; haemolytic anaemia due to antibody (usually Coombs-positive)
'Spur' cells	Cells with long, irregularly-spaced, sharp projections	Liver disease, normal infants, uraemia, microangiopathic haemolytic anaemia, disseminated intravascular coagulation, thrombotic thrombocytopenic purpura, carcinoma, pyruvate kinase deficiency (splenectomized)
Target cells	Cells with a dark centre and periphery and a clear ring in between	Liver disease, thalassaemia haemoglobinopathies, post-splenectomy
Teardrop cells	Shaped like a teardrop	Myeloproliferative disorders myelofibrosis (1° or 2°), extra-medullary haemopoiesis, megaloblastic anaemia

White cell morphology

The distribution of leucocytes on a blood film is not uniform, with larger cells (monocytes and granulocytes) concentrated on the edges and end of the film. If there is a profound leucopenia, it may be necessary to prepare a buffy coat (see p. 22). An estimation of the approximate number of white cells should be made to verify the total white cell count. Differential white cell counts are of limited value, as the confidence limits when counting 100 cells make statistical analysis worthless. Much of the most important information comes from looking around the blood film for the presence of abnormal forms. The presence of right or left shifted neutrophils, the presence or absence of granulation in the neutrophils, toxic granulation, or other inclusion bodies (e.g. Döhle bodies), often provides valuable clues to underlying problems. Nuclear abnormalities like the Pelger-Huet anomaly (dumb-bell or spectacle-shaped nuclei) may be inherited or appear in myelodysplastic syndromes or granulocytic leukaemias.

Lymphocytes, the preponderant white cell in childhood, are abnormal in glandular fever, cytomegalovirus and other virus infections, with the outline of the cytoplasm being distorted by the adjacent red cells. There may be a lymphocytosis as well, and this is often so in whooping cough and the rule in chronic lymphocytic leukaemia. Smear cells, the result of damage to the cells in preparing the film are seen commonly in children and in chronic lymphocytic leukaemia. Some of these abnormalities are set out in Table 1.16.

Vacuolation of the nucleus and cytoplasm occurs whenever there has been a delay in making blood films with EDTA-blood and is worse if the ambient temperature is high, so-called sequestrene change. It is seen in the monocytes first and then the neutrophils, budding or clover-leaf lymphocyte nuclei may occur. Vacuolation may also be seen with bacterial infection (particularly

Table 1.16 White cell abnormalities.

Abnormality	Description	Associated disorders
Atypical lymphocytes	Lymphocytes usually larger than normal, with cytoplasm which often stains deep blue	Infectious mononucleosis and viral infections, toxoplasmosis, drug reactions, post-transfusion syndrome
Auer rods	Rodlike (sometimes round) red inclusions in blast cells	Acute myeloid leukaemia (especially promyelocytic type)
Chédiak-Higashi	Large grey inclusions	Chédiak-Higashi syndrome
Döhle bodies	Small blue cytoplasmic inclusions in neutrophils	Infectious and inflammatory diseases, burns, myeloproliferative disorders
Leucoerythroblastic	Early red and white cell (granulocyte) forms	Myelofibrosis, malignant disease in marrow, acute haemorrhage or haemolysis
Leucocytosis	WBC $> 11 \times 10^9/l$	Physiological or pathological stress, corticosteroids
Lupus erythematosus, (LE) phenomenon	Neutrophils with a homogenous pink inclusion	Lupus erythematosus and collagen diseases, drug reactions
Lymphocytosis	Lymphocytes $>4 \times 10^9/l$ adults $>7 \times 10^9/l$ children	Chronic lymphocytic leukaemia, infectious mononucleosis, pertussis, viral infections, hyposplenism
May-Hegglin anomaly	Basophilic cytoplasmic inclusions in white cells	May-Hegglin syndrome (with thrombocytopenia and giant platelets)
Neutrophil leucocytosis	Neutrophils $>7.5 \times 10^9/l$	Infection, tissue necrosis, myeloproliferative disorders, chronic granulocytic leukaemia, acute haemorrhage/haemolysis, leukaemoid reaction
Pelger-Huët anomaly	Neutrophils with bilobed non-segmented nucleus. Coarse chromatin	Hereditary, myeloid leukaemias, myelodysplasia
Plasma-Türk cells	Plasma cells in blood	Severe bacterial, viral or protozoal infections, multiple myeloma and plasma cell leukaemia, drug reactions
'Shift to the left'	Presence of metamyelocytes and earlier granulocytic forms	Infections, tissue necrosis, diabetic ketoacidosis, leukaemoid reactions, chronic granulocytic leukaemia, myeloproliferative disorders
'Shift to the right'	Hypersegmented neutrophils (5 or more lobes)	Megaloblastic anaemias, iron deficiency, uraemia and hereditary
Smear cells	Disintegrated lymphocyte	Chronic lymphocytic leukaemia, normal babies
Toxic granulation	Coarse purple granules	Infections and inflammatory diseases

in neonates), and is often marked in desperately ill, septicaemic patients.

Another effect of EDTA, seen rarely, is the phenomenon of neutrophil, or eosinophil aggregation, which may lead to a spuriously low total white cell count.

Platelets

The first indication of a low or high platelet count may be through examination of the blood film. In EDTA-anticoagulated blood, the platelets should be evenly dispersed on the film, so it is easy to see what their relative numbers are, but it is important for the film to be made within two hours of collection and to be well stained. 'Thrombocytopenia' whether seen on the film, or with a direct platelet count, is commonly due to a poorly collected blood sample. In any case of thrombocytopenia examine the whole film, and the tail in particular, for platelet clumps and/or fibrin strands. A complete absence of platelets on a film is virtually always due to their loss in the collection process.

Two other causes of a low platelet count are the phenomena of platelet satellitism, when large numbers of platelets adhere closely to the neutrophils, and platelet clumping. These are anticoagulant-related, time-related phenomena leading to a spuriously low platelet count, and are usually of no significance. Platelet counts from blood collected directly from the patient, or from blood which has been in contact with EDTA for only a few minutes, will always provide a true platelet count. Rarely, these phenomena may be associated with platelet antibodies.

Abnormalities of platelet size and shape are prominent in myeloproliferative disorders such as myelofibrosis or thrombocythaemia, when giant forms and megakaryocyte fragments are common. Platelets slightly larger than normal (1–2 μm) are usually seen in immune thrombocytopenia, or after haemorrhage. Unusual giant platelets with dense central condensation of the granules are characteristic of the Bernard-Soulier syndrome (sometimes with thrombocytopenia). The grey platelet syndrome is a condition often associated with thrombocytopenia, with a lack of alpha storage granules.

In films made directly from the patient or from the syringe, platelets will appear in clumps.

BUFFY COAT PREPARATION

Purpose

In some cases of leucopenia, leukaemia or carcinoma, the white cells can be concentrated, stained and examined for the presence of abnormal or immature forms. As such, the buffy coat preparation has in many laboratories been superseded by the cytospin technique (p. 179). It may also be used to demonstrate the lupus erythematosus (LE) phenomenon.

Test sample

Venous blood collected in EDTA.
For LE cells, defibrinated blood.

Equipment

○ Microhaematocrit tubes and centrifuge.
○ Wintrobe haematocrit tube, and bench centrifuge.
○ Pasteur pipette (long-stemmed).
○ Plasticine.
○ Diamond pencil.

Method

Microhaematocrit
1. Fill the tube by capillary action, and seal the 'dry' end of the tube by heating or with plasticine.
2. Centrifuge for four or five minutes.
3. Make a diamond scratch on the tube just below the buffy coat layer. The tube can then be snapped quite easily, and the buffy coat with some plasma expelled on to a microscope slide, and a smear made in the usual way.

Wintrobe tube
1. The tube is filled by means of a long-stemmed pipette. Sufficient blood should be taken up into the pipette to fill the tube in one operation, starting from the bottom of the tube, raising the pipette as filling occurs.
2. The filled tube should be centrifuged in a laboratory centrifuge at 3000 rpm for ten minutes.
3. Remove plasma with a pipette, and then
4. Carefully aspirate with the same pipette the buffy coat layer, and place a drop onto two slides; add a drop of the plasma, mix the buffy coat and plasma with the corner of the 'spreader' and spread films in the usual way.
5. Stain the slides by whatever method(s) is appropriate to the problem being investigated.

BONE MARROW ASPIRATION

Purpose

Bone marrow examination is used to assess the composition, cellularity and maturation of haemopoietic cells in the marrow. It is a useful means of confirming a suspicion of a haematological diagnosis, or to provide further information when examination of the peripheral blood fails to provide sufficient clues. It is a mandatory investigation whenever there is an unexplained cytopenia, and in the follow-up of patients receiving antileukaemia (or anti-malignant disease) therapy. It provides a source of dividing cells for chromosome analysis and it may, on infrequent occasions, provide a positive bacteriological result when all else fails.

Always look at the peripheral blood before doing a bone marrow to decide if additional material is required for chromosome marker studies or bacteriology and whether a trephine biopsy may be required at the same time.

Principle

To penetrate the cortical bone and extract a small sample of marrow from the medullary bone. The sternum and the iliac crest are the most widely used sites for performing bone marrow aspiration; in infants and young children the medial aspect of the upper end of the tibia may be used. The vertebral spinous processes are biopsied very infrequently. Sites of radiological bone abnormality can be specifically sampled.

Equipment

○ Skin cleaning solution (70% ethanol, 0.5% chlorhexidine).
○ 2% lignocaine without adrenaline (2–5 ml).
○ Syringes (2 ml, 5 ml) and needles (21, 22 and 25 gauge).
○ Marrow aspiration needle with sliding or screw guard.
○ EDTA bottle (a paediatric plastic bottle is ideal).
○ Clean microscope slides, 10–12.

Method

1. An explanation should be given to the patient as to why the investigation is being done; most patients will co-operate much more readily if they know the reason for the investigation. Tell the patient what to expect, and talk to him or her throughout the procedure.

2a. Sternal aspiration. It is usually much more comfortable for the patient to have the upper chest and head raised on some pillows rather than being absolutely flat; this position makes it easier for the operator. For women, it is not necessary to expose the whole thorax, and if the woman has very large breasts, this reclining position allows the breasts to fall out of the way. Men with very hairy chests should have a small area shaved. The body of the sternum at the level of the second interspace is the most satisfactory site for a bone marrow aspiration, but the third interspace or the manubrium sterni may be used.

2b. Iliac crest. A position anywhere between the anterior superior and posterior superior iliac spines of the innominate bone can be used. Most haematologists take marrow from the posterior iliac crest (the bone is less hard) with the patient lying on his side with the plane of the pelvis leaning just beyond the vertical. The legs should be pulled up so that the body is curled. Place a supportive pillow behind the upper chest. Some haematologists prefer the patient to be prone with a pillow beneath the pelvis.

3. Cleanse the skin.

4. Infiltrate the skin with 2% lignocaine; warn the patient that it will sting for a few moments.

5. With syringe at a right angle to the skin surface, advance the needle forwards, infiltrating the subcutaneous tissues until needle contacts bone and continuing to inject the local anaesthetic. There will be a momentary period of discomfort when contact is made. After the first shot of lignocaine into the periosteum, proceed outwards in each direction injecting further local anaesthetic until an area of 1 cm^2 is anaesthetised. This occurs very quickly. Withdraw needle/syringe; cover with gauze swab. The depth of penetration needed to touch bone is a guide for setting the guard on the marrow needle.

6. Whilst waiting for the local anaesthetic to take effect (about one minute) make sure that the marrow aspirating needle is functional, test that the stylet fits properly, that the guard is easily operated, and that the syringe for withdrawing the marrow sample fits the marrow needle.

7. With the bevel of the marrow needle uppermost, insert needle through the skin. Bring needle to a position at right angles to the bone surface, and advance until bone is touched. Lower the guard until it is 1 cm above the skin surface. Holding the needle firmly in your hand, with the hub against base of forefinger and tip of index finger against the guard, with firm pressure, push and rotate the needle down through the cortex. There will be a sudden 'give' in resistance when the needle enters the medullary cavity. Warn the patient to expect this. Advance the needle until the guard comes up against the surface of the skin.

8. Withdraw stylet and attach a 2 ml syringe. Warn the patient that some discomfort can be expected, and slowly withdraw plunger. As soon as fluid enters the syringe, cease the suction. Withdraw needle and syringe together; apply gauze swab and ask nurse or the patient to apply pressure at the position you indicate. Apply a plaster.

9. Disconnect syringe from needle, and rapidly place a small drop of marrow fluid 1 cm from the end of the prepared slides. In the manner of peripheral blood films, spread the marrow; these are 'pushes' and a trail of cells is left behind the marrow particles. It is quite useful to squash some of the drops of marrow as this allows the particle cellularity to be assessed more easily.

10. Write the patient's name at the thick end of the preparation with a 4B pencil or on the frosted section if such slides are used, or use a diamond pencil to label the glass slide.

11. Select a number of slides for Romanowsky staining (p. 18) and at least one for iron staining.

Unless it is known what diagnosis is expected, a number of slides should be left unfixed until a preliminary examination is made; additional staining techniques can be performed if needed as an aid to diagnosis.

Comments

— If the patient is very nervous, intravenous diazepam (10 mg) is very effective, if available use Diazemuls.
— The initial explanation to the patient is best given by the doctor looking after the patient; any additional information and reassurance is given by the doctor performing the marrow examination.
— A sternal aspirate is alarming to some patients and the iliac crest should be used.
— Talk to the patient throughout the procedure; you can tell them what to expect and it is soothing (for most!).
— Marrow clots very quickly and speed is essential in preparing the fresh marrow films.
— Don't take more than 0.2 ml of marrow. More is unnecessary (except for culture or chromosome analysis); the sample becomes too diluted with blood. With this small amount there is no need to aspirate or blot excess blood from the slides to get satisfactory preparations.
— Once the slides are made, put the remaining marrow into an EDTA bottle in case more films need to be made. Alternatively, it can be put into a suitable fixative for histological processing (or allowed to clot in the syringe before transferring).
— Fresh peripheral blood films taken at the completion of the marrow aspiration provide invaluable additional information. The blood and marrow should be interpreted together.
— If marrow is required for culture or chromosome analysis, a two syringe technique is advisable. The first, small sample is kept for the morphological examination, and the second, larger sample for any other tests.
— What size syringe? Haematologists vary widely in their choice from 2 ml to 20 ml. I prefer a 2 ml syringe and this is quite sufficient for 99% of marrow collections. It is much easier to 'seek' marrow with a small syringe. If marrow is not obtained immediately, replace stylet, advance the marrow needle and aspirate gently again; this can be repeated a number of times until marrow is (or is not) obtained; a 20 ml syringe would be valueless in such cases, and the excessive suction causes more pain.
— 'Squash' preparations are favoured by some haematologists. In this technique, another slide is placed at right angles on the drop of marrow fluid until it spreads out between the two slides; the top slide is then drawn *down* the length of the bottom slide, thereby spreading out the marrow particles into a single cell layer. Pressure should not be required for normal particles to spread out. This is most valuable for assessing particle cellularity and screening slides for clusters of abnormal cells.
— Look at a skeleton if in doubt about the curves and contours of a particular site. The aspirating needle should always be perpendicular to the bone surface.
— Some bruising may occur in the thrombocytopenic patient; direct pressure over the biopsy site will usually make bruising minimal.
— In young healthy adults, the cortical bone is tough, but in elderly people or in pregnancy, and particularly in myeloma, the bone becomes much softer. There may be uncertainty that the marrow has been penetrated. Setting the guard at 1 cm will always ensure that the needle point is in the cavity.
— The aspirated material represents only a minute fraction of a very large organ, and may not be representative. However, in the vast majority of cases, a bone marrow aspirate provides a great deal of useful information.

Appearance of bone marrow

The stained marrow films, and particularly the fragments, should be scanned under the low ($\times$ 10) objective to assess the overall cellularity (increased in children and the pregnant woman, and decreasing with age, especially samples obtained from the iliac crest), the approximate distribution of haemopoietic cells, assessment of megakarocyte numbers, and looking for any clusters of abnormal cells. The fat content of an aspirated marrow is not assessed easily, although in 'squash' preparations it is easier to observe. Fibroblastic activity cannot be assessed. In starvation disorders (anorexia nervosa) a homogenous pink-staining material is often prominent.

Observations on the maturation of the erythroid and granulocytic components are particularly important, and whether maturation is normal, megaloblastic or dysplastic as well as making an assessment of the relative proportions. The normal ratio of granulocytic/erythroid cells is from 2.5/1–8/1. Decide if any change is due to an increase or a decrease in each type. A differential count of the nucleated cells is done infrequently, but there are occasions when it is necessary, particularly if comparing the blast cell count in patients being treated for acute leukaemia.

Lymphocytes are present in large numbers in children, and numbers decrease with age. In adults, about 10 $\pm$ 5% of the nucleated cells are lymphoid. It is quite possible, in scanning a number of films from a normal adult, to find one slide with an excess of lymphocytes, particularly if a squash preparation is examined. This may well be a normal lymphoid 'island'; if present in more than one film, suspicions of an underlying lymphocytic disorder should be considered, and a trephine biopsy performed.

Other cells present in smaller numbers, megakaryocytes, plasma cells and macrophages should all be looked at for both their numbers and their morphology. With macrophages, the presence of inclusions (cells, debris, pigment or parasites) may be an important clue to the underlying process. Any assessment of a marrow should include a Prussian Blue stain and be examined for the presence of iron and its distribution in the macrophages and erythroblasts.

BONE MARROW TREPHINE

Purpose

Abnormal cells, particularly neoplastic cells, may easily be missed on marrow aspirate films or they may not actually be aspirated, as samples are usually taken only from the one site punctured. Tumour cells are found more easily when a core of bone is removed and processed histologically; this now forms the basis for 'staging' of many neoplastic disorders prior to therapy. Information on the pattern and cellular type in lymphomas is often possible, and with the arrival of specific monoclonal antisera, lymphocytes can be typed on trephine samples. In the myeloproliferative diseases, the degree of fibroblastic involvement can only be assessed on such specimens. In some cases, a marrow trephine biopsy is done to look at the bone architecture, particularly in osteoporosis. Whenever a 'dry tap' occurs with a bone marrow aspirate, a trephine biopsy should be performed to determine whether the marrow is empty or packed with cells (normal or abnormal).

Equipment

See bone marrow aspirate.
○ Trephine biopsy — Jamshidi, Islam, Sacker-Nordin (very rarely used).
○ Swann-Morton Noll surgical blade.

Reagents

Formal saline, 10% or other fixatives.

Method

The trephine should be done on the iliac crest, the posterior part is better and will provide a longer core. Place the patient in the lateral position as described above or prone with a pillow under the pelvis.

1. Skin preparation and local anaesthetic infiltration as for a bone marrow aspirate.

2. Make a small 3 mm incision in the skin with the surgical blade.

3. Insert the trephine through the skin and proceed down to the anaesthetised area of bone; make sure, by asking the patient if it hurts when you touch the bone. Gently push the biopsy needle and trocar into the cortical bone, and once it is fixed (about 0.5 cm) withdraw the trocar.

4. Slowly advance the biopsy needle into the medullary cavity by rotating it back and forth through 90°. This will cause some discomfort, but continue to advance as far as possible. When you think it is at least 2 cm into the cavity, replace the trocar (the distance can be checked by seeing how much projects).

5. The sample has to be 'broken' off from its attachment inside the bone. This can be done in several ways, but probably the best is to rotate the trephine in one direction for several turns and then in the reverse direction. In addition, withdrawing the needle a few millimetres and then wiggling it up and down, from side to side, will break off the core. Withdraw the needle by rotating it in one direction only. Ask the patient or the nurse to press on the needle entry site.

6. The biopsy needle is provided with a probe. Insert this into the biopsy entry end and push the biopsy out through the top of the needle.

7. Dress the biopsy needle area and ask the patient to lie on the site, thus applying localized pressure to it to prevent bleeding, particularly in the thrombocytopenic patient.

Handling the specimen

1. Make touch (imprint) preparations. Monolayer preparations can be made easily by rolling the biopsy down between two slides — you get two preparations with this method; these can be stained by Romanowsky techniques.

2. Place the specimen in formal-saline for processing by the Histopathology Department. But different fixatives may be necessary if immunoglobulin detection techniques are required.

Comments

— The apprehensive patient will benefit by being given 10 mg Diazemuls intravenously.
— There will be occasions when the biopsy fails to come out even though your technique has not changed. Repeat the process in a different spot within the anaesthetised area.
— Some of the biopsy needles come with a 'comfort' knob to assist getting through the bone. These slow the procedure down and, except in some cases of myelofibrosis, are quite unnecessary. If you are hurting your hand in the pushing process, cover the

head of the biopsy needle with a piece of sterile gauze; it works just as well, and saves having to screw the comfort knob on and off.

— A bone marrow aspirate can be done first through the Jamshidi after the needle has been advanced into the medullary cavity. After withdrawing marrow fluid, the needle can then be advanced further as described above to obtain the biopsy sample. However, it is more satisfactory to do a separate marrow aspirate through a standard bone marrow needle.

— If the biopsy is for bone histology, make this quite clear on the histology request form; the processing is different.

— Plastic embedding is becoming more widely used now; it is excellent for cellular detail, but it does not give good results with immunofluorescence techniques, when paraffin preparations are preferable. To obtain the best of both worlds the specimen can be slit longitudinally in a special template. The alternative is to take two biopsies in those cases where different techniques of preparation need to be applied.

— There may be some discomfort at the biopsy site, which can last for several days. Paracetamol will usually offer relief.

Normal appearance

Plastic embedding gives excellent cellular detail as the sections are $2\mu m$ in thickness. Haematoxylin and Eosin, a Romanowsky-stained film and a section ($4\mu m$) stained for reticulin are the histological preparations needed to cover most diagnostic requirements. (Toluidine blue staining is excellent for nuclear cytology).

The slides should be examined under the low power, looking at the general distribution of cellular and fatty spaces, and the trabecular pattern; in addition, clumps of haemopoietic or foreign cells are easily recognised.

The morphology of the normal haemopoietic cells can be more closely looked at under a higher magnification, and with the thin sections now available, even oil immersion objectives can be used.

The occasional lymphoid aggregate is seen in normal people, but two or more should make one suspicious of a lymphoid neoplasm, especially if the aggregate is closely aligned to the trabeculae.

The general texture of the bone trabeculae should not be excluded, as increased number and thickness is often observed in the myeloproliferative disorders, or in carcinomatous involvement. In some tumours, increased osteoclastic activity and bone resorption may be identified.

Reticulin in the normal marrow trephine is not marked, usually consisting of a few fine, scattered strands with no particular distribution.

Composition of reagents

10% Formal saline

40% formalin	10 ml
Normal saline (0.9% NaCl)	90 ml

PLASMA HAEMOGLOBIN

Purpose

In conditions causing intravascular red cell destruction, or when the rate of haemolysis is severe, free haemoglobin will appear in the plasma (haemoglobinaemia).

Principle

Quantitation of haemoglobin in plasma is based on the peroxidase activity of haem bringing about the oxidation of benzidine by hydrogen peroxide. This produces a violet colour which can be measured in a photoelectric colorimeter and compared with the colour produced by a standard haemoglobin solution. It is carried out at room temperature.

Test samples

Citrated blood; nine volumes of blood added to one volume of sodium citrate (32 g/l).

Reagents

- Benzidine 1 g%. CAUTION (see comments).
- Hydrogen peroxide 1%, prepare freshly, dilute 1 volume of '10 vols' H_2O_2 with 2 volumes distilled water.
- Standard haemoglobin solution.
- Diluent. 10% (v/v) glacial acetic acid in distilled water.

Equipment

○ Plastic 'universal' bottles or 15 ml test tubes (iron-free).
○ Photoelectric colorimeter, with a green filter (Ilford 624) or a spectrophotometer, set at 515 nm.

Standards

Haemoglobin solution of known haemoglobin content (10 g/dl). Dilute 20 μl in 10 ml normal saline (= 200 mg/l)

Method

1. To three tubes (Table 1.17), labelled blank, standard and test, add 1 ml benzidine solution.

2. Add to the blank 20 μl distilled water; to the standard, 20 μl known haemoglobin solution and to the tube labelled test, 20 μl plasma.

3. Add 1 ml 1% H_2O_2 to each tube.

4. Mix well, and leave for 20 minutes for colour change to develop completely. (It will be green initially).

5. Add 10 ml of the diluent, 10% glacial acetic acid to each tube.

6. Mix and leave for ten minutes.

7. Transfer the solutions to cuvettes, and read in the photoelectrical colorimeter or spectrophotometer using the blank to zero the machine.

Calculation

1. Plasma haemoglobin mg/l =

$$\frac{\text{absorbance test}}{\text{absorbance std}} \times \frac{\text{conc standard} \times \text{dilution}}{1000}$$

2. Plot optical Density v concentration, connecting reagent blank ('0') to standard (= 200 mg/l)

Normal <40 mg/l

Table 1.17 Estimation of plasma haemoglobin.

	Blank	Standard	Test 1 et.
Benzidine solution	1 ml	1 ml	1 ml
Haemoglobin	—	20 μ 1	—
Water	20 μl	—	—
Plasma	—	—	20 μl
H_2O_2	1 ml	1 ml	1 ml

Mix immediately and leave for 20 minutes for colour change to develop completely.

Acetic acid solution	10 ml	10 ml	10 ml

Mix and leave for 10 minutes.
Read.

Comments

— The avoidance of haemolysis in the collection of blood is the most important factor in achieving worthwhile results. Blood should be drawn off slowly and through a relatively wide-bore needle, which must be removed from the syringe before adding the blood to the sodium citrate.

— Let the blood settle for 60 minutes before centrifuging. Use a new pipette for separating each plasma sample. They remain stable if frozen.

— The small sample, 20 μl, means that a turbid plasma will not interfere with the colorimetric measurement.

— If the haemoglobin content of the test plasma is greatly increased it should be diluted until it is tinged pink.

— The reagent blank should be colourless; its optical density against water is less than 0.02.

— CAUTION Benzidine base is thought to be potentially carcinogenic and it may not be available. Mouth pipetting must be avoided. There are substitutes, but they are not as reliable as benzidine, which should be kept locked up.

Interpretation

If haemolysis is avoided by careful collection and separation of the plasma, very low levels for plasma haemoglobin are found in normal subjects, even after violent exercise. If these criteria have been met, a raised plasma haemoglobin is a reliable sign of recent intravascular haemolysis (e.g. haemolytic transfusion reaction, paroxysmal nocturnal haemoglobinuria, mechanical haemolytic anaemias, etc.). The benzidine method measures methaemoglobin, methaemalbumin as well as plasma haemoglobin.

Composition of reagents

Benzidine reagent 1%

Benzidine base	1 gm
Glacial acetic acid	90 ml
Distilled water	to 100 ml

Dissolve the benzidine base in the glacial acetic acid (keep stoppered) and make up to 100 ml with the distilled water. Store at 4°C in a dark bottle; stable for 1 month.

Plasma haemoglobin diluent

Glacial acetic acid	10 ml
Distilled water	90 ml

Standard haemoglobin solution

Wash 1 to 2 ml of red cells three times with normal saline. After the last wash, add an equal volume of distilled water to the red cells. Add a half volume of carbon tetrachloride and shake hard to haemolyse the red cells. Centrifuge at 3000 rpm for 15 minutes and decant haemolysate into a clean tube. Measure the haemoglobin content.

ERYTHROCYTE SEDIMENTATION RATE

Principle

The erythrocyte sedimentation rate (ESR) is a measure of the rate at which red cells subside when resuspended in autologous plasma and is widely used as a screening test for acute or chronic inflammatory disease and for monitoring the response to therapy. The selected method of the International Committee for Standardization in Haematology (1977) is that of Westergren.

The rate of subsidence of erythrocytes in the 200 mm calibrated area of the Westergren ESR tube is largely determined by the rouleaux-inducing effect of the larger molecular weight plasma proteins, in particular fibrinogen. This effect overcomes the electrostatic repulsive force conferred by the erythrocytes' zeta potential.

There are three phases of erythrocyte sedimentation — an initial lag phase in which erythrocyte aggregation occurs, followed by rapid sedimentation of rouleaux, and terminating in slow packing of erythrocytes towards the bottom of the tube. Dilution of the blood sample, and thus of plasma protein, by the citrate anticoagulant of the Westergren ESR prolongs the lag phase and reduces test sensitivity at low ESR values in comparison with the alternative Wintrobe ESR. The long (200 mm) calibrated area of the Westergren tube prolongs the sedimentation phase, however, to give a more accurate ESR at higher values.

It is not possible to apply a formula to correct accurately for the effect of anaemia, which accelerates sedimentation of rouleaux, but adjustment of the initial blood sample to a standard packed cell volume of 0.35, using autologous plasma, reduces dependence on anaemia (Moseley & Bull 1981). In practice, this is too laborious a procedure for routine use.

Test samples
— Venous blood (4 volumes) may be taken directly into 1 volume of filtered (0.22 μm pore diameter) 109 mmol/l trisodium citrate dihydrate ($Na_3C_6H_5O_7.2H_2O$) as anticoagulant/diluent. This dilution must be accurate. The ESR should then be set up within two hours.
— Venous blood may alternatively be taken first into dry edetic acid (3.4–4.8 mmol/l blood) as anticoagulant and thereafter diluted in citrate in the above proportions. Overnight storage at 4°C of blood anticoagulated with edetic acid results in a false low (approximately 20%) ESR value and is not recommended.
— Other anticoagulants should not be used.

Equipment
Disposable glass or plastic ESR tubes should be used but it is important to establish that the selected tubes give ESR results that are comparable with the ICSH method (International Committee for Standardization in Haematology 1977). This stipulated tubes of 300 ± 1.5 mm overall length (200 mm calibrated length) and 2.55 ± 0.15 mm internal diameter, the bore requiring to be uniform throughout to ± 0.05 mm.

Standards
No suitable standard erythrocyte suspension has yet become available. A British Standard for Westergren tubes is available (British Standards Institution 1987).

Method
1. It is important to thoroughly mix the diluted blood sample before it is aspirated, using a mechanical suction device, up to the 0 mm mark of the Westergren tube.
2. This tube must be located exactly vertically (± 1°) throughout the 60 min test and protected from direct sunlight, draughts, and vibration.
3. At 60 min, the distance between the bottom of the surface (plasma) meniscus to the top of the column of sedimented erythrocytes should be read to the nearest mm and expressed as ESR (Westergren, 1 h) = x mm.

Comments
— The range of ambient temperature at which the test is performed should not exceed 18–25°C.
— There must be no leakage of blood from the ESR tube during the test.
— The trisodium citrate anticoagulant/diluent may be stored for several months at 4°C if filtered (0.22 μm pore diameter) into a sterile container. Commercially available blood sample vials containing predispensed sodium citrate should similarly be stored at 4°C until used.
— Safety aspects of the test must be remembered, and mechanical suction, rather than mouth pipetting always used to fill the ESR tubes. Patient blood sample vials prefilled with citrate and with pierceable caps that allow a disposable ESR tube to be pushed through without opening the vial, are widely used. The test should not normally be performed on potentially infectious 'high risk' blood specimens.
— This simple to perform and frequently requested test suffers from lack of satisfactory quality assurance, although a proposed method has recently been described (Moseley & Bull 1981).

Interpretation
Different reference ranges are quoted but an 'intermediate' range (Lewis 1980) appears to offer highest test efficiency with a satisfactory balance between sensitivity and specificity (Kenny et al 1981):

Males	Upper limit of reference range (mm/h)
17–50 years	10
51–60 years	12
>60 years	14
Females	
17–50 years	12
51–60 years	19
>60 years	20

Higher ESR values than these may be obtained for apparently healthy elderly individuals but, in the age range 60–89 years, an ESR of >19 mm (males) or >22 mm (females) probably warrants investigation (Griffiths et al 1984).

An increase in the ESR above these reference limits indicates an acute-phase, or more chronic, increase in the concentration of plasma proteins, particularly those of larger molecular size such as fibrinogen. An increase in hepatic synthesis of acute-phase proteins occurs in response to any tissue inflammation or other injury that stimulates the local release of humoral mediators, such as interleukin-1, from monocytes/macrophages. Examples include surgery or other trauma, ischaemic infarction, immunological injury, infection, malignancy, collagen vascular disease, and pregnancy. Sedimentation in an ESR tube is also affected, however, by the number and deformability of erythrocytes so that a false high ESR occurs in anaemia and a false low value in polycythaemia or sickle cell disease.

PLASMA VISCOSITY

Principle
The measurement of plasma viscosity is a test of the resistance of plasma to flow deformation. Resistance to flow is determined by the concentration of various macromolecules, fibrinogen in particular. Since plasma behaves as a Newtonian fluid, flow is usually measured at high shear in a capillary viscometer (Harkness 1971, International Committee for Standardization in Haematology 1984) but it may also be measured in a rotational viscometer. An increase in plasma viscosity reflects, as does the erythrocyte sedimentation rate (ESR), any acute-phase or more chronic increase in plasma protein concentration. Advantages of measurement of plasma viscosity over the ESR include independence from erythrocyte count and abnormalities of erythrocyte deformability, calibration against a reference material of known viscosity, low coefficient of variation, and the need for only a small (0.5 ml) plasma test sample that can be stored for up to 6 days.

Test samples
Venous blood anticoagulated with edetic acid (K_2 or Na_2 salt at a concentration of 3.4–4.8 mmol/l blood) should be centrifuged at 1500 g for 5 minutes in a stoppered tube to prevent evaporation. The blood should be centrifuged as soon as possible (and not later than 6 hours) after venepuncture but, once separated, the plasma may be stored for up to one week in a stoppered tube at room temperature. Refrigeration must be avoided. Slight haemolysis has little effect on the result.

Equipment
The 1984 selected method of the International Committee for Standardization in Haematology (1984) was that of Harkness, the principle of which has been described in detail (Harkness 1971). In this method, the glassware of a Harkness capillary viscometer is filled with a priming fluid (36 g/l NaCl) and connected to a mercury manometer which applies a constant head of pressure to a glass capillary tube of precision bore

(0.38 mm internal diameter). The test plasma sample is sucked along this capillary as the mercury returns to equilibrium. The mercury passes along a horizontal section of tubing where there are two electrodes 6.4 cm apart. An electronic timer is activated and stopped as the mercury meniscus passes the electrodes. The working temperature of the instrument is usually set at 25°C ($\pm$ 0.05°C). Commercial viscometers based on this principle, and of manual or semi-automated type, are now available. Rotational viscometers may also be used to measure plasma viscosity.

Standards
A solution of 36 g/l NaCl (chemically pure and filtered), giving a viscosity of 0.943 mPa.s at 25°C, has been recommended for calibrating the Harkness type of capillary viscometer (International Committee for Standardization in Haematology 1984). This standard solution has a specific gravity similar to that of plasma and it also helps to prevent build-up of protein in the capillary tube and specimen cup.

Method
1. A vacuum pump is used to adjust the mercury meniscus in a manometer to give the required head of pressure (1.5–2.0 cm Hg). As soon as air has entered the capillary tube, 0.5 ml of NaCl standard solution should be pipetted into the specimen cup. When the air bubble and a small amount of standard have passed through the capillary, the tap connecting the vacuum line should be closed, the timer set to zero, and the flow time of the mercury between the two electrodes measured as a corresponding volume of standard is sucked along the capillary tube.

2. The flow time of the test plasma sample (0.5 ml) is then measured in the same way.

Calculation
Viscosity of test plasma (mPa.s) =

$$\frac{\text{viscosity of standard x flow time of plasma}}{\text{flow time of standard}}$$

Comments — capillary tube viscometers
— Plasma viscosity is highly dependent on the working temperature (25°C or 37°C) which should be maintained within $\pm$ 0.05°C.
— Introduction of an air bubble between samples helps to clean the capillary tube. Partial blockage, with fibrin for example, may also occur and the capillary tube should then be removed, flushed and recalibrated using NaCl standard solution. Use of plastic, rather than glass, Pasteur pipettes for handling samples will help to reduce blockages of the capillary tube.

— The capillary tube should be flushed, and refilled, with standard solution at the end of each batch of test plasmas. Disinfectant (sodium hypochlorite or glutaraldehyde) can be used to clean the apparatus when required.

— Anticoagulants other than edetic acid should not be used.

Interpretation

Normal reference range (both sexes) at 25°C:

Adults — 1.50–1.72 mPa.s.

Elderly — slightly higher values may be obtained owing to the higher plasma fibrinogen concentration

Pregnancy (last trimester) — up to 1.80 mPa.s

Measurement of plasma viscosity has a low coefficient of variation (<1%) so that an increase of 0.03–0.05 mPa.s or more indicates an abnormality of plasma protein concentration. Plasma hyperproteinaemia may occur as part of the acute-phase response (e.g. acute inflammation or acute tissue damage) or in response to a more chronic stimulus (e.g. chronic inflammation or the haematological stress syndrome [Reizenstein, 1979].

BLOOD VISCOSITY

Principle

The viscosity of a fluid is a measure of its resistance to change in shape, which is determined by the internal friction between adjacent layers of fluid. The velocity gradient between these layers is called the shear rate (measured in reciprocal seconds) and the force per unit area required to produce the velocity gradient is called the shear stress (measured in Pascals). Viscosity is defined as the ratio of shear stress to shear rate and is measured in milli Pascal seconds (mPa.s).

Newtonian fluids, such as plasma, show a constant ratio of shear stress to shear rate whereas whole blood is non-Newtonian, requiring a proportionately greater force to make it flow at low shear rates. Measurement of blood viscosity is therefore more complex than that of plasma, usually requiring a rotational viscometer that can operate at low, as well as at high, shear rates. This type of instrument has two concentric surfaces, one of which rotates, thus shearing the blood sample between them. Viscosity is a measure of the resistance to rotation caused by the blood.

The viscosity of whole blood is determined by its packed cell volume (PCV), plasma protein concentration, and erythrocyte deformability.

Test samples

Solid anticoagulants should be used to avoid haemo-dilution. Either edetic acid (3.4–4.8 mmol/l blood) or lithium heparin (15 IU/ml blood) may be used, although heparinised samples sometimes contain small strands of fibrin and microaggregated platelets. Viscosity measurements should be made within four hours of venepuncture, the sample being stored at ambient temperature.

Equipment

A variety of instrument manufacturers have adapted industrial viscometers for biological studies. Rotational viscometers usually comprise a temperature-controlled sample cup that can be rotated at various speeds to alter the shear rate. A small bob is lowered into the test blood sample in the rotating cup. The rotational torque transmitted by the blood sample can be measured as, for example, the electrical current required to prevent rotation of the bob and plotted as a function of rotational speed on an x-y plotter.

Continuously varying shear rates can be applied using a programmer, and different bob and cup combinations can also be used. These instruments operate, with a coefficient of variation of 3% or less, down to a shear rate of less than $1 \ s^{-1}$ (Inglis et al 1981).

Standards

The Expert Panel on Blood Rheology of the International Committee for Standardization in Haematology has recently made recommendations on the measurement of blood viscosity (International Committee for Standardization in Haematology 1986). Commercially available oils of known viscosity are also available and should be used to check the accuracy of viscometers and to calibrate x-y recorders.

Method

1. The instrument should be mounted on an anti-vibration table and a perspex windshield used to exclude air currents.

2. An external water bath with circulator is usually required to maintain the desired temperature, to ± 0.5°C, in the sample cup. Measurements should be made at 37°C (preferably) or 25°C.

3. The instrument must be levelled so that the bob is in the centre of the cup.

4. Well-mixed anticoagulated blood, sufficient to cover the bob, is pipetted into the cup while avoiding any air bubbles. The bob must then be centred again.

5. Viscosity should be measured at high (~200 s^{-1}) and at low (~1 s^{-1}) shear rates. Measurements at high shear should precede measurements at low shear (International Committee for Standardization in Haematology 1986).

Comments

— The bob and cup must be scrupulously clean and dry.

— Any time delay after pipetting the test sample into the cup may cause an erroneous result owing to settling of erythrocytes. The bob must therefore be adjusted to its central position and rotation started within one minute of adding blood to the cup (Inglis et al 1981). Use of a guard ring, to eliminate surface tension artefacts, may induce greater sedimentation artefacts owing to the time required to fit the ring. When the bob is completely immersed in the test blood sample, surface tension effects are in any case minimised. Use of a guard ring is therefore not recommended for measurements on whole blood.

— Since viscosity is critically dependent on temperature the blood sample should be prewarmed to the operating temperature. It is also recommended that the temperature of 1 ml of water placed in the sample cup be checked to ensure that the water-jacket temperature is sufficiently high.

— Any fibrin strands in the blood sample will grossly distort the result.

— A measurement of erythrocyte deformability, independent of plasma effects, can be obtained by suspending washed erythrocytes in buffer and measuring viscosity at a high shear rate ($\sim$200 s^{-1}). An accurately measured and standardised erythrocyte count is required.

Calculation

A plot of torque reading against rotational speed is obtained on the x-y recorder, the torque being converted to viscosity using manufacturers' tables. Since there is a linear relationship between PCV and the logarithm of whole blood viscosity it is necessary, if variation in PCV is not to be studied, to correct the viscosity reading to a standard PCV (usually 0.45). This can be done using a regression line for the log viscosity-PCV relationship based on normal blood manipulated in vitro to give a PCV range corresponding to that of the patient group (Inglis et al 1981). An alternative is to adjust each test blood sample to a standard PCV or erythrocyte count prior to measurement of viscosity.

Interpretation

A reference range should be determined for each laboratory owing to inter-laboratory differences in shear rate, temperature of measurement, and method of correction for PCV.

If uncorrected for PCV, whole blood viscosity measurements at all shear rates are predominantly determined by the erythrocyte count of the sample. When corrected for PCV, a raised whole blood viscosity value at a low shear rate ($\sim$1 s^{-1}) usually reflects the rouleaux-inducing effect of the larger molecular size plasma proteins, in particular fibrinogen. At high shear rates ($\sim$200 s^{-1}), rouleaux are dispersed so that erythrocyte deformability then influences the result.

When a standard erythrocyte count is used for viscosity studies, patients with a raised mean cell volume (MCV) may give a high viscosity reading (Bareford et al 1985).

PRUSSIAN BLUE STAIN FOR IRON (PERLS)

This method demonstrates iron granules in marrow macrophages, erythroblasts (sideroblasts) and in erythrocytes (siderocytes).

Principle
Ionized iron reacts with acid ferrocyanide to give a blue-green colour.

Test samples
Air-dried marrow, peripheral blood films or other material.

Equipment
Coplin jars.

Reagents
- Potassium ferrocyanide 20 g/l   A
- Hydrochloric acid — 19 : 64 ml concentrated HCl added to water and made to 1 litre   B

Mix equal volumes of A and B immediately before use.
- Methyl alcohol — anhydrous
- Safranin — aqueous 1g/l

Standards
A marrow film known to contain iron is always processed with the test samples.

Method
1. Fix films in anhydrous methyl alcohol for 20 minutes.
2. Place acid ferrocyanide solution (equal parts A and B) in the Coplin jar and immerse slides for 10 minutes at room temperature.
3. Wash slides well in running tap water for 20 minutes.
4. Rinse thoroughly in distilled water.
5. Counterstain with safranin for 5–10 seconds.
6. Mount in neutral mountant.

Comment
All glassware should be soaked in 2 mol/l HCl to remove extraneous iron and finally rinsed in glass distilled water.

Interpretation
In a marrow look for iron in the fragments and at a higher power confirm that these are discrete iron-

staining granules in marrow macrophages. Absence of iron can only be accepted when iron is present in the control slides.

About 50% of normal erythroblasts contain one or two iron granules. An abnormal erythroblast may have several iron granules and in a ringed sideroblast these are distributed as a ring or half-ring about the nucleus.

REFERENCES

X_B Calibration and control of multichannel haematology analysers

Bull B S 1975 A Statistical Approach to Quality Control. In: Lewis S M, Costar J F (eds) Quality Control in Haematology. Academic Press, London. p 111–121

Bull B S, Elashoff R M, Heilbron D C, Couperus J 1974 A Study of various Estimators for the Derivation of Quality Control Procedures from Patient Erythrocyte Indices. American Journal of Clinical Pathology 61: 473–481

Bull B S, Hay K L 1985 Are Red Blood Cell Indexes International? Archives of Pathology and Laboratory Medicine 109: 604–606

Bull B S, Hay K L 1988 Intralaboratory Quality Control using Patients' Data. In: Cavill I (ed) Methods in Hematology Quality Control. Churchill Livingstone, New York. In press

Levy W C, Bull B S, Koepke J A 1986 The incorporation of RBC index mean data into quality control programs. American Journal of Clinical Pathology 86: 193–199

Erythrocyte sedimentation rate

British Standards Institution 1968 Specification for Westergren tubes and support for the measurement of erythrocyte sedimentation rate. British Standard, 2554.

Griffiths R A, Good W R, Watson N P, O'Donnell H F, Fell P J, Shakespeare J M 1984 Normal erythrocyte sedimentation rate in the elderly. British Medical Journal 289: 724–725

International Committee for Standardization in Haematology 1977 Recommendation for measurement of erythrocyte sedimentation rate of human blood. American Journal of Clinical Pathology 68: 505–507

Kenny M W et al 1981 Efficiency of haematological screening tests for detecting disease. Clinical and Laboratory Haematology 3: 299–305

Lewis S M 1980 Erythrocyte sedimentation rate and plasma viscosity. Association of Clinical Pathologists, Broadsheet 94: 1–6

Moseley D L, Bull B S 1981 A comparison of the Wintrobe, the Westergren and the ZSR erythrocyte sedimentation rate (ESR) methods to a candidate reference method. Clinical and Laboratory Haematology 4: 169–178

Plasma viscosity

Harkness J 1971 The viscosity of human blood plasma; its measurement in health and disease. Biorheology 8: 171–193

International Committee for Standardization in Haematology 1984 Recommendation for a selected method for the measurement of plasma viscosity. Journal of Clinical Pathology 37: 1147–1152

Reizenstein P 1979 The haematological stress syndrome. British Journal of Haematology 43: 329–334

Blood viscosity

Bareford D, Stone P C W, Caldwell N M, Meiselman H J, Stuart J 1985 Comparison of instruments for measurement of erythrocyte deformability. Clinical Hemorheology 5: 311–322

Inglis T C McN, Carson P J, Stuart J 1981 Clinical measurement of whole-blood viscosity at low-shear rates. Clinical Hemorheology 1: 167–177

International Committee for Standardization in Haematology 1986 Guidelines for measurement of blood viscosity and erythrocyte deformability. Clinical Hemorheology 6: 439–453

2

Haemoglobin analysis

The haemoglobinopathies include both structurally abnormal haemoglobins (usually the result of a single amino acid substitution in one of the globin chains) and the thalassaemias, a group of disorders characterised by a deficit in the production of one of the globin chains. As a whole the haemoglobinopathies are by far the most common of the human genetic disorders, believed to be maintained at a high frequency in many populations as a result of the relative protection of the heterozygous carriers against *P. falciparum* malaria. Their natural distribution covers a broad belt across the old world including the Mediterranean, western and central Africa, the Middle East, India and SE Asia. However, with the world-wide dispersal of immigrants from these regions, haemoglobinopathies turn up in haematology laboratories everywhere. In addition, isolated cases may occur in any population as a result of a relatively recent mutation.

The techniques for the differential diagnosis of a potential haemoglobinopathy are well-established. A clinical history should be taken from the patient, together with their geographical origins and a family history, including the availability of relatives for family study. A full blood count and a blood film are essential and haemoglobin electrophoresis should also be mandatory in the initial work-up. Structurally abnormal haemoglobins with an altered charge will be detected by electrophoresis; abnormal haemoglobins with a similar electrophoretic migration to HbA may still be suspected if there are functional consequences e.g. abnormal oxygen affinity or unstable haemoglobins. The presence of a thalassaemia will normally be indicated by the abnormal red cell indices and altered morphology; measurement of HbA_2 and HbF should indicate whether α, β or $\delta\beta$ thalassaemia is involved. In doubtful cases, this may be confirmed by measuring globin chain synthesis ratios, which are also useful in those forms with little or no phenotypic effect. It must also be borne in mind that since several different haemoglobinopathies may be present in the same population, interactions of several different disorders may initially present an atypical picture which can often be best sorted out by family studies.

STARCH GEL ELECTROPHORESIS OF HAEMOGLOBINS

Haemoglobin electrophoresis is the main method for the detection of haemoglobin variants and it may also be of importance in the differential diagnosis of the various thalassaemia syndromes. Electrophoretic mobility alone cannot conclusively identify a particular abnormal haemoglobin, but if such information is combined with the clinical and haematological characteristics and the racial background of the patient it may well lead to an adequate presumptive diagnosis.

Electrophoresis is normally carried out at alkaline pH, using one of a number of support media. For large-scale screening purposes, cellulose acetate membranes are probably the most convenient, while many specialist laboratories have retained starch gel as the medium because the combination of its resolving power and larger sample volume improves the detection of minor components.

Test samples
Electrophoresis is normally carried out on haemolysates containing about 80–100 g/l haemoglobin.

1. Centrifuge the anticoagulated blood sample and remove the plasma.

2. Wash the red cells three times in normal saline (8.5 g NaCl/l distilled water).

3. Lyse the cells by mixing with two volumes of distilled water.

4. To two volumes of lysed cells add one volume of carbon tetrachloride and mix thoroughly.

5. Centrifuge at 3000 g for 30 minutes and remove the clarified lysate from above the stromal layer.

6. For storage, add 1–2 drops of a 1% KCN solution; store for up to 4 weeks at 4°C.

Reagents

Hydrolysed potato starch (BDH), stored at room temperature, has a shelf life of several months. More prolonged storage, particularly at high ambient temperatures, may lead to a decline in its gelling properties.

Stock TEB buffer solution, pH 8.6, is stable for six weeks at room temperature.

Protein stains such as Amido Black or Naphthalene Black are reusable for several weeks.

Haemoprotein stains such as o-tolidine or o-dianisidine can be stored at 4°C in a darkened glass bottle for no longer than one month.

Equipment

○ Perspex electrophoresis trays may be purchased commercially or made in a workshop.
○ A voltage regulated D.C. power source, capable of supplying 250 v, is necessary.
○ Since the gels should be run at 4°C, a cold room or domestic refrigerator is required.

Method

1. The starch gel is prepared by heating 60–65 g of hydrolysed starch in 500 ml of TEB buffer diluted 1 in 20 with distilled water in a conical sidearm flask. As the starch begins to boil, the opaque gel becomes clearer and less viscous, at which stage it is degassed by attachment of the sidearm to a vacuum system. When all the air bubbles have been removed, the molten starch is poured into the electrophoresis tray containing the detachable combs, with usually 8 teeth which protrude into the gel and leave the sample slot when removed. A glass plate is used to cover the gel which, when cool, is refrigerated for at least 3 hours.

2. The slot formers are removed and the samples (∼10 μl) loaded using a Pasteur pipette. Molten paraffin wax is used to seal the slots.

3. The gel is placed in the electrophoresis apparatus with the samples at the upper, cathodal end, using filter paper or gauze wicks to connect the gel to the buffer chambers. The cathode chamber (top) contains stock TEB buffer diluted 1:7 with distilled water while the anode (bottom) chamber contains a 1:4 dilution of the stock buffer.

4. Connect the power supply and electrophorese for ∼16 hours (overnight is convenient) at 4°C at 220 v.

5. Remove the gel tray from the electrophoresis equipment and slide out the gel from the tray.

6. Slice the gel horizontally into two halves using a taut-wire gel slicer (Buchner Instruments) and lift each half into separate staining dishes.

7. For protein staining, cover the gel with Naphthalene Black stain and leave for at least one hour. Remove the stain and add destaining solution, agitating gently and replacing the solution as necessary. The gel should be sufficiently destained to read after about 2 hours. When blotted dry, the gel can be wrapped in clingfilm for long-term storage.

8. For haem-protein staining the gel is covered with the o-tolidine solution and a few drops of 100 vols hydrogen peroxide added. Blue staining of the haemoglobin bands develops rapidly, after which the stain is poured off and the gel is rinsed in distilled water.

Comments

— The amount of starch necessary to give a gel of the right consistency (firm but flexible) may vary slightly from batch to batch.
— Incomplete removal of stroma will tend to lead to smearing of the samples during electrophoresis.
— Do not overload the slots.
— The anode and cathode buffers should be changed frequently; prolonged use leads to reduced migration of the samples in the gel.

Interpretation

Figure 2.1 illustrates a typical starch gel containing various abnormal haemoglobins. Under the conditions described above, HbA$_2$ migrates about 1.5 cm towards the anode while HbA will have moved about 4.5 cm. Of the common variants, Hbs C,E and O run with HbA$_2$ while Hbs S,D,G and Lepore migrate about half-way between HbA$_2$ and HbA. HbF moves between HbS and HbA while 'fast' variants, such as HbJ, migrate ahead of HbA, as do the γ and β chain tetramers, Hb Bart's and HbH respectively.

In identifying unknown samples, α chain variants can be distinguished from β chain variants by the presence of not only an abnormal major band ($\alpha_2^x\beta_2$) but also an abnormal HbA$_2$ band ($\alpha_2^x\gamma_2$). Variants of the α chain also tend to comprise a lower proportion of the total haemoglobin (20–25%) than β chain variants (35–55%); this can make detection of the abnormal HbA$_2$ band difficult.

Of the common variants which migrate together, the suspected presence of HbS can be confirmed either by a Hb solubility test (Itano 1953, Schmidt & Wilson 1973) or induction of sickling in whole blood by sodium metabisulphate (see below). Alternatively, agar gel electrophoresis at pH6.0 (Robinson et al 1957, Schneider & Barwick 1982) can be used to distinguish HbS from Hbs D or G. In patients of African origin, HbS is by far the most common variant in this position; among those whose cells do not sickle, the most frequent alternative variant is HbG Philadelphia, an α chain variant.

Both Hbs S and D reach polymorphic frequencies in

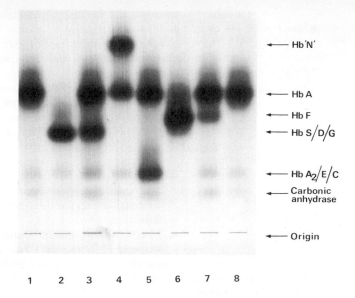

Fig. 2.1 Starch gel electrophoresis, illustrating the relative migration of various abnormal haemoglobins (Amido Black Stain).

some Indian populations. If a sickling test is negative, HbD Punjab (also known as HbD Los Angeles) is the most likely diagnosis.

The other major variants which migrate together on alkaline electrophoresis are Hbs C and E, both of which are associated with significant target cell formation. The geographical range of HbC is largely restricted to West Africa and populations derived therefrom, while HbE is mainly found in SE Asia, from Bangladesh eastwards. Thus knowing the racial origins of the patient is a significant pointer to a diagnosis, although where the two populations have intermixed, as in E Africa, this assumption is less reliable. The two haemoglobins can be distinguished by their susceptibility to oxidation by dichlorophenolindophenol (Frischer & Bowman 1975).

Composition of solutions

Stock TEB buffer, pH 8.6

Tris (hydroxymethyl) aminomethane (tris)	109.00 g
Ethylenediaminetetraacetic acid (EDTA)	5.84 g
Boric acid	30.30 g
Distilled water	to 1 litre

Destaining solution

Glacial acetic acid	100 ml
Methanol	450 ml
Distilled water	450 ml

Protein stain

Napthalene Black	0.8 g
Destaining solution	1.0 litre

o-tolidine stain

o-tolidine	1.0 g
Sodium nitroprusside	1.0 g
5% acetic acid	1 litre

CELLULOSE ACETATE MEMBRANE HAEMOGLOBIN ELECTROPHORESIS

Principle

The separation of different haemoglobins depends mainly on the charge on the haemoglobin molecule at alkaline pH. Since this technique allows good separation to be obtained quickly between Hbs A, F, S, and C it is very useful as part of the primary screen for sickle haemoglobin and other common haemoglobin variants.

Test sample

Any anticoagulant may be used.

Adult and cord blood

Centrifuge sample (3000 rpm for 5 min) and then dilute 20 μl of packed red cells with 150 μl of the haemolysing reagent. Mix gently and leave for at least 5 minutes.

Adult haemolysate

Dilute 40 μl of 100 g/l haemolysate with 150 μl of haemolysing reagent.

Controls

Always include AS and Cord (AF) samples on each plate.

Equipment

○ Cellulose acetate membranes with plastic backing (such as Helena Titan III-H plates, No 3022) are particularly easy to use.
○ Electrophoresis tank.
○ Power unit to supply at least 10 mA at 350 v.
○ Sample applicator.

Method

1. Prepare the electrophoresis tank by placing equal volumes of buffer in the anode and cathode compartments. Set the bridge gap to 7 cm. Wet two electrode wicks in the buffer and place one along each wick support ensuring that they make good contact with the buffer.

2. Lower the cellulose acetate plates slowly into a reservoir of buffer and leave them to soak for at least five minutes before use.

3. Fill the sample well plate with 5 μl of each sample and cover with a 6 cm coverslip or glass slide to prevent evaporation. Load a second sample well plate with diluted wetting agent.

4. Clean the applicator tips by loading with the diluted wetting agent and then applying them to a blotter. Tips should be cleaned in this way immediately prior to use.

5. Remove the cellulose acetate strips from the buffer and blot twice on two layers of clean blotting paper. Do not allow the cellulose acetate to dry. Load the applicator by depressing the tips into the sample wells several times and apply this first loading onto some clean blotting paper. Reload the applicator and apply the samples to the cellulose acetate for approximately five seconds. The actual time required will depend on the type of applicator and the way it is used. The applicator should be used within 15 seconds of being loaded.

6. Apply the samples to the cellulose acetate, positioning the origin 2 cm from the cathodal end of the cellulose acetate.

7. Place the cellulose acetate plates across the bridges, with the plastic side uppermost, so that they make good contact with the electrode wicks. Place two glass slides lengthwise across each plate to ensure good contact but not allowing the slides to touch the wicks, and then electrophorese at 350 v for 25 minutes. Rinse the applicator with distilled water as soon as possible

after use and dry the applicator tips by applying them to blotting paper.

8. After 25 minutes quickly transfer the cellulose acetate to Ponceau S and then leave the strips to fix and stain for 5 minutes.

9. Decolourise the cellulose acetate strips by washing well in three changes of 3% acetic acid. Decolourisation is satisfactory when the cellulose acetate appears white. Blot once with clean blotting paper and leave to dry.

Comments

— If cellulose acetate sheet is used instead of cellulose acetate plates (where the cellulose acetate is bound to a plastic backing) it is better to place the sample side uppermost.

— The separation obtained after 25 minutes is such that the HbA and HbF are separated by approximately 3 mm, HbA and HbS by 8 mm, and HbA and HbC by 16 mm.

Interpretation

Some common haemoglobins migrate as shown:

```
                              Anode
                              − N
                              − J

                              − A
                              − F
                              − S,D,G,Lepore

                              − C,E,O,A₂
        carbonic anhydrase −
                              + + + + + origin
                              Cathode
```

Composition of solutions

Buffer Tris/EDTA/borate (pH 8.5)

Tris	10.2 g
EDTA (disodium salt)	0.6 g
Boric acid	3.2 g
Distilled water	to 1 l

This buffer may be used up to ten times without significant deterioration.

Haemolysing solution

0.5% Triton X-100 in 10 mg/100 ml potassium cyanide (1 ml of 10 g/l KCN in 100 ml solution).

Stain

0.5% Ponceau S in 7.5% trichloroacetic acid (20 g Ponceau S and 300 g TCA in 4 l of distilled water).

3% *acetic acid* (dilute 120 ml glacial acetic acid to 4 l with distilled water).

Wetting agent, such as Helena Zip-prep solution.

CITRATE AGAR HAEMOGLOBIN ELECTROPHORESIS

Principle
The separation of different haemoglobins depends partly on the charge on the haemoglobin molecule at acid pH and partly on its solubility in agar. Purified agar, such as agarose, should not be used since the separation in agarose is different (and usually less helpful) than that obtained in agar. Citrate agar electrophoresis is used because it provides separation of HbS from HbD and HbC from HbE. It also provides clear separation between HbA and HbF.

Test sample
Any anticoagulant may be used.

Adult blood
Centrifuge samples (3000 rpm for 5 min) and then dilute 20 μl of packed red cells with 300 μl of the haemolysing reagent. Mix gently and leave for at least 5 minutes.

Cord blood
Centrifuge samples (3000 rpm for 5 min) and then dilute 30 μl of packed red cells with 150 μl of the haemolysing reagent. Mix gently and leave for at least 5 minutes.

Adult haemolysate
Dilute 20 μl of 100 g/l haemolysate with 150 μl of haemolysing reagent.

Controls
Always include AS, AC and Cord (AF) samples on each plate.

Equipment
○ Difco Bacto-agar.
○ Gel Bond.
○ Electrophoresis tank.
○ Ice packs to keep the buffer and agar cool (if unavailable run in a refrigerator).
○ Power unit to supply at least 40 mA at 150 v.
○ Sample applicator.

Preparation of gel
1. Add 0.5 g agar to 50 ml working buffer. Heat to approximately 95°C stirring gently until the agar has dissolved.

2. Allow the agar to cool to 50°C, pour approximately 10 ml into each of four 80 × 100 × 2 mm perspex trays and allow to set. These plates may then be kept at 4°C for 1 week.

Method
1. Dilute 50 ml stock buffer to 250 ml with distilled water. Prepare the electrophoresis tank by placing equal volumes of this diluted buffer in the anode and cathode compartments. Set the bridge gap to 7 cm. Wet two sponge wicks in the buffer and place one in each buffer compartment. Just before use place a frozen 'ice pack' in each buffer chamber directly under the agar plate.

2. Fill the sample well plate with 5 μl of each sample and cover with a 6 cm coverslip or glass slide to prevent evaporation. Load a second sample well plate with diluted wetting agent.

3. Clean the applicator tips by loading with the diluted wetting agent and then applying them to a blotter. Tips should be cleaned in this way immediately prior to use. Load the applicator by depressing the tips into the sample wells several times and apply this first loading onto some clean blotting paper. Reload the applicator and apply the samples to the agar gel for approximately 5 seconds. The applicator should be used within 15 seconds of being loaded. The application line should be across the centre of the gel.

4. Place gel plate in an inverted position in the electrophoresis tank so that the gel is in contact with sponge wicks and run at a constant voltage of 50 volts for 45 minutes (see comments). Rinse the applicator tips with distilled water as soon as possible after use. Some applicator tips are very delicate and should only be dried by applying them to blotting paper.

5. After 45 minutes transfer the gel to a tray and apply the stain solution by layering onto the agar using a Pasteur pipette. Allow to stain for 10 minutes at room temperature and then wash three times in 3% acetic acid, leaving the gels in the last wash overnight.

6. After overnight soaking in wash solution, float off onto Gel Bond and leave to dry (see comments). These mounted gels may then be kept indefinitely.

Comments
— o-dianisidine is a potentially dangerous reagent and the dry powder should be handled with caution. Gloves should be worn when making up and using the stain mixture.
— The separation obtained is such that HbA and HbF are usually separated by 5 mm, HbA and HbS by 6 mm and HbA and HbC by 10 mm.
— It is very important that the agar is kept cool during the electrophoresis run by the use of ice packs or by

carrying out the run in a cold room or refrigerator. This is especially important if filter paper wicks are used instead of sponges since it is then usually necessary to use a higher voltage to obtain a satisfactory current and this will produce more heat.

- If Gel Bond is not available paper card may be used but it is less satisfactory.
- Other stains, such as Naphthol Black, may also be used.

Interpretation
Some common haemoglobins migrate as follows:

	Anode
	– C
	– S
	– A, A_2, D, E, G, Lepore
origin	+++++
	– F
	Cathode

Composition of solutions

Citrate buffer, pH 6.2
Stock buffer

Trisodium citrate dihydrate	73.5 g
0.5 M citric acid	34.0 ml
Distilled water	to 1 l

Working buffer
Dilute stock buffer 1 in 5 with distilled water.

Dianisidine stain

3% Hydrogen peroxide (10 volumes)	1.0 ml
1% Sodium nitroprusside (nitroferricyanide)	1.0 ml
3% Acetic acid	10.0 ml
0.2% o-dianisidine in methanol	5.0 ml

N.B. Prepare the stain mixture just before use.

Wetting agent such as Helena Zip-prep.

Acetic acid wash
3% solution of glacial acetic acid in distilled water.

QUANTITATION OF HbA_2 USING CELLULOSE ACETATE

Quantitation of the proportion of HbA_2 is an essential technique in the diagnosis of suspected cases of thalassaemia. With very few exceptions, the proportion of HbA_2 is increased above the normal range in cases of heterozygous β thalassaemia, a finding which is totally specific for this condition.

Methods for separating HbA_2 from HbA are either based on column chromatography techniques (Huisman et al 1975) or by electrophoresis in a medium from which the haemoglobin fractions can be recovered. Cellulose acetate strips are suitable (Marengo-Rowe 1965) for the latter and a simple method for HbA_2 quantitation is described below.

Test samples
Normal strength haemolysate (80–100 g/l), as used for haemoglobin electrophoresis and HbF estimation is suitable. Samples are normally run in duplicate.

Equipment
- ○ An electrophoresis tray suitable for cellulose acetate strips.
- ○ A power source supplying 250 v.
- ○ A spectrophotometer for readings at a wavelength of 415 nm.

Method
1. The cellulose acetate strips are dipped in buffer and blotted dry before being stretched taut across the bridges of the electrophoresis tray. Filter paper wicks connect the strips to the chambers containing the TEB buffer.
2. 10 μl of haemolysate is applied to each strip via a microcapillary pipette to give a smooth and even line across the width of the strip, about 1 cm from the cathodal end.
3. Electrophoresis is carried out at 220 v for about 1.5 hours or until there is a clear separation visible between the HbA and the minor HbA_2 bands.
4. The strips are removed and the HbA and HbA_2 zones are cut into narrow strips and eluted in tubes containing 15 ml and 1.5 ml of the buffer respectively.
5. When elution is complete (~20 min) the tubes are inverted to mix the contents and the OD 415 nm of the haemoglobin solutions is determined.

Calculation

Percentage HbA_2

$$= \frac{OD^{415}HbA_2}{OD^{415}HbA_2 + (OD^{415}HbA \times 10)} \times 100$$

Comments
- Smooth and even sample application is important and requires practice.
- Occasional batches of cellulose acetate strips have been found to release particles of cellulose acetate during the elution stage. If the haemoglobin solution

looks slightly cloudy after elution, these particles can be removed by centrifugation in a bench centrifuge.

— The resolution of the HbA and HbA_2 bands is temperature sensitive; under high ambient temperatures some form of cooling (e.g. fan) may be advantageous.

— The haemoglobin concentration of the lysate should not exceed 10 g/dl (poor separation) or fall below 5 g/dl (inaccurate OD measurements).

Interpretation

The proportion of HbA_2 in normal individuals (>6 months of age) is 2.0–3.2%. A batch of known normal samples should be run regularly to check this. The standard deviation of replicate measurements of the same sample should be less than 10% of the mean, and similar figures should be obtained with repeat sampling of the same individual over a period of time. Some variability may occur depending on exactly where the strip is cut but this should not be great enough for the normal values to overlap with the range in β thalassaemia heterozygotes of 3.9–6.5%.

Values much below 2.0% are uncommon; severe iron deficiency has been reported to reduce HbA_2 levels and well-documented cases of δ thalassaemia have been described in which heterozygotes may have HbA_2 levels of 1.0–1.5%.

Samples falling between 3.2 and 3.9% are also rare and should always be repeated. Samples which remain in this range on repeated measurements are of unknown significance and may warrant further investigations, such as family studies, globin chain synthesis, etc.

Composition of solutions

TEB buffer pH 8.9

Tris (hydroxymethyl) aminomethane (tris)	14.4 g
Ethylenediaminetetraacetic acid (EDTA)	1.5 g
Boric acid	0.9 g
Distilled water	to 1 l

QUANTITATION OF HbA_2 USING CELLULOSE MICROCOLUMN METHOD

Principle

At pH 8.5 haemoglobin binds to the top of the cellulose ion exchange column. The HbA_2 is then eluted from the column with a pH 8.3 buffer, following which the remainder of the haemoglobin is eluted from the column with a pH 7 buffer. HbC and HbE elute with HbA_2 and therefore this technique is not suitable for measuring HbA_2 in the presence of HbC, HbE or other haemoglobin variants which elute with HbA_2. As a general rule, the separation of HbA_2 from haemoglobin variants is similar to the separation obtained using electrophoresis on cellulose acetate or starch gel.

Test samples

Any anticoagulant may be used for blood collection. The haemolysate must be prepared from washed red cells and have a haemoglobin concentration of approximately 100 g/l.

Equipment

o Ion-exchanger.
  Pre-swollen microgranular anion exchange cellulose: DE 52 (Whatman & Co.).

Preparation of cellulose

1. Mix 10 g DE 52 with 200 ml Tris buffer pH 8.5 and allow to settle.

2. Decant the supernatant, resuspend the cellulose in a further 200 ml of buffer, and allow it to settle.

3. Decant the supernatant, resuspend the cellulose in a further 200 ml buffer and then stir gently for 10 minutes.

4. Using 1 M HCl, adjust pH to 8.5 whilst stirring.

5. Allow the cellulose to settle, decant the supernatant, and resuspend the cellulose in approximately 100 ml Tris buffer pH 8.5.

The suspended cellulose may be stored at 4°C for one month.

Method

Note — do each sample in duplicate.

1. Place a very small piece of cotton wool in the constriction of a short-form Pasteur pipette and place the pipette in a support rack.

2. Pack the column by pipetting the DE 52 cellulose slurry into the Pasteur pipette and allowing the contents to settle. Continue to apply cellulose until the cellulose bed is 6 cm in length. Allow all the supernatant buffer to flow through, but do not allow the column to become dry. If necessary, add a little more buffer (pH 8.5).

3. Dilute 1 drop of haemolysate with 4 drops Tris buffer pH 8.5 and then apply the diluted haemolysate to the top of the cellulose bed. Allow the samples to be absorbed and if any haemolysate remains on the sides of the column, wash it on to the top of the cellulose bed with a few drops of pH 8.5 buffer.

4. Attach a 10–15 cm length of polythene tubing to the top of the Pasteur pipette as a reservoir. Elute the HbA_2 fraction by washing the column with approximately 8 ml buffer at pH 8.3 and collect the eluate in a 10 ml volumetric flask.

5. Elute the HbA fraction by washing the column with approximately 10 ml of buffer at pH 7.0. Collect the eluate in a 25 ml volumetric flask.

6. Adjust the volumes of the fractions collected to 10 ml and 25 ml respectively using distilled water.

7. Read the absorbances of the fractions at 415 nm against a distilled water blank.

Calculation

%HbA$_2$

$$= \frac{\text{Absorbance HbA}_2 \times 100}{\text{Absorbance HbA}_2 + (\text{Absorbance HbA} \times 2.5)}$$

Note. The duplicates should be within 0.2% of each other

Interpretation

Normal range 2.2–3.2% (mean ± 2SD).

Most people with β-thalassaemia trait will have HbA$_2$ levels of 4% or above. Some people have a raised level of HbA$_2$ if they are a carrier of one of the unstable haemoglobins. In α-thalassaemia trait, the HbA$_2$ will be normal or low.

Comments

— Potassium cyanide is poisonous. Do not mouth pipette.
— Match cuvettes each day, better still, use the same cuvette for the HbA$_2$ and HbA of each sample.
— Read HbA$_2$ and HbA in that order to minimise the effects of carry over.
— Some pH electrodes are unsuitable for Tris and this may lead to serious errors in measuring pH.
— The first time buffers are made up, the elution pattern should be checked by measuring the absorbance of 1 ml aliquots and making small adjustments to the pH of the buffers until the elution profile is satisfactory.

Composition of solutions

Tris/HCl buffer 50 mM, pH 8.5

Tris (hydroxymethyl) methylamine	12.1 g
Potassium cyanide	0.2 g

1. Dissolve in approximately 1900 ml distilled water.
2. Adjust the pH to 8.5 using 2 M HCl and make up to a final volume of 2 litres with distilled water.

Tris/HCl buffer 50 mM, pH 8.3

Make as given above, but adjust the pH to 8.3 with 2 M HCl.

Tris/HCl buffer 50 mM, pH 7.0

Make as given above but adjust the pH to 7.0 with 2 M HCl.

METABISULPHITE TEST FOR SICKLING

Homozygous sickle cell anaemia can normally be diagnosed from the clinical and haematological picture, together with the changes in red cell morphology. None of these changes occur in the heterozygotes and the presence of an electrophoretic variant in the position of HbS is not conclusive. The presence of HbS can be confirmed either by a test based on its reduced solubility relative to other haemoglobins or by demonstrating the induction of sickle cell formation when whole blood is deoxygenated, as described here.

Test samples

This test should preferably be carried out on fresh blood samples; a normal control should be included.

Method

1. Thoroughly mix equal volumes of whole blood and freshly prepared 2% sodium metabisulphite (0.2 g in 10 ml distilled water).
2. A drop is then placed on a slide and covered with a coverslip, the edges of which are sealed with Vaseline.
3. After one hour, the slide is observed under a light microscope.

Interpretation

Normal cells retain their discoid shape in sodium metabisulphite although some tendency to burr cell formation occurs with stored samples. In sickle cell heterozygotes, the variable but characteristic morphology of sickled cells should be readily apparent.

SICKLE SOLUBILITY TEST

Principle

Sickle cell tests depend on the decreased solubility of HbS in conditions of reduced oxygen concentration. The mixture of HbS in a reducing solution will give a turbid appearance, whereas haemoglobins with normal solubility will give a clear solution.

It is important that both negative and positive controls are included with each test and that all tests are later checked using haemoglobin electrophoresis (CAM at alkaline pH).

Test sample

Any anticoagulant may be used.

Method

1. Pipette 2 ml working solution into a 75 × 12 mm test tube.
2. Add 0.02 ml blood and mix well.
3. Leave for 3–5 minutes and examine for turbidity.

Note. Positive and negative controls should be set up with each test.

Interpretation

Examine the tubes in a good light against a background of printed type or lines. It is important to remember that a positive result only indicates the presence of HbS and does not discriminate between AS, SC, SS or Sβ-thalassaemia

Turbid solution — positive result.
Clear solution — negative result.

Comment

— Before testing samples from anaemic patients, adjust the haematocrit to approximately 50% by the removal of plasma.
— False positives may occur in the presence of abnormal plasma proteins or when patients are having parenteral nutrition.

Compositon of solutions

Stock buffer

Anhydrous potassium dihydrogen phosphate	38.8 g
Anhydrous dipotassium hydrogen phosphate	59.3 g
Saponin	2.5 g
Distilled water	to 250 ml

Working solution

Add 0.2 g sodium dithionite to 20 ml buffer and mix well. The solution is stable for one week and both buffer and working solutions should be stored at 4°C. Sodium dithionite may become oxidised on storage.

QUANTITATION OF HbH AND Hb BART'S

The quantitation of HbH and Hb Bart's can also be carried out by elution from cellulose acetate strips after their separation from other haemoglobins by electrophoresis at neutral pH. At this pH, there is little or no separation of HbA from HbF or most variant haemoglobins.

Test samples

Fresh haemolysates should be used since these abnormal haemoglobins are somewhat unstable on storage.

Equipment

As for HbA$_2$ determination.

Method

1. Strips are prepared as for HbA$_2$ quantitation.

2. 5 μl of sample are loaded ~2 cm from the cathodal end of the strip with a microcapillary pipette and electrophoresis is carried out at 190 v for 15–30 min, until a clear separation of the HbH or Hb Bart's from the remaining haemoglobins is achieved.

3. After electrophoresis, the strip is cut to separate the two bands which are then eluted in 2 ml of distilled water. The optical density of the solutions is then read at 415 nm.

Calculation

Percentage HbH (or Hb Barts)

$$= \frac{OD\ ^{415}HbH}{OD^{415}HbH + OD^{415}\ other\ band} \times 100$$

Composition of solutions

0.1 M phosphate buffer pH 7.0

Potassium dihydrogen phosphate	3.11 g
Disodium hydrogen phosphate. 2H$_2$O	1.87 g
Distilled water	to 1 litre

QUANTITATION OF HbF LEVELS

Fetal haemoglobin (HbF), the major haemoglobin in fetal life, is replaced by adult haemoglobin in the perinatal period. This process begins before birth such that, at term, cord blood contains ~60–80% HbF. This level continues to decline rapidly during the next six months (<5%) and then more slowly throughout childhood; indeed there is evidence that there is a very gradual decline throughout adult life.

Increased levels of HbF are seen in various genetic disorders, including β and δβ thalassaemias and hereditary persistence of fetal haemoglobin, and the level of HbF is often a major factor in the differential diagnosis of these heterogeneous conditions. In addition, raised levels may often appear in acquired disorders e.g. aplastic anaemia, leukaemias, other neoplastic diseases, and its reappearance often accompanies any form of acute erythroid expansion. No prognostic significance has been attached to increased levels in these cases.

No single method is suitable for measuring HbF levels across the whole range from 0–100%. Because of its simplicity, the alkali denaturation method (Betke et al 1959, Pembrey et al 1972) is by far the most widely applied but its tendency to overestimate very low levels and significantly underestimate high levels has to be taken into account.

Principle

The alkali denaturation method relies on the resistance to denaturation by alkali of HbF compared to HbA.

This difference is a relative one, not absolute and the conditions are chosen such that during the time of exposure to alkali, most of the HbA is denatured while the HbF is largely unaffected.

Test samples
Normal haemolysate (80–100 g/l) is required; samples which are too dilute will give falsely high results (Pembrey et al 1972).

Reagents
Drabkin's solution should be stored in a dark bottle and may be used for several weeks, as may the saturated ammonium sulphate solution. NaOH should be freshly prepared.

Equipment
○ A standard visible light spectrophotometer is required.

Method
1. Add 0.6 ml haemolysate to 10 ml Drabkin's solution to convert the haemoglobin to cyanmethaemoglobin.
2. Pipette 2.8 ml of the cyanmethaemoglobin solution into each of two test tubes (duplicates) and add 0.2 ml of 1.2 N NaOH.
3. Agitate gently for exactly 2 minutes.
4. Stop the denaturation by adding 2 ml saturated ammonium sulphate and mixing thoroughly. A brownish precipitate of denatured haemoglobin then forms. Allow to stand for 10–15 minutes.
5. The precipitate is removed from the undenatured haemoglobin by filtration through a double layer of Whatman No. 40 filter paper in a small funnel.
6. A control solution of undenatured haemoglobin is prepared by mixing 1.4 ml cyanmethaemoglobin solution, 1.6 ml distilled water and 2.0 ml saturated ammonium sulphate. This is then diluted 1 in 10 with distilled water to give a suitable optical density.
7. Read the optical densities of the test and control samples at 415 nm.

Calculation
% alkali resistant Hb (HbF)

$$= \frac{OD^{415} \text{ test sample}}{OD^{415} \text{ control} \times 20} \times 100$$

Comment
Variability has been observed in the capacity of batches of filter paper to absorb haemoglobin from the filtrate during filtration. In extreme cases this may significantly reduce the optical density of the test sample and as the amount absorbed is fairly constant and not very concen-tration dependent, samples with low HbF levels will be more significantly affected. If this problem is suspected it can be simply checked by removing the precipitate by centrifugation and then reading the optical density before and after filtration.

Interpretation
In studies of the alkali denaturation technique, intra-laboratory reproducibility is generally good but inter-laboratory variability is very high. It is imperative, therefore, that each laboratory determines its own normal range, preferably with a sample size greater than 50. With the above technique, in our hands, 1.0% can be considered as the upper limit of normal; other laboratories may use a value of 2%.

Values between 1 and 5% are occasionally (<1%) encountered in otherwise normal adults; family studies usually demonstrate a genetic basis for these increased levels although the cause is unknown.

Composition of solutions
Drabkin's solution (see p. 14)

Alkali

Sodium hydroxide	4.8 g
Distilled water	to 100 ml

Ammonium sulphate
Prepare a saturated solution.

TEST FOR UNSTABLE HAEMOGLOBINS BY HEAT PRECIPITATION

Abnormal haemoglobin variants may have reduced stability within the red cell, in extreme cases leading to haemolysis and clinical consequences. In some cases, the abnormal haemoglobin may be detected electro-phoretically but samples suspected of containing an unstable haemoglobin may be tested either by the heat precipitation or the isopropanol instability methods.

Test samples
A fresh blood sample and an appropriate normal control are required.

Method
1. Wash 1 ml whole blood three times in saline.
2. Lyse the red cells with distilled water and make up to 5 ml.
3. Add 5 ml 0.01 M phosphate buffer pH 7.4.
4. Remove stroma by centrifugation (~3000 g) for 10 minutes.
5. Incubate the haemoglobin solution at 50°C in a water-bath for 1 hour.

Comment

Fresh blood is preferable since with some unstable haemoglobins, intracellular precipitation may occur spontaneously on storage and the abnormal component may be lost at the centrifugation stage.

Interpretation

Fresh haemolysates should be stable for one hour at 50°C, remaining as a clear solution. Depending on the degree of instability, abnormal samples may vary from a faint cloudiness to flocculent precipitate.

A quantitative assessment of the amount of precipitated material may be achieved by measuring the optical density at 540 nm of the haemoglobin solution before heating and again after removing the heat precipitate by centrifugation.

Composition of solutions

0.01 M phosphate buffer pH 7.4

1. Sodium dihydrogen phosphate $2H_2O$		156.0 mg
Distilled water		to 100 ml
2. Disodium hydrogen phosphate		284.0 mg
Distilled water		to 200 ml

Titrate solution 2 to pH 7.4 by adding solution 1.

TEST FOR UNSTABLE HAEMOGLOBINS — ISOPROPANOL INSTABILITY TEST (Carell & Kay 1977)

Test samples

A small volume of haemolysate, freshly prepared, together with a normal control lysate are required.

Method

1. Add 2 ml isopropanol buffer to 0.2 ml lysate and mix well.
2. Incubate at 37°C and observe regularly for precipitate formation over 30 minutes.

Comment

False positive results may be obtained with aged samples, those containing an increased amount of methaemoglobin and samples containing more than 5–10% HbF.

Interpretation

With normal haemolysates, the haemoglobin solution should remain clear after 30 minutes, while samples containing unstable haemoglobins should become turbid after 5–10 minutes, the degree depending on the amount and the degree of instability of the haemoglobin variant.

Composition of solutions

0.1 M Tris-HCl buffer pH 7.4

Tris (hydroxymethyl) aminomethane	1.21 g
Distilled water	to 100 ml

pH to 7.4 with conc HCl

Isopropanol/tris buffer

0.1 M Tris-HCl pH 7.4	83 ml
Isopropanol	17 ml

HbH INCLUSION BODIES

Incubation of cells containing haemoglobin H with supravital redox dyes results in oxidation and precipitation of the soluble HbH as inclusion bodies within the cell. This allows the detection of some cases of α thalassaemia (α–/α– or αα/—) who have detectable HbH in a very small proportion of their cells.

Method

1. Mix equal volumes of whole blood and 1% Brilliant Cresyl Blue (dissolved in physiological saline and filtered) and incubate at 37°C for 1–2 hours.
2. Prepare blood films of the incubated cells and examine by light microscopy.

Interpretation

In HbH disease, a high proportion of the cells will contain typical HbH inclusions, regularly distributed throughout the cell to give a characteristic 'golfball' appearance. The punctate arrangement of discrete inclusions evenly distributed thoughout the cell is easily distinguished from the 'stringy' appearance of reticulocytes. In some cases of heterozygous α thalassaemia such cells may occur rarely (1 in 100 to 1 in 10000); their presence is confirmatory for α thalassaemia but their absence does not exclude α thalassaemia.

HEINZ BODY PREPARATION

Principle

Heinz bodies are denatured globin and may be stained supra-vitally using Methyl Violet stain.

Test sample

Fresh EDTA or ACD blood is used.

Method

1. Add 1 volume of blood to 4 volumes of the stain solution.
2. Incubate at 37°C for 20 minutes.
3. Make a wet preparation or a film and examine with a × 50 or × 100 oil immersion objective.

Interpretation

Heinz bodies are seen as particles situated close to the cell membrane. They vary in size from 1–3 μm. Although it is usual to see one large Heinz body per cell, several smaller Heinz bodies may sometimes be seen. The spleen has the capacity to remove Heinz bodies from cells as it removes other inclusion bodies, so the inability to detect Heinz bodies does not necessarily prove their absence *in vivo*. Heinz bodies are typically seen after splenectomy, in association with oxidative haemolysis and in the presence of one of the unstable haemoglobins.

Composition of solutions

Dissolve 0.5 g methyl violet in 100 ml saline (9 g/l sodium chloride). Filter before use.

MEASUREMENT OF GLOBIN CHAIN SYNTHESIS

In the majority of cases, the diagnosis of β thalassaemia does not require measurement of globin synthesis ratios; homozygotes are recognised by their clinical and haematological conditions while diagnosis of heterozygotes is based on red cell indices and a raised HbA$_2$ level. However, there are rare forms of heterozygous β thalassaemia in which HbA$_2$ levels are normal and in some mild cases, red cell indices may also be within the normal range, the so-called silent β thalassaemia. In these cases, usually encountered among relatives of thalassaemia major cases, globin chain synthesis ratios may be necessary for proper diagnosis.

A diagnosis of heterozygous α thalassaemia is often made provisionally in an individual with hypochromia and microcytosis, normal HbA$_2$ levels and lack of response to iron therapy. In many cases, such a provisional diagnosis is adequate, since the condition is innocuous. However, a more definite diagnosis may be required in some cases, particularly if pregnancy is contemplated and there is the possibility that the offspring may be at risk of Hb Bart's hydrops fetalis syndrome. Globin gene analysis by Southern blotting is the most precise method of diagnosis, since most cases of α thalassaemia are due to gene deletions; however in non-deletion forms or when gene analysis is not available, globin chain synthesis measurement may be informative.

Since the geographical distribution of α and β thalassaemia genes shows considerable overlap, it is not uncommon for interactions of both to occur within a family, requiring a combination of techniques, including globin synthesis, to elucidate the particular genotypes of individuals.

Principle

Globin chain synthesis ratios can be measured either in bone marrow erythroblasts, or more commonly in peripheral blood reticulocytes. In normal cells, the synthesis of α and β globin chains is equal; however in thalassaemia there is a deficit of α or β chain synthesis. The chain present in excess does not accumulate within the cell but is largely degraded; therefore in order to detect the imbalanced chain production the ratio of newly synthesised chains must be measured.

Reticulocytes (or marrow cells) are incubated with radioactive amino acids for short periods. Globins (and other proteins) are precipitated from the whole cell lysate with acidified acetone, at which stage the sample may be stored. The globin chains are then separated by column chromatography and the radioactivity incorporated into each is measured in a liquid scintillation counter.

Equipment

○ For sample preparation and incubation, a bench centrifuge and shaking water-bath.
○ For chromatography, 1.5 × 25 cm glass columns with a sintered glass filter.
○ A constant volume pump operating in the 0.1–1.0 ml/minute range.
○ A fraction collector holding ~72 tubes.
○ It is most convenient to monitor the column effluent continuously and a UV spectrophotometer with flow-through cuvette is recommended, although not essential.
○ A liquid scintillation counter is necessary to measure the incorporated radioactivity.

Test samples

1. Peripheral blood samples

In normal peripheral blood and in most thalassaemia heterozygotes, the reticulocyte count is very low and some enrichment of reticulocytes may be necessary to ensure adequate radioactive incorporation. This is most simply achieved by centrifugation. Unfortunately, this also enriches the white blood cells which are also active in protein synthesis, and some white cell proteins chromatograph with the globin chains. It is important therefore to remove the buffy coat. Indeed, for reliable results with low reticulocyte (<2%) samples, a more efficient white cell removal procedure is necessary, for which the cellulose column technique of Beutler et al (1976) is recommended.

Removal of white blood cells

1. 10–20 ml of fresh heparinised blood are centrifuged at full speed in a bench centrifuge (~3000 g) for 30 minutes at room temperature.

2. Prepare a slurry consisting of 2 parts α cellulose

(Sigma) to 1 part microcrystalline cellulose (Sigma) in 30 ml reticulocyte saline (RS), allow to swell for 10 minutes. Pour the slurry into a lightly plugged 10 ml syringe to form a 3–4 ml column; do not allow to dry out.

3. Discard the plasma from the centrifuged blood sample and carefully remove the buffy coat disc with an orange stick.

4. The top 0.5 ml of reticulocyte enriched red cells are removed with a Pasteur pipette and added to 2 ml RS.

5. The red cells suspension is applied to the column, washed through with RS and collected in a total volume of ~20–25 ml. White blood cells are retained by the column.

6. Centrifuge the diluted red cells to obtain packed cells. There should be virtually no lysis during these procedures, which also serve to wash the cells free from plasma.

2. Bone marrow samples

Separation of erythroblasts from total bone marrow cannot be simply achieved and therefore the whole sample is used. Normal marrow aspirates are quite suitable, peripheral blood contamination being minimised by only taking a small volume, <0.5 ml. It is very important that the marrow is not allowed to even partially clot and it is preferable that the syringe (and needle) are heparinised before collection. The sample should be immediately transferred to a container with 100 u heparin in RS or culture medium. The cells should then be washed three times with RS.

Method

Incubation procedure

1. Add 0.5 ml of packed cells to 1.3 ml incubation medium and add $75\mu l$ of 1 mg/ml freshly prepared ferrous ammonium sulphate.

2. Pre-incubate at 37°C in a shaking water-bath for 10 minutes and add 50 μCi ^{3}H leucine.

3. Continue the incubation for the requisite time, normally one hour.

4. Stop the incubation by adding ice-cold RS and wash the cells three times.

5. If it is necessary to store the incubated cells at this stage they should be snap frozen in a dry-ice/acetone mixture and stored at −20°C. Prolonged storage at this stage is not advisable.

Comments

— Although fresh blood should normally be used for incubations, results may be obtained after a few hours in transit, and on occasions a successful outcome has been obtained after 24 hours.

— Variability in batches of incubation medium, presumably due to the human serum component, may affect the amount of ^{3}H leucine incorporation but do not appear to alter the α/β chain ratios obtained. Batches should be dispensed into aliquots and stored at −20°C.

— Occasional problems with large radioactive 'pre'peaks have been ascribed to particular batches of isotope, possibly due to radiochemical degradation products. It is advisable, therefore, to purchase ^{3}H leucine in amounts appropriate to the level of usage and avoid prolonged storage.

— There is an inverse relationship between incubation temperature and the α/β chain synthesis ratio. The temperature of the water-bath should therefore be checked.

— The rate of incorporation of leucine into globin is normally linear for at least 1 hour, and longer in samples with high reticulocyte counts. Beyond this period, when the rate of incorporation declines, differential effects on α and β chain synthesis may occur, distorting the ratio.

— For a more detailed discussion, see Clegg (1983).

Preparation of globin

1. The washed, incubated cells should be lysed by the addition of 2 volumes of distilled water. In the case of bone marrow, three cycles of freezing and thawing should be carried out to ensure lysis.

2. The globin is precipitated from the lysate by the addition of at least 20 volumes of freshly prepared 2% concentrated HCl in acetone, at −20°C, with thorough mixing. The suspension is allowed to stand at −20°C for ~15 minutes to ensure complete precipitation.

3. The precipitate is centrifuged down at a very low speed to avoid compaction and then washed gently three times in acetone at −20°C.

4. The globin is dried by washing once in ether at room temperature, and allowing the residual ether to evaporate by air drying.

5. At this stage the globin powder may be stored in a dry sealed container at −20°C.

Comments

— The ratio of acidified acetone to lysate should not be less than 20:1, otherwise there may be incomplete precipitation and differential loss of α and β chains.

— It is very important to keep the temperature as low as possible, particularly while there is acid around, to prevent deamidation of the globin chains.

— Avoid getting water into the globin (e.g. from a water suction device) as this will prevent it drying as a fine powder and may result in poor chromatographic separations.

Globin chain separation

1. Weigh out 480 g AR grade urea and add distilled water to one litre (8 M); stir at room temperature until dissolved (~1 hour).

2. Filter the urea solution through Whatman no. 3 paper.

3. Add 0.15 g dithiothreitol (1.0 mM) and 1.1 g disodium hydrogen phosphate (0.08 M).

4. Adjust the pH to 6.4 with 20% orthophosphoric acid. This solution is referred to as the starting buffer.

5. Dissolve 15–60 mg globin in 2 ml starting buffer and dialyse against two changes of 50 ml starting buffer.

6. To prepare the column, 2.5 g carboxymethylcellulose (Whatman CM23) are suspended in 50 ml starting buffer and poured into the column, giving a bed height of ~20 cm. Once the resin has settled, do not allow it to dry out but connect it to the reservoir of the gradient marker and wash with starting buffer at a rate of ~0.5 ml/minute, until the sample is dialysed.

7. Remove the buffer head from the column and apply the sample carefully, washing it with 2–3 ml/minutes starting buffer.

8. Reconnect the column to the pump and continue to pump starting buffer through the loaded column for ~30 minutes, until the unbound material has eluted.

9. The effluent from the column should pass through the recording spectrophotometer (reading at 280 nm, if continuous monitoring is available) to the fraction collector which should be set to collect 5 ml fractions.

10. Prepare the limiting buffer by dissolving 0.8 g disodium hydrogen phosphate in 200 ml starting buffer (final conc. 0.036 M) and readjust the pH to 6.4 with 20% orthophosphoric acid.

11. Add the limiting buffer to the gradient maker and, once the unbound material has eluted, adjust the level of the starting buffer chamber to 200 ml and open the connection between the two chambers.

12. At this flow rate, the chromatography should be completed in ~14 hours, so that normally it is allowed to run overnight.

13. 0.4 ml aliquots of each fraction plus 0.1 ml distilled water, are then added to 5 ml scintillation liquid (toluene or xylene based cocktails are suitable) and their incorporated radioactivity measured in a liquid scintillation counter.

14. The radioactivity profile can then be plotted out, together with the optical density profile if available, and the counts in each globin peak determined by summing the counts from the tubes containing the peak. The background level, which is the average count in the area between the peaks, should be subtracted for each tube.

Comments

— Urea should be made freshly since ammonium cyanate, which forms on standing, may react with free amino groups on the globin chains altering their net charge.

— The dialysis step may not be necessary if all the acid has been removed from the globin before drying. However, it is a useful precautionary measure.

— Overloading of the columns may lead to differential globin chain binding, with some chains lost in the unbound material, distorting the chain synthesis ratio. This possibility may be checked by comparing the total counts ratio with the specific activity ratio (see below).

— Contamination of the globin chains with other radioactive proteins, either through incomplete removal of white cells before incubation, or in incubations of bone marrow samples that are not highly erythroid, is usually apparent if the radioactive profile of the fractions does not follow the optical density profile smoothly or has additional small peaks. Furthermore, with contaminated samples the baseline between peaks may not be flat and often slopes, being higher at the start of the profile than at the end. Such contaminated samples can often be cleaned up, either by gel filtration of the globin sample prior to chromatography, or by an extended gradient.

Gel filtration is conveniently carried out on 100 × 2 cm columns of Sephadex G-100 run in 5% formic acid. The recovered globin chain peak can then be freeze dried after dilution 1:4 with distilled water.

A suitable method for extending the gradient is to connect three chambers in series, with the first two containing starting buffer and the third containing limiting buffer, as described above. Many of the contaminants will elute before the β globin chains with this non-linear gradient. Such a gradient is also useful for improving the resolution of γ and β chains if an accurate measure of their relative proportion is necessary.

— Since α and β chains contain the same number of leucine residues (18), no correction is necessary in calculating the relative incorporation. However, if γ chains, with only 17 leucine residues, are present, the total incorporation must be corrected by 18/17 relative to β and α, i.e. multiply the γ chain counts by 1.06.

— In order to check that quantitatively equal recovery from the column of α and β chains has been achieved, the specific activities should be measured. The peak tube of each chain is dialysed against three changes of 0.5% formic acid and the optical density measured at 280 nm and the radioactivity remeasured. The c.m./mg is calculated for each chain, using corrections for the differences in absorbance of 0.56 for α, 0.84 for β and 1.12 for γ. The α/β specific activity ratio should equal the total counts

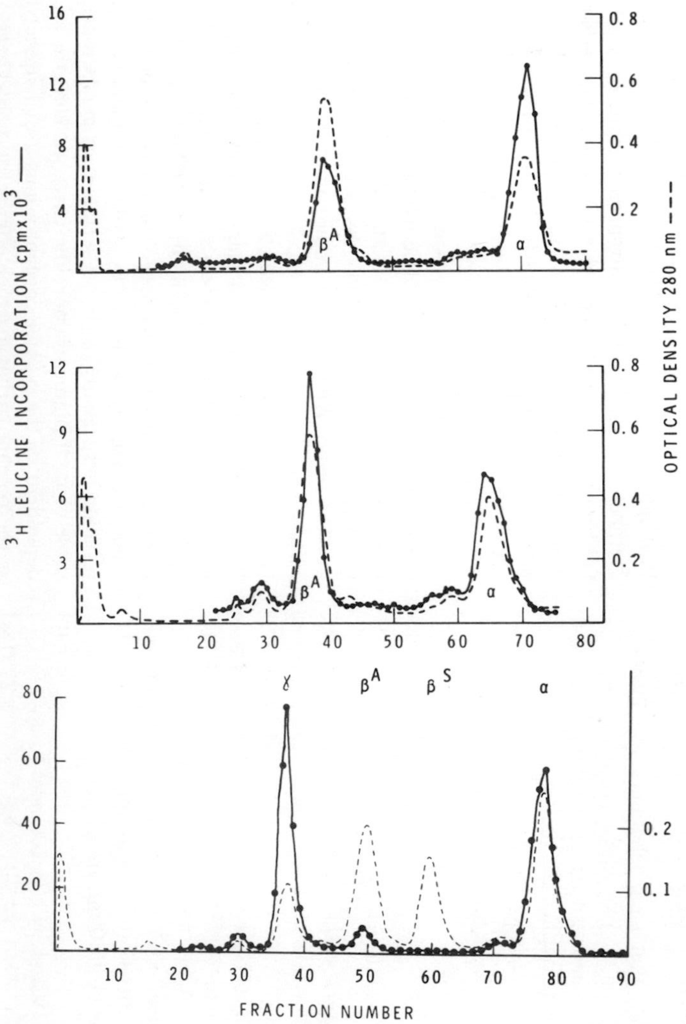

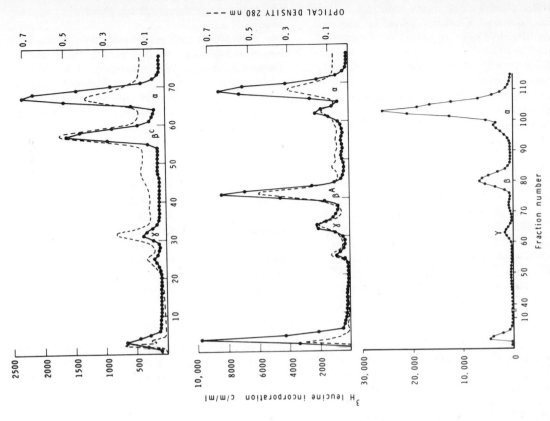

Fig. 2.3 Further chain separation profiles from samples of: top — HbC/β thalassaemia compound heterozygote; middle — mild β thalassaemia intermedia; bottom — a more severe β thalassaemia intermedia, illustrating the improved resolution of γ and β chains obtained with a non-linear, three chambered gradient.

Fig. 2.2 Radioactivity and optical density profiles obtained following CM-cellulose chromatography of: top — β thalassaemia trait; middle — normal adult; bottom — sample from a fetus at risk for sickle cell anaemia to illustrate the separation of γ, βᴬ and βˢ chains. Note the lack of ³H leucine incorporation into the βˢ chain, demonstrating that the fetus was normal.

ratio under conditions of steady state globin chain synthesis, as found in normal individuals and thalassaemia heterozygotes.

Interpretation

Typical chromatography profiles from various samples are shown in Figs. 2.2 and 2.3 and the range of results observed in our laboratory for various combinations of α and β thalassaemia genes is shown in Table 2.1.

Table 2.1 Globin chain synthesis ratios in our laboratory for defined thalassaemia syndromes.

Condition	Genotype		α/β chain synthesis ratio	
			Range	Mean
Normal	$\alpha\alpha/\alpha\alpha$	β^A/β^A	0.9–1.12	1.05
Heterozygous β thal	$\alpha\alpha/\alpha\alpha$	$\beta^A/\beta^{th\star}$	1.6–2.7	2.12
Mild α thal	$\alpha\alpha/-\alpha$	$\beta^A\beta^A$	0.8–1.1	0.87
Severe α thal	$-\alpha/-\alpha$ or $\alpha\alpha/--$	$\beta^A\beta^A$	0.5–0.8	0.70
HbH disease	$-\alpha/--$	$\beta^A\beta^A$	0.2–0.5	0.32
Mild α thal/ β thal heterozygote	$\alpha\alpha/-\alpha$	$\beta^A\beta^{th\star}$	1.1–1.6	1.30
Severe α thal/ β thal heterozygote	$-\alpha/-\alpha$ or $\alpha\alpha/--$	$\beta^A\beta^{th\star}$	0.7–1.0	0.85
HbH disease/β thal heterozygote	$-\alpha/--$	$\beta^A\beta^{th\star}$	0.4–0.6	0.51

$\star$Assorted molecular defects, including β^+ and β^0 thalassaemia.

It is important that each laboratory establishes its own normal range on samples with a near normal reticulocyte count. Intra-laboratory reproducibility on duplicated incubations or duplicated chain separations should be high (α/β synthesis ratios within 0.05) but there appears to be some variability in the ratios obtained between laboratories, probably due to undefined minor technical differences.

Composition of solutions

Reticulocyte saline (RS)

0.13 M NaCl	7.59 g
0.005 M KCl	0.37 g
0.007 M $MgCl_2$ $6H_2O$	1.54 g
Distilled water to	1 litre

Incubation medium

0.25 M $MgCl_2.6H_2O$ (0.5 mg/10 ml) + 10% glucose (1 g/10 ml) in RS	2.7 ml
0.164 M Tris HCl (1.99 g in 100 ml H_2O), pH 7.75	27.0 ml

0.01 M trisodium citrate (73 mg/25 ml) in dialysed AB plasma	21.6 ml
0.01 M $NaHCO_3$ (29.4 mg/35 ml) in dialysed AB plasma	32.0 ml
Amino acid mixture (see below)	54.0 ml

AB plasma (or serum if available) should be dialysed extensively against RS. Sterilise via a 0.45 μ filter and aliquot 1.3 ml fractions. Store at 20°C.

Amino acid mixture

	mg		mg
Alanine	89	Methionine	22
Arginine	44	Phenylalanine	132
Aspartic acid	190	Proline	80
Asparagine	132	Serine	87
Glycine	199	Threonine	101
Glutamine	585	Tryptophan	31
Histidine	230	Tyrosine	72
Isoleucine	20	Cysteine	24
Lysine	131	Valine	187

Each of the above amounts of amino acid dissolved separately in 25 ml RS gives a 20× required final concentration. Combine 3 ml of each and add 6 ml RS. Adjust pH to 7.75 with NaOH. Remainder of amino acid solutions may be stored at −20°C for future batches.

MEASUREMENT OF CARBOXYHAEMOGLOBIN (HbCO)

Principle

Methods for measuring carboxyhaemoglobin in blood fall broadly into two groups: those in which the carbon monoxide is dissociated from haemoglobin and then quantified; and those, mostly spectrophotometric, where the pigment is measured directly.

Spectrophotometric methods make use of the spectral differences between carboxyhaemoglobin and haemoglobin in its various forms. The oxyhaemoglobin spectrum has absorption bands designated alpha, beta, and gamma, whose peak wavelengths are 576, 540, and 414 nm respectively, with a minimum at 560 nm. For carboxyhaemoglobin these wavelengths are shifted to 568, 538, 420 respectively, with a minimum at 558 nm. Reduced haemoglobin has a single broad band with a maximum at 555 nm in place of the alpha and beta bands, and hence no minimum at 560 nm. In those methods comparing carboxy- and oxyhaemoglobin, blood containing a mixture of both pigments will produce a spectrum with peaks intermediate between those of each pigment alone; the exact wavelengths are dependent on the relative concentrations usually defined as the percent carboxyhaemoglobin saturation. Using a preparation of blood saturated with oxygen in the first place, and carbon monoxide in the second, absorbance measurements may be made at two of the above wavelengths, e.g. 576 and 560, or 540 and 560 nm, and a graph of the ratio of these absorbances versus carboxyhaemoglobin saturation may be plotted. The carboxyhaemoglobin saturation of an unknown sample may be determined by measuring its absorbance at the same wavelengths and interpolating the ratio. Alternatively the absorbance difference of the sample can be measured at a single wavelength, before and after the replacement of the carbon monoxide by oxygen, and the carboxyhaemoglobin saturation read from a standard curve, or calculated from an equation taking into account the molar extinction coefficient of carboxyhaemoglobin at the relative wavelength. Methods comparing carboxyhaemoglobin with reduced haemoglobin can be used in a similar manner. Instead of converting reduced haemoglobin to oxyhaemoglobin, oxyhaemoglobin is converted to reduced haemoglobin, avoiding the possibility of displacing carbon monoxide from haemoglobin by oxygen in the preparation of the sample for analysis (see selected method below).

Biochemical basis

Haemoglobin, and other haem-containing proteins, such as cytochrome oxidase and myoglobin, combine with carbon monoxide to form carbonyl-haem pigments. In the case of haemoglobin the carbonyl compound is generally known as carboxyhaemoglobin. Both oxygen and carbon monoxide combine reversibly with haemoglobin, but as the affinity of haemoglobin for carbon monoxide is over 200 times that of oxygen the inhalation of air containing a small but significant concentration of carbon monoxide above the usual level can lead to a substantial increase in the equilibrated level of carboxyhaemoglobin in the blood. The inhalation of gas mixtures containing a large proportion of carbon monoxide can lead to the replacement of oxyhaemoglobin almost entirely, and grossly reduce the transport of oxygen.

Test samples

Collect a sample of blood into a tube containing heparin or EDTA, minimising the air-space above the sample.

Equipment

Absorbance is measured at 540 nm and 555 nm, using a correctly calibrated spectrophotometer with a narrow band-pass (<5 nm).

Standards and controls

Known concentrations of carboxyhaemoglobin may be prepared in a tonometer or, alternatively, 150 ml separating funnels may be used. Add 5 ml of normal blood to 2 separating funnels and allow pure oxygen to flow through one, and pure carbon monoxide to flow through the other, for 15 minutes. The funnels are rotated during this period so that a thin film of blood is in contact with the gas. At the end of this period the taps are closed and the funnels stoppered. The blood is rotated for further 15 minutes. Use the procedure described below to measure the absorbance at 540 nm and 555 nm respectively for each of the two samples and calculate the ratio for 0% carboxyhaemoglobin (RCO_0) and for 100% carboxyhaemoglobin (RCO_{100}). Using a correctly calibrated spectrophotometer there should be a linear relationship between A540/A555 nm ratios within the range of 0% and 100% carboxyhaemoglobin. Intermediate standards are usually made by mixing the two primary standards in different proportions but are difficult to prepare accurately. If the A540/A555 nm ratio (100%) obtained in a correctly calibrated spectrophotometer is close to 1.23 linearity may be assumed.

Method (Tietz & Fiereck 1973, Tietz 1986)

1. Add 50 μl of blood to 10 ml of dilute ammonia reagent. Mix and allow to stand for 2 minutes; at the end of this time a clear haemolysate should be obtained.

2. Add approximately 10 mg of sodium dithionite to 3 ml of the haemolysate. Prepare in a similar way a blank using dilute ammonia solution in place of the haemolysate. Carefully mix each solution.

3. After about 5 minutes read the absorbances in a spectrophotometer at 540 nm and 555 nm — by this time the absorbance values should be stable.

Calculation

Calculate the ratio A540/A555 nm(RU), and obtain the carboxyhaemoglobin value by interpolation from the standard curve or from the equation:

$$\%COHb = \frac{(RU - RCO_0) \times 100}{RCO_{100} - RCO_0}$$

Comments

— To identify the presence of other abnormal pigments dilute aliquots of the blood sample with water and obtain spectra between 400 and 700 nm with and without the presence of dithionite.

— Many spectrophotometric methods may be accurate if only carboxyhaemoglobin and haemoglobin are present in the sample. If the calibration curve for carboxyhaemoglobin has been constructed on the basis of these pigments alone, the presence of other haemoglobin derivatives — such as methaemoglobin, sulphaemoglobin or cyanmethaemoglobin — will lead to inaccuracies since they will contribute to the total absorbance at each wavelength. In these circumstances there will be difficulties in relating the proportion of carboxyhaemoglobin present to the oxygen-carrying pigment, since the latter cannot be measured accurately. One commercial oximeter (Instrumentation Laboratory Ltd.) may provide a partial solution to this problem in that the carboxy- and oxyhaemoglobin fraction can be accurately measured, but the measurement of methaemoglobin is less precise. In any case it is always good practice to obtain an absorbance spectrum of the sample over the range 400–700 nm which may allow the detection of some of these pigments. The identification of these other, non-oxygen carrying pigments can be important in the investigation of cases in which fires or smoke inhalation are potential sources of carbon monoxide poisoning.

— Factors which influence the choice of method include the apparatus which is available to the laboratory, the ease of each method, and the workload. With the virtual disappearance of carbon monoxide in town gas, most laboratories receive few requests for the measurement of carboxyhaemoglobin in cases of poisoning, making the purchase of specialised equipment uneconomic. Most laboratories have a spectrophotometer, and spectrophotometric methods are both fast and simple to perform. In view of this, and despite the objections mentioned above, a spectrophotometric method is recommended. However this method is insufficiently sensitive for the precise measurement of carboxyhaemoglobin in studies of environmental contamination by carbon monoxide e.g. cigarette smoking or traffic pollution, nor is it sensitive enough for the measurement of endogenously-produced carbon monoxide.

Interpretation

Small quantities of carbon monoxide are produced in vivo in the process of the conversion of haem to bilirubin leading to the presence of low levels (less than 1%) of carboxyhaemoglobin in the circulating blood (Coburn et al 1963). As the levels are proportional to the rate of haem catabolism, levels of this pigment are higher in newborn infants than in older children (Ostrander et al 1982). Minimally raised levels have been observed in patients with haemolytic anaemias and in those with ineffective haem synthesis (Coburn et al 1964, Lindahl 1980). The other important variable affecting the blood level is the rate of respiratory excretion of the gas (Ostrander et al 1982).

The carboxyhaemoglobin level in the blood of city dwellers is usually less than 1.5%; the percentage in smokers is usually greater than 6%, but may reach levels of 16% or more (Wald et al 1981). Such levels may also be observed in the blood of subjects in occupational groups exposed to carbon monoxide in the course of their work, such as traffic policemen.

Acute carbon monoxide poisoning may be the result of accidental exposure to air heavily contaminated with the fumes of fuel heaters or central-heating boilers (Thompson & Henry 1983). Another important cause of accidental poisoning is exposure to the combustion gases in burning buildings which contain large quantities of wood or furnishings manufactured from synthetic or natural organic materials. In such circumstances hydrocyanic acid gas may also be produced and may in fact be the cause of death. Cyanide combines principally with methaemoglobin to form the stable pigment, cyanmethaemoglobin (Linden et al 1984). Deliberate self-poisoning may be achieved by the manipulation of space heaters or more commonly by self-exposure to the exhaust gases of a motor car in a poorly ventilated space.

Symptoms of carbon monoxide poisoning are associated with carboxyhaemoglobin levels greater than 20–30%. Prominent among them are headache, dizziness, nausea, vomiting, and dyspnoea on effort. Although such symptoms are commonplace, subsequent disasters may be avoided if the possibility of chronic carbon monoxide poisoning is given careful consideration. Patients with levels above 60–70% with typical cherry-red appearance of the skin are usually found unconscious; death occurs with increasing frequency above these levels. Carboxyhaemoglobin levels observed in patients suffering from carbon monoxide poisoning do not always match the severity of the condition; levels above 15% in smokers and 5% in non-smokers may therefore be of diagnostic importance. Removal of the subject from the carbon monoxide-contaminated environment and his subsequent ventilation before the collection of the blood sample may account for such discrepancies (Clark et al 1981). Blood for the diagnosis of carbon monoxide poisoning should be collected at the earliest opportunity.

Reagents

Ammonia solution — 15.9 ml of concentrated ammonia (SG 0.880) is diluted to 1 litre with distilled or deionised water.

Sodium dithionite — general purpose reagent.

Carbon monoxide — a small cylinder from BDH or another reputable supplier.

Oxygen — a suitable cyclinder from BOC or other reputable supplier.

MEASUREMENT OF METHAEMOGLOBIN (Hi) AND SULPHAEMOGLOBIN (SHb)

Principle

Methaemoglobin and sulphaemoglobin can be measured

simultaneously using their spectral peaks at 630 nm and 620 nm respectively. Sulphaemoglobin is measured at 620 nm, but the contribution of other haem pigments to the absorbance must be allowed for. Cyanide converts methaemoglobin and oxyhaemoglobin to cyanmethaemoglobin without affecting the absorbance of sulphaemoglobin. The difference in absorbance at 630 nm before and after the addition of cyanide is a measure of methaemoglobin. The presence of both of these pigments may be reported in mass units or as proportion of the total haem pigment present in the sample of blood.

Test samples

Venous or capillary blood is collected into a standard tube containing EDTA or heparin as anticoagulant.

Equipment

○ Narrow band-pass spectrophotometer (<5 nm), calibrated for wavelength and accuracy of absorbance.

Standard

Cyanmethaemoglobin standard (see section on haemoglobin) is required for the measurement of total haemoglobin pigments. Standards for methaemoglobin and sulphaemoglobin are not available; factors for each fraction are derived experimentally (see below).

Method (Makerem 1974, Evelyn & Malloy 1938)

1. Add 0.2 ml blood to 10 ml of working phosphate buffer. Mix thoroughly, wait for 5 minutes, then centrifuge. Remove the supernatant and measure its absorbance at 630 nm against a water blank (A1). After measuring the absorbance the contents of the cuvette are returned to the remainder of the supernatant.

2. Add 1 drop of neutralised cyanide solution to the above supernatant, mix, wait 2 minutes then read the absorbance again at 630 nm (A2). Again, return the contents of the cuvette to the remainder of the supernatant.

3. Add 1 drop of ammonia solution to the supernatant obtained in step 2 and mix. Read the absorbance of the solution at 615, 618, 620, 622 and 625 nm. If a definite peak is found at 620 nm the absorbance at this wavelength is recorded as A3. If no peak is detected sulphaemoglobin is not present in the sample in a clinically important quantity.

4. Take 2.0 ml of solution from step 3, and add it to 8.0 ml of working phosphate buffer to which 1 drop of potassium ferricyanide solution has been added. Mix, wait for 2 minutes, then add 1 drop of neutralised cyanide solution, wait a further 2 minutes, and measure the absorbance at 540 nm (A4).

Determination of constants

Obtain a sample of normal blood collected as above. Measure the total haemoglobin concentration (see p. 13). Prepare two dilutions of the sample in phosphate buffer as in step 1 of the method. Using one aliquot, follow the procedure outlined above, readings A3 and A4 only are required. To the second aliquot, add 1 drop of ferricyanide solution, mix, wait for 2 minutes for conversion of oxyhaemoglobin to methaemoglobin and measure the absorbance at 630 nm (D1). Add one drop of the neutralised cyanide solution, mix, wait for 2 minutes for the conversion of methaemoglobin into cyanmethaemoglobin and read the absorbance at 630 nm again (D2). Then add 1 drop of ammonia solution, mix and read the absorbance at 620 nm (D3).

$k1$ = total Hb concn/A4
$k2$ = total Hb concn/D1 − D2
$k3$ = (M.Wt. × d)/(10000 × E × 4)

where: M.Wt. = approximate molecular weight of sulphaemoglobin
d = dilution in the assay
10000 = allows for change of concentration of g/l and g/dl respectively
E = millimolar absorption coefficient

= 64 500 × 51/10000 × 21 × 4
= 3.89

Pure sulphaemoglobin is difficult to prepare, we have therefore used published values for its millimolar absorptivity in calculating $k3$ [Henry 1974].

$k4$ = total Hb concn/A3
$k5$ = Hb concn/D3

Calculation

Total Hb concn = $k1$ × A4 g/100 ml
Methaemoglobin = $k2$ (A1 − A2) g/100 ml
% methaemoglobin = (methaemoglobin concn/total Hb concn) × 100
Sulphaemoglobin = $k3$ (A3 − (Total Hb − MetHb)/k4 − MetHb/k5) g/100 ml
% sulphaemoglobin = (sulphaemoglobin concn/total Hb concn) × 100

Comments

— Turbidity can cause erroneous results. Turbidity may arise either from lipaemia, or precipitation of plasma proteins during the assay. The cuvette contents should be inspected for turbidity at each stage of the assay. Should turbidity occur repeat the assay with erythrocytes that have been washed with saline.

— The presence of bilirubin in high concentration may also affect the absorbance readings. This problem may also be overcome by using saline-washed red cells.

— As there is contradictory evidence concerning the stability of methaemoglobin, it is best to perform the analysis without delay.

Interpretation

Methaemoglobin

In a normal individual up to 1.5% of the circulating haemoglobin may be present in the form of methaemoglobin. Levels greater than 10% may cause obvious clinical cyanosis. Below 25% patients may be symptom-free, but over this level headache and dyspnoea on effort may be observed. Whilst the presence in adequate concentrations of ascorbate and reduced glutathione helps to minimise the level of methaemoglobin in the red cell, the most important mechanism for achieving this is the NAD methaemoglobin-reductase system.

Over-production of methaemoglobin may result directly from ingestion of oxidising agents such as nitrites, nitrates or chlorates; other substances including some drugs such as phenacetin or sulphonamides cause this through some intermediary mechanism. Homozygotes expressing the autosomal inheritance of methaemoglobin-reductase deficiency have methaemoglobin levels of 10–50%. Heterozygotes usually have normal levels but are more sensitive to drugs or oxidising agents than the normal population. Abnormal haemoglobins of type M form methaemoglobin more readily (Bunn et al 1977). A number of reducing agents, including ascorbate, will slowly reduce methaemoglobin to haemoglobin. Methylene Blue is very active in this respect and may be used for the treatment both of secondary methaemoglobinaemia due to over-production, and the enzyme defect (Jaffe 1966).

Sulphaemoglobin

Haemoglobin in the presence of oxygen and hydrogen sulphide will form sulphaemoglobin. This is a stable compound which does not reduce to form haemoglobin as does methaemoglobin. It is not normally present in the circulating blood in relative concentrations greater than 1%. The mechanism for the production of sulphaemoglobin in vivo is not clear but it may be observed in the blood in the patients who have received drugs such as phenacetin or sulphonamides. The pigment may also be formed as a result of absorption of unknown materials from the gastrointestinal tract or following infections with *Clostridium welchii*.

Composition of solutions

Stock phosphate buffer pH 6.6, 0.065 mol/l
Dissolve 1.9 g of anhydrous Na_2HPO_4 and 2.72 g of KH_2PO_4 in distilled water and dilute to 500 ml.

Working phosphate buffer pH 6.6, 0.016 mol/l
Dilute stock buffer 1 in 4 as required.

Potassium ferricyanide, 200 g/l

Stock sodium cyanide, 100 g/l

Working neutralised sodium cyanide
Mix equal volumes of sodium cyanide solution and 10% v/v acetic acid. Use within one hour of preparation.

Ammonia solution SG 0.88

OXYGEN DISSOCIATION CURVE

The amount of oxygen that the haemoglobin molecule will take up for any given oxygen tension is known as the oxygen affinity of haemoglobin. It is usually expressed as the P_{50} or the partial pressure of oxygen required to half saturate the molecule. If one plots a graph of the percentage saturation against the partial pressure of oxygen (pO_2) a sigmoid curve is obtained (Fig. 2.4). This shaping is due to a phenomenon referred to as the 'haem-haem interaction'.

Various systems have been evolved to measure the oxygen dissociation curve of haemoglobin using Gasometric, spectrophotometric and polarimetric techniques.

The use of the Hem-O-Scan Oxygen Dissociation Curve Analyser has proved to be very satisfactory. This machine uses a dual wavelength spectrophotometric technique with oxygen pressure being monitored with a Clark oxygen electrode.

Principle

This is explained in the manufacturer's handbook.

Test samples

Venous blood drawn into lithium heparin and stored on ice until the time of assay, which should be within 2–3 hours of collection.

Control/standard

No standards as such are available, so a sample of comparable age, from a known normal subject, is used and run through in parallel as a control.

Reagents

No reagents as such need to be made up.

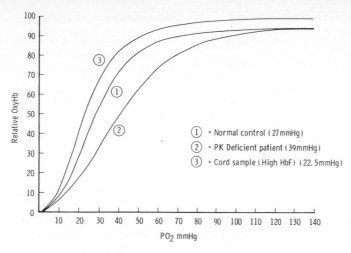

Fig. 2.4 Oxygen dissociation curves.

Method
The method used is that found in the manufacturer's handbook.

Units
The results are expressed in mm Hg 37°C and pH 7.4.

Results
Male P_{50} = 27.4 ± 1.0 mm Hg at 37°C
Female P_{50} = 27.8 ± 1.3 mm Hg at 37°C

Comment
Many factors influence the position of the oxygen dissociation curve such as temperature, pH, 2,3-DPG content, MCHC and base excess. It is important to note that the P_{50} obtained by this method is measured at a fixed temperature of 37°C and pH of 7.4 and therefore does not necessarily relate directly to the in vivo P_{50} of the patient which may well differ when, for example, severe acidosis or hypothermia are present. It will, however, give a fairly accurate result in conditions where the haemoglobin molecule is abnormal or modified. This equipment is expensive to buy but for rapidity of results and technical facility it is highly recommended for use in the routine laboratory.

REFERENCES

Starch gel electrophoresis of haemoglobins
Frischer H, Bowman J 1975 Hemoglobin E, an oxidatively unstable mutation. Journal of Laboratory and Clinical Medicine 85: 531–538
Itano H A 1953 Solubilities of naturally occuring mixtures of human hemoglobins. Archives of Biochemistry and Biophysics 47: 148–159
Robinson A R, Robson M, Harrison P, Zeulzer W W 1957 A new technique for differentiation of hemoglobin. Journal of Laboratory and Clinical Medicine 50: 745–752
Schmidt R M, Wilson S M 1973 Standardization in detection of abnormal hemoglobins: solubility tests for hemoglobin S. Journal of the American Medical Association 225: 1225–1230
Schneider R G, Barwick R C 1982 Hemoglobin mobility in citrate agar eletrophoresis — its relationship to anion binding. Hemoglobin 6: 199–208

Cellulose acetate membrane haemoglobin electrophoresis
International Committee for Standardisation in Hematology 1978 Recommendations of a system for identifying abnormal hemoglobins. Blood 52: 1065–1067

National Committee for Clinical Laboratory Standards 1986 Detection of abnormal hemoglobin using cellulose acetate electrophoresis. NCCLS 6: No 9, H8-A Villanova
Schneider R G 1973 Developments in laboratory diagnosis. In: Abramson (ed) Sickle cell disease. p 230–243

Citrate agar haemoglobin electrophoresis
International Committee for Standardisation in Hematology 1978 Recommendations of a system for identifying abnormal hemoglobins. Blood 52: 1065–1067
Milner P F, Gooden H M 1975 Rapid citrate-agar electrophoresis in routine screening for hemoglobinopathies using a simple hemolysate. American Journal of Clinical Pathology 64: 58–64
National Committee for Clinical Laboratory Standards 1981 Proposed Guidelines for citrate agar electrophoresis for confirming identification of mutant hemoglobins. NCCLS 1: 461–480

Quantitation of HbA₂ using cellulose acetate
Marengo-Rowe A J 1965 Rapid electrophoresis and quantitation of haemoglobin on cellulose acetate. Journal of Clinical Pathology 18: 790–792

Quantitation of HbA$_2$ using microcolumn method

Huisman T H J, Schroeder W A, Brodie A R, Mayson S M, Jakway J 1975 Microchromatography of hemoglobins III. A simplified procedure for the determination of hemoglobin A$_2$. Journal of Laboratory and Clinical Medicine 86: 700–702

International Committee for Standardisation in Hematology 1978 Recommendations for selected methods for quantitative estimation of Hb A$_2$ and for Hb A$_2$ reference preparation. British Journal of Haematology 38: 573–578

Sickle solubility test

Lehmann H, Huntsman R G 1974 Man's haemoglobins, 2nd edn. North Holland, Amsterdam, p 388–399

Quantitation of HbF levels

Betke K, Marti H R, Schlicht I 1959 Estimation of small percentages of foetal haemoglobin. Nature 184: 1877–1878

Pembrey M E, McWade P, Weatherall D J 1972 Reliable routine estimation of small amounts of foetal haemoglobin by alkali denaturation. Journal of Clinical Pathology 25: 738–740

Heinz body preparation

Beutler E, Dern R J, Alving A S 1955 The Hemolytic effect of Primaquine VI. J Lab Clin Med, 45, 40–50

Webster S H 1949 Heinz body phenomenon in erythrocytes, A Review. Blood 4: 479–497

Test for unstable haemoglobins — isopropanol instability test

Carrell R W, Kay R 1977 A simple method for the detection of unstable haemoglobins. British Journal of Haemotology 23: 615–619

Measurement of globin chain synthesis

Beutler et al West C, Beume K G 1976 The removal of leucocytes and platelets from whole blood. Journal of Laboratory and Clinical Medicine 88: 328–333

Clegg J B 1983 Hemoglobin synthesis. In: Weatherall D J (ed) The thalassaemias. Methods in Hematology Vol 6: 54–73. Churchill Livingstone, Edinburgh

Measurement of carboxyhaemoglobin

Clarke C J, Campbell D, Reid W H 1981 Blood carboxyhaemoglobin and cyanide levels in fire survivors. Lancet 1: 1332–5

Coburn R F, Blakemore W S, Forster R E 1963 Endogenous carbon monoxide production in man. Journal of Clinical Investigation 42: 1172–8

Coburn R F, Danielson G K, Blakemore W S, Forster R E 1964 Carbon monoxide in blood: analytical method and sources of error. Journal of Applied Physiology 19: 510–15

Huffner J G, Weber J P, Savoie J Y 1981 Quantitative determination of carbon monoxide in blood by head-space gas chromatography. Journal of Analytical Toxicology 5: 264–6

Lindahl J 1980 Quantification of ineffective erythropoesis in megaloblastic anaemia by determination of endogenous production of ^{14}CO after administration of glycine-2-^{14}C. Scandinavian Journal of Haematology 24: 281–191

Linden C H, Kulig K, Rumack B H 1984 In: Edlich R F, Spyker D A (eds) Current emergency therapy. Appleton-Century and Crofts, Connecticut, 756

Ostrander C R, Cohen R S, Hopper A O, Cowan B E, Stevens G B, Stevenson D K 1982 Paired determinations of blood carboxyhaemoglobin concentration and carbon monoxide excretion rate in term and preterm infants. Journal of Laboratory and Clinical Medicine 100: 745–55

Tietz N W, Fiereck E A 1973 The spectrophotometric measurement of carboxyhaemoglobin. Annals of Clinical and Laboratory Science 3: 36–42

Tietz N W 1986 Textbook of Clinical Chemistry. W B Saunders Philadelphia, 1699–1703

Thompson N, Henry J A 1983 Carbon monoxide poisoning: poisons unit experience over five years. Human Toxicol 2: 335–8

Wald N J, Idle M, Boreham J, Bailey A 1981 Carbon monoxide in breath in relation to smoking and carboxyhaemoglobin levels. Thorax 36: 366–9

Wigfield D C, Hollebone B R, MacKeen J, Selwin J C 1981 Assessment of the methods available for the determination of carbon monoxide in blood. Journal of Analytical Toxicology 5: 122–5

Measurement of methaemoglobin (Hi) and sulphaemoglobin (SHb)

Bunn H F, Forget B G, Ranney H M 1977 Human hemoglobins. WB Saunders, Philadelphia

Evelyn K A, Malloy H T 1938 Microdetermination of oxyhemoglobin, methemoglobin, and sulfhemoglobin in single sample of blood. Journal of Biological Chemistry 126: 655–662

Jaffe E R 1966 Hereditary methemoglobinemias associated with abnormalities in the metabolism of erythrocytes. American Journal of Medicine 41: 786–98

Makarem A 1974 In: Henry R J, Cannon D C, Winkelman J W (eds) Clinical chemistry: Principles and technics, 2nd edn. Harper and Row, New York, p 1149–1154

Oxygen dissociation curve

American Instrument Company (AMINCO), Silver Spring, Maryland, USA

Antonini E, Bunon M 1971 In: Neuberger A, Tatum E L (eds) 'Heamoglobin and Myoglobin in their interaction with ligands.' p 169

Bellingham A J, Lenfant C 1971 'Hb affinity for O$_2$ determined by O$_2$-Hb dissociation analyser and mixing technique. Journal of Applied Physiology 30: 903–904

Benesch R, MacDuff G, Benesch R E 1965 'Determination of oxygen equilibria with a versatile new tonometer.' Analytical Biochemistry 11: 81–87

Imai K, Morimoto H, Kontani M, Watari H, Hirata W, Kunoda M 1970 'Studies on the function of abnormal haemoglobin. 1. An improved method for automatic measurement of the oxygen equilibrium curve of haemoglobin'. Biochimica et Biophysica Acta 200: 189–196

Rossi-Fanelli A R, Antonini E, Caputo A 1958 'Studies on the structure of haemoglobin. 1. Physiochemical properties of human globin'. Biochimica et Biophysica Acta 30: 608–615

Torrance J D, Lenfant C 1969 'Methods for determination of O$_2$ dissociation curves, including Böhr effect.' Respiration Physiology 8: 127–136

Wiseman L 1981 Evaluation of Haem-o-Scan Oxygen Dissociation Curve Analyser for Fellowship of IMLS

3

Radionuclides in haematology

A combination of the full blood count, blood film, reticulocyte count, and bone marrow examination usually allows an adequate assessment of haemopoiesis, and whether any abnormalities are likely to be due to impaired cell production or to an increased rate of cell destruction. In occasional cases the use of radionuclide tracers can provide more quantitative data about overall activity of the erythroid marrow and about red cell lifespan. In addition, the use of surface organ counting and/or scanning allows data to be obtained concerning the predominant sites of erythropoiesis or of cell destruction. Oral administration of compounds which have been trace-labelled with radionuclides (e.g. iron salts or vitamin B_{12}) can be used to assess gastrointestinal absorption, while abnormal losses from the body (e.g. of iron or red cells due to bleeding from the gut) can be measured after parenteral injection of suitable radionuclide labels. Radionuclide dilution techniques also provide the simplest methods for measuring red cell and plasma volumes. The latter are the radionuclide tests most frequently used by haematology laboratories in the investigation of possible polycythaemia and of anaemias in which plasma volume expansion may be a contributory factor.

PRACTICAL CONSIDERATIONS IN THE USE OF RADIONUCLIDES

Radionuclides have been used in haematology since the earliest days of their use in diagnostic medicine and the first work published in this field, in 1939, concerned the use of a radioisotope of iron to study iron metabolism. Since then, of course, while the use of radioisotopes of iron for this purpose remains one of the most universally performed radionuclide investigations in haematology, the range of tests using radionuclides and the number of different radionuclides which are used have both expanded enormously. In nearly all laboratory haematology tests using radionuclides, however, the test depends ultimately on the measurement of the quantity of radioactivity in the specimen under investigation and

the comparison of this with a standard. Thus, for instance, in a Schilling test the quantity of radioactive vitamin B_{12} excreted in the urine over 24 hours is compared with the quantity administered to the patient; in a red cell survival test the quantity of radioactivity remaining on the red cells in the circulation is measured over a period of days or weeks and compared with the quantity present shortly after injection of the labelled cells; and in a radioassay the quantity of radioactivity bound to the sample is compared with the quantity bound to standard preparations of the substance being assayed. In all these cases these measurements are achieved by detecting and measuring the β, γ or X rays which are emitted by the radionuclide as a result of its decay process.

Table 3.1 lists the most commonly used radionuclides in haematology along with their physical properties which are most relevant to their use. From this it can be seen that the mode of radioactive decay, the radioactive half-life, and the type, energy and number of the emissions all vary widely from one radionuclide to another. Because of this it is necessary to use different types of counting equipment and different equipment settings to accurately measure the quantity of radioactivity present in a specimen depending on which radionuclide is present in the sample.

In this chapter the basic physics of the radionuclides used in haematology is presented together with a brief description of the instrumentation employed to measure the radioactivity present in a sample and, in addition, the general steps which are necessary to ensure that the result obtained is accurate and of known precision are covered.

Basic physics of radionuclides

Radioactive decay
When the nucleus of an atom does not contain a stable combination of neutrons and protons it will, at some time, undergo radioactive decay. Although there are several ways in which this can occur, all involve the emission of a charged particle, or the capture of an

Table 3.1 The radionuclides most commonly used in haematology, their decay modes, radioactive half-lives and principal emissions with their relative abundance.

Radionuclide	Decay mode	Half-life	Max. β energy (MeV)	Principal X & γ ray energies (MeV)
^{3}H	β$^-$	12.3 years	0.02(100)	—
^{14}C	β$^-$	5730 years	0.16(100)	—
^{32}P	β$^-$	14.3 days	1.71(100)	—
^{51}Cr	EC	27.8 days	—	0.320(9)
^{52}Fe	EC, β$^+$	8.2 hours	0.80(57)	0.511(114),0.165(94)
^{59}Fe	β$^-$	45.6 days	1.57(100)	1.29(43),1.09(56)
^{57}Co	EC	270 days	—	0.122(87),0.136(10)
^{58}Co	EC, β$^+$	71.3 days	0.48(15)	0.811(99),0.511(30)
^{99m}Tc	IT	6.05 hours	—	0.140(88)
^{111}In	EC	2.81 days	—	0.173(89),0.247(94)
^{113m}In	IT	99.8 mins.	—	0.393(65)
^{125}I	EC	60.2 days	—	0.035(7),0.027(112)
^{131}I	β$^-$	8.05 days	0.81(100)	0.364(83)

Key to decay modes: β$^-$ decay by emission of a β$^-$ particle, EC decay by capture of an orbiting electron, β$^+$ decay by emission of a positron, IT isomeric transition.

orbiting electron, by the nucleus. This results in a change in the number of protons present in the nucleus and therefore the transformation of the atom from one element into another.

The nucleus of the new (daughter) atom is then usually left in a so-called 'excited state' with excess energy which is immediately lost by the emission of one or more photons of radiation known as gamma (γ) rays. In addition X-ray photons are also emitted in electron capture decays as a result of the changes in the electron orbits around the nucleus. There are, however, two important special cases. First, if the nucleus decays directly to its ground state, as is the case for ^{3}H, ^{14}C and ^{32}P in Table 3.1, then there is no γ-ray emission. Second, if the excited state is itself sufficiently stable for the daughter nucleus to remain in it for a measurable length of time, then, when it does eventually lose its excess energy and drop to the ground state a γ ray will be emitted but without being associated with either particle emission or electron capture. This is known as an isomeric transition and in diagnostic medicine metastable radionuclides such as ^{99m}Tc which undergo this process are increasingly being used since when administered to patients they generally result in a lower absorbed radiation dose to the patient than is obtained from comparable radionuclides that do not decay by isomeric transmission.

The charged particle that is emitted or captured by the nucleus in the original decay process is, for all the radionuclides in common use in haematology, either a beta (β) particle or an electron. A β particle has a mass and electrical charge numerically equal to that of an electron but may be either negatively or positively charged. The negatively charged particle is known as a β$^-$ particle and the positively charged particle as a β$^+$ particle or positron. The β$^+$ particle however itself only has an extremely short lifespan, as when it has lost its kinetic energy it will combine with an electron and be transformed into two photons of radiation of energy 0.511 MeV known as annihilation radiation.

Thus, in practice, as a result of the decay of all the commonly used radionuclides in haematology either β$^-$ particles or γ or X ray photons will be emitted from the atom and can be detected in order to measure and compare the quantity of radioactivity present in different samples. However, since it is much simpler to detect X and γ rays than β$^-$ particles it is usual to detect these when they are produced in the decay process and only to measure the β particle emission when there is an absence of photon emission or when these are of very low energy (< 0.01 MeV). Thus for all the radionuclides listed in Table 3.1 with the exception of ^{3}H, ^{14}C and ^{32}P it is the photon emissions of X and γ rays which are normally detected rather than the β particles. However it is also important to appreciate that the ease with which a certain radionuclide can be detected will also depend on the relative abundance of the X and γ rays emitted. Thus although ^{51}Cr and ^{113m}In emit γ rays of similar energy, as is shown in Table 3.1, since the ^{51}Cr γ ray is only emitted in 9% of its decays while the ^{113m}In γ ray is emitted in 65% of its decays, the count rate from ^{113m}In will be approximately seven times higher than that from ^{51}Cr per unit of radioactivity present.

Radioactivity measurement units
In the past the quantity of radioactivity present in a source or sample has been specified in a unit called the curie (Ci) which, for historical reasons, is defined as that amount of radioactive material in which the number of radioactive nuclei undergoing decay in each second is 3.7×10^{10}. However, although this unit is still in

limited use it is being replaced by the SI unit of radio-activity, the becquerel (Bq). One becquerel corresponds to one disintegration every second and hence there is a conversion factor of 3.7×10^{10} for converting curies into becquerels.

In practice in the laboratory the quantity of radio-activity in samples and stock solutions will generally range between about 500 Bq in low activity samples being assayed in a counter to 5×10^7 Bq in stock solutions or, in conventional notation, from 0.5 KBq to 50 MBq.

Radioactive half-life

The rate at which the nuclei of any given radionuclide undergo radioactive decay is a characteristic property of that radionuclide and is unaffected by any physical or chemical condition, and the greater the instability of the nucleus the greater is the probability that it will decay in any time interval. This probability therefore is also characteristic of the radionuclide and although it is not possible to make any prediction about when any indi-vidual nucleus will actually decay, in practice, as we have seen above, we are normally faced with relatively large numbers of decays per second. Thus, despite the fact that the individual decays occur at random, the rate of decay of the group as a whole can be mathematically described and measured with a high degree of accuracy.

The law of radioactive decay is that the average number of decays occurring in one second in a sample of a radionuclide at any time is proportional to the number of nuclei of that radionuclide in the sample at that time.

Mathematically, the fraction of the parent nuclei remaining at time t is given by the expression in equa-tion 1, where $\varkappa$ is called the radioactive decay constant (and represents the fraction of atoms undergoing decay in unit time), N(o) is the number of nuclei present at time t = o and N(t) is the number remaining after time t.

1. $$N(t)/N(o) = e^{-\lambda t}$$

The radioactive half-life is the time taken for the number of parent nuclei to be reduced by one half and this is related to the decay constant by the expression in equation 2 (where $T_{\frac{1}{2}}$ is the radioactive half-life).

2. $$\lambda = 0.693/T_{\frac{1}{2}}$$

Therefore equation 1 can be rewritten in the form of equation 3, and it is this form which is normally used since the half-life is usually a more informative and easily remembered entity than the decay constant,

3. $$N(t) = N(o).e^{-0.693t/T_{\frac{1}{2}}}$$

and in terms of the quantity of radioactivity present (A(t) at time t and A(o) at time t = o) this equation 3 becomes equation 4.

4. $$A(t) = A(o).e^{-0.693t/T_{\frac{1}{2}}}$$

In practice a correction to a measurement for the decay of the radionuclide will only be needed occasionally. For instance, in a red cell survival meas-urement using ^{51}Cr-labelled cells, provided all the blood samples taken over the course of the study are counted at the same time, even though approximately 2.5% of the radioactivity will have been lost through radioactive decay every 24 hours, it is not necessary to make a correction for the radioactive decay since the same correction factor would need to be applied to all the counts. However, if say ^{99m}Tc has been used as a red cell label for a blood volume measurement and it takes one hour to count all the samples and standards, then by the end of that hour if the first sample was counted again, because of its measurable decay over this time period, the count would appear to be reduced by approximately 11%. Therefore, in this case, because of the measurable radioactive decay during the time taken to count the samples, it would be necessary to make a correction for this, and, assuming all subsequent meas-urements are corrected to the time of counting the first sample, an increasing correction factor would need to be applied to each count.

The other main time when a correction for radioactive decay is necessary is when allowance needs to be made for the time difference between the measurement or reference time of a stock solution and its use in order to ensure that the correct quantity of radioactivity is used. Thus, using ^{111}In as an example, let us assume that a stock solution of 75 MBq is available, from which we need 10 MBq to label a patient's platelets for platelet survival studies. Normally the reference activity date and time marked on the stock vial will not be the same as that when the radioactivity is needed and therefore there will be either more or less radioactivity in the stock solution depending on whether the reference date and time is in the future or in the past. Assuming the reference time is 24 hours in the future, since ^{111}In will decay to 78% of its initial value over 24 hours, the actual quantity of ^{111}In in the stock vial will be 75/0.78 or 96.1 MBq, or alternatively if the reference time was 24 hours prior to use, the quantity in the stock vial would be 75×0.78 or 58.5 MBq. Thus, in the first case, in order to obtain 10 MBq it would be necessary to with-draw 10.4% of the vial contents, and in the second case it would be necessary to withdraw 17.1%, and therefore use a much larger volume of the solution.

Instrumentation

It has already been noted that for the majority of the radionuclides used in haematology it is the γ or X rays emitted as a result of the radioactive decay process which are detected and counted rather than the β particles and only when these photon emissions are absent or of very low energy that the β particles are counted instead. The well scintillation counter or gamma counter is now the universally accepted instrument for general X and γ ray sample counting, and for β particle counting special liquid scintillation counters (β counters) are normally used.

Both these types of counter work in essentially the same way and rely on a photomultiplier tube to detect scintillations produced in the detector scintillator and to produce an electrical pulse output whose number and amplitude is proportional to the number and energy of the absorbed photons or β particles producing the scintillations. These pulses are then amplified, passed through an energy analyser and then counted. The purpose of the analyser is best shown with reference to Figure 3.1. This shows a spectrum of the number of pulses detected from a ^{51}Cr source as a function of the amplitude of the pulse. As can be seen there is a distinct peak (known as the photopeak) corresponding to the detection of the 0.32 MeV energy γ rays of ^{51}Cr but in addition to this there are also other γ rays detected which are either lower energy scattered γ rays or background γ rays and it is necessary, in order to achieve the maximum precision in counting, to reduce the influence of these non-photopeak events as much as possible. This is achieved by using the energy analyser, which is set so that only photopeak events are counted, and

typically the effective width of this counting window will be about 20% of the photopeak energy.

Thus for the case illustrated in Figure 3.1 the only events counted would be those detected within the marked 20% window between 0.288 and 0.352 MeV. The β particle spectrum is, however, rather different as the β particles emitted do not all have the same energy and usually are in most abundance at about one third of the maximum energy given in Table 3.1. Thus the analyser window settings used in β counters are generally much larger than those used in gamma counters, though when spectral changes are used to correct for quenching (see below) narrower windows of similar size to those used in gamma counters are used.

Most counters also have more than one counting channel and this makes it possible to set the counter up so that two or sometimes more separate radionuclides in the same sample may be counted simultaneously by setting the counting window for each radionuclide over the photopeak for its photon emission. However, when this is done for samples containing more than one radionuclide it is usually necessary to correct for the crosstalk between the two radionuclides and in order to do this it is necessary to count a pure sample of each radionuclide in all channels and then use the ratio of the counts in each channel to correct the sample counts.

Gamma counters — special considerations

Most gamma counters use a sodium iodide crystal as the detector and this has a well cut into it into which the sample to be counted is placed, and typically these are large enough to accept sample volumes of up to several millilitres. Systems for counting larger samples such as

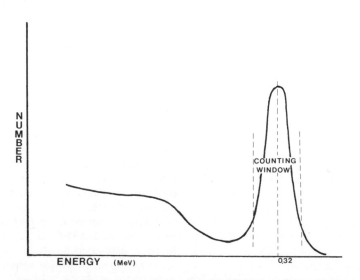

Fig. 3.1 An energy spectrum for the γ rays emitted by ^{51}Cr measured with a sodium iodide detector showing the limits of the analyser counting window that would be used in practice.

24 hour urine collections or faecal samples are however available, though in this case the sample is generally placed between two opposed detectors or within a large well made from a plastic scintillator, since very large sodium iodide crystals are extremely expensive. One problem with all these counters is that of the change in sensitivity with the volume of the sample being counted and this needs to checked carefully for every counter, since only the part of the sample in the centre of the detector crystal will be counted with maximum efficiency.

Another important point when considering the suitability of any scintillation counter for counting particular radionuclides is the size of the detector crystal. In general, the higher the energy of the photons that are to be detected, the larger the size of the detector crystal will need to be. For example, 10 mm of sodium iodide will absorb 99% of the X and γ rays emitted by ^{125}I and 92% of the γ rays emitted by ^{99m}Tc but only about 18% of the γ rays emitted by ^{59}Fe. Thus the sensitivity of a small counter designed specifically for counting ^{125}I would be totally inadequate for counting ^{59}Fe, for which even 75 mm will only be 75% efficient. It is therefore necessary to use much larger detector crystals for counting the radionuclides emitting higher energy γ rays. However it must also be pointed out that a large crystal will not be ideal for low energy radionuclides. This is because the background count increases with increasing crystal size and will hence unnecessarily increase the error in the sample count for low energy radionuclides, for which the sample count will not increase with the larger crystal.

A further important point concerns the use of multiple well counters. In these there are normally up to 16 separate crystal detectors, allowing up to 16 samples to be counted simultaneously. With these counters care needs to be taken to ensure firstly, that the sensitivity is the same for each detector and, secondly, that there is adequate shielding between the detectors, the latter point being particularly important if samples emitting high energy γ rays are being counted, since the majority of these counters are designed specifically for ^{125}I.

Beta counters — special considerations

Conventional scintillation counters cannot be used for β particle counting as the aluminium casing which is necessary around the sodium iodide detector crystal absorbs all except the highest energy β particles so that they never reach the detector. In liquid scintillation counters this problem is overcome by using the sample to be counted itself in the place of the detector crystal, the sample being suspended or dissolved in a liquid scintillator based on an organic solvent. However,

because the energy of the β particles from ^3H in particular is very low, the size of the signal pulses is also very small and these are often comparable with the random electrical 'noise' pulses which are generated in the photomultiplier tube itself. This results in very high background counts which effectively reduce the accuracy of the measurement.

This problem is usually solved using two complementary methods. Firstly, by refrigerating the system, the temperature of the photomultiplier tube can be reduced and this reduces the noise level; secondly, by using two photomultiplier tubes operated in coincidence so that a scintillation is only counted if it is observed by both tubes simultaneously, most of the remaining 'noise' contribution to the background can be eliminated.

The major problem with liquid scintillation counting is the reduction in efficiency due to chemical and colour quenching. Chemical quenching is caused by the chemical absorption of the energy released during the decay process before it can be transferred to the scintillator, and colour quenching is caused by the absorption of the emitted light before it reaches the photomultiplier tubes. The general effect of quenching is to change the energy spectrum of the detected β particles as shown in Figure 3.2 by reducing both their apparent energy and their number. Sample preparation methods are therefore much more important and critical in beta counting than they are in gamma counting.

Three main methods are used to correct for quenching, and facilities for making these corrections are normally incorporated in commercial equipment. The primary method involves counting each sample twice, once normally and once after the addition of a known small quantity of the radionuclide being counted. Then, from the increase in the measured counts, the relative counting efficiency can be calculated for each sample and used to correct the original count. The second method makes use of the change in the spectral shape caused by quenching and involves dividing the spectrum into two counting channels covering different parts of the spectrum. Because the quantity of quenching alters the ratio of the counts detected in each channel, measurement of this ratio provides a measure of the severity of quenching — and hence a correction factor — provided a calibration has been previously obtained using the primary method. The third method utilises a γ ray source which is positioned close to the sample. The γ rays from this source interact with the liquid scintillator and the increase in the number of counts recorded gives a measure of the relative amounts of quenching present in each sample. As with the second method this also has to be calibrated against the primary method, however in practice, once the calibration curves have been

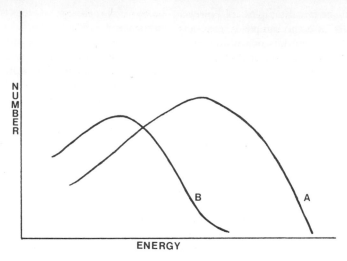

Fig. 3.2 Typical unquenched (A) and quenched (B) beta particle spectra from a liquid scintillation counter.

obtained for each radionuclide, either the second or the third methods of correction are normally used.

Statistical factors and measurement precision

As has already been noted, nearly all measurements involve comparison of the quantities of radioactivity in different samples. However, since radioactive decay is a random process, repeated measurements on the same sample will not give identical results and it is therefore important to be able to determine the likely error in the result obtained.

The standard deviation of a single measurement of the number of γ, X or β particles detected in a given time is simply equal to the square root of that number, thus the larger the number detected or counted, the smaller the error in the measurement becomes when expressed as a percentage of the result. In practice, therefore, if a count of N is recorded, then the true count has approximately a 68% probability of lying between $N - \sqrt{N}$ and $N + \sqrt{N}$, a 95% probability of lying between $N - 2\sqrt{N}$, and $N + 2\sqrt{N}$, and a 99.7% probability of lying between $N - 3\sqrt{N}$ and $N + 3\sqrt{N}$. Thus, if a count of 10 000 is obtained, the true count has a 99.7% probability of lying between 9700 and 10 300, or is 10 000 $\pm$ 300.

This, however, is only the error in a single count and in practice it is usually necessary to correct this count for the background count measured over the same period of time when no sample or a blank sample is in the counter. In this case the result is given by $N - B$ where B is the background count, but a single standard deviation in this result is now given by $\sqrt{N + B}$ so that the error in the result is increased. Thus if the sample count is again 10 000 and the background count is 6000,

the true sample count will have a 99.7% probability of lying between 4000 $\pm$ 1200 — a much larger error than that in a single uncorrected count.

Often it is also necessary to divide (or multiply) one count by another, and in this case the relative standard deviation needs to be used. This is the standard deviation expressed as a percentage of the count. The relative standard deviation in the result is then given by $\sqrt{(v_1{}^2 + v_2{}^2)}$ where v_1 and v_2 are the relative standard deviations in the two counts.

For example, if in a given counting time 10 000 counts are obtained from sample A, 2000 counts from sample B and 500 counts from the background, then, working in this case to just one single standard deviation, the true count from sample A is likely to lie within the range 9500 $\pm$ $\sqrt{10\ 500}$ or 9500 $\pm$ 102, and the true count from sample B is likely to lie within the range 1500 $\pm$ $\sqrt{2500}$ or 1500 $\pm$ 50. Now, to calculate the standard deviation of the ratio of the counts it is necessary to convert these standard deviations in the sample counts to relative standard deviations. Thus, for sample A the relative standard deviation is $100 \times 102/9500$ or 1.08 and for sample B is $100 \times 50/1500$ or 3.33, so that the relative standard deviation in the result is given by $\sqrt{1.08^2 + 3.33^2}$ or 3.50. Thus one standard deviation in the value of the ratio of the counts A/B is given by $(9500/1500) \times (3.50/100)$ or 0.22 so that the measured ratio of 6.33 has a 68% probability of lying within the range 6.33 $\pm$ 0.22 or a 99.7% probability of lying between 6.33 $\pm$ 0.66.

From the above it can be seen that the error in a result can be significantly larger than simple inspection of the initial sample count might suggest, and the error in the final result will be dominated by the error in the least precisely measured component of the calculation. In addition, of course, it must always be appreciated that, even if the error is calculated to three standard deviations, there is still a small probability that the true result will lie outside this range.

Conclusion

All diagnostic radionuclide procedures in haematology involve the measurement of the quantity of radioactivity in samples and, generally, the comparison of a sample count with that obtained from a standard in order to calculate a result from the test. A large range of different radionuclides is now used for these tests and it is important that suitable and accurately set-up instrumentation is used to make the measurements. Radioactive decay corrections to the measured counts are sometimes necessary as may also be corrections for differing sample volumes, counting sensitivities and quenching effects. Finally the statistical error in the sample counts and result must be determined so that the likely accuracy of the final result can be calculated and the confidence with which the result can be given a clinical interpretation assessed.

RED CELL AND PLASMA VOLUME — GENERAL COMMENTS

The demonstration of an absolute increase in red cell volume is essential for the diagnosis of polycythaemia. Increases or decreases in plasma volume can give rise to apparent anaemia or polycythaemia. Where this is suspected, combined measurements of red cell and plasma volume will identify discrepancies between estimates of peripheral blood haemoglobin concentration and total red cell volume. Minor extension of the procedure makes it possible to estimate the volume of blood held in an enlarged spleen.

Principle

A small volume of radiolabelled red cells or plasma is injected intravenously and sufficient time allowed for uniform mixing with the circulating blood. Plasma volume can then be calculated directly by dividing the total injected plasma radioactivity by the radioactivity in unit volume of plasma. Red cell volume can be calculated by measuring the dilution of the red cell label in whole blood together with the patient's PCV.

For red cell labelling the most commonly used radionuclides are ^{51}Cr (as sodium chromate) and ^{99m}Tc (as sodium pertechnetate), though ^{113m}In or ^{111}In are occasionally used as alternatives to ^{99m}Tc. The tracer used for plasma volume measurements is usually ^{125}I (or ^{131}I)-labelled human serum albumin. If ferrokinetic measurements using ^{59}Fe-labelled plasma transferrin are

carried out, these can also provide an estimate of plasma volume (see p. 73).

Selection of radionuclide

The use of the dilution technique for blood volume measurements depends upon firm binding of the radionuclide label to the blood component and an absence of loss of the component from circulation during the time of the measurement. The choice of radionuclide will be governed by how closely these ideal characteristics are approached, upon the ease of the labelling procedure, and upon the radiation characteristics of the radionuclide (e.g. half-life and ease of counting, particularly if two different radionuclides are to be counted simultaneously).

Red cell labelling

^{51}Cr labels globin within red cells. The labelling procedure is simple. Elution (loss of label from the cells) is negligible over the time (1 h) required for red cell volume measurement, but becomes significant where red cell survival studies over several weeks are carried out (see p. 66). The relatively long radioactivity half-life (28 d) of ^{51}Cr is a disadvantage in terms of radiation dose where only blood volume measurements are to be made, but is essential if there are to be additional measurements of red cell survival and/or prolonged surface counting measurements.

^{99m}Tc labels the β globin chain of haemoglobin in undamaged cells, but labels red cell stroma in heat-damaged cells (see p. 78). The red cells must be pretreated with stannous ion to enable stable binding of ^{99m}Tc. Spontaneous elution in vivo is slight over the first 10–20 minutes but thereafter amounts to 4–10% per hour. This is a disadvantage in red cell volume measurements if the mixing time is likely to be prolonged (e.g. in cases of cardiac failure or gross splenomegaly). With a half-life of only 6 hours ^{99m}Tc is likely to be chosen where repeated measures of red cell volume are planned. It is a much better γ emitter than ^{51}Cr and may therefore be more suitable where short-term surface counting and/or scanning is also required.

^{111}In (half-life 2.8 d) or ^{113m}In (half-life 100 min) label both red cell stroma and haemoglobin. Ionic indium is not taken up by cells and has to be mixed with a suitable ligand (e.g. oxine, acetylacetone, tropolone) to form a lipid soluble complex which enters cells. Elution is much less than with ^{99m}Tc during the first hour in vivo, and In is therefore more suitable where delayed mixing is expected.

Plasma labelling

^{125}I-labelled human serum albumin is commonly used (^{125}I is readily distinguished from ^{51}Cr, ^{99m}Tc and ^{113m}In and is therefore normally preferred to an ^{131}I-label).

Albumin is slowly lost from circulating plasma to extravascular fluids, and allowance for this has to be made in calculating the plasma volume.

Equipment

The same equipment is needed for each of the various methods for red cell and plasma labelling. Labelling procedures should be carried out using sterile techniques, preferably in a laminar flow hood. All solutions must be sterile and pyrogen free.

○ Bench centrifuge
○ Sterile disposable syringes (1 ml, 10 ml, 20 ml) and needles
○ Volumetric flask (100 ml)
○ Laboratory balance
○ Precision micropipettes
○ Well-type gamma scintillation counter

RED CELL VOLUME (ACD ^{51}Cr METHOD)

Reagents

● NIH-A acid citrate dextrose.
  Trisodium citrate dihydrate 22 g
  Citric acid (monohydrate) 8 g
  Dextrose (hydrous) 25 g
  Water to 1 litre
  Sterilise by autoclaving at 126°C for 30 minutes as 1.5 ml aliquots in 30 ml screw capped bottles.
● ^{51}Cr as sodium chromate (e.g. Amersham, UK). The stock (1 or 2 mCi, 37 or 74 MBq) is conveniently diluted in isotonic saline and dispensed in amounts of 100–200 μCi/ml using individual vials which can be sterilised by autoclaving. The specific activity should be not less than 20 μCi (740 kBq) per μg at the time of use.
● Isotonic sterile saline (9 g/litre).

Method

Cell labelling

1. Collect 10 ml of blood and add to 1.5 ml sterile NIH-A ACD solution.
2. Centrifuge (1000 g for 5–10 min).
3. Remove and discard supernatant. Take care not to remove any red cells.
4. Add sodium chromate solution 0.1–0.2 μCi/kg (3.7–7.4 kBq/kg) body weight, dropwise with constant mixing. The volume should be at least 0.2 ml (dilute in isotonic saline if necessary). The specific activity should be such that less than 2.0 μg of chromium is added per ml of packed cells.
5. Stand for 15 minutes at room temperature.

6. Wash the labelled cells twice in 4–5 volumes (20 ml) of isotonic saline (where there is increased red cell osmotic fragility, e.g. in hereditary spherocytosis, use 12 g/litre NaCl).
7. Resuspend the cells to a final volume of about 10 ml. Draw cells up into a 10 ml syringe and attach the needle (plus protective cap) to be used for injection. The protective cap should be labelled with a marker pen to allow easy identification for later reweighing.

Preparation of standard

1. Weigh full syringe, needle and cap (W_1) to the nearest mg.
2. Ensure cells are well mixed in syringe and inject, through the needle, approximately 1 ml into a volumetric (100 ml) flask. Replace marked needle cap.
3. Reweigh syringe needle and cap (W_2).
4. Make standard flask to volume (V) with 0.4 g/l NH_4OH.

Administration of labelled red cells

1. The patient should be rested in a recumbent state for 15 minutes prior to injection, and should remain resting for blood sampling (changes in posture may alter the plasma volume).
2. Inject the labelled cells intravenously over approximately 30 seconds.
3. At the end of the injection apply constant pressure to the syringe plunger to ensure no flow back into the syringe before the needle is withdrawn from the vein. Replace the marked needle cap.
4. Weigh empty syringe, needle and cap (W_3).

Blood samples

1. Obtain a baseline blood sample before injection of the labelled cells as a check for any background patient radioactivity (e.g. from previous radionuclide tests). Thereafter samples should be taken at 10, 20 and 60 minutes, the latter being essential if mixing is likely to be delayed (e.g. with splenomegaly or cardiac failure).
2. Each 5 ml blood sample should be taken from a vein other than that used for injection of the labelled cells, and mixed with solid EDTA anticoagulant.
3. Measure the PCV of each sample.
4. Deliver known volumes (e.g. 3 ml) into counting tubes and lyse with a small amount of saponin (to allow uniform distribution of the ^{51}Cr throughout the counting sample).
5. Measure the radioactivity of each sample, together with an equal volume of the standard and a background count. The coefficient of variation due to counting statistics should not exceed 2%.

Calculation

1. Calculate total radioactivity injected =

$$C_S \times V \times \frac{(W_2 - W_3)}{(W_1 - W_2)} \text{ counts per second (cps)}$$

where

C_S = cps (corrected for background counts) per ml of diluted standard.

V = volume of flask containing diluted standard.

W_1 = weight (g) of full syringe, needle and cap.

W_2 = weight (g) of syringe, needle and cap after removal of standard.

W_3 = weight (g) of empty syringe, needle and cap after injection.

i.e. $(W_2 - W_3)$ = weight of labelled cells injected, and

$(W_1 - W_2)$ = weight of labelled cells in the standard.

2. Then red cell volume =

$$\frac{\text{total radioactivity injected (cps)}}{C_t} \times PCV_t$$

where C_t = cps (corrected for background counts) per ml of whole blood at time t.

and PCV_t = packed cell volume of the sample at time t.

Comments

— A mean of values for red cell volume obtained from the test samples at 10 minutes and 20 minutes may be used provided mixing is complete by 10 minutes. Otherwise use the value obtained from the 60 minute sample if this is substantially greater.

— PCV measurements should be by electronic counter or by a direct centrifugation method corrected for trapped plasma.

— In the equally satisfactory ^{51}Cr 'citrate wash' method, the ACD solution in step 1 of the cell labelling procedure is replaced by 30–40 ml of citrate phosphate dextrose solution (trisodium citrate dihydrate, 3.0 g; sodium dihydrogen phosphate, 0.015 g; dextrose, 0.2 g; water to 100 ml).

Interpretation (see p. 65).

RED CELL VOLUME (^{99m}Tc METHOD)

Reagents

- Freshly prepared stannous chloride ($SnCl_2.2H_2O$) solution.

- ^{99m}Tc sodium pertechnetate — freshly generated from a ^{99m}Tc sterile generator (e.g. Amersham, UK).
- Isotonic sterile saline for injection.

Method

Cell labelling

1. Collect 5 ml of blood in a preheparinised syringe, add to 20 ml saline, centrifuge at 1000 g for 5 minutes and remove supernatant to leave approximately 2.0 ml packed red cells.

2. Dissolve 2 mg $SnCl_2.2H_2O$ in 20 ml saline, within 10 minutes of use. Filter (0.22 μm Millipore) into a sterile container. Transfer 0.2 ml into 100 ml sterile saline, mix and withdraw 0.3 ml to add to the 2 ml packed red cells (approximately 0.015 μg tin/ml red cells).

3. Stand 'tinned' red cells at room temperature for 5 minutes.

4. Add 25 μCi (925 kBq) of freshly generated ^{99m}Tc in approximately 0.2 ml saline, with constant mixing.

5. Stand at room temperature for 5 minutes.

6. Centrifuge and wash once in 20 ml cold saline.

7. Resuspend cells in approximately 10 mls saline and draw up into a syringe prior to preparation of standard and injection of the patient.

Carry out further procedures and calculation as for ^{51}Cr method, except that test blood samples should be taken at 10 and 30 minutes.

Comments

— Elution of the ^{99m}Tc label increases after 30 minutes and the method is therefore less satisfactory when there is delayed mixing (60 minute samples give unreliable results).

— An alternative method of pre-tinning the cells is to do this in vivo, using a preliminary intravenous injection of Pyrolite (sodium pyrophosphate, sodium trimetaphosphate and stannous chloride mixture: New England Nuclear) or Amerscan Stannous Agent (sodium medronate and stannous fluoride mixture: Amersham, UK).

— Arrangements should be made to count the blood samples on the day of the study since the half-life of ^{99m}Tc is only 6 hours.

Interpretation (see p. 65)

RED CELL VOLUME (INDIUM METHOD)

Indium is available as ^{111}In chloride (in 0.04 M HCl), ^{111}In oxine isotonic solution (in 100 μg/ml Polysorbate 80, 6 mg/ml HEPES buffer and 0.75% sodium chloride), or may be produced as ^{113m}In chloride by elution from a ^{113m}In sterile generator (Amersham, UK). Cell labelling using ^{113m}In as an acetylacetone complex is described.

Reagents

- Acetylacetone (Sigma, BDH or E. Merck). Store at 4°C but bring to room temperature and dilute to 1.9 g/litre in HEPES buffer (pH 7.6) prior to use.
- Freshly generated ^{113m}In.
- Isotonic sterile saline.

Method

Cell labelling

1. Collect 5 ml blood in a sterile container with 100 IU heparin.
2. Centrifuge and wash cells once in 20 ml isotonic saline.
3. Add 10 ml 1.9 g/l acetylacetone and mix gently for 1 minute.
4. Add ^{113m}In (approximately 1 μCi, 37 kBq, per kg body weight).
5. Roller mix for 5 minutes.
6. Centrifuge and wash twice in sterile saline.
7. Resuspend cells in approximately 10 mls saline and draw up into a syringe prior to preparation of standard and injection of the patient.

Carry out further procedures and calculations as for the ^{51}Cr method.

Arrangements should be made to count the samples immediately since the half-life of ^{113m}In is only 100 minutes.

Interpretation (see p. 65)

PLASMA VOLUME

Reagents

Human albumin (not less than 20 g/litre) labelled with ^{125}I (e.g. 50 μCi ^{125}I and 20 mg albumin/ml; Amersham, UK).

Method

1. Collect 20 ml of blood in a syringe containing a few drops of heparin.
2. Transfer to a sterile screw cap bottle and centrifuge (1000 g for 5–10 minutes).
3. Transfer approximately 7 ml plasma to a second sterile container.
4. Add ^{125}I-labelled human serum albumin (0.05 μCi, 1.8 kBq, per kg body weight, mix and draw up labelled plasma into a 10 ml syringe. Attach needle (plus protective cap) to be used for injection — mark the protective cap for easy identification for later weighings.

Preparation of standard and *administration of the*

labelled plasma to the patient should be carried out as for red cell volume measurements (p. 62), with the following differences:

1. The known weight of plasma added to the volumetric flask should be diluted to volume with saline.
2. A stopwatch should be started at the midpoint of the injection into the patient (or the exact time carefully noted) in order to time the later blood samples.

Blood samples

1. Collect 5–10 ml blood into bottles containing solid heparin (from a vein other than that used for injection of the labelled plasma) at 10, 20 and 30 minutes (record actual time).
2. Centrifuge and separate the plasma.
3. Count an equal volume (e.g. 3.0 ml) of each sample in a gamma counter, together with the same volume of the standard and a background count. The coefficient of variation attributable to counting statistics should not exceed 2%.

Calculation

1. After subtracting background counts, plot the counts/ml for each plasma sample (y axis) against time (x axis) on semilogarithmic paper. Extrapolate the line obtained to zero time to estimate the radioactivity of the plasma at zero time (Fig. 3.3).
2. Calculate total radioactivity injected =

$$C_S \times V \times \frac{(W_2 - W_3)}{(W_1 - W_2)} \quad \text{counts per second (cps)}$$

where

C_S = cps (corrected for background counts) per ml of diluted standard

V = Volume of flask containing diluted standard

W_1 = Weight (g) of full syringe, needle and cap

W_2 = Weight (g) of syringe, needle and cap after removal of standard

W_3 = Weight (g) of empty syringe, needle and cap after injection

3. Then plasma volume =

$$\frac{\text{Total radioactivity injected (counts per second)}}{C_0}$$

where C_0 = cps per ml of plasma at zero time.

Comment

— Thyroidal uptake of radioiodine may, if desired, be blocked by oral administration of stable iodine,

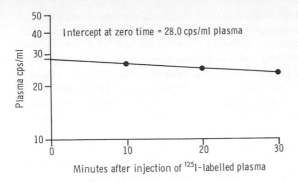

Fig. 3.3 Determination of plasma volume with extrapolation back to zero time plasma counts. In this example a total of 74 284 ^{125}I cps had been injected into the patient, giving a plasma volume of 74 284 ÷ 28.0 = 2653 ml.

60 mg potassium iodide daily starting 1 day before injection and continuing for 2–4 weeks.

Interpretation (see p. 65)

TOTAL BLOOD VOLUME

This is the sum of red cell and plasma volumes which can be measured simultaneously using two radionuclides (e.g. ^{51}Cr red cells and ^{125}I-labelled plasma). Results calculated from a single measure (either red cell or plasma volume) and the PCV are less reliable.

Simultaneous measurements

It is convenient to inject the two labels sequentially through a single butterfly needle, flushing with 10 ml saline after each dose to ensure that no residual radio-activity is left in the butterfly tubing. A proportion of any ^{51}Cr counts will be cross-counted into the ^{125}I channel. However, the reverse is not true and since whole blood is used only to obtain the ^{51}Cr counts of the red cells and separated plasma is counted for ^{125}I, no cross-counting corrections are needed, provided separate plasma and red cell standards are used.

An alternative is to add the ^{125}I-labelled albumin directly to the ^{51}Cr-labelled red cells prior to injection, to prepare a single standard, and to count only whole

blood samples (at 10, 20, 30 and 60 minutes). In this case the ^{125}I channel has to be corrected for crossover of ^{51}Cr counts. In addition, the PCV of each sample is needed to calculate the ^{125}I counts per ml of plasma and hence the plasma volume.

Calculated total blood volume

This is derived from

a. $$\frac{\text{Red cell volume}}{0.9 \times \text{PCV}}$$

or b. $$\frac{\text{Plasma volume}}{1 - (0.9 \times \text{PCV})}$$

where 0.9 is a mean ratio of whole body haematocrit to the venous haematocrit (corrected for plasma trapping). In addition to a considerable variation in normal subjects, this ratio may be lower in cardiac failure and higher with splenomegaly, where results are particularly likely to be inaccurate.

Interpretation

There is no ideal expression of the results of blood volume measurements which gives a clear indication of normality or otherwise in every case. Results are usually expressed as ml/kg body weight and compared with a normal range.

Normal (95%) range

		ml/kg
Red cell volume	Men	25–35
	Women	20–30
Plasma volume		40–50
Total blood volume		60–80

However, since fat is relatively avascular the result may be distorted by using the weight alone, and give rise to an underestimate (e.g. in obese patients).

Predicted volumes (Retzlaff et al 1969)

An alternative is to compare the measured values with those predicted from the patient's height and weight, or from their surface area (Table 3.2).

Table 3.2 Blood volume from surface area, height and weight

	S = Surface area (m^2)		Ht = Height (cm), wt = weight (kg)
Red cell volume			
Men	1100 S	or	8.2 Ht + 17.3 wt − 693
Women	840 S	or	16.4 Ht + 5.7 wt − 1649
Plasma volume (ml)			
Men	1630 S	or	23.7 Ht + 9.0 wt − 1709
Women	1410 S	or	40.5 Ht + 8.4 wt − 4811

Only measured values which vary from the predicted volumes by at least 25% should be considered definitely abnormal (Hurley 1975).

The volume of circulating leucocytes and platelets is usually negligible. However, in occasional patients in whom these cells are increased in number (e.g. in chronic myeloid leukaemia) the calculation of total blood volume as the sum of red cell and plasma volumes will be an underestimate.

Calculation of the ratio of 'whole body PCV' (red cell volume: total blood volume) to peripheral PCV may sometimes be helpful. The normal mean value (0.9) has a wide variation, but an increased ratio may indicate an increased pool of red cells in the spleen. Furthermore, in patients with gross splenomegaly delayed mixing of the labelled cells with pooled splenic red cells may lead to an apparent increase in measured red cell mass between 10 minutes and 60 minutes: this increase may be used as a rough guide to the size of the splenic red cell pool.

RED CELL SURVIVAL

Red cell survival studies are used to demonstrate and quantify a reduction in the lifespan of the patient's own red cells. They are frequently combined with surface counting studies (see p. 74) in an attempt to identify major site(s) of red cell destruction.

Principle
Red cell survival is measured by one of two main techniques:

Cohort labelling
A population of newly formed red cells is labelled (e.g. by ^{14}C-glycine) over a restricted period of time. The release, and subsequent removal from circulation, of this population is then monitored to determine mean cell lifespan. Because the study has to be continued for the entire lifespan of the cohort it can be very prolonged. Combined with the need for tedious β counting techniques this means that cohort labelling is impractical for routine clinical use.

A variant of this technique uses ^{59}Fe in an attempt to measure effective red cell production, and from this calculates the mean red cell survival in patients who are assumed to be in steady state (see p. 71).

Random labelling
A sample of circulating red cells of all ages is labelled using ^{51}Cr (as sodium chromate) or di-isopropyl phosphofluoridate (DFP) labelled with ^{32}P or ^{3}H. ^{51}Cr, being a γ emitter, is easy to use and may also be used for surface counting. However it has the disadvantages

of variable rates of elution from the circulating red cells, particularly during the first 1–3 days, and of possible selective labelling of young red cells (i.e. non-random labelling). Although this makes accurate determination of red cell lifespan impossible, this is rarely critical in clinical use where labelling with ^{51}Cr is usually the method of choice. DFP shows less elution after the first 24 hours, but as a β emitter requires more elaborate counting procedures, and is rarely used except for research purposes (for method see ICSH 1971).

The ^{51}Cr random labelling method will be described here.

Reagents and equipment
As for ^{51}Cr method for red cell volume (p. 62).

Method

Cell labelling and administration to patient
The procedure is identical to that used for determination of red cell volume (p. 62). However, use a larger dose of ^{51}Cr [0.5 μCi (19 kBq)/kg body weight, or 1.0 μCi(37 kBq)/kg if surface counting is also to be carried out].

Prepare a standard only if red cell volume is to be determined simultaneously.

Blood samples
1. Take 5 ml venous blood into solid anticoagulant (e.g. EDTA) from a vein other than that used for injection, at 10 minutes and, if mixing is likely to be delayed (e.g. with cardiac failure or splenomegaly) at 60 minutes.

2. A further sample should be taken at 24 h, at least three specimens between days 2 and 7, and thereafter two samples per week for the rest of the study.

3. Measure the Hb or PCV on part of each specimen using an electronic or manual method corrected for plasma trapping.

4. Pipette an accurate volume (e.g. 3 ml) from each well-mixed sample into a counting tube, and lyse with a small amount of saponin powder.

5. Count all the samples together at the end of the study to avoid the need to correct for radionuclide decay.

6. The coefficient of variation attributable to counting statistics should not exceed 2%. If there is more than 2% difference between the 10 minute and 60 minute samples the latter should be used to calculate the red cell survival.

Calculation
1. For each sample subtract the background counts and calculate the count rate (e.g. counts per second, cps) per ml of whole blood. If the samples have been

counted at different times against a ^{51}Cr standard, correct also for radioactive decay.

2. Where the patient is in steady state (Hb or PCV constant, reticulocyte count constant, no blood transfusions for 2 months before and during the study) correct for minor day-to-day variations in PCV by calculating for each sample the cps per ml of red cells (or g of Hb).

$$\text{e.g. cps/ml red cells} = \frac{\text{cps/ml of whole blood}}{\text{PCV}}$$

3. Where, as is more common in clinical practice, the patient is not in steady state, it is not possible to measure red cell lifespan accurately. However a reasonable estimate can be obtained by assuming that total blood volume remains constant and using the cps/ml of whole blood from step 1. If the patient receives a blood transfusion during the study the blood volume can be assumed to have returned to its pretransfusion level by 24 hours.

4. Express counts from steps 1 or 2 as a percentage of the day 0 (10 minute or 60 minute) counts:

^{51}Cr survival on day t

$$= \frac{\text{cps/ml whole blood (or RBCs) on day t}}{\text{cps/ml whole blood (or RBCs) on day 0}} \times 100\%$$

5. Multiply the percentage ^{51}Cr survival from step 4 by the elution correction factors shown in Table 3.3 to obtain the percentage red cell survival.

6. Plot the % red cell survival against time on arithmetic and semilogarithmic axes for visual inspection.

Table 3.3 Elution correction factors for converting ^{51}Cr survival to true red cell survival (ICSH 1980).

Day	Correction factor	Day	Correction factor
0	1.00	16	1.22
1	1.03	17	1.23
2	1.05	18	1.25
3	1.06	19	1.26
4	1.07	20	1.27
5	1.08	21	1.29
6	1.10	22	1.31
7	1.11	23	1.32
8	1.12	24	1.34
9	1.13	25	1.36
10	1.14	26	1.38
11	1.16	27	1.40
12	1.17	28	1.42
13	1.18	29	1.45
14	1.19	30	1.47
15	1.20		

Interpretation

1 a. If the data appear to be fitted by a straight line on the arithmetic plot it is likely that red cell destruction is largely the result of senescence (i.e. all cells are surviving to about the same age before being destroyed). A straight line may then be fitted using a least squares procedure and the mean cell lifespan is given by the time at which extrapolation of the fitted line reaches zero activity.

b. If the plot appears curvilinear on arithmetic, but linear on semilogarithmic axes an exponential survival function is likely, corresponding to a random red cell destruction mechanism. The best straight line should be fitted to the semilogarithmic plot, and mean cell lifespan is then the time corresponding to 37% survival.

c. It is frequently not obvious which plot gives the best fit, particularly where clinical considerations limit the duration of the study in patients with only modest shortening of the red cell lifespan. In these circumstances use of a statistical fitting criterion may be helpful.

d. If the plot appears curvilinear on both arithmetic and semilogarithmic axes, draw the best smooth curve through the data points and construct a tangent to the curve at zero time. An estimate of the mean cell lifespan is then given as the time at which the tangent cuts the time axis.

2. Occasionally the points on day zero are significantly above what is otherwise a good fit straight line on either the arithmetic or semilogarithmic plot. This may be due to early elution of ^{51}Cr from viable cells or may indicate a subpopulation of cells undergoing rapid destruction. If the latter is felt to be clinically unlikely use the line of best fit through the later points to determine mean cell lifespan, recalibrating the point of interaction of the line with the y (% surviving) axis as 100%. In order to demonstrate a subpopulation of rapidly destroyed cells, more frequent initial blood samples should be taken and analysis for a dual population carried out (see note 3 below).

3. In some haemolytic anaemias (e.g. paroxysmal nocturnal haemoglobinuria, sickle cell disease) or after blood transfusion there may be two populations of cells with widely varying lifespans. In these cases it is necessary to separate the two components of the survival curve before analysis (Fig. 3.4).

a. Extrapolate the tail of the curve plotted on arithmetic axes back to the time of injection to obtain the % of longer lived cells (% L). From this, by subtraction, calculate the % of shorter-lived cells (% S).

b. Estimate the mean red cell lifespan of the longer-lived population (MCL$_L$) as the time when the extrapolated line cuts the time axis.

c. Estimate the mean cell lifespan of the total population of red cells (MCL$_T$) as the time at which a

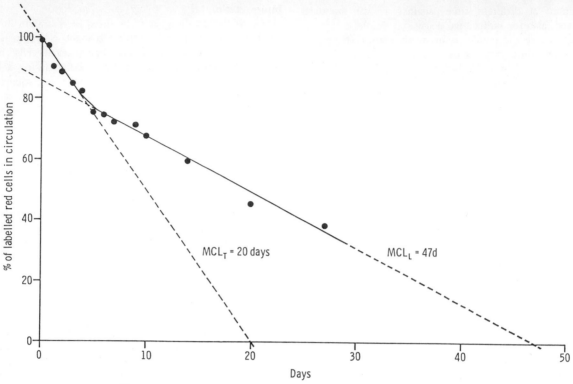

Fig. 3.4 Arithmetic plot of ^{51}Cr red cell survival in a patient with haemolysis due to homozygous haemoglobin Constant Spring, analysed as a double population of cells. Extrapolation of the less steep slope to the ordinate indicates the proportions of longer-lived cells (L, 84.4%) and of shorter-lived cells (S, 15.6%). The overall mean cell lifespan (MCL$_T$) of 20 days is made up from the MCL$_L$ of the long-lived cells (47 days), and the MCL$_L$ of the shorter-lived cells (5 days), the latter being calculated as shown in the text. (Figure modified from Derry S, Wood W G, Pippard M, et al 1984 Journal of Clinical Investigation 73: 1673–1682.)

tangent to the initial steep slope of the curve cuts the time axis.

d. The mean cell lifespan of the short-lived population is then given as:

$$MCL_S = \frac{\% \, S}{\dfrac{100}{MCL_T} - \dfrac{\% \, L}{MCL_L}}$$

Where
    S = shorter-lived population,
    L = longer-lived population,
    T = total red cells,
    MCL = mean cell lifespan.

Comments

— In the past it was usual to plot the % ^{51}Cr survival *without* the elution correction and to determine the T$_{50}$Cr (i.e. the time taken for the concentration of ^{51}Cr in the circulating blood to fall to 50% of its initial value). However, the T$_{50}$Cr bears no consistent relationship to the mean cell lifespan, and gives no information as to the mechanism of red cell destruction (e.g. senescent or random).

— The rate of elution of ^{51}Cr varies with red cell labelling techniques but is about 1% in normal subjects with the ACD or citrate wash methods. However, this rate may vary considerably more in patients with haematological disorders and lead to unpredictable errors in red cell survival studies. Table 3.3 gives correction factors for ^{51}Cr elution.

— Mathematical computer modelling may be applied to the red cell survival data, with the use of functions to fit the survival curves. These functions may be based on physiological models or may be arbitrary (e.g. ICSH 1980). It is doubtful whether these have much to add to the simple procedures described above, particularly in view of the potential errors which may arise from the use of ^{51}Cr and unpredictable rates of elution.

— Where there is significant external blood loss (>20 ml/day) the mean cell life may be artificially shortened. A correction for this can be applied:

$$\text{True MCL} = L \times \frac{RCV}{RCV - (L \times V)}$$

where L = apparent mean cell life, RCV = red cell volume (measured at the start of the red cell survival study), and V is the volume (ml) of red cells lost/day.

Normal values

Mean cell lifespan	110 ± 40 (2SD) days	
$T_{50}Cr$	25–33	days

^{51}Cr IN VIVO COMPATIBILITY TEST

To determine whether or not survival of donor red cells is normal in cases where:

1. in vitro serological tests suggest all normal donors are incompatible with the recipient or

2. the recipient has a haemolytic transfusion reaction despite negative serological tests, and requires a further transfusion.

Method

1. Under sterile conditions remove 1 or 2 ml of blood from the donor bag (anticoagulant ACD or CPD).

2. Label 0.5 ml red cells with ^{51}Cr (10–20 μCi, 370–740 kBq) using standard procedure (p. 62), and make up to a final volume of approximately 10 ml in sterile saline.

3. Note the time of the midpoint of the i.v. injection into the recipient.

4. Using a different vein, take blood samples into solid anticoagulant (e.g. EDTA) at 3, 10 and 60 minutes, and, if the degree of urgency allows, after 5 or 6 hours and at 24 hours. Take sufficient blood at 10 and 60 minutes (10 ml) to allow plasma to be counted separately in addition to whole blood.

5. Pipette an accurate volume (e.g. 3 ml) of whole blood and separated plasma into counting vials, and lyse red cells with saponin (p. 62).

6. Count the samples and express the radioactivity as a percentage of the counts in the 3 minute blood sample.

Interpretation

1. With compatible cells the counting rate at 60 minutes is >97% of that of the 3 minute sample.

2. In emergency, donor cells may be transfused with minimal hazard when red cell survival at 60 minutes is greater than 70% and the amount of radioactivity in plasma at both 10 and 60 minutes is not more than 3% of that of the 3 minute whole blood sample. (This is because the concentration of offending antibody is likely to be low, and destruction of the much larger volume of transfused cells is likely to be negligible or very slow).

3. When survival is significantly lower at 10 minutes than 3 minutes, but does not change further by 60 minutes, a two component curve involving an IgM antibody is likely. There may well be no immune response and good survival after transfusion of a larger volume of the donor cells.

4. When the survival shows a single exponential decline the antibody is likely to be IgG and an immune response may well occur. A delayed haemolytic transfusion reaction is likely if a large volume of the donor cells is transfused.

5. If time is available the additional samples up to 24 h will make it clear whether there is any substantial destruction of donor cells.

Comments

— In patients whose serum is known to contain haemolytic antibodies, the volume of labelled red cells should be reduced to 0.1–0.2 ml to reduce the risk of provoking shivering and fever.

— In most cases in which there is doubt about the survival of donor cells there will have been little destruction by 3 minutes, and the counts at this time are a valid 100% survival reference value. However, where red cell destruction is very rapid, labelled cells may have already been destroyed during the allowed mixing time of 3 minutes. For precise estimation of survival under these circumstances an independent measure of red cell volume is needed, and a standard should be prepared from the labelled donor cells (see p. 62) to allow calculation of total ^{51}Cr injected. Then the '100% survival' reference value

$$= \frac{\text{total } ^{51}Cr \text{ injected (cps)}}{\text{red cell volume (ml)}} \quad \text{cps/ml of red cells}$$

The red cell volume may be estimated from the recipient's height and weight, and PCV (see p. 65), or measured by simultaneous injection of recipient cells labelled with ^{99m}Tc.

FERROKINETIC ASSESSMENT OF ERYTHROPOIESIS

The use of radio iron to quantitate erythropoiesis has a limited role in clinical practice in the investigation of anaemias whose aetiology (e.g. hypoplastic, haemolytic, or ineffective erythropoiesis) is not clear from simple measures of reticulocyte count and bone marrow examination. Such studies may also be useful in monitoring the effect of treatment e.g. in patients with marrow hypoplasia.

Principle

Iron bound to the plasma transport protein, transferrin, is taken up by transferrin receptors which are normally located predominantly on erythroid precursors within the bone marrow (Fig. 3.5). Within the erythron the iron is incorporated into haem, the transferrin being released back to the circulation. Attempts have therefore been made to assess the size of the erythron by measuring the rate at which injected ^{59}Fe bound to transferrin is cleared from circulation. This rate, in combination with the plasma iron concentration, allows calculation of the plasma iron turnover rate (PIT). In addition, the extent to which the ^{59}Fe is incorporated into haem and appears in the circulating red cells (e.g. at 14 days) has been used to provide some measure of effective erythropoiesis.

Unfortunately there are a number of serious objections to such a simple analysis:

1. Total plasma iron turnover includes iron delivered to non-erythroid tissues, particularly the liver cells (Fig. 3.5). Such non-erythroid iron uptake may predominate in those cases of hypoplastic anaemia in which an accurate measure of the severity of the disorder may be particularly desirable.

2. Although the initial part of the curve of plasma ^{59}Fe clearance (usually the first hour or two) can be fitted with a single exponential decline, there are subsequent refluxes of ^{59}Fe back into circulation. These include an early reflux (around 10 h) of transferrin-bound ^{59}Fe which has entered extravascular fluids, and a later reflux (around 8 d) which includes ^{59}Fe recycled via macrophages from wastage, ineffective erythropoiesis (Fig. 3.5). The former, extravascular, flux (about 8% in normals) will increase the initial rate of plasma ^{59}Fe clearance independently of the size of the erythron. The later reflux ^{59}Fe (about 26% in normals) will have a second chance of being taken up by transferrin receptors and of appearing in viable circulating red cells: this means that simple measurements of the product of the PIT and percentage utilisation of ^{59}Fe in red cells will normally overestimate the amount of effective erythropoiesis. By contrast, the percentage utilisation of ^{59}Fe in red cells will underestimate effective erythropoiesis in conditions in which there is marked early haemolysis of circulating red cells.

3. More recently it has been recognised that a transferrin molecule that is fully saturated with iron (diferric transferrin) is a much more efficient donor of iron to tissues bearing transferrin receptors than monoferric transferrin. Patients with a high plasma transferrin saturation will therefore have a higher plasma-iron turnover than patients with a low saturation even if the number of transferrin receptors, and size of the erythron, is the same in both cases.

There have been a number of different approaches to dealing with these problems. Detailed analysis of the plasma ^{59}Fe clearance curve, with multiple samples usually over 2 weeks, has enabled measurement of the early and late reflux components. One group (Cook et al 1970) used the results of such studies in subjects

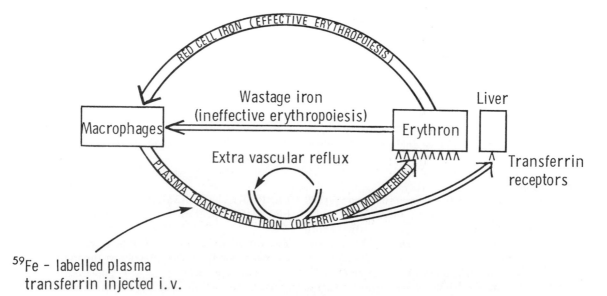

Fig. 3.5 Major pathways of iron metabolism and the features, in addition to erythron transferrin uptake, which influence the rate of plasma iron turnover.

without significant haemolysis or ineffective erythropoiesis to derive a simple function of the plasma iron concentration which could be applied more generally and enabled calculation of non-erythron iron turnover. Thus, by measurement of the total PIT and subtraction of the non-erythron iron turnover, total erythron iron turnover (EIT) could be calculated after measurements of plasma ^{59}Fe clearance completed within a few hours. Other groups (e.g. Ricketts et al 1975, Barosi et al 1978) have emphasised the prolonged study of the plasma ^{59}Fe clearance curve and the use of computer curve fitting programmes and compartmental analysis in an attempt to quantitate effective and ineffective erythropoietic iron turnover. Unfortunately the assumptions underlying this kind of approach tend to break down in those very conditions of haemolysis or ineffective erythropoiesis in which the analysis might be most useful. By calculating the red cell utilisation of ^{59}Fe as a fraction of the total ^{59}Fe that had passed through the plasma up to the time of measurement, and multiplying this fraction by the total PIT, it was possible to calculate effective red cell iron turnover (RCIT), but this was valid only if there had been no early destruction of mature labelled red cells due to haemolysis. As a by-product, mean red cell lifespan could be estimated from the RCIT: this calculation assumed that the measurement obtained at a single time corresponded to the average red cell production in a patient otherwise in steady state (i.e. with a constant total amount of iron in red cell haemoglobin). Calculations of total erythropoiesis (marrow iron turnover, MIT) required that all 'wastage iron' resulting from ineffective erythropoiesis or haemolysis was made visible for analysis by refluxing to the plasma, with no retention of ^{59}Fe by the macrophages (Fig. 3.3). This assumption may break down, e.g. in iron-loading, dyserythropoietic anaemias such as the thalassaemia disorders. Here any fraction of the ^{59}Fe which is retained and stored in macrophages would be wrongly interpreted as non-erythroid tissue iron turnover (TIT) rather than iron turnover due to ineffective erythropoiesis (IIT). A complete description of the amounts of effective and ineffective erythropoiesis therefore seems an unrealistic goal for studies based solely on analysis of the clearance curve for plasma [59]Fe.

The above analyses did not take account of the effects on PIT of variable proportions of diferric and monoferric transferrin. A recent simple approach (Cazzola et al 1985, 1987a) allows for this factor by using the percentage saturation of the TIBC to convert the PIT into a measure of erythron transferrin uptake. This method, which has the practical advantage that it can be completed in a single day, gives a useful evaluation of total erythroid activity in both hypoplastic and hyperproliferative anaemias and will be described below.

Reagents

- [59]Fe as ferric citrate injection BP. This is supplied by Amersham, UK as a sterile solution containing 1% w/v sodium citrate dihydrate, made isotonic with sodium chloride, at a concentration of 100 μCi (3.7 MBq)/ml. Specific activity should be greater than 5 μCi/μg iron at the time of use. Immediately before use prepare a working solution (3–4 μCi/ml) using sterile isotonic saline in 0.01 N HCl (pH 2) as diluent. (An alternative, preferred by some authorities, is sterile [59]FeSO$_4$ diluted with pH 2 isotonic saline before use).
- Heparin for injection 1000 units/ml.

Equipment

○ Sterile Vacutainer tube (10 ml).
○ Volumetric flask (100 ml).
○ Laboratory balance.
○ Well-type gamma counter.
○ Selection of 1, 2, 5, 10 and 20 ml syringes and needles.

Method

1. [59]Fe Labelling of plasma

a. Take 15–20 ml of patient's blood in a syringe containing a few drops of heparin. Centrifuge at 1000 g for 5–10 min to separate plasma.

b. Transfer 7–10 ml plasma to a sterile Vacutainer tube. N.B. The patients serum iron and TIBC should be measured within 1–2 days of the study to confirm an unsaturated iron binding capacity greater than 18 μmol/litre. Where the UIBC is less than this, plasma from an ABO compatible donor (hepatitis B surface antigen and HIV antibody negative) should be used.

c. Draw up 0.4–0.6 ml ^{59}Fe solution (1.5–2.0 μCi, 55–74 kBq) and inject this slowly through the top of the Vacutainer, drop by drop, with constant mixing of the plasma.

d. Incubate at room temperature for 30 minutes.

e. Draw up the labelled plasma into a 10 ml syringe, and fit a 20 g needle and cap (mark with a marker pen to ensure easy identification for later reweighings).

2. Preparation of standard

a. Weigh (W_1) full syringe, needle and cap to the nearest mg.

b. Inject 1–2 ml of labelled plasma into a volumetric flask (100 ml) and bring to volume with 0.01 N HCl.

c. Reweigh syringe, needle and cap (W_2) to determine the weight of labelled plasma used to prepare the standard.

3. Administration of ^{59}Fe-labelled plasma

a. Insert an intravenous 19 g Butterfly-type needle

and take baseline blood samples (10 ml in heparin and 5 ml in EDTA anticoagulant). Keep the cannula patent with heparinised sterile isotonic saline in between subsequent sampling times.

b. Inject the ^{59}Fe-labelled plasma into a different vein over about 1 minute, recording the time at the midpoint of the injection. Hold the plunger firmly down while withdrawing the needle to prevent any flow back.

c. Replace the needle cap and reweigh the syringe, needle and cap (W_3) to determine the weight of injected ^{59}Fe-labelled plasma.

4. Blood sampling

a. Samples should be taken at around 5, 10, 20 and 30 minutes with a further 4 samples over the next 2 hour, samples being collected earlier if the anticipated clearance rate is rapid.

b. Collect 5 ml blood at each time (after discarding the first 2 ml from the heparinised cannula) and anticoagulate in tubes containing solid heparin. Record the exact time of sampling.

c. Where red cell utilisation of ^{59}Fe is to be measured, collect a further 5 ml blood in EDTA at 14 days. If the entire curve of red cell utilisation is required, collect additional 5 ml EDTA samples daily for 3 days and thereafter on alternate days.

5. Processing of samples

a. Centrifuge the baseline and subsequent heparinised blood samples and pipette 2.0 ml of plasma from each into counting tubes.

b. Pipette 2.0 ml ^{59}Fe standard (in duplicate) into counting tubes.

c. Count the plasma samples and standard, as well as background counts, in a well-type scintillation counter.

d. If red cell ^{59}Fe utilisation is to be measured, pipette 4 ml of each well-mixed EDTA sample into counting tubes, and count against 4 ml ^{59}Fe standard.

e. Obtain sufficient counts to give a coefficient of variation due to counting statistics of less than 3%.

f. Measure the plasma iron and TIBC (see p. 84) on the baseline heparinised plasma.

g. Measure the PCV (by a method which corrects for plasma trapping) on the baseline EDTA sample and on any subsequent samples taken for red cell ^{59}Fe utilisation measurements.

Calculations

Plasma ^{59}Fe clearance

1. Plot the count rate/ml of plasma against time on semilogarithmic paper (Fig. 3.6).

2. Fit a line to the initial data points which fall on a straight line — ignore any later points which fall above this line as a result of reflux of plasma ^{59}Fe.

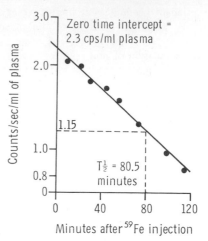

Fig. 3.6 Typical clearance of ^{59}Fe from plasma showing derivation of the zero time intercept and $T_{\frac{1}{2}}$.

3. Determine the extrapolated zero time plasma radioactivity and the half-clearance time ($T_{\frac{1}{2}}$) from the graph. Bias in drawing the line may be eliminated by using a least squares method to fit the data to a simple exponential function, $C_t = C_o e^{-0.693t/T_{\frac{1}{2}}}$, (where C_t = count rate/ml of plasma at time t after injection, C_o = is the value of C_t at the time of injection assuming instantaneous mixing, and 0.693 is the natural logarithm of 2). In any event the data should always be plotted for visual inspection, to exclude any outlying points.

Plasma iron turnover (PIT)

1. The amount of iron passing through the plasma in unit time (PIT) is the product of the fractional clearance rate of iron and the plasma iron concentration. The plasma iron concentration is measured on the baseline blood sample, and the fractional clearance is calculated by dividing the natural logarithm of 2 (0.693) by $T_{\frac{1}{2}}$ (minutes) and converting from minutes to days. In addition, it is usual to express the result in relation to unit volume of whole blood. Thus:

PIT (μmol/litre whole blood/24h) =

$$\frac{\text{Plasma iron}}{(\mu\text{mol/litre})} \times \frac{0.693 \times 60 \times 24}{(T_{\frac{1}{2}} \text{ (min)})} \times \frac{\text{plasma volume}}{\text{total blood volume}}$$

This expression can be simplified, to a very close approximation, as

PIT (μmol/litre whole blood/24h)

$$= \text{Plasma iron } (\mu\text{mol/litre}) \times \frac{1000}{T_{\frac{1}{2}}} \times (1 - 0.9 \text{ PCV})$$

where 0.9 is the assumed relationship between peripheral and whole body PCV.

Erythron transferrin uptake (ETU)

Three additional simple calculations are needed to convert PIT to uptake of transferrin-iron complex by the erythron (a measure of the number of transferrin receptors and thus the size of the erythron).

1. Subtraction of extravascular flux (EVF). EVF (that portion of plasma iron which escapes to the extravascular space before its early reflux back into circulation) is calculated as a function of the plasma iron concentration on the basis of the data of Cook et al 1970:

EVF (μmol/litre whole blood/24h)
= Plasma iron (μmol/litre) $\times$ (1–0.9 PCV) $\times$ 1.5

After subtracting the extravascular flux from the PIT, the remainder is assumed to leave the blood by binding to tissue transferrin receptors. Thus tissue iron uptake (IU) is given by the expression:

IU (μmol/litre whole blood/24 h) = PIT − EVF

2. Conversion of tissue iron uptake (IU) to tissue transferrin uptake (TU). This takes into account a 4.2-fold advantage of diferric over monoferric transferrin in reacting with membrane transferrin receptors, and uses the percentage saturation of the plasma TIBC (S) to predict the relative proportions of di - and mono-ferric transferrin in the individual patient (Cazzola et al 1985).

TU (μmol/litre whole blood/24h)
$$= IU \times \frac{(200 + 2.2S)}{(200 + 6.4S)}$$

3. Subtraction of the mean normal value for transferrin uptake by non-erythroid tissues. Transferrin uptake by non-erythroid tissues is derived from the product of [100 − mean normal % red cell ^{59}Fe utilisation (85%)] and mean normal TU (71 μmol/litre whole blood/24 h) and is 11 μmol/litre whole blood/24 h.

Erythron transferrin uptake (ETU),
(μmol/litre whole blood/24h) $= TU - 11$

Plasma volume

1. Calculate total ^{59}Fe radioactivity injected.

Total injected ^{59}Fe (cps)
$$= standard (cps/ml) \times \frac{(W_2 - W_3)}{(W_1 - W_2)} \times V$$

where $(W_1 - W_2)$ = weight (g) of standard made to volume V (100 ml),

and $(W_2 - W_3)$ = weight (g) of labelled plasma injected.

2. Plasma volume $= \dfrac{\text{total injected } ^{59}\text{Fe (cps)}}{C_O}$

where C_o = cps/ml of plasma at zero time (Fig. 3.6).

3. The red cell volume, needed to calculate percentage red cell ^{59}Fe utilisation, may be estimated indirectly from plasma volume and the zero time PCV (assuming a ratio of 0.9 of whole body to peripheral PCV):

Red cell volume (ml)
$$= \frac{\text{plasma volume (ml)} \times 0.9 \text{ PCV}}{(1 - 0.9 \text{ PCV})}$$

This calculation is sufficiently accurate for most clinical purposes, except in cases of gross splenomegaly, but where greater precision is needed a direct measure of red cell volume (e.g. using ^{51}Cr or ^{99m}Tc — see p. 62) should be made on the 14th day of the study.

Red cell ^{59}Fe utilisation

1. Calculate for each whole blood sample the count rate/ml of red cells

cps/ml red cells
$$= \frac{\text{cps/ml of whole blood sample}}{\text{PCV of that sample}}$$

2. Calculate the ^{59}Fe present in the total red cell volume as a percentage of total injected ^{59}Fe.

Red cell utilisation (%)
$$= \frac{\text{cps/ml red cells} \times \text{red cell volume (mls)}}{\text{total injected } ^{59}\text{Fe (cps)}} \times 100$$

3. To obtain the red cell utilisation curve, plot the percentage utilisation values for each sample against time on arithmetic graph paper.

4. The marrow transit time is the time taken to reach 50% of maximum red cell utilisation.

Comments

— It has been suggested that the ^{59}Fe-labelled plasma should be passed through an exchange resin to ensure that no non-transferrin bound iron is present prior to injection (Cavill 1971). With the use of ^{59}Fe as described (the slow addition of very small amounts of ^{59}Fe of high specific activity in patients with a UIBC > 18 μmol/litre) this does not appear to be necessary. (Any unbound ^{59}Fe is cleared rapidly by the liver and would lead to errors in the calculation of plasma volume and red cell ^{59}Fe utilisation.)

— In patients with reticulocyte counts in excess of 5% all blood samples should be placed on ice, and centrifugation to separate the plasma should be at 4°C, to prevent in vitro uptake of plasma ^{59}Fe by reticulocytes.

Normal values ($\pm$ *2 SD*)

T$_{\frac{1}{2}}$ plasma ^{59}Fe clearance	80 $\pm$ 30 minutes
PIT	127 $\pm$ 60 μmol/litre whole blood/24h
ETU	60 $\pm$ 24 μmol/litre whole blood/24h
Red cell utilisation	85 $\pm$ 8%
Marrow transit time	approximately 80 hours

The T$_{\frac{1}{2}}$ alone provides no clinically useful information about the amount of erythropoiesis, except that when grossly prolonged (>200 minutes) erythroid marrow hypoplasia is virtually certain. A very rapid clearance (T$_{\frac{1}{2}}$ < 30 minutes) indicates that extraction of plasma iron by the marrow is maximal. This may occur in iron deficiency or with gross erythroid marrow expansion (e.g. in some cases of β thalassaemia intermedia) where demand can outstrip what would otherwise be an adequate iron supply.

In patients with aplastic anaemia or pure red cell aplasia the PIT is a poor guide to erythropoietic activity being only slightly reduced, with the remaining iron turnover going to non-erythroid tissues. By contrast, the ETU gives a good indication of the extent of erythropoiesis, and the red cell utilisation of ^{59}Fe is at very low levels (e.g. 10–15%).

In patients with haemolytic or dyserythropoietic anaemias both the PIT and ETU are typically increased, and the ETU may reach 10–15 times normal. The ETU indicates transferrin uptake by the erythron, and it is assumed that this is directly related to the number of erythroid precursors in the bone marrow. However, in the conditions associated with very rapid plasma clearance of ^{59}Fe (see above), the shortened T$_{\frac{1}{2}}$ may indicate that the transferrin receptors on the erythron are not fully saturated: under these circumstances the advantage of diferric over monoferric transferrin in delivering iron is lost (Cazzola et al 1987b) and ETU may underestimate the size of the erythron. In dyserythropoietic anaemias red cell utilisation of iron is reduced (e.g. to 30–50%) and the marrow transit time is increased. In haemolytic anaemias, percentage red cell utilisation is suboptimal and may begin to decline even within 14 days because of early destruction of labelled red cells.

The marrow transit time has been used to estimate the degree of stimulation by erythropoietin, which speeds the release of labelled red cells. However, in general, little extra information is obtained for the effort required to obtain the full red cell utilisation curve.

ASSESSMENT OF SITES OF RED CELL DESTRUCTION AND OF ERYTHROPOIESIS BY SURFACE COUNTING USING ^{51}Cr-LABELLED RED CELLS

This is done in order to identify the main sites of red cell destruction in haemolytic states particularly with reference to liver and spleen and as a guide to the possible benefits of splenectomy.

Principle

^{51}Cr-labelled red cells are injected, often as part of a red cell survival study (see p. 66), and surface counts are collected over liver, spleen and heart over the next few days. In the absence of any lysis or red cell sequestration to deposit ^{51}Cr in the spleen or liver, counts over these organs would be expected to fall at the same rate as those of the heart (representing the blood pool). Conversely, accumulation of excess counts over one or other organ implies red cell destruction at that site.

Equipment and reagents

○ As for ^{51}Cr red cell labelling procedure (p. 62).
○ A lead-shielded scintillation detector (at least 75 mm in diameter and 37 mm thick) with a single hole collimator. Improved uptake curves are obtained using two opposing detectors with the patient placed between them.

Method

1. Label a sample of the patient's red cells with 1 μCi (37 kBq)/kg ^{51}Cr as sodium chromate using standard procedure (p. 62).

2. Prepare a standard prior to injecting the patient if simultaneous red cell volume measurements are to be made or if the surface counts are to be calibrated at the end of the study to give quantitative data (see Comments).

3. The patient should be supine, in the same position, for each successive set of surface counts.

4. Mark the counting points on the skin with non-water-soluble marking ink, and cover with transparent plastic dressing:

Heart — in the midline at the level of the third interspace.
Liver — half-way between the right midclavicular and anterior axillary lines, 3–4 cm above the costal margin.
Spleen — the point of highest counting rate (found by preliminary counting for a few seconds over adjacent sites on the first occasion after injection of the labelled red cells).

The detector should be placed vertically over heart and liver and horizontally over the spleen, with the collimator just touching the skin. The exact position must be reproduced as exactly as possible for each successive count.

5. The first set of counts should be carried out 60 minutes after injection of the ^{51}Cr- labelled cells, and thereafter counts should be made daily in a severe haemolytic state, or at least 6 times over the next 2 weeks where the haemolytic rate is less rapid.

6. At least 2500 counts should be recorded at each site, preferably taking the mean of duplicates — the measurements should be repeated if they differ from each other by more than 5%.

7. On each counting day a ^{51}Cr standard (approximately 50 kBq) must be counted under identical conditions and the background counting rate of the detector must also be recorded.

Calculation (see Table 3.4)

1. Correct counts over each organ for background and, using the standard counts on each day, for radioactive decay and day-to-day changes in instrument performance.

2. In order to compare results in different patients 'normalise' the counts over the heart on day 0 to 1000 and adjust all other counts at every site proportionately to give the 'normalised' observed counts.

3. Using the changes in normalised heart counts, calculate the counts at the other sites which would be predicted at each time in the absence of excess ^{51}Cr deposition.

4. Plot any excess counts (observed minus predicted) over liver and spleen against time (e.g. Fig. 3.7).

5. Calculate the spleen:liver count ratios as a measure of the relative accumulation of ^{51}Cr in spleen and liver. The ratio on day 0 may be taken as 1 and the subsequent ratios expressed proportionately. These 'normalised' ratios are also plotted against time (Fig. 3.7).

Comments

— Count rates may be affected significantly by minor changes in positioning of the detector, and isolated readings may therefore be misleading.

— Count rate is dependent upon (i) the volume of the organ counted in relation to its total volume, (ii) the distance of the organ from the body surface, and (iii) the loss of ^{51}Cr from the organ after cells have been destroyed in it (about 6%/day). The data obtained are therefore qualitative in nature.

Table 3.4 Analysis of ^{51}Cr surface counting data in a patient with hereditary elliptocytosis.

Day of study	0	1	2	3	6	8	10
'RAW' COUNTS (cps)							
Background	1.0	1.0	1.1	1.1	1.1	1.0	1.0
^{51}Cr standard	237.6	234.0	219.9	222.1	207.9	197.6	186.7
Corrected for background	236.6	233.0	218.8	221.0	206.8	196.6	185.7
Standard correction factor	1.00	1.02	1.08	1.07	1.14	1.20	1.27
Heart							
Corrected for background	123.9	109.7	106.0	89.2	81.0	64.2	66.2
Corrected for standard	123.9	111.4	114.6	95.5	92.6	77.2	84.3
Liver							
Corrected for background	46.8	47.0	44.7	37.1	34.1	32.3	30.1
Corrected for standard	46.8	47.7	48.3	39.7	39.0	38.8	38.4
Spleen							
Corrected for background	107.9	113.0	116.6	124.4	123.2	124.6	142.3
Corrected for standard	107.9	114.7	126.1	133.2	140.5	149.9	181.2
NORMALISED COUNTS							
Heart — observed	1000	899	925	771	748	623	680
Liver — observed	377	385	390	320	315	313	310
— expected	377	339	349	291	282	235	257
— excess	—	46	41	29	33	78	53
Spleen — observed	871	926	1018	1075	1164	1210	1462
— expected	871	783	806	671	651	543	593
— excess	—	143	212	404	513	667	869
SPLEEN: LIVER RATIO							
— observed	2.31	2.41	2.16	3.36	3.69	3.86	4.72
— normalised	1.00	1.04	1.13	1.45	1.60	1.67	2.05

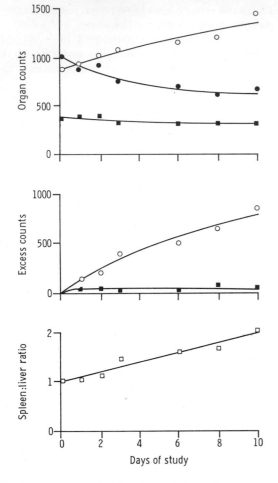

Fig. 3.7 Normalised data from Table 3.4 showing excess ^{51}Cr counts over the spleen in a patient with hereditary elliptocytosis ($\bullet$ = heart, $\bigcirc$ = spleen, $\blacksquare$ = liver). Excess counts of over 300 (speen) or 200 (liver) may be considered abnormal.

— Quantitative imaging, e.g. after a second injection at the end of the study of a known amount of either ^{51}Cr–labelled heat damaged red cells or ^{113}In colloid, may be used to calibrate the external counting equipment and thus to quantify splenic red cell uptake. However, the extra information obtained is rarely of clinical importance.

Interpretation

Four main patterns of ^{51}Cr surface counting may be identified:

1. Little or no excess accumulation in either spleen or liver (e.g. in paroxysmal nocturnal haemoglobinuria).

2. Excess accumulation in spleen only (e.g. hereditary spherocytosis, hereditary elliptocytosis, and some cases of auto-immune haemolysis).

3. Excess accumulation in liver only (e.g. in sickle cell disease).

4. Excess accumulation in both organs (e.g. in some cases of auto-immune haemolysis).

Splenectomy is most likely to be of benefit with patterns 2 or 4, though the magnitude of ^{51}Cr accumulation correlates poorly with the response.

ASSESSMENT OF SITES OF ERYTHROPOIESIS BY SURFACE COUNTING USING ^{59}Fe-LABELLED PLASMA

The sites of erythropoiesis, particularly in patients who may have extramedullary erythropoiesis (e.g. in the spleen in myelofibrosis) can be determined with ^{59}Fe.

Principle
^{59}Fe-labelled plasma is injected, often as part of a determination of the rate of plasma ^{59}Fe clearance, and a collimated scintillation detector is used to make surface counts over liver, spleen, sacrum (bone marrow) and heart (blood pool).

Equipment and reagents
$\bigcirc$ As for ^{59}Fe plasma labelling (p. 71).
$\bigcirc$ Collimated scintillation probe as for ^{51}Cr surface counting method (p. 74).

Method
1. Label a sample of the patient's plasma with 5 μCi (185 kBq) ^{59}Fe using standard procedure (p. 71).

2. Prepare a standard prior to injection if plasma volume is to be measured at the same time.

3. Mark the counting points over heart, liver and spleen as previously described for ^{51}Cr surface counting, and an additional point in the midline against the posterior surface of the upper one-third of the sacrum with the patient lying prone.

4. The first set of counts should be started at about 5 minutes. Repeat at 30 minutes, and then hourly for 5–6 hours. Thereafter count at 24 hours and on alternate days for 10–14 days.

5. On each counting day a ^{59}Fe standard (approximately 50 kBq) must be counted under identical conditions and the background counting rate of the detector must be recorded.

Calculation
1. Correct counts over each organ for background and, using the standard counts on each day, for radioactive decay and changes in instrument performance.

2. Express the counts over each organ as a ratio to the initial counts over that organ and plot the ratios against time on arithmetic graph paper (Fig. 3.8).

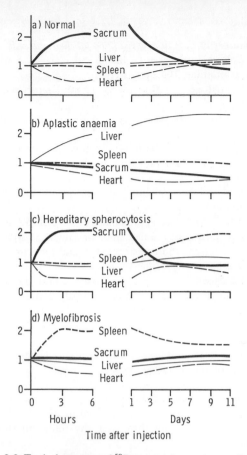

Fig. 3.8 Typical patterns of ^{59}Fe external counting. a. In the normal, ^{59}Fe leaves the blood (heart counts) and enters the bone marrow (sacrum). Marrow activity then falls as the ^{59}Fe enters the haemoglobin of newly formed red cells in the blood. Liver and spleen show little change. b. In aplastic anaemia, ^{59}Fe leaves the blood more slowly to enter the parenchymal liver cells rather than the marrow, and little appears in the circulating red cells. c. In hereditary spherocytosis, ^{59}Fe is cleared rapidly to the marrow, and there is a suboptimal later appearance in circulating red cells as the latter are sequestered in the spleen. d. In the case of myelofibrosis shown, ^{59}Fe is initially cleared to the spleen rather than marrow, and its subsequent release to circulating red cells is evidence that erythropoiesis within the spleen is largely effective.

Comments

— ^{59}Fe surface counting is laborious, and the data obtained are qualitative.
— Direct rectilinear scanning may be used to obtain more quantitative data on the sites of erythropoiesis. Alternatively, a quantitative image may be obtained by scintillation scanning at a known time after injection of plasma labelled with the short-lived radionuclide ^{52}Fe. This measurement of the uptake of ^{52}Fe can be used to calibrate the ^{59}Fe surface counts

that were present at the same time after radio iron injection. The amount of effective erythropoiesis, (e.g. in the spleen in myelofibrosis) may then be calculated from the fall in the ^{59}Fe external counts over the subsequent days.

Interpretation

1. As a general rule the clearance of ^{59}Fe from the blood (heart) during the first few hours, and the reciprocal increase in surface counts at another site, indicate uptake of transferrin-bound ^{59}Fe by transferrin receptors at that site.

2. Typical ^{59}Fe surface counting patterns are shown in Figure 3.8. They demonstrate the main alternative pathways for the initial uptake of transferrin iron as sacrum (bone marrow) and liver, the former route predominating normally, but the latter being uncovered in aplastic anaemia.

3. There may be abnormal early clearance from the blood (heart) to the spleen where there is extramedullary erythropoiesis. This contrasts with the more delayed accumulation of surface counts (e.g. over the spleen and/or liver) which is characteristic of excessive destruction of young, ^{59}Fe-containing red cells in haemolytic anaemias.

Combined ^{51}Cr and ^{59}Fe surface counting

Combined ^{51}Cr and ^{59}Fe surface counting may occasionally be useful to assess both red cell destruction and production at particular sites, e.g. in myelofibrosis with hypersplenism. Difficulties with cross-counting of ^{59}Fe into the ^{51}Cr counting window can be avoided by completing the ^{51}Cr study before starting the ^{59}Fe study. However, this is time consuming and rarely convenient, and it is possible to combine the two measurements. In this case the ^{59}Fe study should be started 24 hours earlier to allow measurement at each site of the fraction of ^{59}Fe counts appearing in the ^{51}Cr window. The fraction is then used to calculate the contribution of ^{59}Fe counts to all the subsequent ^{51}Cr counts obtained at that site, and to make the appropriate correction to the ^{51}Cr counts.

^{52}Fe scanning for erythropoietic activity

Approximately 100 μCi (3.7 MBq) of ^{52}Fe (half-life 8 h) may be used to label plasma in the standard way (p. 71) and to determine plasma iron clearance as described on page 72. Because it has somewhat lower γ ray energy than ^{59}Fe it can also be used to image the marrow and any abnormal splenic extramedullary erythropoiesis, usually at 3–4 hours after injection. With the use of appropriate phantoms to calibrate the imaging equipment, the scans can be used to quantitate the percentage splenic ^{52}Fe uptake. Because of the short half-life of ^{52}Fe, assessment of the effectiveness of such splenic erythropoiesis requires an additional ^{59}Fe surface counting study (see p. 69). The use of ^{52}Fe is limited by its poor availability as it can be produced only in a cyclotron.

SPLENIC RED CELL VOLUME

This can be used in patients with significant splenomegaly to determine the size of the splenic red cell pool which, if increased, may contribute to an anaemia.

Method
1. Label the patient's red cells with approximately 4 mCi (148 MBq) ^{99m}Tc or 1mCi (37 MBq) ^{113}In, and determine the red cell volume using standard procedures (p. 62).
2. Obtain a quantitative scan of the splenic area about 30 minutes later (more if there is delayed mixing due to gross splenomegaly).
3. To define the boundary separating the spleen from the blood pool in the heart it may be necessary to carry out a second scan using heat damaged red cells to delineate the spleen.
4. The radioactivity in the spleen is expressed as a percentage of the total radioactivity injected (calculated from a standard) and converted to a volume in ml from the measurement of total red cell volume.

Interpretation
The normal red cell pool is <5% of the total red cell volume (<70 ml in an adult).

In the absence of scanning facilities, a qualitative assessment of splenic red cell pooling may be obtained from the difference in red cell mass calculated at 10 minutes (partial mixing) and 60 minutes (full mixing) after injection of labelled red cells (p. 62).

ASSESSMENT OF SPLENIC FUNCTION USING HEAT-DAMAGED RED CELLS

The injection of heat-damaged labelled red cells may be used to demonstrate splenic enlargement or accessory splenic tissue on scintillation scanning, or to assess possible hyposplenism by measuring the rate of clearance of the damaged cells from circulation.

Equipment and reagents
○ As for ^{99m}Tc method for red cell volume (p. 63).
○ 12 g/litre sterile NaCl.
○ Water bath strictly controlled at a temperature of 49.5–50°C.

Method

Preparation of heat damaged ^{99m}Tc-labelled red cells
1. Collect 5 ml patient's blood and place in a sterile bottle containing 100 units heparin.
2. Centrifuge (1200 g for 5–10 min) and remove the plasma.
3. Transfer 2 ml packed cells to a 30 ml sterile screw capped glass bottle.
4. Heat in water bath (49.5–50°C) for exactly 20 minutes with occasional gentle mixing.
5. Wash cells twice in l2 g/litre saline.
6. Add 0.3 ml stannous chloride (p. 63) and stand for 5 minutes.
7. Add ^{99m}Tc. Use approximately 150 μCi (5.6 MBq) for blood clearance studies alone or 1mCi (37 MBq) if spleen imaging is to be performed. Stand for 5 minutes.
8. Wash once in 12 g/litre saline.
9. Resuspend the cells in about 10 ml 12 g/litre saline and inject without delay, recording the time of the midpoint of the injection.

Scanning
Scintillation scanning is usually started 1 hour after injection of the damaged cells.

Clearance of damaged red cells
1. Take a first blood sample (5 ml in solid EDTA or heparin) exactly 3 minutes after the midpoint of the injection.
2. Further 5 ml blood samples should be taken at 10, 20, 30 and 60 minutes.
3. Pipette a known volume (e.g. 3 ml) of each sample of whole blood into counting tubes and count in a well-type scintillation counter.
4. Express each count as a percentage of the radioactivity in the 3 minute sample.
5. Plot the results on semilogarithmic graph paper against time and determine the T_{50} (time taken to reach 50% of the 3 min value).

Comment
— ^{51}Cr may also be used to prepare labelled heat-damaged red cells. The cells are labelled with 0.5 μCi (19 kBq)/kg for clearance studies or 2.0 μCi (74 kBq)/kg for spleen imaging, using standard techniques (p. 62). The cells are then damaged as described for ^{99m}Tc, rewashed and resuspended in saline for injection.

Interpretation

Normal range
$T_{50} = 5$–15 minutes.
The T_{50} is prolonged in thrombocythaemia, coeliac

disease and other disorders associated with splenic atrophy.

MEASUREMENT OF BLOOD LOSS USING ^{51}Cr-LABELLED RED CELLS

Quantitation of blood loss, particularly into the gastrointestinal tract, may be helpful in the investigation of unexplained iron deficiency anaemia.

Principle
^{51}Cr-labelled autologous red cells are injected, and since ^{51}Cr is neither excreted into the gut or reabsorbed, measurement of faecal radioactivity in comparison with blood radioactivity gives a reliable measure of haemorrhage into the gastrointestinal tract.

Equipment
As for red cell volume measurement (p. 62) with the addition of a large volume sample counter.

Method
1. Label the red cells from 10 ml patient's blood with ^{51}Cr (100 μCi, 3.7 MBq) using the standard method (p. 62) and inject intravenously.
2. There is no need to prepare a standard from the labelled cells or to calculate the total ^{51}Cr injected unless red cell volume is to be measured simultaneously.
3. Collect all stools in suitable plastic cartons, usually for 10 days.
4. Collect a 5 ml blood sample in solid anticoagulant (e.g. EDTA) on each day of the study. A measured volume (e.g. 4 ml) of each blood sample should be diluted in about 100 ml of water in the same type of container as is used for the stool collection.
5. Count stools and diluted blood samples in a large volume counter.

Calculation
Calculate the volume of blood in the faecal samples of each day (t) of the study

$$= \frac{\text{count rate in day t faeces} \times \text{volume (ml) of day t blood}}{\text{count rate in day t blood sample.}}$$

Comments
— Blood losses from other sources, including menstruation, can be measured in a similar way by counting pads placed in a carton.
— It is important to ensure that there is no urine contaminating faecal or menstrual collections since any ^{51}Cr eluted from red cells is excreted in the urine.

Interpretation
Blood losses of over 2 ml/day may be considered abnormal.

^{59}Fe TOTAL BODY COUNTER METHOD FOR ASSESSING BLOOD LOSS

Principle
Iron is conserved by the human body and turnover is normally slow (up to 0.1% of total body iron/day). Thus serial total body counting over weeks or months after an i.v. dose of ^{59}Fe may allow abnormal rates, though not the source, of iron loss (i.e. bleeding) to be identified.

Equipment
Total body counter.

Method
1. Determine the 'machine' background counts, the counts in the patient prior to ^{59}Fe administration (if any), and counts in a suitable ^{59}Fe standard to be used throughout the study.
2. Inject intravenously 1 μCi (37 kBq) ^{59}Fe citrate, diluted to 1 ml in sterile pH 2 saline. The injection should be given slowly over 2 minutes to ensure binding to plasma transferrin, and thus transport to the erythron. (Studies are rarely done in any but iron deficient patients who have more than sufficient UIBC to ensure transferrin binding of the ^{59}Fe.)
3. Count the patient in the total body counter immediately after injection to give the 100% reference value.
4. Repeat measurements of machine background, total body counts and counts of the reference ^{59}Fe standard (to allow correction for radionuclide decay) at intervals over several weeks.

Calculation
1. 100% reference value = $P_1 - P_0$
2. % Retention of ^{59}Fe on day t

$$= \frac{P_t - B_t(P_0 \div B_0)}{P_1 - P_0} \times \frac{S_0 - B_0}{S_t - B_t} \times 100$$

3. % Remaining ^{59}Fe lost between day t and a later day, t_1,

$$= \frac{\% \text{ retention}_t - \% \text{ retention}_{t1}}{(\% \text{ retention}_t + \% \text{ retention}_{t1})/2} \times 100$$

where P_0, P_1 and P_t = patient count rates immediately before, immediately after, and at t days after ^{59}Fe injection, respectively.

B_0 and B_t = machine background on day 0 and day t respectively.

S_0 and S_t = standard count rates on day 0 and day t respectively.

Comments

— It is sometimes convenient to combine radioiron measures of iron absorption (see p. 80) with blood loss studies in the investigation of unexplained iron deficiency. In such cases the 10–14 day retention of an oral dose of ^{59}Fe may be taken as the 100% reference value.

— In premenopausal women it may be convenient to count immediately before and after each period to assess menstrual blood loss and determine whether there is any additional blood loss from other sources between periods.

— The ^{59}Fe method, being carried out over a longer time than ^{51}Cr stool collection, may be better suited to identifying intermittent blood loss, and assessing long-term rates of blood loss, than the ^{51}Cr stool collections. However, the latter are much more sensitive in the short-term detection of relatively small daily blood losses.

Interpretation

1. Nearly all the ^{59}Fe will be incorporated into red cells, particularly in those iron deficient subjects in whom the test is most likely to be carried out. If an assumption is made that at any time after injection 100% of the ^{59}Fe is present in red cells, the percentage of the remaining total body ^{59}Fe which is lost becomes equivalent to the percentage total blood volume loss. The blood volume may be estimated from height and weight (see p. 65) to allow calculation of blood loss in ml between successive measures of total body counts.

2. Where greater precision is required, a standard from the ^{59}Fe injected should be prepared. By counting whole blood samples (collected at each visit to the total body counter) against this standard, the percentage of total injected counts remaining per ml of blood can be calculated. Since the total body counts immediately after injection of the ^{59}Fe also represent the total ^{59}Fe counts injected, any changes in percentage total body ^{59}Fe retention can be converted to mls of blood lost:
Blood loss (ml) between days t and t_1

$$= \frac{(\% \text{ retention } ^{59}\text{Fe})_t - (\% \text{ retention } ^{59}\text{Fe})_{t1}}{(\% \text{ injected counts per ml blood}_t + \% \text{ injected counts per ml blood}_{t1})/2}$$

IRON ABSORPTION

Measurements of iron absorption are rarely indicated clinically, but they may be helpful in occasional cases of iron deficiency in determining whether a failure of response to oral iron therapy is due to malabsorption or, more commonly, failure to take the medication (where absorption is normal or increased).

Principle

A test dose of ^{59}Fe-labelled iron is given by mouth, and since once iron is absorbed there is minimal physiological iron excretion, the percentage retention after 10–14 days is equivalent to percentage iron absorption.

Reagents

- Ferrous sulphate ($FeSO_4.7H_2O$)
- Ascorbic acid
- ^{59}Fe as ferric chloride in 0.01 mol/litre HCl (Amersham, UK).

Test dose: prepare immediately before use by dissolving 15 mg $FeSO_4.7H_2O$ (i.e. 5 mg iron) and 50 mg ascorbic acid in 25 ml water. Add 2 µCi (74 kBq) ^{59}Fe.

Equipment

Total body counter.

Method

1. Fast patient overnight.

2. Determine machine background and patient background counts and count a suitable ^{59}Fe standard to be used throughout the study.

3. Administer test dose of oral iron in the morning and recount the patient.

4. Fast patient for a further 2 hours.

5. Repeat the patient's total body count, together with background and standard counts at 10–14 days.

Calculation

1. 100% Reference value = $P_1 - P_0$

2. % Retention (= absorption) of ^{59}Fe on day 10–14

$$= \frac{P_2 - B_2(P_0 \div B_0)}{P_1 - P_0} \times \frac{S_0 - B_0}{S_2 - B_2} \times 100$$

where P_0, P_1, and P_2 = patient's total body counts immediately before, immediately after, and at 10–14 days after the oral ^{59}Fe, respectively.

B_0 and B_2 = machine background on day 0 and on day 10–14, respectively.

S_0 and S_2 = standard counts on day 0 and day 10–14, respectively.

Comment
— Faecal excretion of ^{59}Fe is prolonged by the shedding of mucosal cells containing some of the ^{59}Fe initially taken up — this is why a counting interval of 10–14 days in needed.

Interpretation
The normal range for percentage iron absorption is very wide, but normal subjects usually fall within the range 10–35%. In iron deficiency much higher values (up to 80%) are expected, and values below 10% in these circumstances may indicate malabsorption.

The test uses a ferrous iron salt to assess the absorptive mechanism: it provides no information as to the availability and absorption of iron from the patient's diet.

Plasma iron tolerance
Where a total body counter is unavailable, or the use of radioisotopes is to be avoided (e.g. in children) changes in plasma iron concentration after a large dose of oral inorganic iron can provide evidence as to the ability to absorb iron in iron deficient subjects.

The patient is fasted overnight and 5 ml heparinised blood is taken immediately before, and 3 hours after, an oral dose of 100 mg of iron given as ferrous sulphate.

The plasma is separated for iron estimation.

Failure of the plasma iron to increase by more than 18 μmol/litre suggests the possibility of intestinal malabsorption.

USE OF RADIOLABELLED PLATELETS AND WHITE CELLS

It has been possible to label platelets with ^{51}Cr for many years and, more recently, with ^{111}In. However, only with the advent of ^{111}In has there been a satisfactory γ emitting label for leucocytes. The use of ^{111}In has enabled an extension of conventional studies of ^{51}Cr-labelled platelet survival to a variety of imaging studies, including quantitative scanning of both platelet and leucocyte distribution.

Platelets
The use of labelled platelets is set out in Chapter 30.

Leucocytes
Granulocyte kinetic studies have little clinical relevance at present, but the use of scanning with ^{111}In-labelled leucocytes to detect inflammatory bowel disease and local sepsis is now widely accepted and has a high degree of sensitivity and specificity.

REFERENCES

Practical considerations in the use of radionuclides
Bowring C S 1981 Radionuclide tracer techniques in haematology. Butterworths, London
Lewis S M, Bayly R J (eds) 1986 Radionuclides in haematology (Methods in Hematology, Vol. 14). Churchill Livingstone, Edinburgh

Red cell and plasma volume
Hurley P J 1975 Red cell and plasma volumes in normal adults. Journal of Nuclear Medicine 16: 46–52
International Committee for Standardization in Haematology 1980 Recommended methods for measurement of red-cell and plasma volume. Journal of Nuclear Medicine 21: 793–800
Peters A M, Osman S, Reavy H J, Chambers B, Deenmamode M, Lewis S M 1986 Erythrocyte radiolabelling: in vitro comparison of chromium, technetium, and indium in undamaged and heat damaged cells. Journal of Clinical Pathology 39: 717–721
Retzlaff J A, Tauze W N, Kielly J M, Stroebal C F 1969 Erythrocyte volume, plasma volume and lean body mass in adult men and women. Blood 33: 649–667

Red cell survival
International Committee for Standardization in Haematology 1971 Recommended methods for radioisotope red-cell survival studies. British Journal of Haematology 21: 241–250
International Committee for Standardization in Haematology 1980 Recommended method for radioisotope red-cell survival studies. British Journal of Haematology 45: 659–666
Mollison P L 1983 Blood transfusion in clinical medicine, 7th edn. Blackwell Scientific Publications, Oxford, p 606–608
Moroff G, Sohmer P R, Button L N 1984 Proposed standardization of methods for determining the 24-hour survival of stored red cells. Transfusion 24: 109–114

Ferrokinetic assessment of erythropoiesis
Barozi G, Cazzola M, Morandi S, Stefanelli M, Perugini S 1978 Estimation of ferrokinetic parameters by a mathematical model in patients with primary acquired sideroblastic anaemia. British Journal of Haematology 39: 409–423
Cavill I 1971 The preparation of ^{59}Fe-labelled transferrin for ferrokinetic studies. Journal of Clinical Pathology 24: 472–474
Cazzola M, Huebers H A, Sayers M H, MacPhail A P, Eng M, Finch C A 1985 Transferrin saturation, plasma iron turnover and transferrin uptake in normal humans. Blood 66: 935–939
Cazzola M, Pootrakul P, Huebers H A, Eng M, Eschbach J, Finch C A 1987a Erythroid marrow function in anemic patients. Blood 69: 296–301
Cazzola M, Pootrakal P, Bergamaschi G, Huebers H A, Eng M, Finch C A 1987b Adequacy of iron supply for erythropoiesis: in vivo observations in humans. Journal of Laboratory and Clinical Medicine 110: 734–739

Cook J D, Marsaglia G, Eschbach J W, Funk D D, Finch C A 1970 Ferrokinetics: a biological model for plasma iron exchange in man. Journal of Cinical Investigation 49: 197–205

Cook J D, Finch C A 1980 Ferrokinetic measurements. In: Cook J D (ed) Methods in Hematology 1 (Iron), Churchill Livingstone, Edinburgh, p 134–147

Ricketts C, Jacobs A, Cavill I 1975 Ferrokinetics and erythropoiesis in man: the measurement of effective erythropoiesis, ineffective erythropoiesis and red cell lifespan using ^{59}Fe. British Journal of Haematology 31: 65–75

Assessment of sites of red cell destruction and of erythropoiesis

Bowring C S 1986 Imaging and quantitative scanning. In: Lewis S M, Bayly R J (eds) Radionuclides in haematology (Methods in Hematology, Vol. 14). Churchill Livingstone, Edinburgh, p 151–172

Dacie J V, Lewis S M 1984 Practical haematology, 6th edn. Churchill Livingstone, Edinburgh

Finch C A, Deubelbeiss K, Cook J D et al 1970 Ferrokinetics in man. Medicine 49: 17–53

Hegde U M, Williams E D, Lewis S M, Szur L, Glass H I, Pettit J E 1973 Measurement of splenic red cell volume and visualisation of the spleen with ^{99m}Tc. Journal of Nuclear Medicine 14: 769–771

International Committee for Standardization in Haematology 1975 Recommended methods for surface counting to determine sites of red-cell destruction. British Journal of Haematology 30: 249–254

Jandl J H, Greenberg M S, Yonemoto R H, Castle W B 1956 Clinical determination of the sites of red cell sequestration in hemolytic anemias. Journal of Clinical Investigation 35: 842–867

Pettit J E, Lewis S M, Williams E D, Grafton C A, Bowring C S, Glass H I 1976 Quantitative studies of splenic erythropoiesis in polycythaemia vera and myelofibrosis. British Journal of Haematology 34: 465–475

Measurement of blood loss

Bannerman R M 1975 Measurement of gastro-intestinal bleeding using radioactive chromium. British Medical Journal 2: 1032–1034

Stack B H R, Smith T, Hywel Jones J, Fletcher J 1969 Measurement of blood and iron loss in colitis with a whole-body counter. Gut 10: 769–773

Iron absorption

Bothwell T H, Charlton R W, Cook J D, Finch C A 1979 Iron metabolism in man. Blackwell Scientific Publications, Oxford, ch 21 (Measurement of iron absorption) p 425–438

Callender S T, Witts L J, Warner G T, Oliver R 1966 The use of a simple whole-body counter for haematological investigations. British Journal of Haematology 12: 276–282

4

Assessment of iron status

In assessing any individual's iron status three main compartments of body iron need to be considered:

1. *Storage iron* — in the form of ferritin and haemosiderin in macrophages throughout the body and in hepatocytes (mean adult iron stores 1.0 g in men and 0.3 g in women).

2. *Transport iron* — iron in the plasma bound to the transport protein, transferrin (approximately 4 mg in an adult).

3. *Red cell iron* — mainly haemoglobin and accounting for most of the body's iron (approximately 2.5 g in an adult).

Storage iron

Serum ferritin concentrations are closely related to tissue non-haem iron concentrations, and can be used to provide an indirect assessment of total iron stores. This is because intracellular iron is a major stimulus to ferritin synthesis and small amounts of the newly-synthesised protein are secreted into the circulation, probably by both macrophages and hepatocytes. The amount of urine iron excretion after a test dose of an iron-chelating agent (e.g. desferrioxamine) has also been used as an indirect measure of iron stores. Though largely superseded by serum ferritin assay, urine iron measurements are still used to plan iron chelation therapy in iron-loaded patients. The synthesis of transferrin within the liver is inversely related to iron stores so that the serum total iron binding capacity (TIBC) is typically increased by iron deficiency and reduced by iron overload. As will be discussed with the individual assays, all these indirect measures of iron stores are affected by factors other than iron status. Direct tissue biopsy may thus still be needed — a bone marrow aspirate stained for iron (p. 31) may help in the differential diagnosis of iron deficiency and the 'anaemia of chronic disorders', whereas estimation of the iron content of a liver biopsy gives the most accurate assessment of the degree of potentially toxic, parenchymal iron overload.

Transport iron

The concentration of serum iron, and more particularly the saturation of the TIBC, gives a measure of the current iron supply to the tissues. Values for the small amount of iron in plasma are liable to wide fluctuations in normal individuals, but tend to stabilise in disorders of iron metabolism. The percentage saturation of the TIBC gives the best guide to the availability of iron to the tissues since upon this depends the relative proportions in circulation of diferric as opposed to monoferric and apotransferrin — diferric transferrin donates iron more efficiently to the tissues than monoferric transferrin. Values persistently below a 16% saturation of the TIBC in adults give rise to iron-deficient erythropoiesis. Values maintained above 70% imply a risk of excess iron deposition in parenchymal tissues, especially hepatocytes.

Red cell iron

Any assessment of total body iron must consider the large fraction normally present in red cell haemoglobin. For example, apparently 'normal' iron stores in an anaemic patient are likely to mean a substantial reduction in total body iron. Iron supply may then be limiting in any subsequent response to treatment of the underlying cause for the anaemia.

Two further measures provide information about the amount of iron which has been supplied to red cell precursors during their development. Where iron supply is limited (whether by true iron deficiency or in association with the anaemia of chronic disorders), the immediate precursor of haem, protoporphyrin, accumulates in the red cell precursors. It is lost only very slowly from mature red cells after their release into the circulation. Increased concentrations of red cell protoporphyrin (which can be rapidly assessed by direct fluorimetry of zinc protoporphyrin) thus provide evidence for a reduced iron supply over the preceding few weeks. The other measure is the amount of ferritin synthesised within developing red cells. Red cell ferritin is increased in iron overload, and reduced where iron supply to the bone marrow has been inadequate. Its measurement has been suggested as an assessment of tissue iron loading which is less influenced by other variables than the serum ferritin (see p. 87). However, the disorders of haemoglobin synthesis (e.g. thalassaemia) most liable to be associated with iron loading also lead independently to increased red cell ferritin concentrations, limiting the value of the measurement for this purpose. Red cell protoporphyrin and ferritin measurements remain largely research tools and have not been widely used in routine laboratories. Those seeking further details should consult the references by Labbe & Finch 1980 (red cell protoporphyrin) and Cazzola et al 1983 (red cell ferritin).

Clinical use

There is no single measurement of iron status that is ideal for all clinical circumstances. In severe uncomplicated iron-deficiency anaemia, the finding of either a combination of reduced serum iron and increased TIBC or a low serum ferritin serves to confirm the diagnosis. In hospital practice, where anaemia complicating other illnesses frequently has to be distinguished from early iron deficiency anaemia, assessment of both iron stores and transport iron is likely to be necessary, since the 'anaemia of chronic disorders' characteristically shows increased iron stores in the presence of reduced amounts of transport iron. Screening for iron overload (e.g. in first degree relatives of patients with idiopathic haemochromatosis, or others at risk of excessive dietary iron absorption such as patients with β thalassaemia intermedia) should include both the percentage saturation of the TIBC and serum ferritin assays, since changes in iron supply to the tissues commonly precede any increase in parenchymal iron stores. Where these tests are abnormal, and there is no obvious source of iron loading (e.g. regular blood transfusions), liver biopsy is usually needed to quantify the iron load and assess possible tissue damage.

SERUM IRON AND TOTAL IRON BINDING CAPACITY (TIBC)

Measurement of the serum (or plasma) iron and TIBC and calculation of the percentage saturation of the TIBC provides information about the current iron supply to the tissues. This can be helpful in identifying iron-deficient erythropoiesis and is an essential part of any screen for iron overload.

Principle

Serum iron
The method is based on the ICSH recommended assay.

A mixed acid reagent is used to release the transferrin-bound iron, reduce the ferric iron to ferrous, and to precipitate the serum proteins. The ferrous iron in the remaining supernatant is colour-developed using buffered bathophenanthroline sulphonate, and the absorbance of the resulting pink solution is read at 535 nm. A standard iron solution and a 'blank' (iron-free water) are treated similarly.

Serum TIBC
Sufficient iron is added to saturate the serum TIBC, any excess is removed by adsorption using solid magnesium carbonate, and after centrifugation the supernatant is assayed for iron as above. This method can be modified by using radioactive (^{59}Fe) saturating iron to measure the unsaturated iron binding capacity (UIBC).

Test samples

Stop any oral iron therapy (or desferrioxamine therapy) at least 12 hours before sampling.

Either serum or heparinised plasma is suitable (EDTA, oxalate or citrate anticoagulants interfere with the assay).

Avoid haemolysis during collection and separate from the red cells as soon as possible (especially if the reticulocyte count is high).

Samples may be kept at 4°C up to 1 week and indefinitely at −20°C.

Equipment

Wash all glass ware in detergent and then soak at least 6 hours in HCl (2 mol/litre) before rinsing with iron-free water (see p. 86). This is to remove any contaminating iron, a potential source of serious error.

Disposable plastic tubes (e.g. 12 × 75 mm) are convenient for the sample assays. Random tubes from each batch should undergo 'blank' iron analysis to check for possible iron contamination.

Use of a semi-automatic dispenser (e.g. Oxford pipetter) speeds up addition of mixed acid and chromagen reagents.

Reagents

For both serum iron and TIBC assays
- *Mixed acid reagent* (1 mol HCl, 0.6 mol trichloracetic acid and 0.4 mol thioglycollic acid per litre). (See p. 86).
- *Chromagen solution* (1.5 mol sodium acetate and 0.5 mmol bathophenanthroline sulphonate per litre). (See p. 87).

Additional reagents for TIBC assay
- *Saturating iron solution* (100 μmol iron/litre in 5 mmol HCl/litre). 10 ml stock ferric chloride

solution (see p. 87) made to 100 ml with iron-free water in a volumetric flask.

- *Light magnesium carbonate*, reagent grade (approximate formula $3MgCO_3$, $Mg(OH)_2$, $3H_2O$) e.g. as supplied by Mallinckrodt or BDH.

Standards and controls

Working iron standard (40 μmol/litre in 5 mmol HCl/litre). Take 2.0 ml stock iron standard (p. 87), add 400 ml iron-free water, and make to 1 litre with 5 mmol HCl/litre.

Internal control

Pooled fasting human serum, taken with care to avoid haemolysis. Aliquots should be stored frozen at $-20°C$.

Method
Serum Iron

1. Set up 2 test tubes for each sample.
2. Place 1.0 ml test sample or 1.0 ml working iron standard or 1.0 ml iron-free water (blank) in the first tube.
3. Add 1.0 ml mixed acid reagent. Vortex mix, and stand for 15 minutes.
4. Centrifuge at 1000 g for 10 minutes to sediment protein precipitate.
5. Pipette 1.0 ml of the optically clear supernatant into the second test tube.
6. Add 1.0 ml chromagen solution to each supernatant, mix, and stand for at least 15 minutes.
7. Measure absorbances at 535 nm against distilled water in a spectrophotometer. (The colour is stable for several hours).

Calculation

$$\text{Serum iron } (\mu\text{mol/litre}) = \frac{A_T - A_B}{A_S - A_B} \times 40$$

A_T = Absorbance of test sample
A_S = Absorbance of standard (40 μmol iron/litre)
A_B = Absorbance of blank.

Comments
— If the supernatant after centrifugation remains turbid, heat at 56°C for 15 minutes before centrifugation.
— Absorbance of reagent blank should be less than 0.015 in a 1 cm pathway against water. Higher values suggest reagent contamination with iron (see p. 84).
Normal range 11–28 μmol/litre in adults. Higher in neonates (27–45 μmol/litre in cord blood), and lower in children aged less than 12 years (where values as low

as 5 μmol/litre may occur with no other evidence of iron deficiency).

Method
Serum TIBC

1. Set up 4 test tubes for each sample.
2. Place 1.0 ml of test sample in the first tube.
3. Add 1.0 ml iron saturating solution and vortex mix. Stand for 15 minutes at room temperature.
4. Add approximately 0.15 g light magnesium carbonate using a previously calibrated tube or scoop. Stopper the tube with Parafilm, vortex mix, and place on a rotating turntable for 30 minutes.
5. Centrifuge at 1000 g for 15 minutes, transfer the supernatant to a fresh tube and repeat the centrifugation to remove any last traces of magnesium carbonate.
6. Transfer 1.0 ml of the final supernatant to the third test tube and assay for iron as described under serum iron.

Calculation

1. $\text{TIBC } (\mu\text{mol/litre}) = \dfrac{A_T - A_B}{A_S - A_B} \times 40 \times 2$

A_T = Absorbance of test sample
A_S = Absorbance of standard (40 μmol/litre)
A_B = Absorbance of blank
2 = Dilution due to addition of equal volume of iron saturating solution in step 3.

2. Saturation of the TIBC (%) =

$$\frac{\text{serum iron } (\mu\text{mol/litre})}{\text{serum TIBC } (\mu\text{mol/litre})} \times 100$$

Comments
— Inefficiency of adsorption by magnesium carbonate is about 3% of the unbound excess iron and is thus greatest in samples where the transferrin saturation is 100%. In addition, adsorption of sample water leads to an approximate 5% increase in concentration of plasma proteins. TIBC will therefore be overestimated, particularly at high levels of transferrin saturation, though this is not usually of clinical significance.
— It is usual to take the TIBC assay to the point of separation of the supernatant from the $MgCO_3$, before continuing with the iron assay in parallel with the serum iron assay on the same sample.

Normal ranges:
TIBC 47–70 μmol/litre
Saturation of the TIBC 16–60%

Method
Serum UIBC

1. Sufficient $^{59}FeCl_3$ (approx 10 μCi/100 ml) is added

to the saturating iron solution (otherwise identical to that used in the TIBC assay) to provide about 20000 cpm/ml on the gamma counter to be used.

2. The exact concentration of iron in the saturating solution is determined by the serum iron method above.

3. Test samples are prepared as in the serum TIBC method (steps 1–5) using ^{59}Fe-labelled iron saturating solution in step 3.

4. 1.0 ml of the final supernatant (step 6) is counted for gamma radiation against 1.0 ml of a 1 in 2 dilution of the ^{59}Fe-labelled iron saturating solution (standard) and 1.0 ml of water (blank).

Calculation

1. UIBC (μmol/litre) $= \dfrac{C_T - C_B}{C_S - C_B} \times Fe_S$

C_T = counts in test sample
C_S = counts in standard
C_B = background counts
Fe_S = iron concentration (μmol/l) of iron saturating solution.

2. TIBC = Serum iron + UIBC

Comments

— The overall precision of estimates of the TIBC by the colorimetric assay and from the radioactive UIBC determination is comparable.

— Original descriptions of these methods used 2.0 ml sample volumes. Scaling down to 1.0 ml involves no significant loss of precision for clinical use.

— Automated methods for serum iron include those based on the assay described here. A manual method for saturation of the TIBC is needed before the same automated assay can be used for the TIBC.

Interpretation

In normal subjects serum iron concentrations show wide fluctuations from day to day and a diurnal variation (highest in morning and lowest in evening). However, these fluctuations tend to disappear in iron deficiency or overload. The serum iron concentration and especially the percentage saturation of the TIBC reflect the iron supply to the tissues at the time of sampling. They give little guide to the state of iron stores. For example, in the progressive development of iron deficiency the serum iron concentration is unaffected until iron stores are exhausted; conversely, increased iron stores associated with the 'anaemia of chronic disorders' are usually accompanied by a reduction in serum iron concentration. The serum iron and TIBC also vary independently from each other, and consideration of the pattern of change of both measures, together with the

Table 4.1 Interpretation of serum iron and TIBC.

Measurement	Increased	Decreased
Serum iron	Iron overload Liver disease Chronic alcoholism Hypoplastic anaemia Haemolysis/ineffective erythropoiesis	Iron deficiency Infection/inflammation 'Anaemia of chronic disorder'
Serum TIBC	Iron deficiency Pregnancy Oral contraceptive	Iron overload Infection/inflammation 'Anaemia of chronic disorder'

percentage saturation of the TIBC, gives the most clinically useful information.

The factors which may influence the measures of transport iron are shown in Table 4.1. Apart from in iron deficiency, a reduction of serum iron concentration is most commonly due to systemic illness where the serum TIBC is also characterstically low and the percentage saturation of the TIBC is thus less severely reduced than in iron deficiency anaemia. Increases in serum iron concentration and percentage saturation of the TIBC are most commonly due to liver disease, or to failure of the bone marrow to utilise iron effectively. Nevertheless, persistently high values for the percentage saturation of the TIBC may be the first indication of a risk of increased uptake of iron by parenchymal tissues and of developing pathological iron overload.

Reagents

All chemicals must be of the lowest possible iron content.

● *Iron-free water* must contain less than 0.2 μmol iron/litre: glass distilled water may be satisfactory, but deionisation may be necessary.

● *Stock iron standard* (20 mmol iron/litre in 1.0 mol HCl/litre).
   1. 0.1117 g (2 mmol) dry, polished iron wire (greater than 99.5% purity).
   2. Dissolve in 15 ml HCl (7 mol/litre) in a 100 ml volumetric flask. Solution is hastened by heating in a boiling water bath.
   3. Make to volume with iron-free water.
   4. Keep indefinitely with flask tightly stoppered.

● *Mixed acid reagent* (1 mol HCl, 0.6 mol trichloracetic acid and 0.4 mol thioglycollic acid per litre).
   1. Dissolve 98 g trichloracetic acid* in 300 ml iron-free water in a 1 litre volumetric flask.

*Redistillation may be needed if iron content is greater than 0.00003%.

2. Add 28 ml thioglycollic acid (97% purity) and 500 ml hydrochloric acid (2 mol/litre).
3. Make to volume with iron-free water.
4. The solution is stable for at least 3 months if stored in a dark brown bottle.

- *Chromagen solution* (1.5 mol sodium acetate and 0.5 mmol bathophenanthroline sulphonate per litre).
  1. Dissolve 204 g sodium acetate trihydrate* (123 g anhydrous salt) in 900 ml iron-free water.
  2. Add 0.268 g bathophenanthroline sulphonate (4:7-diphenyl–1:10-phenanthroline) dissolved in 50 ml iron-free water.
  3. Make to volume with iron-free water in a 1 litre volumetric flask.
  4. The reagent is stable for at least 2 weeks if kept in a dark brown bottle.

- *Stock ferric chloride solution* (1 mol iron/litre and 50 mmol HCl/litre).
  1. Dissolve 0.27 g ferric chloride ($FeCl_3.6H_2O$) in 50 ml HCl (1 mol/litre).
  2. Make to volume with iron-free water in a 1 litre volumetric flask.
  3. The reagent is stable indefinitely and is used to prepare the iron-saturating solution for serum TIBC assay.

SERUM FERRITIN

Measurement of the serum (or plasma) concentration of ferritin can provide a non-invasive assessment of iron stores, useful in the diagnosis of both iron deficiency and iron overload.

Principle
There are two main types of immunoassay used to detect the tiny amounts of ferritin in human serum.

Non-competitive assays

Immunoradiometric assays (IRMA) In a two-site (sandwich) IRMA, unlabelled antibody to human ferritin is attached to a solid phase (e.g. plastic tubes coated with antibody to human spleen ferritin). A diluted test sample, or ferritin standard, is added, and ferritin is bound to the solid phase antibody in an amount which is proportional to its concentration in the serum. After washing, the bound ferritin is detected by incubation with excess ^{125}I-labelled antibody to ferritin. A second wash then removes any excess ^{125}I-labelled antibody and the solid phase is counted in a gamma

*Iron content should be less than 0.00002%.

counter. The amount of radioactivity is directly proportional to the amount of ferritin present in the test samples. It is essential to assay at two dilutions because of the high-dose hook effect, whereby it is possible to obtain false normal values using sera containing very high ferritin concentrations. In addition, the pH and protein concentration of the diluted samples has to be carefully controlled since these factors influence the binding of the ferritin to the solid phase antibody.

Enzyme-linked assays. In these two-site labelled antibody assays the ferritin in test samples (or known standards) is first attached, as above, to unlabelled antiferritin antibodies coating a solid phase. However, detection of the bound ferritin utilises an antiferritin antibody labelled with an enzyme, e.g. horse radish peroxidase or alkaline phosphatase, rather than [125]I. After washing away unbound labelled antibody, the enzyme activity remaining is detected by reacting with suitable substrate to yield a coloured product which can be measured spectrophotometrically. The optical density is then proportional to the amount of ferritin bound by the solid phase antibody. A sensitive enzyme-linked assay using microtitre plates as the solid phase and a monoclonal antibody to human liver ferritin has been described by Flowers et al 1986.

Competitive radioimmunoassay (RIA)
In an RIA there is competition for the binding sites on limited amounts of an antiferritin antibody between ferritin in the test sample or standard and added ^{125}I-labelled ferritin. The amount of ^{125}I-labelled ferritin which is bound is inversely related to the concentration of ferritin in the unknown sample. The antibody-bound ferritin is precipitated by a second antibody directed against immunoglobulin, separated from any unbound ferritin by centrifugation, and counted in a gamma counter. A standard curve is constructed from the counts derived from standards containing known concentrations of ferritin, and used to determine the ferritin concentrations of the unknown samples. Most commercial kit assays use the RIA principle.

Biochemical basis
Ferritin (M.Wt. 450 000) is found in all body cells and consists of a spherical protein shell (within which ferric iron is stored) made up from 24 subunits. There are at least two types of subunit, H (M.Wt. 22 000) and L (M.Wt. 19 000). Varying admixtures of these subunits account for the wide range of ferritins of different iso-electric points (isoferritins) found in different tissues e.g. liver and spleen ferritin is more basic, and richer in L subunits than acidic, H-rich, heart ferritin. Plasma ferritin consists almost entirely of L subunits, though it is heterogeneous on isolectric focusing due to varying degrees of glycosylation of the protein. As a result,

although antibodies raised against different ferritin preparations are likely to have variable specificities to different isoferritins, this is unlikely to affect the immunoassay of plasma ferritin in which only the antibodies to L-rich basic ferritins will contribute.

Test samples

Either heparinised plasma or serum are suitable. Storage is satisfactory at 4°C for up to one week but thereafter should be at −20°C. Repeated freezing and thawing prior to assay should be avoided. If samples are to be sent through the post, 10 μl of 2% sodium azide can be added as a preservative to each ml of serum or plasma. Most assays require 50–200 μl of serum.

Reagents and equipment

Preparation of reagents requires complex techniques. These include:

1. The isolation and purification of human spleen (or liver) ferritin. This involves homogenisation of the tissue, precipitation of other proteins by limited exposure to heat, ammonium sulphate precipitation of ferritin, partial purification of the redissolved ferritin by ultracentrifugation (100 000 g for 2 hours), and gel filtration on Sepharose 6B. Purity is then examined by polyacrylamide gel electrophoresis and the protein concentration determined by the method of Lowry.

2. The preparation of antibodies to human ferritin. Polyclonal antibodies are raised in rabbits (sheep or goats are also suitable) and extracted from the antiserum by immunoabsorption (using horse spleen ferritin bound either to aminocellulose or cyanogen bromide activated Sepharose 6B).

3. Iodination with ^{125}I, either of the antiferritin antibodies (IRMA), or of the purified human ferritin (RIA).

Preparation of these reagents (detailed by Worwood 1980) is beyond the scope of most routine laboratories. As a result many will use one of the commercial kits available for ferritin assay. These have the disadvantage of being expensive, and the consequent need to batch test means that where limited numbers of tests are required there may be considerable delay in assaying samples. The equipment required includes:

○ Precision micropipettes.
○ Plastic assay tubes.
○ Water-bath for incubation.
○ Centrifuge.
○ Gamma counter.

Standards and controls

A control pool of serum, collected from about 12 normal subjects (discard any haemolysed serum) should be stored in aliquots of 0.5 ml for up to 2 years at −20°C.

Commercial kits provide their own range of ferritin standard solutions. A reference, lyophilised preparation of human ferritin is now available (ICSH 1984). This is intended for calibration of local preparations of human ferritin for use as secondary standards.

Methods

Most commercial kits (e.g. Ferritin RIA Kit, Amersham) provide simple methods which can be completed within a single working day. Test samples and the control serum should be assayed in duplicate. Dilution is necessary for sera containing high concentrations of ferritin. Detailed descriptions of suitable IRMA and RIA procedures are given in the comprehensive review by Worwood 1980.

Comment

— Comparisons of commercial kits have shown considerable variation in results between the kits (e.g. Grail et al 1982). However, results were internally consistent and provided a reliable guide to iron stores. Variation between assays is likely to be reduced with the use of a reference standard for human ferritin.

Interpretation

Normal range. Normal concentrations of serum ferritin fall within the range 15–300 μg/litre, but are dependent on age and sex. Values are relatively high at birth (mean 125 μg/litre), increase to a peak of around 250 μg/litre by one month (as haemoglobin iron moves to iron stores), and thereafter decrease to a mean of around 20–30 μg/litre during infancy, childhood and adolescence. In men, values then increase throughout life to a mean of around 100 μg/litre (range 30–300 μg/litre) after the age of 30 years. In women values remain around 30 μg/litre (range 15–200 μg/litre) until after the menopause, when concentrations begin to increase and eventually approach those of men of the same age. In pregnancy, in the absence of iron supplements, serum ferritin concentrations decline until around 32 weeks before levelling off, usually at concentrations indicating very low or absent iron stores.

Factors influencing the serum ferritin concentration are shown in Table 4.2.

Serum ferritin concentrations <15 μg/litre invariably indicate storage iron depletion. However, where iron deficiency coexists with diseases such as rheumatoid arthritis, inflammatory bowel disease or renal failure, serum ferritin concentrations of up to 50 or even 100 μg/litre may still indicate exhausted iron stores. This is because the serum ferritin behaves as an acute phase protein and is disproportionately raised in patients with inflammatory or infective disorders. These disorders are frequently associated with a secondary anaemia in which a further increase in serum ferritin may be expected as iron is shifted from circulating

Table 4.2 Interpretation of serum ferritin.

Increase	Decrease
1. *Increased body iron stores* Primary (idiopathic) haemochromatosis Secondary iron overload (e.g. transfusion-dependent anaemias)	*Reduced body iron stores* Iron deficiency Pregnancy
2. *Increased ferritin protein synthesis* Inflammation/infection Malignant disease (e.g. AML, hepatoma, carcinoma of pancreas) Hyperthyroidism	*Decreased ferritin protein synthesis (rare)* Vitamin C deficiency
3. *Release of tissue ferritins* Hepatic necrosis Chronic liver disease Spleen or bone marrow infarction (e.g. sickle cell disease) Malignant disease	

haemoglobin to iron stores. As a result of these changes, the finding of a normal or increased serum ferritin concentration can help to distinguish an anaemia of chronic disorders from true iron deficiency anaemia, both disorders in which there is evidence of a reduced iron supply to the marrow (low saturation of the TIBC and development of microcytic red cells).

In contrast to the unequivocal evidence of storage iron depletion provided by a low serum ferritin, elevated concentrations are most commonly due to causes other than increased iron stores (Table 4.2). Very high concentrations may be seen with cell necrosis affecting ferritin-rich tissues. When the liver is affected increased serum enzyme concentrations may give a clue to the source of the ferritin. Increased ferritin-protein synthesis is seen with inflammatory disease (see above) and possibly with various malignancies. However, the suggestion that there may be specific 'tumour ferritins' released into the serum remains unproven, and in most cases raised levels of serum ferritin in cancer are likely to be due to redistribution of iron to stores in anaemic patients and to cellular damage e.g. by metastatic disease. Serum ferritin concentrations are usually greater than 1000 μg/litre in symptomatic idiopathic haemochromatosis. In transfusional iron overload ferritin concentrations may reach up to 20 000 μg/litre, but values greater than 4000 μg/litre often reflect liver damage as well as increased liver iron stores. In screening for iron overload a serum ferritin assay must be combined with measurement of the transferrin saturation (see p. 84). Although a normal serum ferritin provides good evidence against the presence of iron overload, there have been occasional patients (e.g. with β thalassaemia intermedia) who have values lower than

expected from the liver iron content, possibly as a result of accompanying ascorbate deficiency.

Sequential measurements of serum ferritin are useful in monitoring long-term iron balance in patients at risk of iron deficiency (e.g. those receiving chronic haemodialysis for renal failure) and in those being treated with phlebotomy or iron chelation for iron overload. There is a considerable day-to-day variation in serum ferritin concentration even in normal individuals (coefficient of variation of repeated samples is approximately 20%), and this may be even greater in iron-loaded subjects: attention should, therefore, be focused on long-term trends in serum ferritin values rather than transient fluctuations.

URINE FERRIOXAMINE IRON

Measurement of urine iron after a test dose of the iron chelating agent desferrioxamine is occasionally used as a screening test for parenchymal iron overload. In addition, the response to different doses given as s.c. infusions can be used to plan the optimum long-term treatment for patients with iron-loading anaemias, such as the thalassaemia disorders.

Principle
The method is based on, and uses the same reagents and equipment as the serum iron method (p. 84). The ferrioxamine iron is reduced by a mixed acid reagent before colour development with buffered bathophenanthroline sulphonate. The absorbance at 535 nm is read against a standard iron solution with correction for reagent and urine 'blanks'.

Test samples
24-hour urine collections are made in acid-washed, iron-free plastic containers. Record the total volume and retain a sample for assay (store at −20°C if this is to be delayed more than a few days).

The test dose of desferrioxamine may be a single i.m. injection of 500 mg in 2 ml water for injection, followed by a single 24-hour urine collection. However, for assessment of a dose-response curve, s.c. infusions of approximately 25, 50, 75 and 100 mg/kg body weight may be given over a period of 12 hours using a small infusion pump (use multiples of 500 mg desferrioxamine — the amount in a single vial). 24-hour urine collections should then begin with the start of each infusion: urine ferrioxamine iron excretion is largely complete by the end of 24 hours, but if time permits the most accurate estimates of iron excretion are obtained by continuing the urine collection for a second 24 hours after each dose.

Equipment.
As for serum iron assay (p. 84).

Reagents
- *Mixed acid reagent.* 1 mol HCl, 0.6 mol trichloracetic acid and 0.4 mol thioglycollic acid per litre. See p. 84.
- *Chromagen solution.* 1.5 mol sodium acetate and 0.5 mmol bathophenanthroline sulphonate per litre. See p. 84.
- *'Blank chromagen' solution.* 1.5 mol sodium acetate/litre: as above but with omission of bathophenanthroline sulphonate.

Standard
Working iron standard (40 μmol iron/litre in 5 mmol HCl/litre). Take 2.0 ml stock iron standard (p. 85), add 400 ml iron-free water, and make to 1 litre with 5 mmol HCl/litre.

Method
1. Set up 3 test tubes for each sample.
2. Disperse any urine sediment by vortex mixing and pipette 2.0 ml into the first tube.
3. Add 2.0 ml mixed acid reagent, mix and stand for 15 minutes.
4. Centifuge at 3000 g for 10 minutes to remove any sediment or protein precipitant.
5. Place 2 separate 1.0 ml aliquots of the supernatant in each of the remaining 2 test tubes.
6. To one add 1.0 ml chromagen solution (urine test) and to the other 1.0 ml 'blank chromagen' solution (urine blank). Mix and stand for at least 30 minutes.
7. An iron standard and reagent blank are prepared by taking 1.0 ml working iron standard solution or 1.0 ml iron-free water respectively, and adding 1.0 ml mixed acid reagent followed by 2.0 ml chromagen solution to each tube. Mix well.
8. Measure absorbances in a spectrophotometer against distilled water at 535 nm.

Calculation
Total urine iron (μmol)

$$= \frac{A_T - (A_{UB} + A_{RB})}{A_S - A_{RB}} \times 40 \times V$$

A_T = Absorbance of urine test
A_{UB} = Absorbance of urine blank
A_{RB} = Absorbance of reagent blank
A_S = Absorbance of standard (40 μmol iron/litre)
V = 24 h urine volume in litres.

Comments
— Where urine iron concentration exceeds 180 μmol (10 mg)/litre, suitable dilution of the urine should be made in iron-free water before the test.
— Up to 25 g desferrioxamine/litre in the urine has no effect on the iron estimation provided the waiting period for colour development in step 6 is not reduced.
— Absorbance of the reagent blank should not exceed 0.015 in a 1 cm pathway against water.
— The method will underestimate any spontaneous excretion of haemosiderin iron in the urine, though this is usually less than 18 μmol (1.0 mg) even in heavily iron-loaded thalassaemic patients. This consideration is therefore unimportant in assessing the reponse to desferrioxamine.

Interpretation
In subjects with normal iron stores, 24-hour urine iron excretion after a single test dose of 500 mg desferrioxamine is less than 20 μmol (1.1 mg), whereas in subjects with symptomatic haemochromatosis it usually exceeds 80 μmol (4.5 mg). However, values are influenced by factors besides iron load and are lower in the presence of ascorbate deficiency or immediately after a blood transfusion. A dose-response curve designed to aid planning of long-term iron chelation therapy should therefore be obtained after ascorbate repletion and at a fixed point in the blood transfusion cycle in transfusion-dependent subjects. The optimum dose is usually taken as that at which greatest iron excretion is obtained before the response curve begins to flatten significantly.

LIVER IRON CONCENTRATION

This provides the most definitive guide to the extent of iron overload. When combined with histological assessment of the liver biopsy it also provides information about possible tissue toxicity (e.g. fibrosis).

Principle
The liver biopsy is dried to constant weight and completely digested in acid. The iron content of the resulting solution is determined by colour development using buffered bathophenanthroline sulphonate and absorbance readings at 535 nm against a known iron standard.

Test sample
Rinse approximately 1 cm of a percutaneous liver biopsy specimen with saline and dry to constant weight in an oven at 120°C. Small samples of wedge liver biopsies can be processed in the same way.

Equipment

○ Digestion mantle.
○ 30 ml Kjeldahl flasks.
○ 13 × 100 mm screw capped plastic test tubes.

All glass ware must be rendered iron-free as described under serum iron method (p. 84).

Reagents

All chemicals should be of the lowest possible iron content.

- *Acid mixture.* Equal volumes of concentrated sulphuric (98%) and nitric (70%) acids.
- *Hydrogen peroxide*, analar, 30% solution.
- *Sodium acetate buffer.* Dissolve 3.3 mol (450 g) sodium acetate trihydrate (iron content <0.00002%) in 1000 ml iron-free water. Adjust pH to 4.75 with glacial acetic acid.
- *Chromagen solution.* Dissolve 0.4 mmol (0.214 g) bathophenanthroline sulphonate in 50 ml iron-free water in a 100 ml volumetric flask. Add 14 mmol (1 ml) thioglycollic acid (97% purity) and make to volume with iron-free water. The solution is stable in a dark brown bottle for up to 14 days.

Standard

Working iron standard (40 μmol iron/litre in 5 mmol HCl/litre). Take 2.0 ml stock iron standard (p. 87), add 400 ml iron-free water, and make to 1 litre with 5 mmol HCl/litre.

Method

1. Place the weighed dry liver biopsy in a 30 ml Kjeldahl flask and add 0.15 ml acid mixture.
2. Heat gently on digestion mantle until a pale yellow oily residue is obtained (after approximately 15 mins). Cool.
3. Add 0.15 ml hydrogen peroxide and heat for a further few minutes until the solution is water clear. Cool.
4. Pipette 15 ml iron-free water into the flask, seal with Parafilm, and mix.
5. A blank digest (no biopsy sample) should be treated in the same manner.
6. Prepare 4 test tubes each containing 1.0 ml sodium acetate buffer.

7. To these add 5.0 ml water (reagent blank) or 5 ml standard containing 0.04 μmol iron (1 ml working iron standard plus 4.0 ml iron-free water) or 5 ml sample digest, or 5 ml blank digest.

8. Add 0.2 ml chromagen solution to each tube, mix and stand at least 30 minutes.

9. Measure absorbance in a spectrophotometer at 535 nm against water. If the absorbance is greater than 0.5 with the sample digest, a smaller volume of the latter should be used in step 7, making up to 5.0 ml with iron-free water before repeating the colour development.

Calculation

Iron content (μmol/g dry liver)

$$= \frac{A_D - A_B}{A_S - A_{RB}} \times 0.04 \times \frac{15}{V} \div W$$

A_D = absorbance of sample digest
A_B = absorbance of blank digest
A_S = absorbance of 0.04 μmol iron standard
A_{RB} = absorbance of reagent blank
15 = final volume (ml) of sample digest
V = volume of sample digest which was colour-developed
W = dry weight (g) of liver sample.

Comments

— This assay measures total iron content, including any haem iron. However, in iron overload conditions the latter is insignificant compared with the much larger iron stores, and the method gives an accurate assessment of iron overload.

— Dry liver iron concentration is about 4 times that of wet liver.

Interpretation

Normal range. 6–24 μmol iron/g dry liver (0.03–0.13% of the dry weight). Symptomatic haemochromatosis is usually accompanied by liver iron concentrations >1.0% of the dry weight. Total liver iron burden also depends on the liver size, which may be increased in, for example, the thalassaemia disorders.

REFERENCES

Barry M, Sherlock S 1971 Measurement of liver-iron concentration in needle-biopsy specimens. Lancet 1: 100–103

Cazzola M, Arosio P, Barosi G, Bergamaschi E, Dezza L, Ascari E 1983 Ferritin in the red cells of normal subjects and patients with iron deficiency and iron overload. British Journal of Haematology 53: 659–665

Finch C A, Bellotti V, Stray S et al 1986 Plasma ferritin determination as a diagnostic tool. Western Journal of Medicine 145: 657–663

Flowers C A, Kuizon M, Beard J L, Skikne B S, Covell A M, Cook J D 1986 A serum ferritin assay for prevalence studies of iron deficiency. American Journal of Haematology 23: 141–151

Grail A, Hancock B W, Harrison P M 1982 Serum ferritin in normal individuals and in patients with malignant lymphoma and chronic renal failure measured with seven different commercial immunoassay techniques. Journal of Clinical Pathology 35: 1204–1212

International Committee for Standardization in Haematology 1978 The measurement of total and unsaturated iron-binding capacity in serum. British Journal of Haematology 38: 281–90

International Committee for Standardization in Haematology 1978 Recommendations for measurement of serum iron in human blood. British Journal of Haematology 38: 291–4

International Committee for Standardization in Haematology (Expert Panel on Iron) 1984 Preparation, characterization and storage of human ferritin for use as a standard for the assay of serum ferritin. Clinical and Laboratory Haematology 6: 177–191

Koerper M A, Dallman P R 1977 Serum iron concentration and transferrin saturation in the diagnosis of iron deficiency in children: normal developmental changes. Journal of Pediatrics 91: 870–874

Labbe R F, Finch C A 1980 Erythrocyte protoporphyrin: application in the diagnosis of iron deficiency. In: Cook J D (ed) Methods in Hematology 1 (Iron). Churchill Livingstone, Edinburgh, p 44–58

Pippard M J 1983 Iron loading and chelation therapy. In: Weatherall D J (ed) Methods in Hematology 6 (The Thalassemias). Churchill Livingstone, Edinburgh, p 103–113

Worwood M 1980 Serum ferritin. In: Cook J D (ed) Methods in Hematology 1 (Iron). Churchill Livingstone, Edinburgh, p 59–89

5

Haemolytic anaemia

Haemolytic anaemia may be suspected in an anaemic, slightly icteric patient, but firm diagnosis can only be made in the laboratory. The findings arise from increased red cell destruction, from increased red cell regeneration and from evidence of an immunological mechanism.

A blood count shows anaemia, often with a raised MCV. In acute haemolysis the white cell count is raised. There is almost invariably a marked increase in reticulocytes unless there is an accompanying arrest of haemopoiesis, usually due to a parvovirus infection or accompanying severe folic-acid deficiency. The plasma is yellow. Anaemia and reticulocytosis can be due to gastrointestinal haemorrhage, but in such cases jaundice is unusual unless there is liver disease.

The stained peripheral blood film is usually very helpful, showing either spherocytes (common both to hereditary spherocytosis and to auto-immune haemolytic anaemia), or agglutination usually by cold antibodies. More bizarre red cell morphology is seen in some severe enzyme deficiencies or in sickle cell anaemia, but in other cases of non-spherocytic haemolytic anaemias polychromasia may be the only abnormal finding. White cells may be increased and atypical lymphocytes may be seen in infectious mononucleosis, and increase in lymphocytes is present in chronic lymphatic leukaemia.

Haemolysis may be confirmed by absence of haptoglobins as well as by carrying out a red cell survival study. Suspicion of spherocytes can be explored by osmotic fragility and auto-haemolysis tests.

An important subdivision is in the presence or absence of antibody on the red cell surface and in plasma. When spherocytosis is absent, the direct antiglobulin test is negative and there are no cold agglutinins, the disorders constituting non-spherocytic haemolytic anaemia are considered, including paroxysmal nocturnal haemoglobinuria (acid-lysis or Ham's test, sucrose-lysis and acetylcholinesterase estimation), and enzyme deficiencies including glucose-6-phosphate dehydrogenase deficiency and pyruvate kinase deficiency and, rarely,

other deficiencies. In inherited red cell abnormalities the red cell membrane structure can be looked at.

The second major group is auto-immune haemolytic anaemia due to an antibody on the red cell surface or to high thermal amplitude cold agglutinins — almost invariably IgM, rarely anti-i. This is dealt with on page 428.

SERUM HAPTOGLOBIN (Hp)

Haptoglobins are a group of genetically inherited α_2 globulins, synthesised in the liver, whose function is specifically to bind free haemoglobin in the plasma. The molecular weight of the Hp/Hb complex is such that it will not pass through the renal tubules, and the haemoglobin-haptoglobin complex is carried to the reticulo-endothelial system for degradation. The release of free haemoglobin to plasma as occurs in a haemolytic anaemia results in rapid saturation of the haptoglobin system and the disappearance of free haptoglobin since the restoration of plasma levels of haptoglobin is relatively slow. It is thus a useful test when the presence of minor degrees of haemolysis is suspected.

Principle

A known amount of haemoglobin, in the form of a haemolysate, is added to the unknown serum to be tested. The haemoglobin-haptoglobin complex is electrophoresed, and after separation of the complex from free haemoglobin has been achieved, the fractions are eluted off the cellulose acetate and the concentration determined using a spectrophotometer. Alternatively the strips can be scanned by densitometry. The haemoglobin-haptoglobin complex migrates with the α_2 globulin complex whereas free haemoglobin migrates in the β globulin position. Haptoglobins can be presumed to be absent when no band is present in the α_2 position.

Test samples

Allow whole blood to clot in glass and, after centrifuging the sample, remove the serum with a Pasteur pipette ensuring that no red cells are included. Store at −20°C until required for assay.

Controls
An aqueous solution of haemolysate (see below) is run in parallel as a reference sample.

Reagents
- *0.012 M Tris buffer, pH 8.9.* Dissolve 14.5 g Tris (hydroxymethyl)-methylamine, 1.5 g EDTA (free acid) and 0.9 g boric acid in 900 ml deionised distilled water. Adjust pH accordingly and make up to 1 litre.
- *Haemolysate.* Prepare as for haemoglobin electrophoresis (p. 33) and adjust to concentration of approximately 4.0 g/dl.

Method
1. Add 1 volume of haemolysate to 1 volume of serum and mix (giving final Hb concentration 20 mg/ml).
2. Allow to stand for 20 minutes.
3. Soak cellulose acetate strips in buffer, remove and blot dry.
4. Place the strips in the electrophoresis tank and apply 20 μl of the serum/lysate across the centre of the strip ensuring that the line is straight, even and does not come too near the edge of the paper.
5. Set at constant voltage of 200 volts and switch on power.
6. Allow to run for up to 2 hours or until good separation of the bands occurs.
7. Switch off power and remove strips.
8. Cut strips into the segments containing the free haemoglobin and the haptoglobin-haemoglobin complex.
9. Place the segments into tubes and add 3.0 ml of deionised distilled water to each.
10. Allow the haemoglobin to elute off the segments and then read the optical density at 412 nm.

Calculation

$$\text{Haptoglobin g/l} = \frac{\text{OD Hp/Hb Complex} \times 100}{\text{OD free Hb} + \text{OD Hp/Hb Complex}} \times \text{Hb in lysate g/l}$$

Normal range
Results are expressed as haemoglobin binding capacity in mg/dl or g/l of serum. Haptoglobin = 30 − 250 mg/dl (0.30 − 2.5 g/l).

Comment
— In most routine laboratories the demand for haptoglobin determination is low, and if large numbers of tests are to be run it is advisable to use a commercial radioimmunodiffusion test. In addition, this technique may be used as a screening method by which the electrophoretic strip can be stained with Ponceau S (0.2% in 3% trichloracetic acid) for the presence of the haemoglobin-haptoglobin complex without the need for actual measurement.

Interpretation
The haemoglobin-haptoglobin complex is cleared from the plasma at a rate of 15 mg/100 ml/hour. Thus minimal amounts of haemolysis will cause the complete disappearance of haptoglobin from the circulation. The practical usefulness of the test is also limited by the fact that there is a wide normal range and some individuals have genetically inherited low levels. Ideally the patient's pre-haemolysis levels should be known for exact interpretation of results but this is rarely possible. In addition haptoglobin levels are modified by other conditions such as infection, malignancy and liver disease.

OSMOTIC FRAGILITY

This test may be required to confirm a suspicion of spherocytosis in a blood film. Red cells that are spherocytic take up less water in hypotonic solution before rupturing than normal red cells. This difference is used as a test of red cell shape.

Principle
The osmotic fragility of freshly taken erythrocytes reflects their ability to absorb water without rupturing and producing lysis. This feature is determined by the volume to surface area ratio of the cells, and with normal biconcave cells the volume may increase by up to 70% before lysis may occur.

Test samples
Venous or capillary blood collected into lithium heparin. Alternatively defibrinated blood may be used. To defibrinate blood quickly and easily a few paper clips are placed in a plain glass universal container, venous blood added and the bottle gently rotated until, after about 5 minutes, a complete fibrin clot has formed on the paper clips which can then be easily removed. The osmotic fragility test should preferably be carried out within 2 hours of blood collection.

Standards and controls
No standards as such are available. A sample from a

Table 5.1 Preparation of NaCl dilutions for red cell osmotic fragility.

NaCl %	0.10	0.20	0.30	0.35	0.40	0.45	0.50	0.55	0.60	0.65	0.70	0.75	0.80	0.90
Working NaCl solution ml	5.0	10.0	15.0	17.5	20.0	22.5	25.0	27.5	30.0	32.5	35.0	37.5	40.0	45.0
Distilled water ml	45.0	40.0	35.0	32.5	30.0	27.5	25.0	22.5	20.0	17.5	15.0	12.5	10.0	5.0

known normal individual is collected at the same time as the test sample and run in parallel as a control.

Reagents

Stock solution

1.71 M Buffered sodium chloride (AR) pH 7.4. This is known as the 10% stock solution and contains the equivalent of 100 g/l sodium chloride.

Dissolve NaCl 90 g; Na_2HO_4, 13.65 g and $Na_2H_2PO_42H_2O$, 2.34 g in approximately 500 ml of distilled water. Adjust the final volume to 1 litre. As the accuracy of the test depends crucially on having correct solutions of NaCl, some prefer to buy in this stock solution (BDH).

Working solution

Dilute the stock solution 1:10 with distilled water and use this to make a series of hypotonic solutions ranging in concentration from 1.0 g/litre (0.1%) to 9.0 g/litre (0.9%) sodium chloride as in Table 5.1

Method

1. Allow working hypotonic solutions to reach room temperature and dispense 5.0 ml volumes into suitable stoppered tubes.

2. Add 0.05 ml of well-mixed whole blood to each tube and mix gently by inversion.

3. Leave at room temperature for 30 minutes.

4. Remix by inversion and centrifuge at 1200 g for 10 minutes.

5. Read optical density of supernatants at 540 nm using that of the 9.0 g/l NaCl as a blank, and that of the 1.0 g/l as a 100% lysis control.

6. Calculate the percentage haemolysis at each concentration of NaCl as follows:-

$$\% \text{ haemolysis} = \frac{\text{OD Test}}{\text{OD } 0.10\% \text{ Solution}} \times 100$$

7. Plot a graph of % haemolysis against concentration of NaCl (Fig. 5.1).

Units

The result of the osmotic fragility may be expressed as the concentration of NaCl causing 50% haemolysis — i.e. the median corpuscular fragility (MCF).

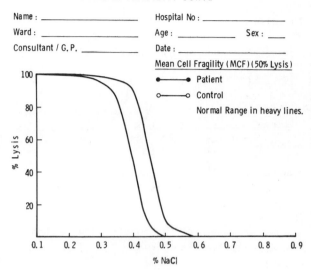

Fig. 5.1 Osmotic fragility graph.

Normal range of MCF at pH 7.4 and 20°C is 4.0–4.45 g/l. NaCl in fresh samples.

INCUBATED OSMOTIC FRAGILITY

Principle

When blood is incubated at 37°C the red cells continue to metabolise glucose for energy to maintain their normal shape and size. When cells are defective and have increased energy requirements this period of incubation will stress the abnormal cells more than those of the control and result in increased susceptibility to osmotic lysis.

Test sample

Duplicate samples of the freshly drawn whole blood are dispensed aseptically into sterile screw capped bottles and placed in an incubator at 37°C. After 24 hours, inspect the samples and if no infection is evident, mix, and pool them. Estimate the fragility of the blood as stated above.

Standards/controls

As for immediate osmotic fragility, and treated as for test sample.

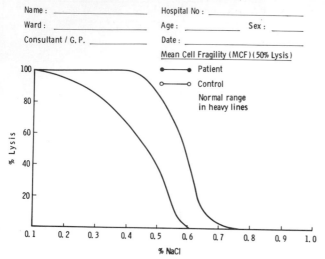

Fig. 5.2 Incubated osmotic fragility graph.

Reagents

As for immediate osmotic fragility, but include a 10.0 g/l NaCl to act as a blank.

Method

As for immediate osmotic fragility. Plot graph as in Figure 5.2.

Units

As for immediate osmotic fragility.

Normal range

MCF = 4.65 − 5.9 g/l NaCl after incubation at 37°C for 24 hours.

Comment

— The stock NaCl solution will keep for many months at 4°C in a well-stoppered bottle. The working NaCl solution will keep for some weeks at 4°C but if it appears cloudy it should be discarded.
— Pre-weighed vials of buffered sodium chloride, giving a solution osmotically equivalent to 10% w/v NaCl, are available commercially.
— The main problem with the incubation of blood at 37°C for 24 hours is the possibility of bacterial contamination; this is not always easy to detect but infected blood often has an offensive odour.

Interpretation

The osmotic fragility curve may be shifted either to the left or the right, and the MCF be above or below the normal range but these alterations are not diagnostic of any specific condition and merely reflect the ability of certain types of cells to resist osmotic lysis. For example reticulocytes are more resistant to lysis than normal cells, whereas in conditions where spherocytes are present in the blood the curve may show a right shift and elevated MCF. The test is mostly used to help in the diagnosis of hereditary spherocytosis, when the curve usually shows a right shift which is further exacerbated after incubation of the blood at 37°C for 24 hours. However, in mild cases the shift in the curve may be slight and other tests required to help in the diagnosis.

AUTOHAEMOLYSIS TEST

When fresh normal blood is incubated at 37°C for 24 hours little or no lysis takes place, and after 48 hours incubation the amount of lysis present is still small. If excess sterile glucose is added to the blood before incubation the amount of lysis present after 48 hours is markedly reduced.

The metabolic activity of the red cell and the cellular membrane play an important role in determining the amount of lysis which may occur after 48 hours incubation with or without the presence of excess added glucose.

Test samples

Venous blood collected with sterile precautions into lithium heparin or defibrinated as described on page 94 is used and the test should be set up within a few hours of collection of the blood.

Controls

No standards as such are available, so a sample collected from a known normal individual at the same time as the test sample is run in parallel as a control.

Reagents

• 10% Sterile glucose solution (100 mg/ml), made up in sterile distilled water.
• 0.04% Aqueous ammonia solution.

Method

1. Dispense four 1 ml or 2 ml aliquots of whole blood into separate sterile screw-capped bottles.
2. Keep at least 1 ml of whole blood to use as a 100% lysis control and store at 4°C.
3. Spin down remainder and keep plasma/serum to use as a blank. Store at 4°C.
4. To two of the original four bottles add aseptically 100 μl of the sterile glucose solution.
5. Place the series of bottles in a 37°C incubator.
6. After 24 hours gently mix the contents of the bottles by inverting at least ten times.

7. After 48 hours incubation, inspect the bottles for infection★. If none is evident, pool the contents of each pair of bottles.

8. Estimate the haematocrit of each and record.

9. Centrifuge the remainder to obtain the supernatant plasma/serum.

10. Dilute the pre- and post-incubation serum 1:10 with 0.04% ammonia solution.

11. Read the optical density at 540 nm of the post-incubation plasma/serum using the diluted pre-incubation plasma/serum as a blank.

12. Dilute the whole blood kept at the beginning 1:200 with 0.04% ammonia solution and use as the 100% lysis control.

★See incubated osmotic fragility (p. 95).

Calculation

Using the following formula, calculate the amount of lysis which has occurred.

$$\frac{R_T}{R_O} \times \frac{D_O}{D_T} \times (1\text{-Hct}_T) \times 100$$

Where R_T = OD diluted serum/plasma at 48 hours
R_O = OD diluted whole blood
D_T = dilution of serum (i.e. 1/10)
D_O = dilution of whole blood (i.e. 1/200)
Hct_T = haematocrit at 48 hours.

Units

Expressed as a percentage

Normal range

Lysis after 48 hours incubation at 37°C:-
Without added glucose = 1.75 ± 0.75%
With added glucose = 0.5 ± 0.25%

Comment

— It has been suggested that it would be more accurate when small amounts of haemoglobin have been released, to measure the lysis by a chemical method in preference to the photometric method described. However, this would be much more time consuming and possibly to no advantage.

— It is important to perform this test under strictly aseptic conditions as bacterial contamination will produce excess lysis.

Interpretation

Many laboratories consider that the autohaemolysis test has outlived its usefulness. It is not diagnostic of any specific disease and abnormal results are given in a variety of conditions. In the investigation of congenital haemolytic anaemias all that can be inferred is that, when excess lysis is present, which can be corrected by glucose, the cell 'probably' has a normal glycolytic pathway and that a biochemical defect is present elsewhere.

ACIDIFIED GLYCEROL LYSIS TEST (AGLT)

The lipid composition of the cell membrane is a major determinant of its permeability to glycerol and hence the rate at which cells lyse when exposed to glycerol.

Principle

The rate of entry of the water molecule into the red cell is slowed down by the presence of added glycerol. This allows the time taken for lysis to occur to be measured. As with the osmotic fragility test, the same principles apply in that spherocytes which have a raised volume to surface area are unable to resist swelling and consequently lyse in a shorter time.

Test samples

Venous or capillary blood collected into EDTA. Blood up to 24 hours old gives satisfactory results.

Controls

No standards as such are available, so a sample collected from a normal individual at the same time as the test sample is run in parallel as a control.

Reagents

● *0.1 M Phosphate buffer*
  a. Weigh out 7.45 g of Na_2HPO_4 dissolve in approximately 300 ml of distilled water in a volumetric flask and adjust final volume to 500 ml.
  b. Weigh out 6.8 g of KH_2PO_4, dissolve in approximately 300 ml of distilled water in a volumetric flask and adjust final volume to 500 ml.
  Add 2 volumes of solution (a) to 1 volume of solution (b).

● *0.154 M Sodium chloride*
  Weigh out 9.0 g of NaCl and dissolve in 1 litre of distilled water.

● *Isotonic phosphate buffered saline (PBS)*
  Add 9 volumes of the 0.154 M NaCl solution to 1 volume of the 0.1 M phosphate buffer. Adjust pH accurately to 6.85 ± 0.05.

● *0.3 M Glycerol (AR)*
  Add 23 ml (27.65 g) of glycerol to 300 ml of PBS and adjust to 1 litre with distilled water.

Method

1. Dispense 5.0 ml of PBS into a test tube.

2. Add 20 μl of anticoagulated whole blood and mix gently.

3. Transfer 1 ml of this suspension to a cuvette with a 1.0 cm light path and place in the well of a recording spectrophotometer, set at wavelength 625 nm. Start the recorder.

4. Add 2.0 ml of the glycerol reagent rapidly from a syringe pipette and mix well. At the same moment as the glycerol reagent is added start a stop watch.

5. Measure the time taken for the optical density to fall to half the value of that before the addition of the glycerol reagent. Stop the stop watch at this point.

Units

The results are expressed as the time taken for the optical density to fall to half of its original value ($AGLT_{50}$).

Normal value

Normal > 1500 seconds (Patients with HS = 50 ± 15.0 s).

Comment

— The AGLT requires less blood than the osmotic fragility test and can be performed more rapidly. However, the pH and volumes of red cell suspensions and glycerol are critical. Depending on the type of pipette used it is important to ensure that no red cells remain adherent to the sides when delivering blood into the PBS.

Interpretation

This test is mainly used as an aid to the diagnosis of hereditary spherocytosis and has a higher detection rate in symptomless relatives of known affected individuals than the conventional osmotic fragility curve. However, as with the latter, positive results occur in other causes of spherocytosis, such as auto-immune haemolytic anaemia. It is particularly useful as a screening test in large family studies and population surveys.

DEMONSTRATION OF RED CELL MEMBRANE PROTEINS BY SODIUM DODECYL SULPHATE POLYACRYLAMIDE GEL ELECTROPHORESIS (SDS-PAGE)

Principle

Abnormally-shaped red cells in patients with haemolytic anaemia can be the result of deficient amounts or total absence of certain red cell membrane proteins. The SDS-PAGE technique separates proteins on the basis of molecular weight and allows visual analysis of stained protein bands. This test should be used for analysing red cells from patients in whom red cell defects are suspected, generally in hereditary spherocytosis, ellipto-

cytosis and pyropoikilocytosis. Before performing this test, other possible sources for the anaemia (nutritional deficiencies, haemoglobinopathies, enzyme deficiencies) should be eliminated.

Reagents

Sample preparation reagents

- N-saline
- Lysing buffer (5 mM $NaPO_4$, pH 7.6, 1 mM EDTA, 1 mM phenylmethylsulphonyl fluoride (PMSF)).
- Solubilising buffer
  Mix as follows:

0.5 M Tris-Cl, pH 6.8	1.2 ml
10% SDS	1.2 ml
Glycerol	1.2 ml
Dithiothreitol	231 mg

  Store frozen in 0.5 ml aliquots

Gel-forming reagents

- 1.5 M Tris-Cl, pH 8.8
- 0.5 M Tris-Cl, pH 6.8
- Acrylamide stock solution containing 30 g acrylamide, 0.8 g bis-acrylamide per 100 ml. Filter through Whatman No. 1 filter paper and store at 4°C in a dark bottle.
- 10% SDS
- 10% ammonium persulphate (freshly prepared)
- N, N, N, N-tetramethylethyldiamide (TMED)
- Electrode buffer (24.0 g Tris base, 115.2 g glycine, 4 g SDS to a final volume of 4 litres with water).

Stain and analysis reagents

- Staining solution (0.05% Coomassie Brilliant Blue R-250 in 25% insopropanol, 10% acetic acid).
- 10% acetic acid
- 25% pyridine

Equipment

○ High-speed centrifuge (at least 20 000 g).
○ Commercial slab gel apparatus.
○ Spectrophotometer and/or densitometer.

Method

Preparation of membrane samples

1. Wash blood equivalent to 1 ml of 40% haematocrit 3 times with N-saline 1000 g or for 5 minutes.

2. Add 40 ml of ice-cold lysing buffer to each sample. Allow to sit 10 minutes on ice.

3. Pack membranes by centrifuging at 20 000 g for 10 minutes

4. Aspirate supernatant and adjust volume of pellet to 0.5 ml.

5. Add 0.5 ml solubilising buffer to pellet and boil for 5 minutes.

Preparation of slab gel

1. Separating gel solution (designed for 10 × 14 cm glass plates with a 1.5 ml wide spacer).

    a. Mix as follows:

Water	1.5 ml
Acrylamide stock solution	7.0 ml
1.5 M Tris-Cl, pH 8.8	7.5 ml
10% SDS	0.3 ml
10% Ammonium persulphate	0.1 ml
TMED	7.5 μl

2. Transfer separating gel solution to assembled slab gel apparatus. Overlay separating gel solution carefully with water to prevent meniscus formation. Allow to polymerise several hours, or overnight.

3. Remove overlay water.

4. Prepare stacking gel.

    a. Mix as follows:

Water	6.3 ml
0.5 M Tris-Cl, pH 6.8	2.5 ml
Acrylamide stock solution	1.0 ml
10% Ammonium persulphate	0.1 ml
TMED	7.5 μl

5. Apply sufficient stacking gel solution to top of separating gel to cover comb. Insert comb and let stacking gel polymerise for 1 hour.

Running sample

1. Place gel in electrode buffer.

2. Carefully and slowly remove comb by pulling straight up.

3. Add 6 μl sample per mm of well width.

4. Electrophorese at 25 v, constant voltage, until dye front just reaches bottom of gel — approximately 15 hours.

5. Stain gel in staining solution for at least 8 hours.

6. Destain with 10% acetic acid with gentle shaking until background is clear. This can be facilitated by the addition of a small piece of commercial polyurethane foam packing material which will absorb the dye.

Analysis

1. Perform scanning densitometry on intact gel.

2: Colour elution technique: cut out protein bands of interest in both patient sample and control. Add 1 ml of 25% pyridine. Shake overnight at room temperature to elute colour. Read OD at 605 nm.

Comment

— If proteolytic damage to membrane proteins is suspected, 1.0 mm diisopropylfluorophosphate (DFP) can be cautiously added when performing initial cell lysis instead of PMSF. DFP is more effective than PMSF; however, it is also more toxic.

— The water used for preparation of the gel itself should be at least double-glass distilled. Trace contaminants reduce the resolution of the bands.

— The glass plates should be absolutely clean and free of scratches. Soaking plates in Chromerge is recommended.

— Scanning densitometry for comparison of protein band areas can be performed on either dried or wet gels. If the appropriate apparatus is available, wet gels provide better resolution and less distortion.

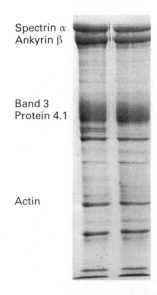

Spectrin α
Ankyrin β

Band 3
Protein 4.1

Actin

Fig. 5.3 SDS-PAGE analysis of normal (left) and protein 4.1-deficient (right) erythrocyte membranes.

Interpretation

SDS-PAGE patterns may be abnormal both qualitatively and quantitatively. Qualitative differences such as the appearance of new bands or loss of definition of bands are apparent from comparison with control samples. Quantitative changes can also be detected by inspection if marked. Modest quantitative differences are best appreciated by comparing the ratio of the band in question with some other contrast band such as band III. In general, we feel that quantitative changes must be more than 15% different from control samples before they are considered significant when using densitometry. However, utilising the pyridine method, Agre has recently suggested that, at least for spectrin, biologically significant differences of even 5–10% can be detected (Agre et al 1985). A decrease in the amount of any of the major membrane proteins can result in decreased membrane stability. In hereditary spherocytosis, quantitative differences in spectrin content can be expected in more than 50% of the patients.

Composition of solutions

1.5 mM Tris-Cl, pH 8.8

Tris base	18.15 g
Water	50 ml

Adjust to pH 8.8 with 1 N HCl. Make up to 100 ml.

0.5 M Tris-Cl, pH 6.8

Tris base	6.0 g
Water	50 ml

Adjust to pH 6.8 with 1 N HCl. Make up to 100 ml.

0.2 M Tris-Cl, pH 7.4

Tris base	24.2 g
Water	800 ml

Adjust to pH 7.4 with 1 N HCl. Make up to 1 litre.

TBS

NaCl	8.2 g
0.2 M Tris-Cl, pH 7.4	25 ml

Make up to 1 litre.

0.1 M EDTA, pH 7.4

Ethylenediamine tetra-acetic acid tetra-sodium salt	3.8 g
Water	50 ml

Adjust to pH 7.4 with 1 N HCl. Make up to 100 ml.

0.1 M EGTA, pH 7.4

Ethyleneglycol tetra-acetic acid	3.8 g
Water	50 ml

Adjust to pH 7.4 with 1 N NaOH. Make up to 1 litre.

0.1 M KCl

KCl	7.45 g

Make up to 1 litre with water.

150 mM PMSF

Phenylmethylsulphonyl fluoride	260 mg

Make up to 10 ml with isopropanol.

Lysing buffer

0.2 M Tris-Cl, pH 7.4	25 ml
0.1 M KCl	70 ml
0.1 M EGTA or 0.1 M EDTA	10 ml
0.15 M, PMSF	16.7 ml

Make up to 1 litre.

RED CELL MEMBRANE STABILITY ASSAY

Principle

The mechanical stability of the red cell membrane is analysed by measuring the resistance of the red cell membrane to fragmentation under shear stress in either a shaking assay or with an Ektacytometer. The former simply measures the morphological transformation of discs to fragments which occurs when red cells are shaken vigorously. The latter measures changes in red cell deformability which occur when the cells are maximally stressed in a coaxial cylinder viscometer. Under this stress, the cells are stretched out to ellipses and then lose membrane fragments, becoming indeformable spheres. This loss of deformability is monitored over time by measuring the laser diffraction pattern of the dextran-suspended cells and a half-time for the loss of deformability is derived. This test should be used for analysing red cells from patients in whom cell membrane defects are suspected, generally in hereditary spherocytosis, elliptocytosis and pyropoikilocytosis. Before performing this test, other possible sources for the anaemia (nutritional deficiencies, haemoglobinopathies, enzyme deficiencies) should be eliminated.

Reagents

- 5 mM Tris-Cl, 140 mM NaCl, pH 7.4 (TBS)
- 5 mM Tris-Cl, 7 mM KCl, 1 mM EGTA, pH 7.4 (lysing buffer)
- 37% Dextran T-40 (Pharmacia) in 180 mOsm PBS, pH 7.4, 90 cps
- 1% Uranyl acetate
- 3% Triton X-100 in 5 mM $NaPO_4$, 1 mM mercaptoethanol, pH 7.4 (Triton reagent)

Equipment

- Pipette shaker (Clay-Adams, 1550 oscillations/min).
- 0.7 by 7 cm test tubes.
- Ektacytometer (Technicon Corp., Model 152, or suitable equivalent).
- High-speed centrifuge (at least 20 000 g).

Preparation of samples

Shaking assay

1. Wash red cells three times in TBS. Pack at 1000 g for 5 minutes.
2. Lyse red cells with 20 volumes of ice-cold lysing buffer. Pack membranes by centrifuging at 20 000 g for 10 minutes.
3. Incubate packed ghosts for 15 minutes at 25°C with 2 volumes of Triton reagent.

Ektacytometry

1. Repeat steps 1 and 2 of shaking assay.
2. Incubate packed membranes in 10 volumes of TBS for 1 hour at 37°C.
3. Centrifuge 20 000 g for 5 minutes.

Method

Shaking assay

1. Transfer 200 μl of skeleton suspension to small test tubes (0.7 by 7 cm) mounted horizontally on a pipette shaker.

2. Shake at 1550 oscillations per minute for 40 minutes at 4–6°C.

3. Take 5 μl of skeleton suspension and apply to siliconised microscope coverslip and examine morphology. Fragile membranes will appear disintegrated in comparison to intact controls.

Ektacytometry

1. Mix 50 μl of packed red cell membranes per 1 ml of 37% dextran solution.

2. Perform ektacytometry in a Technicon Ektacytometer Model 152 as follows:

a. Add the suspension to Ektacytometer bowl and apply maximal stress of 750 dynes/cm^2.

b. Plot the deformability index versus time curve off the machine (Fig. 5.4).

3. The deformability index will decay more rapidly with fragile membranes in comparison to controls. Patient versus control curves can be directly compared, or half-times for the change from maximal to minimal deformability can be derived.

Interpretation

The interpretation of the morphological effects of the shaking assay is self evident. The interpretation of the Ektacytometer curves depends upon comparison with contemporaneous controls and a normal value for fragility half-times if this parameter is used.

Composition of solutions

As for SDS-PAGE electrophoresis.

HAM'S TEST (ACIDIFIED-SERUM TEST)

In paroxysmal nocturnal haemoglobinuria (PNH) a proportion of red blood cells are susceptible to lysis by complement so that the condition presents as a haemolytic anaemia. In the laboratory these cells can be detected by exposing them to complement in acidified sera, and although normal cells are not lysed, a proportion of those from PNH patients are lysed, especially by the patient's own serum. Should the patient's own serum be low in complement, ABO compatible donor sera can be used.

Other agents can also be used to activate either the classical or alternative complement pathways and so demonstrate sensitivity to lysis.

Principle

The patient's red cells are incubated at 37°C with a selection of fresh compatible acidified sera including the patient's own serum and then examined for any traces of haemolysis which may have occurred.

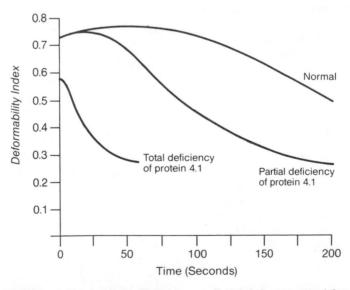

Fig. 5.4 Red cell membrane stability as measured in the Ektacytometer. Resealed ghosts prepared from normal and protein-deficient cells were exposed to 750 dynes/cm^2 in the Ektacytometer, and decline of the deformability index (DI) was measured as a function of time. The rate of DI decline is a measure of membrane stability. Membranes totally deficient in protein 4.1 fragmented more rapidly than did normal membranes. Partially deficient membranes showed intermediate reductions in membrane stability.

Test samples

Venous blood is drawn from the patient. The red cells required are obtained from defibrinating the sample or by placing it into heparin, oxalate, citrate or EDTA anticoagulant. The serum is best obtained by using a defibrinated sample but may be collected by allowing blood to clot spontaneously at 37°C or room temperature.

Control/standard

It is important if possible to include known PNH cells or artificially created 'PNH-like' cells in each batch. These 'PNH-like' cells can be produced by treating normal red cells with chemicals such as sulphydryl compounds, like L-cysteine, reduced glutathione and 2-amino ethylisothiouronium (AET).

Reagents

- 0.5 M HCl
- 0.154 M NaCl. Dissolve 9 g of sodium chloride in one litre of deionised distilled water.

Method

1. ABO and Rhesus group the patient's red cells (see Section 4).
2. Select compatible non-haemolysed sera from samples collected the same day/time as patient sample.
3. Number eight (75 × 10 mm) glass tubes accordingly.
4. Place ten drops of individual selected sera into appropriate tubes numbered 1–6.
5. Into tubes 7 and 8 place ten drops of patient's serum.
6. Add one drop of 0.5 M HCl to tubes 1–7.
7. Add one drop of normal saline to tube 8.
8. Mix well.
9. Add one drop of patient's washed 20% cell suspension to each tube.
10. Mix and incubate at 37°C for one hour.
11. Re-mix and centrifuge.
12. Examine for haemolysis, using tube 8 and the original serum samples for comparison.

Results

If the tubes above show any haemolysis the test is positive. Select the serum which has encouraged the most haemolysis and use it in the controlled Ham's test.

CONTROLLED HAM'S TEST

Principle

As for screening test.

Test samples

As for screening test.

Controls/standard

As for screening test.

Reagents

- 0.2 M HCl
- 0.154 M NaCl. Dissolve 9 g of sodium chloride in one litre of deionised distilled water.

Method

1. Deliver 0.5 ml of the serum selected from the screening test into a 75 × 12 mm glass tube.
2. Place in water bath at 56°C for 20 minutes.
3. Whilst this is proceeding wash Group O normal cells three times with normal saline.
4. After final wash make up to a 20% cell suspension.
5. To each of four tubes add the following mixtures of serum, acid and cells. (Table 5.2)
6. Mix well and incubate at 37°C for one hour.
7. After incubation, mix and centrifuge.
8. Examine for haemolysis.

Table 5.2

	FNCS*	0.2M HCl	Inactivated FNCS*	20% patient cells	20% normal cells
Tube 1	10 drops	1 drop	—	1 drop	—
Tube 2	10 drops	1 drop	—	—	1 drop
Tube 3	—	1 drop	10 drops	1 drop	—
Tube 4	10 drops	—	—	1 drop	—

*FNCS = fresh normal compatible serum

Results

Marked lysis occurring in tube 1 with or without a trace of lysis in tube 4 denotes the PNH abnormality. A positive result in any other tube indicates a false result except possibly in a case of a rare congenital dyserythropoietic anaemic, CDA Type II or HEMPAS whose cells will give a negative result with their own acidified serum.

SUCROSE-LYSIS TEST

Principle

When placed in low-ionic strength solution, erythrocytes adsorb complement from serum, and PNH cells — because of their increased sensitivity to complement lysis — will be affected whereas normal cells will not.

Test samples

Venous blood is drawn from the patient and one sample

allowed to clot and the other placed in anticoagulant as in the Ham's test.

Control/standard
As for Ham's test.

Reagents
- *5 mM Sodium dihydrogen orthophosphate* (Na$H_2PO_42H_2O$). Dissolve 0.78 g in 100 ml deionised distilled water.
- *5 mM Disodium hydrogen orthophosphate* (Na_2HPO_4). Dissolve 0.71 g in 100 ml deionised distilled water.
- *0.27 M Sucrose*. Dissolve 9.24 g sucrose in 91.0 ml of first reagent and 9.0 ml of second reagent. Adjust pH to 6.1 if necessary.

Method
1. To each of four labelled tubes (75 × 10) add the following. (Table 5.3)
2. Incubate at 37°C for 30 minutes.
3. Centrifuge.
4. Examine for lysis.

Table 5.3

Tube	Sucrose	Saline	Patient's serum	FNCS	Patient's cells
1	0.85 ml	—	0.05 ml	—	0.1 ml
2	—	0.85 ml	0.05 ml	—	0.1 ml
3	0.85 ml	—	—	0.05 ml	0.1 ml
4	—	0.85 ml	—	0.05 ml	0.1 ml

Result
A positive result is denoted by lysis occurring in the sucrose-containing tube (tube 1).

ACETYLCHOLINE ESTERASE (ACHE)

Paroxysmal nocturnal haemoglobinuria (PNH) is an acquired haemolytic disorder in which the patient's red cells become susceptible to haemolysis by complement. The site of the abnormality has been shown to be on the cell membrane which acquires an increased affinity for complement components.

Principle
The hydrolysis of acetylthiocholine to thiocholine is catalysed by acetylcholine esterase. The rate of formation of thiocholine is measured by its interaction with 5,5-dithiobis (2 nitrobenzoic acid) (DTNB) which produces a yellow chromophore which can be measured at 412 nm.

Test samples
Venous or capillary blood collected into ACD, EDTA or lithium heparin may be used. The samples should be stored at 4°C until required.

Standard/controls
A sample collected at the same time from a known normal individual is run in parallel as a control.

Reagents
- *1.0 M Tris-HCl buffer, EDTA (5 mM), pH 8.0.* 12.1 g of Tris (hydroxymethyl) methylamine and 168 mg of EDTA (disodium salt) are dissolved in 80 ml deionised distilled water. The pH is adjusted with HCl and the final volume made up to 100 ml.
- *3.4 mM Sodium citrate (1%).* Dissolve 1 g of sodium citrate (trisodium salt) in 100 ml deionised distilled water
- *0.75 mM 5,5-Dithiobis (2-nitrobenzoic acid) (DTNB).* Dissolve 30 mg of DTNB in 100 ml of 3.4 mM sodium citrate.
- *15 mM Acetylthiocholine iodine.* Dissolve 43.4 mg in 10 ml of deionised distilled water.

Method
Sample preparation
1. Thoroughly mix the samples to be assayed.
2. Add 1.0 ml of whole blood to 10.0 ml of 0.154 M saline in a graduated glass centrifuge tube. Mix well and centrifuge for 10 minutes at 1500 g.
3. Decant supernatant and remove buffy coat with a Pasteur pipette. Repeat the process twice more.
4. After final wash, resuspend the packed red cells in 0.154 M saline (2 volumes of saline to 1 volume of packed cells). Mix well. Retain an aliquot of the suspension for a Coulter count determination.
5. Prepare a 1 in 20 haemolysate by adding 1 volume of suspended washed cells to 19 volumes of deionised distilled water. Freeze the haemolysate in acetone/dry ice and keep frozen until required. To thaw place the haemolysate in a beaker of water at RT°C just before assay.

Assay method
1. Dilute the thawed haemolysate 1:10 with water.
2. Pipette the following reagents into suitable tubes:

	Test	Reagent blank
Tris buffer	0.3 ml	0.3
DTNB	0.1 ml	0.1
Distilled water	2.4 ml	2.5
Haemolysate	0.1 ml	0.1

3. Mix well and place tubes in water bath set at 37°C for 10 minutes.
4. Add 0.1 ml of acetylthiocholine iodide to Test only.
5. Mix and transfer contents to a 3 ml cuvette and record the increase in optical density at 412 nm for 10

minutes of both the test and the reagent blank against a water blank.

Calculation

Using the millimolar extinction coefficient (13.6) of the yellow chromophore produced:

Acetylcholine esterase activity =

$$\frac{OD_T - OD_B/min}{RBC} \times 4412 \text{ IU}/10^{10} \text{ RBC}$$

To convert to IU per gm Hb multiply activity per 10^{10} RBC by $\dfrac{100}{MCH}$

Normal range

Acetylcholinesterase activity = 10.25 ± 1.9 IU/10^{10} RBC
= 34.3 ± 7.0 IU/gm Hb

Comments

— For storage of reagents see under G6PD and GSH assay.
— If butyryl-thiocholine iodide is substituted for acetylthiocholine iodide there is no activity in normal red cells.

Interpretation of results

Low levels of activity are found in paroxysmal nocturnal haemoglobinuria (PNH). The activity in Type III cells is very low, but because the proportion of abnormal cells in PNH may be variable, the activity of ACHE may be normal or only slightly reduced, making the test of limited diagnostic value. The activity is also markedly influenced by red cell age and will therefore be higher when there is a young cell population.

Levels lower than the adult normal range are found in cord blood.

GLUCOSE-6-PHOSPHATE DEHYDROGENASE (G6PD)

Glucose-6-phosphate dehydrogenase (G6PD) deficiency is the commonest genetically inherited sex-linked enzyme deficiency. Most individuals are entirely symptom-free and only haemolyse when exposed to oxidant compounds, intercurrent disease or, with some variants, the fava bean. Others have a non-spherocytic haemolytic anaemia. G6PD deficiency is an important cause of neonatal jaundice and can even lead to kernicterus. For this reason it is important to know if a deficiency is present in order that appropriate medical advice concerning the avoidance of haemolytic agents can be given.

Several methods for detecting G6PD deficiency are set out — two are suitable for screening, another is a cytochemical test, and finally a quantitative assay method is described.

All haematology laboratories should be able to perform simple screening tests for the identification of this common enzyme deficiency. Various methods are available for screening for G6PD by fluorescence, reduction of methaemoglobin, catalase inhibition by cyanide and dye reduction tests.

Two methods will be described — use of the reduction of Nitro Blue Tetrazolium (NBT), and the fluorescent spot test recommended by the International Committee for Standardization in Haematology (ICSH).

G6PD SCREENING TEST (NBT SPOT TEST)

Principle

Whole blood or haemolysate is incubated with an excess of glucose-6-phosphate, which in the presence of a sufficient amount of G6PD will convert NADP to produce NADPH. This in the presence of phenazine methosulphate (PMS), which behaves as an electron transfer agent, will cause the soluble NBT dye to be reduced to blue insoluble formazan particles.

Test samples

Venous or capillary blood collected into lithium heparin or EDTA. Stable for up to two weeks if kept at 4°C.

Controls/standards

No standards as such are available, so a sample of comparable age from a known normal individual is run in parallel as a control. If possible a negative and a positive control should also be run in parallel, but this is not always convenient, so a reagent blank can be used as a screen for zero activity.

Reagents

- *0.75 M Tris (2 amino-hydroxy-methyl propane 1–3 diol) buffer, pH 8.5.* 8.95 g of Tris dissolved in about 90 ml of distilled water. Adjust pH with concentrated HCl and make up to a final volume of 100 ml. Stable at 4°C.
- *Buffer/substrate solution.* To 20 ml distilled water add:
- Glucose-6-phosphate   40 mg
  NADP   25 mg
  Nitro Blue Tetrazolium   25 mg
  Tris buffer   5 ml
  Stable at 4°C for up to one month.
- *Phenazine methosulphate.* 1 mg/ml in distilled water. Prepare freshly for use.

Method

1. Pipette 0.9 ml buffer/substrate solution into tube.
2. Add 0.01 ml whole blood.
3. Add 0.05 ml PMS solution.
4. Mix by vortex.
5. Leave at room temperature, away from direct sunlight, for 30 minutes.
6. Read macroscopically for colour change.

Results (see Fig. 5.5)

Normal individuals show a dark brown coloration with possibly a blue precipitate. Deficient males or homozygous females show little or no change. Heterozygote females may show a tan colour, little change or near normal result.

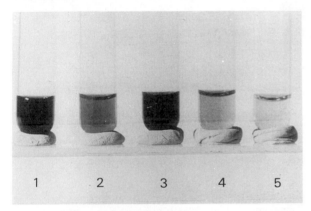

Fig. 5.5 NBT spot test. 1. Normal control. 2. Heterozygote female. 3. Normal male. 4. Homozygote male. 5. Blank.

Interpretation of screening tests

See notes on fluorescent spot test.

G6PD SCREENING TEST (FLUORESCENT SPOT TEST)

Principle

This is a mini-enzyme assay which is based on the fluorescence of NADPH under UV light. In G6PD deficiency the inability to produce adequate NADPH results in lack of fluorescence.

Test/samples

As for NBT screening test. In addition blood may be spotted onto Whatman No 1 filter paper by the finger prick technique. Label clearly. This method is useful for population screening as several patient blood samples can be spotted onto one piece of filter paper and travel satisfactorily by post.

Reagents

- *0.75 M Tris HCl buffer pH 7.8.* Dissolve 9.1 g of Tris in 80 ml of deionised distilled water. Adjust pH to 7.8 with HCl and make up to 100 ml.
- *0.02 M Glucose-6-phosphate.* Dissolve 120 mg in 20 ml deionised distilled water.
- *Saponin 1%.* Dissolve 0.4 g in 40 ml of deionised distilled water.
- *7.5 mM NADP.* Dissolve 120 mg in 20 ml of deionised distilled water.
- *8 mM oxidised glutathione (G-S-S-G).* Dissolve 96 mg in 20 ml of deionised distilled water.

Mix the above reagents as follows:

Buffer	60 ml
Glucose-6-phosphate	20 ml
Saponin	40 ml
NADP	20 ml
Glutathione	20 ml
Distilled water	40 ml

Dispense 2.0 ml aliquots into stoppered plastic tubes and store at −20°C until use. This reagent is stable for 2 years in the frozen state.

Method

1. To 0.1 ml of thawed screening reagent add 0.01 ml of whole blood or an 0.8 cm^2 punch of dried blood from the filter paper.
2. Mix well and allow to stand at RT°C for 15 minutes. Switch on the UV light.
3. Spot 0.01 ml of the mixture around the edge of Whatman No 1 filter paper. Label clearly and allow to dry.
4. Examine for fluorescence under long-wave UV light.

Results

Normal individuals show a bright fluorescence. Deficient males and homozygous females show little or no fluorescence. Heterozygote females may show low, intermediate or normal fluorescence.

Interpretation

It must be remembered that these are screening tests, and individuals showing doubtful or low fluorescence must have their activity confirmed by enzyme assay. In addition, if a haemolytic crisis has just occurred with consequent reticulocytosis or the patient has received a recent blood transfusion, the results may be invalidated by these populations of cells.

CYTOCHEMICAL DEMONSTRATION OF G6PD DEFICIENCY

This test is used for the qualitative determination of G6PD deficiency. Some female heterozygotes give normal results in both the screening test and the direct assay because of the degree of random inactivation of one X chromosome and this test will help diagnose the carrier state.

Principle

In the test, methaemoglobin formation is prompted by incubating red cells with sodium nitrite. The cells are then incubated with Nile Blue sulphate to stimulate the hexose-monophosphate pathway along with added glucose as substrate. Following this initial incubation a tetrazolium compound is added and the cells further incubated. During this time the soluble tetrazolium salt will be converted to its insoluble form which will appear within the cells as purple-black granules. Cells unable to reduce the methaemoglobin back to oxyhaemoglobin because of G6PD deficiency will remain free of granules.

Test samples

Venous or capillary blood collected into lithium heparin, EDTA or ACD and tested within eight hours of collection. Store at 4°C until testing.

Controls and standards

No standards as such are available, so a sample of comparable age is run through, in parallel, to act as a control. Ideally a negative and positive control should be run but this is not always convenient.

Reagents

- *0.18 M Sodium nitrite.* Dissolve 1.25 g/100 ml distilled water. The solution is stable for one month in a darkened bottle at 4°C.
- *0.154 M Isotonic saline.* Dissolve 9.0 g NaCl/l distilled water.
- *Incubation medium*

0.154 M Isotonic Saline	4.0 ml
0.28 M Glucose (5.0 g/100 ml)	1.0 ml
0.3 M Phosphate buffer (pH 7.0)	2.0 ml
Nile Blue sulphate (11 mg/100 ml)	1.0 ml
Distilled water	2.0 ml

- *MTT tetrazolium.* Dissolve 50 mg of 3-(4,5-di-methylthiazolyl-1-2)-2,5-diphenyl tetrazolium bromide in 10 ml of isotonic saline.
- *0.103 M Hypotonic saline.* Dissolve 60 mg NaCl in 10 ml distilled water.

Method

1. Centrifuge whole blood at 1200 g for minutes, discard supernatant and mix packed cells by vortex.

2. Add 0.25 ml cells to centrifuge tube containing 4.5 ml isotonic saline and 0.25 ml sodium nitrate. Incubate at 37°C for 20 minutes.

3. Centrifuge at 1200 g for 10 minutes.

4. Discard supernatant and wash cells three times in isotonic saline and after final wash remove buffy coat and mix remaining cells well by vortex action.

5. Transfer 0.05 ml of mixed packed cells to tube containing 1.0 ml of incubation medium and incubate at 37°C for 30 minutes.

6. Add 0.20 ml of MTT solution. Mix gently and incubate at 37°C for 60 minutes.

7. Resuspend cells and place one drop adjacent to one drop of hypotonic saline on a glass slide; thoroughly mix the drops.

8. Cover with coverslip and examine with an oil-immersion objective for the presence of formazan granules within the cells.

Units

No units as such are used.

Interpretation

Normal red cells will contain abundant granules. G6PD-deficient cells will be devoid of granules although a few cells may contain one or two small granules. In a female heterozygote with G6PD deficiency, some cells will be devoid of granules and the remainder show an abundance.

QUANTITATIVE ASSAY FOR GLUCOSE-6-PHOSPHATE DEHYDROGENASE

Principle

G6PD is the first enzyme on the pentose phosphate pathway and converts glucose-6-phosphate (G6P) to 6-phosphogluconate (6PGA) which in turn is converted to ribulose-5-phosphate (R5P) by the enzyme 6-phosphogluconic dehydrogenase (G6PD). At both stages NADP is converted to NADPH and the rate of formation of the latter is followed spectrophotometrically. The reaction is stoichiometric i.e. 1 mole of G6P converted results in the reduction of 1 mole of NADP.

$$1. \ \text{G-6-P} + \text{NADP}^+ \xrightarrow{\text{G6PD}} 6\text{PGA} + \text{NADPH}$$

$$2. \ 6\text{PGA} + \text{NADP}^+ \xrightarrow{\text{6PGD}} \text{R5P} + \text{NADPH}$$

The results can be expressed using reaction 1 as recommended by the WHO but most laboratories now link reactions 1 and 2 in the assay and subtract the result of reaction 2 from the total activity which gives a more accurate measurement of the amount of G6PD present and is recommended by ICSH (International Committee for Standardization in Haematology).

Test samples

Lithium heparin, EDTA, ACD or CPD can be used as anticoagulants. Assay should be performed as soon as possible following blood collection but the enzyme is stable at 4°C for up to three weeks if delay is inevitable.

Controls

Blood from a known normal individual, collected at the same time, should be run in parallel together with blood from a known deficient patient if available.

Reagents

- *1 M Tris HCl, 0.5 mM EDTA, pH 8.0.* 12.1 g of Tris (hydroxymethyl) methylamine and 168 mg of disodium EDTA are dissolved in 80 ml of deionised distilled water. The pH is adjusted with HCl and the final volume made up to 100 ml.
- *18 mM G6P* (disodium salt). Dissolve 55 mg G6P in 10 ml deionised distilled water. Store in 1.0 ml aliquots in plastic containers at −20°C.
- *18 mM PGA* (trisodium salt). Dissolve 68 mg in 10 ml deionised distilled water. Store in 1.0 ml aliquots in plastic containers at −20°C.
- *6 mM NADP* (disodium salt). Dissolve 48 mg in 10 ml deionised distilled water. Store in 1.0 ml aliquots in plastic containers at 4°C.
- *0.3 M Magnesium chloride.* Dissolve 6.1 g of magnesium chloride in 100 ml of deionised distilled water. Store at 4°C.

Method

Preparation of haemolysate

1. Add 1.0 ml well-mixed whole blood to 9.0 ml of ice-cold 0.154 M saline (0.9%) and centrifuge at 1500 g for 10 minutes at 4°C.

2. Decant supernatant and remove buffy coat but do not disturb reticulocyte rich top layer of the red cells. Wash twice more with ice-cold isotonic saline.

3. Resuspend the packed cells in an equal volume of saline. Mix well and take aliquot for Coulter count and reticulocyte count.

4. Add 1 volume of red cell suspension to 9 volume of deionised distilled water.

5. Freeze the haemolysate in acetone/dry ice mixture and keep frozen at −20°C until assay, which should be as soon as possible.

6. Just prior to assay thaw the lysate in a beaker of water at room temperature.

Assay

1. All specimens should be assayed in duplicate.

2. To 3 tubes labelled A, B and C add the following reagents (ml).

	Tube A	Tube B	Tube C
Tris/EDTA buffer	0.3	0.3	0.3
NADP	0.1	0.1	0.1
MgCl₂	0.1	0.1	0.1
Haemolysate	0.1	0.1	0.1
Water	2.3	2.2	2.3

3. Mix and incubate at 37°C for 10 minutes.

4. Just prior to assay add (ml)

	Tube A	Tube B	Tube C
G6P	0.1	0.1	—
6PG	—	0.1	0.1

5. Transfer to 3.0 ml cuvettes and record the increase in OD for 5 to 10 minutes at 340 nm and 37°C against a blank of 0.1 ml haemolysate in 2.9 ml water.

6. Using only the linear part of the recording calculate the increase in OD/min for each sample.

Calculation

Using the millimolar extinction coefficient (6.22) of NADPH:

1. Activity, as recommended by WHO

$$\text{G6PD IU}/10^{10} \text{ RBC} = \frac{\Delta\text{OD/min}_A \times 482}{\text{RBC (in millions)}}$$

2. Activity, as recommended by ICSH

$$\text{G6PD IU}/10^{10} \text{ RBC} = \frac{\Delta\text{OD/min}_B - \Delta\text{OD/min}_C}{\text{RBC (in millions)}} \times 482$$

Normal range at 37°C
WHO G6PD IU/10¹⁰ RBC = 3.6 ± 0.6
ICSH G6PD IU/10¹⁰ RBC = 2.5 ± 0.5

To convert to activity/g Hb multiply by $\dfrac{\text{MCH}}{100}$

Comments

— It is essential that high quality substrates and co-enzymes are purchased from reliable firms. Read the manufacturer's instructions carefully regarding the recommendations for storage. Most made-up reagents keep well at −20°C with the exception of NADP which is more stable at 4°C (N.B. The reduced forms of these coenzymes are unstable and should be prepared freshly for use).

— Ideally leucocytes should be removed from the blood (see PK method, p. 110) but we have found this makes little difference to the final results of the assay if the buffy coat is removed with a Pasteur pipette.

— Do not try to weigh out substrates and coenzymes accurately but weigh out an approximate amount and adjust the volume of solvent accordingly.

— The method described uses 3.0 ml cuvettes of 1 cm light path as these are always available. However it is slightly more expensive on reagents, and the method can be scaled down for use with 1.0 ml cuvettes.

— If a spectrophotometer with a constant temperature housing unit is not available, take the temperature of the reaction mixture in the cuvette at the end of the assay. Tables are available for correction of activity according to temperature.

— On no account must the haemolysate be refrozen and used for further assay. If a repeat is required then a fresh haemolysate must be prepared from the whole blood. Also discard vials of thawed substrates and coenzymes at the end of the day's run.

— It is important when pipetting red cell suspensions that no cells are left adhering to the pipette. With automatic plastic tipped pipettes this is not a problem.

— All laboratories should establish their own normal range.

Interpretation

Males and homozygous females with G6PD deficiency give low results, the level depending on the type of variant, but usually it is below 30% of the adult normal range. Heterozygote females can present a problem as they may have low, intermediate or normal levels depending on the degree of inactivation of the abnormal X chromosome. If a normal result is found in a suspected female heterozygote her carrier status can be confirmed by the cytochemical staining technique (p. 105).

G6PD-deficient patients who have had a recent haemolytic episode with subsequent reticulocytosis or a blood transfusion may have apparently near normal results, but they never reach the level that would be expected if a normal individual had a reticulocytosis of similar degree. The assay should be repeated at a later stage when the reticulocyte count is back to normal.

Raised values are found in normal cord blood. There are over 100 different variants of G6PD, and if exact characterisation of the enzyme is required the patient should be referred to a specialist centre.

REDUCED GLUTATHIONE (GSH)

Reduced glutathione (GSH) constitutes virtually all of the non-protein sulphydryl compounds present within the mature erythrocyte. Its function is primarily as a source of reducing potential for the cell.

Principle

5,5^1-Dithiobis (2-nitrobenzoic acid) (DTNB) is a disulphide agent which is readily reduced by sulphydryl compounds, forming a highly yellow coloured anion which can be measured spectrophotometrically. This method has been modified for use with modern spectrophotometers with slit widths of less than 2 nm. These are generally available in most modern laboratories. The accuracy of the method cannot be guaranteed if less sophisticated spectrophotometers or colorimeters are used.

Test samples

Whole blood collected into EDTA, lithium, ACD or CPD may be used. The assay should be performed as soon as possible after blood collection but if storage is necessary GSH is stable for up to 20 days in ACD or CPD and up to 5 days in lithium or heparin at 4°C. On no account should specimens collected into EDTA or lithium be allowed to stand at room temperature for any length of time as there will be considerable loss of activity within 24 hours.

Standards/controls

A standard solution of glutathione is run through with each batch of tests.

Reagents

- *1.0 mM Reduced glutathione (GSH)*. Dissolve 30 mg of glutathione in 100 ml of 0.154 M saline immediately prior to assay.
- *Precipitating solution*. 1.67 g of glacial metaphosphoric acid, 0.2 g of disodium EDTA, and 30 g of sodium chloride are dissolved in 100 ml of deionised distilled water.
- *0.3 M Na_2HPO_4*. Dissolve 21.24 g of the anhydrous salt in 500 ml of deionised distilled water.
- *0.034 M Sodium citrate pH 8.0*. Dissolve 1 g of sodium citrate (trisodium salt) in 100 ml deionised distilled water.
- *0.5 mM 5,5^1-dithiobis (2-nitrobenzoic acid) (DTNB)*. Dissolve 20 mg of DTNB in 100 ml of 0.034 M sodium citrate solution.

Method

1. Measure the haematocrit of the whole blood on the Coulter counter.
2. Add 0.2 ml of whole blood to 1.8 ml of deionised distilled water. Add 0.2 ml of the standard glutathione solution to 1.8 ml of distilled water.
3. Allow to stand for no more than 3 minutes.
4. Add 3.0 ml of precipitating solution to test and standard and mix well. At the same time prepare a reagent blank by adding 3.0 ml of precipitating solution to 2.0 ml of deionised distilled water.
5. Allow to stand for 10 minutes.

6. Filter test, standard and blank solutions through Whatman No 1 Paper.

7. Add 0.5 ml filtrate to 2.0 ml of 0.3 M Na_2HPO_4 and place in 3 ml cuvettes of 1 cm light path.

8. Read the OD of the test and standard solution at 412 nm against the reagent blank (OD_1).

9. Add 0.25 ml of DTNB solution to blank, standard and test samples. Mix well by inversion and immediately take a second OD reading against the reagent blank (OD_2).

Calculation

Using the standard solution of glutathione:
Glutathione mg/100 ml RBC

$$= \frac{OD_2 - OD_1 \text{ Test}}{OD_2 - OD_1 \text{ Std}} \times \frac{3000}{\text{Hct \%}}$$

or using the millimolar extinction coefficient of the yellow anion produced when glutathione reacts with DTNB, which is 13.6.
Glutathione mg/100 ml RBC

$$= \frac{OD_2 - OD_1 \text{ Test} \times 31040}{\text{Hct \%}}$$

To convert results to μ moles GSH/gHb multiply GSH mg/100 ml RBC by

$$\frac{1000}{\text{MCHC} \times 307}$$

where 307 is the molecular weight of glutathione.

Normal range

GSH mg/dl RBC	88.3 ± 11.8
GSH μ moles/gHb	8.6 ± 1.3

Comments

— Glutathione oxidises very readily when exposed to air, and the solutions should not be allowed to stand for more than a few minutes after the water addition in stage 2 of methodology.
— The reaction temperature is not critical and the test can be performed at room temperature.
— The development of the yellow colour after the addition of DTNB is fairly rapid, but the colour begins to fade after 10 minutes so the second OD reading should be within this period.
— The precipitating solution should be prepared freshly every 28 days.

Interpretation

Glutathione may be reduced or absent in rare congenital defects of glutathione synthesis. Its use in the diagnosis of glucose-6-phosphate dehydrogenase deficiency is described in the glutathione 'stability' test. Increases have been described in various conditions such as dyserythropoiesis, myelofibrosis, pyrimidine-5-nucleotidase deficiency and other rare congenital haemolytic anaemias of unknown cause.

GLUTATHIONE STABILITY TEST

The incubation of red cells from normal subjects with the oxidant compound acetylphenylhydrazine has little or no effect on the glutathione content of the cells, since such oxidation is reversed by the normal reducing potential. This reduction is primarily brought about by NADPH formed during the conversion of glucose-6-phosphate dehydrogenase (G6PD) in the first two steps of the pentose phosphate pathway (see p. 106). In defects of the pentose phosphate pathway the glutathione is not protected from oxidation i.e. 'stabilized' and the content of the cells is reduced after such incubation.

Principle

After prior incubation of blood with acetylphenylhydrazine the test is performed as for the reduced glutathione assay.

Test samples

As for the reduced glutathione assay.

Standards/controls

A normal control sample of blood is run through with each batch of assays.

Reagents

0.67 M Acetylphenylhydrazine. 100 mg of acetylphenylhydrazine are dissolved in 1.0 ml of acetone and 5 μl volumes are transferred to 75 mm × 12 mm test tubes. The tubes are placed in an incubator and the contents allowed to dry out. The tubes are stoppered and stored in the dark until required.

All other reagents are as for the reduced glutathione assay.

Method

1. 1.0 ml of whole blood is added to a tube containing acetylphenylhydrazine and 1.0 ml of whole blood is added to a second tube not containing acetylphenylhydrazine.

2. Mix well and incubate at 37°C for one hour.

3. Remix the contents of each tube and incubate further for one hour at 37°C.

4. Repeat steps 2 and 3 until the samples have had a total of 3 hours incubation.

5. After incubation, estimate the glutathione content in both samples of blood by the method described on page 108.

Comment
— As for the reduced glutathione assay.

Interpretation
Normal subjects show a decrease in glutathione content of not more than 20% of the original value, whereas in males suffering from G6PD deficiency the decrease is much greater and occasionally be total. Heterozygote G6PD-deficient females show decreases up to about 50% of the original value. The test is not specific for G6PD deficiency and other rare defects of the pentose phosphate pathway will give abnormal results.

Normal and G6PD-deficient neonates give a positive test but the former attain normal values by the age of one week or less.

PYRUVATE KINASE

Pyruvate kinase (PK), the penultimate enzyme in the Embden-Meyerhof pathway, catalyses the phosphorylation by phosphoenol pyruvate (PEP) of adenosine diphosphate (ADP) to adenosine triphosphate (ATP). Congenital loss of PK activity is an important, though rare, cause of congenital haemolytic anaemia.

Principle
The rate of the formation of pyruvate in reaction 1 is linked to the lactic dehydrogenase reaction,

1. $PEP + ADP \xrightarrow[Mg^{2+}, K^+]{PK} Pyruvate + ATP$

and the oxidation of reduced nicotinamide adenine dinucleotide (NADH) is measured at 340 nm as shown in reaction 2.

2. $Pyruvate + NADH + H^+ \xrightarrow{LDH} Lactate + NAD^+$

The method described as used in this laboratory with good success for a number of years is one based on a modification of the method of Bucher & Pfleiderer (1955) by Krebbs & Eggleston (1965).

Test samples
Venous or capillary blood collected into ACD or lithium heparin may be used. The samples should be stored at 4°C until the time of assay which, preferably, should be as soon as possible after collection.

Standards/controls
A sample from a known normal individual is collected at the same time as the test sample and assayed in parallel as a control.

Reagents
- *0.1 M Potassium phosphate buffer pH 7.0.* Dissolve 1.07 g K_2HPO_4 and 0.53 g KH_2PO_4 in 70 ml deionised distilled water and make up to 100 ml. Check the pH.
- *0.1 M Magnesium chloride.* Dissolve 2.03 g of $MgCl_26H_2O$ in 100 ml deionised distilled water.
- *0.025 M Phosphoenol pyruvate (PEP).* Dissolve 11.6 mg/ml of the tri-cyclohexyl ammonium salt in deionised distilled water. For the low substrate assay, dilute 1 in 20 with deionised distilled water.
- *0.04 M Adenosine diphosphate.* Dissolve 19.7 mg/ml of the trisodium salt in deionised distilled water.
- *0.004 M Reduced nicotinamide adenine dinucleotide* (NADH). Dissolve 2.7 mg/ml in deionised distilled water.
- *Lactate dehydrogenase* (LDH). Dilute stock commercial preparation down to 5 units per ml with deionised distilled water.

Method
Removal of leucocytes

1. Equal amounts of α-cellulose and dry microcrystalline cellulose are mixed with 0.154 M NaCl to form a slurry.

2. Place approximately 2.0 ml in the barrel of 5.0 ml plastic syringe held vertically in a clamp.

3. Wash with 5.0 ml saline.

4. Immediately layer 1.0 ml of well-mixed test sample on top of slurry.

5. Collect effluent containing red cells.

6. Wash with 1.0 ml saline and collect effluent.

Preparation of haemolysate

1. Wash the red cell suspension three times at 4°C with ice-cold saline.

2. Reconstitute the packed red cells with two volumes of isotonic saline and mix well.

3. Take aliquot and perform red cell count on Coulter counter and reticulocyte count.

4. Add 1 volume of accurately measured red cell suspension to 9 vols of deionised distilled water (1:10 haemolysate).

5. Freeze immediately in acetone/dry ice.

6. Just before assay completely thaw by placing in a beaker of water of room temperature.

Assay

1. Set up two pairs of duplicates for each sample, one pair for normal substrate concentration, and one pair for reduced substrate concentration.

2. Add the reagents to the tubes as follows:

	Normal substrate	*Low substrate*
Buffer	2.0 ml	2.0 ml
MgCl$_2$	0.3 ml	0.3 ml
ADP	0.1 ml	0.1 ml
NADH	0.1 ml	0.1 ml
LDH	0.1 ml	0.1 ml
Water	0.2 ml	0.2 ml
Haemolysate	0.1 ml	0.1 ml

3. Invert, or vortex, to mix the contents and then place in a water-bath set at 30°C and allow to equilibrate for 10 minutes.

4. Add 0.1 ml of PEP to reaction mixture. Mix and transfer the contents to a cuvette and place in spectrophotometer.

5. Record the change in absorbance at 340 nm over 10 minutes against a blank of 0.1 ml haemolysate and 2.9 ml distilled water at 30°C.

6. There is no need to run a 'reagent blank'.

Calculation

For each molecule of PEP dephosphorylated, one molecule of NADH is oxidised. (The millimolar extinction coefficient of NADH is 6.22.)

$$\frac{OD/min \times 485}{RBC \text{ in millions}} = IU \text{ PK}/10^{10} \text{ RBC at 30°C}$$

To convert IU/10^{10}RBC to IU/gHb multiply by 100/MCH (pg).

Normal range PK = 2.2–4.2 IU/10^{10} RBC at 30°C
= 7.2–14.0 IU/gHb at 30°C
Low substrate PK = 39.7% ± 10.0%

Comments

— See G6PD assay for general comments on quality and storage of reagents.

— Whole blood can be stored satisfactorily at 4°C for up to 20 days but once the haemolysate has been prepared the assay must be performed as soon as possible.

— The quantities described in this method are for 3.0 ml 1 cm light path cuvettes. The method can be scaled down for use with 1.0 ml cuvettes.

— It is essential that white cells and platelets are removed from the blood before preparation of the haemolysate as otherwise falsely high results will be obtained.

— It is also essential to know the reticulocyte count of the blood after passage through the cellulose column

as young red cells have high PK activity and their presence may mask a deficiency. Further tests can be performed on young and old cells by differential centrifugation.

— Enzyme activity is proportional to temperature. If a spectrophotometer with a temperature controlled housing unit is unavailable, take the temperature of the reaction mixture at the end of the assay whilst still in the cuvette to ensure that there has been no marked fall.

— It is essential when expressing results as 10^{10} RBC that the volume of red cell suspension used to prepare the 1:10 haemolysate be measured as accurately as possible.

— Small amounts of fructose-1,6-diphosphate present in the haemolysate have a stimulatory effect on the enzyme and it is suggested that the haemolysate should be dialysed before assay. We have found this procedure to be time-consuming and to make little difference to the final results.

Interpretation

Pyruvate kinase deficiency is inherited as an autosomal recessive condition. Low values are found in the homozygous state and intermediate levels in heterozygote carriers. However, there is considerable biochemical heterogeneity in the types of abnormal pyruvate kinase and, except in the case of consanguinity, the propositus is likely to be a compound heterozygote, and normal values are occasionally found in the routine assay in patients with abnormal pyruvate kinase. The use of the low substrate assay may detect some cases if the results are normal at both concentrations and there is supporting evidence for suspected PK deficiency, such as a shifted oxygen dissociation curve and raised 2,3 DPG levels, referral to a specialised centre is recommended.

2,3 DIPHOSPHOGLYCERATE (DPG)

The most abundant organic phosphate compound within the red cell is 2,3 DPG, being present in approximately the same molecular concentration as haemoglobin. It is produced as an intermediate of anaerobic glycolysis via the Rapaport Luebering shunt and its main physiological importance is its ability to react stoichiometrically with deoxyhaemoglobin. This reaction lowers the oxygen affinity of haemoglobin and shifts the position of the oxygen dissociation curve.

Principle

The method is based on that of Keitt (1971) and uses a linked enzyme system. By adding excess enzyme and coenzymes, the stoichiometric conversion of 2,3 DPG

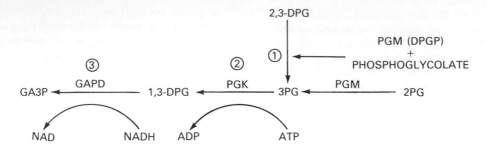

Fig. 5.6 2,3 Diphosphoglycerate assay.

to GA3P is measured using the oxidation of NADH to NAD in step 3 to calculate the activity (Fig. 5.6). DPGP is present in commercially available PGM and phosphoglycolate is added to stimulate this phosphatase activity in step 1.

Test samples

Venous blood collected into lithium heparin. The sample should be kept at 4°C until extraction with perchloric acid, which should be as soon as possible. If the specimen has to travel, or be kept for some time before extraction, collection into CPD is recommended.

Standards/controls

A control sample should be run through with each batch of tests. A suitable preparation is available from the Sigma Chemical Company.

Reagents

- *Perchloric acid (6% w/v)*. Dilute 5.0 ml of 70% perchloric acid (or 6.5 ml of 60%) to 100 ml with deionised, distilled water.
- *2 M Potassium bicarbonate*. Dissolve 20 g $KHCO_3$ in 100 ml deionised, distilled water and store at 4°C.
- *0.032 M Imidazole buffer, pH 7.6*. Dissolve 2.2 g imidazole in 800 ml deionised distilled water. Adjust the pH with normal HCl and make up to final volume of 1 litre. Store at 4°C.
- *0.15 M Magnesium chloride*. Dissolve 3.1 g of $MgCl_26H_2O$ in 100 ml deionised distilled water and store at 4°C.
- *0.15 M Hydrazine sulphate*. Dissolve 19.6 mg/ml deionised distilled water. Prepare freshly for use.
- *0.03 M Adenosine triphosphate (Di-sodium salt)*. Dissolve 18.3 mg/ml deionised, distilled water. Prepare freshly for use.
- *0.03 M 2-Phosphoglycolate (Tricyclohexylammonium salt)*. Dissolve 13.6 mg/ml deionised distilled water. Prepare freshly for use.
- *0.075 M Reduced glutathione*. Dissolve 23.3 mg/ml deionised, distilled water. Prepare freshly for use.

- *0.0024 M NADH*. Dissolve 1.6 mg/ml deionised, distilled water. Prepare freshly for use.
- *GA3PD (rabbit muscle: 800 iU/ml)*. Dilute solution 1: 15 for use.
- *PGK (yeast: 4500 IU/ml)*. Dilute solution 1:130 for use.
- *PGM (rabbit muscle : 2000 IU/ml)*. Dilute solution 1:32 for use.

Method

Specimen preparation

1. Thoroughly mix the sample and measure the haematocrit of the whole blood.
2. Add 1.0 ml of whole blood to 2.0 ml of ice-cold 6% perchloric acid and mix well.
3. Centrifuge for 10 minutes at 1500 g.
4. Decant 0.9 ml of clear supernatant to a stoppered tube and add 0.3 ml of 2M $KHCO_3$. Mix well.
5. Once effervescence has ceased the sample can be deep frozen until assay.

Assay method

1. Set up each assay in duplicate.
2. For each batch set up duplicate tubes for a control and a blank.
3. Pipette the following reagents into the tubes:

	Test	Blank
Imidazole buffer	1.9 ml	1.9 ml
MgCl₂	0.1 ml	0.1 ml
Hydrazine sulphate	0.1 ml	0.1 ml
ATP	0.1 ml	0.1 ml
Phosphoglycolate	0.1 ml	0.1 ml
GSH	0.1 ml	0.1 ml
NADH	0.1 ml	0.1 ml
PGA Extract	0.2 ml	—
Water	—	0.2 ml
GA3PD	0.1 ml	0.1 ml
PGK	0.1 ml	0.1 ml

4. Mix well and equilibrate at room temperature.
5. Record absorbance at 340 nm and 25°C using 3 ml cuvettes of 1 cm light path.

6. Add 0.1 ml PGM to tests and blanks.

7. Mix and leave at room temperature for 25 minutes.

8. Return to spectrophotometer and record absorbance.

9. Calculate the fall in OD which has occurred. (ΔOD Test)

Calculation

$$\frac{(\Delta OD\ Test - \Delta OD\ blank)}{HCT\ \%} \times 965$$
$$= 2,3DPG\ mM/l\ RBC$$

Normal range

2,3DPG = 4.0–5.0 mmoles/l RBC

Comment

— Storage of reagents is as for G6PD deficiency (p. 106).

— All phosphorylated glycolytic intermediates continue to be metabolised when blood is withdrawn and protein precipitation should be immediate. If any length of time is to elapse between withdrawal of blood and extraction it is essential to store in a nutrient medium.

Interpretation

The 2,3 DPG value of red cells is altered in a wide variety of physiological and pathological conditions which are beyond the scope of this book to deal with. Generally, elevated values are found in anaemia, hypoxia, alkalosis and defects in the glycolytic pathway beyond the Rapaport-Luebering shunt. Pyruvate-kinase deficient patients often have very high values — up to 12 mM/l RBC. In conditions where the 2,3 DPG is elevated the oxygen dissociation curve shows a right shift and consequently a facilitation of oxygen release to the tissues.

Conversely, in conditions such as severe acidosis, the 2,3 DPG level is lowered but the exact extent to which the patient suffers by this reduction has yet to be evaluated.

REFERENCES

Serum haptoglobin
Bernier G M 1967 A method for the rapid estimation of serum haptoglobin levels. Clinica Chemica Acta 18: 309–312
Owen J A, Better F C, Hoban J 1969 A simple method for the determination of serum haptoglobins. Journal of Clinical Pathology 13: 163–164
Ratcliffe A P, Hardwicke J 1964 Estimation of serum haemoglobin-binding capacity (haptoglobin) on Sephadex G-100. Journal of Clinical Pathology 17: 676–679

Osmotic fragility
Murphy J R 1967 The influence of pH and temperature on some physical properties of normal erythrocytes and erythrocytes from patients with hereditary spherocytosis. Journal of Laboratory and Clinical Medicine 69: 758–775
Parpart A K, Lorenz P B, Parpart E R, Gregg J R, Chase A M 1947 The osmotic resistance (fragility) of human red cells. Journal of Clinical Investigation 26: 636–640

Autohaemolysis
Grimes A J, Leets I, Dacie J V 1968 The Autohaemolysis Test: Appraisal of the method for the diagnosis of Pyruvate Kinase deficiency and the effect of pH and additives. British Journal of Haematology 14: 309–322
Selwyn J G, Dacie J V 1954 Autohaemolysis and other changes resulting from the incubation in vitro of red cells from patients with congenital haemolytic anaemia. Blood 9: 414–438

Acidified glycerol lysis test
Demiel R A, Geurts Van Kessel W S M, Van Deenen L L M 1972 The properties of poly-unsaturated lecithins in monolayers and liposomes and the interaction of these lecithins with cholesterol. Biochimica et Biophysica Acta 266: 26–40

Gottfried E L, Robertson N A 1974 Glycerol lysis time as a screening test for erythrocyte disorders. Journal of Laboratory and Clinical Medicine 83: 323–333
Kroes J, Ostwald R 1971 Erythrocyte membrane — effect of increased cholesterol content on permeability. Biochimica et Biophysica Acta 249: 647–650
Zanella A, Izzo C, Rebulla P, Zanuso F, Perroni L, Sirchia G 1980 Acidified Glycerol Lysis Test: a screening test for spherocytosis. British Journal of Haematology 45: 481–486

Demonstration of red cell membrane proteins by SDS-PAGE
Agre P, Casella J, Zinkam W, McMillan C, Bennett V 1985 Partial deficiency of erythrocyte spectrin in hereditary spherocytosis. Nature 314: 380–383
Fenner C, Traut R R, Mason P T, Wikman- Coffelt J 1975 Quantification of Coomassie blue stained proteins in polyacrylamide gels based on analyses of eluted dye. Analytical Biochemistry 63: 595–602
Laemmli U K 1970 Cleavage of structural proteins during the assembly of the head of bacteriophage T4. Nature 227: 680–685
Tchernia G, Mohandas N, Shohet S B 1981 Deficiency of skeletal membrane protein hand 4.1 in homozygous hereditary elliptocytosis. Implications of erythrocyte membrane stability. Journal of Clinical Investigation 68: 454–460

Red cell membrane stability assay
Lui S C, Palek J 1980 Spectrin tetramer- dimer equilibrium and the stability of erythrocyte membrane skeletons. Nature 285: 586–587
Mohandas N, Clark M R, Heath B P, Rossi M, Shohet S B 1982 A technique to detect reduced mechanical stability of red cell membranes: Relevance to elliptocytic disorders. Blood 59: 768–774

Ham's test

Crookson J H, Crookson M C, Burnie K L, Francombe W H, Dacie J V, Davis J A, Lewis S M 1969 Hereditary erythroblastic multinuclearity associated with a positive Acidified-serum test: a type of congenital dyserythropoietic anaemia. British Journal of Haematology 17: 11–26

Verwilghen R L, Lewis S M, Dacie J V, Crookson J H, Crookston M C 1973 HEMPAS: congenital dyserythropoietic anaemia (Type II). Quarterly Journal of Medicine 42: 257–271

Sucrose-lysis test

Hartman R C, Jenkins D E Jnr 1965 The 'sugar-water' test for paroxysmal nocturnal haemoglobinuria. New England Journal of Medicine: 275: 155–157

Acetylcholine esterase

Metz J, Bradlow B A, Lewis S M, Dacie J V 1960 The acetylcholinesterase activity of the erythrocytes in paroxysmal nocturnal haemoglobinaemia in relation to the severity of the disease. British Journal of Haematology 6: 372–380

G6PD screening test (fluorescent spot test)

Beutler E, Blume K G, Kaplan J C, Lohr G W, Ramot B, Valentine W N 1979 ICSH: Recommended screening test for glucose-6-phosphate dehydrogenase (G6PD) deficiency. British Journal of Haematology 43: 465–467

Beutler E, Mitchell M 1968 Special modification of the fluorescent screening method for glucose-6-phosphate dehydrogenase deficiency. Blood 32: 816–818

Brewer G J, Tarlov A R, Alving A S 1962 The methaemoglobin reduction test for primaquin-type sensitivity of erythrocytes. Journal of the American Medical Association 180: 386–388

Darley J H, Personal observation

Fairbanks V F, Beutler E 1962 A simple method for detection of erythrocyte glucose-6-phosphate dehydrogenase deficiency (G-6-PD spot test). Blood 20: 591–601

Jacob H S, Jandl J H 1966 A simple visual screening test for glucose-6-phosphate dehydrogenase deficiency. New England Journal of Medicine 274: 1162–1167

Cytochemical demonstration of G6PD deficiency

Fairbanks V F, Lampe L T 1968 A tetrazolium linked cytochemical method for the estimation of glucose-6-phosphate dehydrogenase activity in individual erythrocytes: application in the study of heterozygote for glucose-6-phosphate dehydrogenase deficiency. Blood 31: 589–603

Quantitative assay for glucose-6-phosphate dehydrogenase

Beutler E ed 1975 Red cell metabolism, a manual of biochemical methods, 2nd edn. Grune and Stratton, New York

Reduce glutathione

Beutler E, Duron O, Kelly B M 1963 Improved method for the determination of blood glutathione. Journal of Laboratory and Clinical Medicine 61:882–888

Glutathione stability test

Beutler E 1957 The Glutathione instability of drug-sensitive red cells. A new method for the in vitro detection of drug sensitivity. Journal of Laboratory and Clinical Medicine 49: 84–95

Zinkham W H 1959 An in vitro abnormality of glutathione metabolism in erythrocytes from normal newborns: mechanism and clinical significance. Paediatrics 23: 18–32

Pyrurate kinase

Beutler E (ed) 1975 Red cell metabolism, a manual of biochemical methods, 2nd edn. Grune and Stratton, New York

Beutler E, Blume K G, Kaplan J C, Lohr G W, Ramot B, Valetine W N 1977 International Committee for Standardization in Haematology: Recommended methods for red cell enzyme analysis. British Journal of Haematology 35: 331–340

Bucher Th, Pfleiderer G 1955 In: Colowick S P, Kaplan N U (eds) Methods in enzymology Volume 1. Academic Press, New York, p 435

International Committee for Standardization in Haematology 1979 Recommended methods for the characterization of red cell Pyruvate Kinase variants. British Journal of Haematology 43: 275–286

Krebs H A, Eggleston L V 1965 The role of pyruvate kinase in the regulation of gluconeogenesis. Biochemistry Journal 94: 3c

2,3 Diphosphoglycerate

Keitt A S 1971 Reduced nicotinamide adenine dinucleotide linked analysis of 2,3-diphosphoglyceric acid: spectrophotometric and fluorometric procedures. Journal of Laboratory and Clinical Medicine 77: 470–475

6

Megaloblastic anaemia

Megaloblastic anaemia is one of the important causes of macrocytic anaemia, and a raised MCV in a blood count is often the first indication of such a process. In an early case with little or no anaemia the peripheral blood film may show little else other than mild macrocytosis. As the disease progresses hypersegmented neutrophils and anisocytosis, poikilocytosis and red cell fragments may appear.

There are many disorders producing macrocytosis with a normoblastic marrow including hypothyroidism, alcoholism, a young red cell population (haemolytic anaemia, response to blood loss), myelodysplastic syndromes, aplastic and hypoplastic anaemia, and as a response to many drugs particularly those used in treatment of neoplasms. For this reason a marrow aspirate is most useful in milder cases. The marrow will show megaloblastic haemopoiesis. In severe cases the diagnosis is more self-evident although confirmation of megaloblastosis in the marrow is desirable. Megaloblasts also appear in some inherited disorders such as orotic aciduria, some cases of Lesch-Nyhan syndrome and after drugs such as cytosine arabinoside, methotrexate and hydroxyurea.

When a marrow aspirate is done a deoxyuridine suppression test can be performed. This can provide rapid confirmation of 'megaloblastosis' and also an indication as to whether the deficiency is that of cobalamin or folate. It should be done in potentially complex cases.

When megaloblastic anaemia is present, serum is sent for B_{12} and folate assay and whole blood for red cell folate assay. Urinary excretion of formiminoglutamic acid after an oral histidine load and of methylmalonic acid after a valine load are not often performed although a note about these tests is appended.

Absorption of B_{12} remains an important step in investigating B_{12} deficiency but folate absorption tests are nowadays confined to experimental medicine with the rare exception of congenital folate malabsorption presenting as severe megaloblastic anaemia in the first few months of life.

On the B_{12} side, tests for intrinsic-factor antibodies and assay of intrinsic factor in gastric juice remain useful as are measurements of B_{12} binding proteins, particularly transcobalamin II.

DEOXYURIDINE SUPPRESSION TESTS

The deoxyuridine suppression test assists in the diagnosis of megaloblastic states by measuring the efficiency of a vitamin B_{12}- and folate-dependent biochemical step within bone marrow cells.

Principle

The ability of deoxyuridine to suppress the incorporation of [^{3}H] thymidine into the DNA of bone marrow cells is impaired in vitamin B_{12} or folate deficiency states.

Biochemical basis

The reaction central to the deoxyuridine suppression test is the methylation of deoxyuridylate (dUMP) to thymidylate (dTMP), a step in the biosynthesis of the thymine moiety of DNA. The methyl donor is 5,10-methylenetetrahydrofolate polyglutamate. Exogenous deoxyuridine (dU) and thymidine (TdR) can also be incorporated into DNA (Fig. 6.1).

When normal cells are incubated with deoxyuridine, the subsequent incorporation of [^{3}H]thymidine ([^{3}H]TdR) into DNA is suppressed (Killman, 1964) — this phenomenon is commonly referred to as deoxyuridine suppression. The exogenous deoxyuridine is phosphorylated and methylated to expand the intracellular pool of thymidine triphosphate (dTTP) which dilutes the specific activity of the [^{3}H]dTTP and inhibits thymidine kinase. Deoxyuridine may also inhibit thymidine kinase directly and other possible mechanisms of deoxyuridine suppression have not been excluded (Pelliniemi & Beck 1980).

In marrow cells from patients with a deficiency of vitamin B_{12} or folic acid, deoxyuridine suppression is less effective. Thymidylate synthesis is impaired so that the deoxyuridine causes a smaller expansion of the

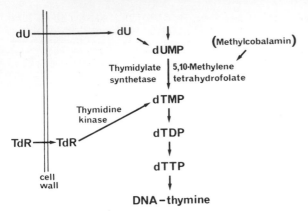

Fig. 6.1 The biochemical reactions involved in the deoxyuridine suppression test. dU, deoxyuridine. dUMP, deoxyuridine monophosphate (deoxyuridylate). dTMP, thymidine monophosphate (thymidylate). dTDP, thymidine disphosphate. dTTP, thymidine triphosphate. TdR, thymidine.

dTTP pool. A reduced supply of 5,10-methylenetetrahydrofolate is thought to cause the impairment of thymidylate synthesis, although the mechanism by which this occurs in vitamin B_{12} deficiency is not yet clear (Chanarin et al 1980).

Folic acid added to the marrow cells in vitro will regularly cause a correction of the abnormal deoxyuridine suppression in both vitamin B_{12} and folate deficiency states, whereas cobalamins will sometimes do so in vitamin B_{12} deficiency (Metz et al 1968, Zittoun et al 1978, Ganeshaguru & Hoffbrand 1978, Deacon et al 1980). Improved efficiency of the methylation of deoxyuridylate is the presumed mechanism. These additions also reduce [^{3}H]TdR incorporation by megaloblastic cells in the absence of deoxyuridine (Wickramasinghe & Saunders 1979).

Reagents
- Tris-Buffered Hanks' Solution (TBHS): Hanks' solution (Gibco Ltd) containing 60 mmol/l Tris, pH 7.4 (Sigma Chemical Co.)
- •* 2' deoxyuridine (thymine- and thymidine-free), 1.0 mmol/l in TBHS (Sigma).
- •* Cyanocobalamin, 10 mg/l in TBHS (Sigma).
- •* Folic acid, 500 mg/l in TBHS (Fisons Scientific Equipment).
- [Me-^{3}H] thymidine, 10 μCi/ml in TBHS (specific activity approximately 40 Ci/mmol: Amersham International plc).

* Reagents are made up weekly and stored at $-20°C$. The deoxyuridine suppression test may be performed either in tubes or in microtitre plates; the same reagents are used with both methods.

- Liquid scintillation fluid: 2.5 l scintillation-grade toluene containing 15 g 2,5-diphenyloxazole (PPO) and 0.3 g 1,4-di-2-(5-phenyloxazolyl) benzene (POPOP) (Fisons Scientific Equipment). Or use commercial equivalent.

A. Tube deoxyuridine suppression test

Equipment
- Syringes (10 ml), and 23- and 25-gauge needles (internal diameters 0.635 mm and 0.508 mm respectively).
- 30 ml plastic Universal containers (Sterilin Ltd.).
- Shaking water-bath (Camlab Ltd.).
- Nucleated cell counter (Coulter Ltd.).
- Whatman filter discs, 2.1 cm diameter, 3 mm grade.
- Pin-board for drying filter discs. Household pins are pushed through a square of corrugated card and a further square of card attached beneath to prevent extrusion of the pins.
- 10 ml scintillation vials with lids.
- Beta particle counter.

Method

Preparation of marrow
1. Aspirate approximately 1 ml of marrow and add 5–10 drops to 2 ml TBHS containing 25 units/ml preservative-free heparin. (Use the remainder of the marrow for the preparation of smears).
2. Fit a 23-gauge needle onto a 10 ml syringe, remove the plunger and pour in the marrow suspension. If necessary, rinse out the container with a small volume of TBHS and add to the syringe. Replace the plunger and expel the suspension through the needle. Repeat this procedure once.
3. Expel the marrow suspension once through a 25-gauge needle using the procedure as in step 2.
4. Centrifuge the marrow suspension in a conical tube at 600 g for 5 minutes. Remove the buffy coat with a Pasteur pipette and disperse it in 1 ml of TBHS.
5. Perform a nucleated cell count using a Coulter counter or other convenient method. Add sufficient TBHS so that the final nucleated cell count is $2.5 - 5 \times 10^9/l$.

The test
1. Place 6 plastic Universal containers in a rack and number them 1–6 (Table 6.1).
2. Add 0.5 ml of the cell suspension to each tube.
3. Add 0.25 ml of autologous serum or TBHS to each tube.
4. To tubes 1 and 2, add 0.1 ml TBHS.
5. To tubes 3 and 4, add 0.1 ml cyanocobalamin solution.
6. To tubes 5 and 6, add 0.1 ml folic acid solution.

Table 6.1 The contents of the tubes in the deoxyuridine suppression test. After 1 hour, 50 μl [^{3}H]TdR is added to all the tubes. The final concentrations of deoxyuridine, cyanocobalamin and folic acid are 0.1 mmol/l, 1.0 mg/l and 50 mg/l, respectively.

Tube number	Marrow cell suspension (ml)	Autologous serum or TBHS (m)	TBHS (ml)	Deoxyuridine, 1 mmol/l in TBHS (ml)	Cyanocobalamin, 10 mg/l in TBHS (ml)	Folic acid, 500 mg/l in TBHS (ml)
1	0.5	0.25	00.2	—	—	—
2	0.5	0.25	0.1	0.1	—	—
3	0.5	0.25	0.1	—	0.1	—
4	0.5	0.25	—	0.1	0.1	—
5	0.5	0.25	0.1	—	—	0.1
6	0.5	0.25	—	0.1	—	0.1

7. To tubes 1, 3 and 5, add 0.1 ml TBHS.

8. To tubes 2, 4 and 6, add 0.1 ml deoxyuridine solution.

9. Replace the lids and incubate all the tubes in a shaking water-bath at 37°C for 1 hour.

10. Add 50 μl [^{3}H]TdR to all tubes, replace the lids and incubate for a further 1 hour at 37°C in the shaking water-bath.

11. Fill each tube with ice-cold phosphate-buffered saline and centrifuge at 1300 g for 5 minutes. Discard the supernatant and repeat.

12. Suspend the cell pellet in 0.5 ml phosphate-buffered saline and mix thoroughly.

13. Perform a nucleated cell count on the suspension in each tube.

14. Number two filter discs in pencil for each tube, and mount on the pin-board. Place 0.1 ml of the appropriate cell suspension on each disc and allow to dry overnight at 37°C, or for 15–20 minutes in the hot air from a hair-dryer.

15. Remove the discs from the pin-board, place them all together in a 250 ml beaker and add approximately 100 ml 10% trichloroacetic acid at 4°C. Keep the beaker at 4°C for 20 minutes.

16. Pour off the trichloroacetic acid and add approximately 100 ml methanol at room temperature. Leave for 10 minutes, pour off the methanol, add a further volume of approximately 100 ml methanol and leave for 10 minutes. Finally pour off the methanol, and rinse the discs briefly in acetone.

17. Dry the discs with a hair-dryer for 10–15 minutes.

18. Place each disc in a scintillation vial, add 4 ml of liquid scintillation fluid, leave for at least 1 hour, and count the radioactivity using a suitable beta particle counter. Measure the background count using scintillant alone.

Calculation

After correcting for background, the mean activity of each pair of discs is expressed as ct/min per 10^3 nucleated marrow cells.

The dU-suppressed value (per cent)

$$= \frac{\text{uptake of [}^3\text{H]-TdR after pre-incubation with dU}}{\text{uptake of [}^3\text{H]-TdR without pre-incubation with dU}} \times 100$$

$$= \frac{\text{ct/min per } 10^3 \text{ cells in tube 2}}{\text{ct/min per } 10^3 \text{ cells in tube 1}} \times 100$$

For the dU-suppressed value in the presence of cyanocobalamin or folic acid, the same calculation is applied to tubes 3 and 4, and to tubes 5 and 6, respectively.

The correction caused by a vitamin is defined as the difference between the dU-suppressed values with and without the vitamin expressed as a percentage of the value without the vitamin. Corrections of 15% or more are regarded as significant.

Comments

— Red cell contamination should be kept as low as possible when preparing the cell suspension, or an unacceptable degree of quenching may occur.

— If the cell count on the washed cell suspension is low ($< 1.0 \times 10^9/1$), 0.2 ml should be spotted onto each filter disc.

— Autologous serum is not essential, and may be replaced by TBHS.

— It has been suggested that phytohaemagglutinin-stimulated peripheral blood mononuclear cells may be used as a substitute for bone marrow cells (Das & Herbert 1978). We find, however, that lymphocytes become folate-deficient in culture (Matthews & Wickramasinghe 1986a), and that in consequence there is no correlation between the deoxyuridine-suppressed value given by bone marrow cells and that given by lymphocytes (Matthews & Wickramasinghe 1988).

Interpretation

The geometric mean and 95% reference interval for the

dU-suppressed value in patients without evidence of B_{12} or folate deficiency in our laboratory are 3.5 and 1.4 — 8.6%, respectively. Each laboratory should establish its own normal range as minor variations in technique may affect the results. The following may cause a raised dU-suppressed value (Wickramasinghe 1983).

1. Deficiency of vitamin B_{12} or folic acid.
2. Treatment with some antimetabolites (e.g. methotrexate and 5-fluorouracil).
3. Nitrous oxide exposure.
4. Congenital abnormality of vitamin B_{12} or folate metabolism.
5. Protein-energy malnutrition.

Since causes 2, 3 and 5 can be readily identified on clinical grounds, and congenital abnormalities of vitamin B_{12} and folate metabolism are rare, in practice a raised dU-suppressed value usually indicates deficiency of vitamin B_{12} or folic acid. This is particularly valuable when investigating a macrocytosis, as causes other than vitamin B_{12} or folate deficiency do not affect the dU-suppressed value. Furthermore, the raised dU-suppressed values given by patients with a deficiency of vitamin B_{12} or folate are usually not completely abolished by a coexistent deficiency of iron, even when the latter reduces the mean cell volume into the normal range. A raised dU-suppressed value occurs early in the course of vitamin B_{12} or folate deficiency, and may precede the development of macrocytosis and morphological megaloblastic change. Nevertheless about 3% of vitamin B_{12}-deficient patients give a dU-suppressed value within the upper part of the normal range; such patients suffer from only a mild degree of deficiency.

The general interpretation of the effects of the addition of vitamins on the deoxyuridine suppression test is that folic acid will significantly reduce the dU-suppressed value in both vitamin B_{12} and folate deficiency, but that cyanocobalamin will do so only in vitamin B_{12} deficiency. Unfortunately, in a substantial proportion of cases of vitamin B_{12} deficiency, cyanocobalamin fails to correct the dU-suppressed value, and conversely, cyanocobalamin has been observed to cause correction of the dU-suppressed value in occasional cases of folate deficiency (Wickramasinghe & Saunders 1977).

B. Plate deoxyuridine suppression test

This method is quicker and easier to perform than the tube test, and large numbers of samples can be readily accommodated. The results are as accurate and precise as those obtained with the tube test (Matthews & Wickramasinghe 1986b).

Equipment

○ Syringes (10 ml) and needles (23- and 25-gauge).

○ Cooke microtitre plates with 12 × 8 U-shaped wells (Sterilin Ltd.).
○ Titertek plate-shaker (Flow Laboratories Ltd.).
○ Cell harvester + filter mats (Multimash 2000; Dynatech Laboratories Ltd).
○ Scintillation vial inserts (Gallenkamp).
○ Beta particle counter.
○ Air incubator.

Method

Preparation of marrow. As for tube test.

The test (Fig. 6.2)

1. Place 80 μl of the marrow cell suspension into the first 9 wells of rows A, B and C of the microtitre plate.
2. Add 10 μl TBHS to the wells in rows A and B, and 10 μl deoxyuridine solution to the wells in row C.
3. Add 10 μl TBHS to the wells in columns 1–3, 10 μl cyanocobalamin solution to those in columns 4–6 and 10 μl folic acid solution to those in columns 7–9.
4. Mix the contents of the wells using the plate-shaker.
5. Cover the plate with plastic film and incubate for 1 hour at 37°C.
6. Remove from the incubator, add 10 μl [^{3}H]TdR to the wells in rows B and C, but *not* row A, and mix on the plate-shaker.
7. Incubate for a further 1 hour under the same conditions as in step 5.
8. Embed the plate in crushed ice until cold (5–10 min), add 10 μl of [^{3}H]TdR to the wells in row A, and proceed immediately to step 9.
9. Place a filter mat in the cell harvester, pre-wet the discs, and harvest the cells from each row using approximately the following sequence: water 10 s, 10% trichloroacetic acid 10 s, methanol 10 s and air 10–15 s.

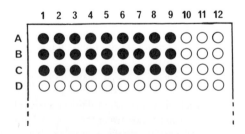

Fig. 6.2 The layout of the microtitre plate for the deoxyuridine suppression test. The wells in row A are used to measure background activity, those in row B the uptake of [^{3}H]TdR in the absence of dU, and those in row C the uptake of [^{3}H]TdR in the presence of dU. The wells in columns 1–3 receive no vitamin supplements, those in columns 4–6 are supplemented with cyanocobalamin, and those in columns 7–9 with folic acid.

10. Dry the filter mat overnight at 37°C, or more quickly (approximately 20 min) with a hairdryer.

11. Place the discs in liquid scintillation vial inserts, add 2 ml scintillant, cap the tubes and count the radioactivity.

Calculation

The mean background count is calculated from the counts in row A, and subtracted from the count relating to each well.

dU-suppressed value (per cent)

$$= \frac{\text{mean ct/min row C wells 1–3}}{\text{mean ct/min row B wells 1–3}} \times 100$$

The dU-suppressed value is calculated similarly for the data obtained in the presence of folic acid and cyanocobalamin.

Comments

— It is important that the filter discs are adequately pre-wetted with water: the time of 2 s recommended by the manufacturer is too short, and we find that approximately 5 s is needed.

— A vacuum of 50 cm mercury is adequate for harvesting the marrow cells.

— The [^{3}H]TdR solution should be kept scrupulously sterile, otherwise a high background count may result.

Interpretation

The correlation between the results with this method and the tube test is good (r=0.9), but the dU-suppressed values obtained tend to be higher. With the plate test, the geometric mean and 95% reference interval determined in our laboratory on 19 adult patients without B_{12} or folate deficiency were 5.1% and 2.0–12.8%, respectively, but it is again important for each laboratory to establish its own normal range. Provided that the appropriate reference range is used, the interpretation is the same as that of the tube test.

SERUM COBALAMIN (B_{12}) LEVEL

The serum cobalamin concentration is important in determining the cause of megaloblastic anaemia, in assessing cobalamin status in patients with disease of the small gut and in those consuming vegetarian diets. Serum cobalamin levels are low in cobalamin deficiency and are raised in myeloproliferative disorders.

Increasingly, laboratories are using commercial kits for assay of serum B_{12} levels. If so, it is imperative that adequate control procedures are used. Three methods for the assay of B_{12} are described.

1. Microbiological assay with *Lactobacillus leichmannii*.
2. Microbiological assay with *Euglena gracilis*.
3. Saturation analysis using a solid phase method.

MICROBIOLOGICAL ASSAY WITH *LACTOBACILLUS LEICHMANNII*

Principle

L. leichmannii requires preformed vitamin B_{12} for growth in culture. If a serum extract is added to a B_{12}-free culture medium the amount of growth of *L. leichmannii* depends on the amount of B_{12} present in the serum extract. The growth is compared with that in media to which known amounts of B_{12} have been added (standard curve).

Test samples

Sera are assayed and stored frozen until required.

Preparation for assay

This process releases B_{12} from its binding proteins and converts B_{12} analogues to cyanocobalamin. To a 25 ml screw capped container add

Serum	2.0 ml
0.4 N Acetate buffer pH 4.5	0.5 ml
0.1% Sodium cyanide	1.0 ml
Water	16.0ml

Autoclave for 10 minutes at 116°C, cool and add 0.5 ml of 0.2 mol-K_2HPO_4 to each container. Remove precipitate by filtration through Whatman No. 1 paper into a 25 ml screw capped container. The clear filtrate is assayed. Extracts can be prepared a day before the assay and left at 4°C.

Reagents

- *L. leichmannii* may be obtained in the U.K. from the National Collection of Industrial and Marine Bacteria, (NC1B 8117), or in the USA from the American Type culture collection (ATCC 7830 or 4797).

- *Culture and assay media* are most conveniently obtained in dehydrated form (Difco) and reconstituted as directed.

- *Bacto B_{12} assay medium USP* (Difco) is prepared by dissolving dry powder in distilled water. 15 ml is required for each serum sample, 150 ml for the standard curve and 45 ml for washing the organism and for a reading blank.

- *Bacto-micro inoculation broth* (Difco) is dissolved as indicated and dispensed in 10 ml aliquots in screw capped containers. These are autoclaved at 121°C for 15 minutes and stored at 4°C.

- *Bacto-micro assay culture agar* (Difco) is prepared as instructed and 5 ml aliquots distributed into screw capped containers. These are autoclaved at 121°C for 15 minutes and stored at 4°C.
- *Cyanocobalamin solution.* A pharmaceutical ampoule containing 250 μg cyanocobalamin (cytamen, Glaxo, or equivalent) is opened, 1.0 ml transferred to 25% ethanol solution in distilled water (v/v) and made up to 50 ml. This contains 5.0 μg B_{12}/ml.

  40 ml of B_{12} solution (5.0 μg/ml) is made up to 1 litre in 25% ethanol. This is the stock solution (200 ng/ml) and is stored at 4°C.
- *Fresh glass-distilled water.*

Equipment
- Pyrex glass tubes 150 × 19 mm.
- Metal racks with lids holding 36 150 × 19 mm tubes.
- 25 ml capacity screw cap glass containers.
- 37°C incubator.
- Autoclave.
- Photometer.
- Pasteur pipettes — 50 drops/ml.
- Vortex mixer.

B_{12}-free serum extract
The growth of *L. leichmannii* is slightly retarded in the presence of serum extract. By adding B_{12}-free serum extract to the standard curve the growth rate becomes similar in tubes with serum extracts.

Obtain a 100 ml serum by pooling laboratory samples and add 875 ml 0.4 N cyanide-acetate buffer pH 4.5 as used for preparing serum extract. Autoclave at 116°C for 100 minutes, add 25 ml 0.2 mol K_2HPO_4 and remove precipitate by filtration through Whatman No 1 paper.

Activate three 5 g aliquots of charcoal by heating at 140°C for 2 hours (p. 140). Add 5 g charcoal to the serum extract, mix for 20 minutes and repeat with 2 further additions of charcoal. Finally remove the bulk of the charcoal by filtration through Whatman No 1 paper and finally by filtration through a mullipore filter.

Standards and controls
Standard curve. These are cyanocobalamin dilutions containing from zero to 200 pg. Make up the following B_{12} working solutions:

Initial solution:	2.0 ml stock solution to 200 ml distilled water (2 ng/ml).
Solution A:	5.0 ml initial solution to 100 ml (100 pg/ml).
Solution B:	20.0 ml solution A to 100 ml (20 pg/ml).
Solution C:	5.0 ml solution A to 500 ml (1 pg/ml).

The standard curve is made up in triplicate in 150 × 19 mm tubes as shown in Table 6.2. In addition a tube containing 3 ml water and 3 ml B_{12}-free serum extract is prepared for setting the photometer to zero. This tube should be capped to avoid inadvertent inoculation.

Wash tubes. Prepare 4 150 × 19 mm tubes each containing 5 ml water and 5 ml assay medium.

Controls

Normal serum. A pool of sera or a donation from an individual is stored in 2.5 ml aliquots at −20°C. Its value is determined in several assays, if possible, in more than one laboratory.

Serum of low B_{12} content. Several 100 ml blood should be taken before specific therapy is given, from patients with low serum B_{12} levels. The value is determined by several assays. Sera are stored at −20°C. These two sera (normal and low B_{12} content) are included in each assay.

Table 6.2 Standard curve for *L. leichmanni assay.*

Tube	Solution/volume (ml)	Water (ml)	B_{12}-free serum extract (ml)	B_{12} content (pg)
1	C 1.0	2.0	2.0	1
2	B 0.25	2.75	2.0	5
3	B 0.5	2.5	2.0	10
4	B 0.75	2.25	2.0	15
5	B 1.0	2.0	2.0	20
6	B 1.5	1.5	2.0	30
7	B 2.5	0.5	2.0	50
8	A 0.7	2.3	2.0	70
9	A 1.0	2.0	2.0	100
10	A 2.0	1.0	2.0	200
Photometer blank	— —	3.0	2.0	0

Recovery. One ml of solution A (100 pg/ml) is added to 2 ml of normal serum. This is prepared for assay as described using 15 ml (instead of 16 ml) water.

In general, all controls should assay with 10% of the expected values.

The organism

Using sterile techniques, the freeze-dried organism is suspended in 10 ml culture medium and incubated at 37°C overnight. The organism is subcultured morning and evening for 8 passages and the final overnight culture distributed in 0.25 ml aliquots into 40 2 ml screw capped sterile ampoules and stored directly in liquid nitrogen without any further manipulation. The culture should be plated out to confirm its purity.

For each assay one ampoule is removed from liquid nitrogen, thawed at room temperature and 10 ml broth inoculated from 1 drop from a sterile 50 drop Pasteur pipette. This is incubated for 6 hours at 37°C, and centrifuged at 1500 g for 5 minutes. The supernatant is decanted and the pellet is washed three times using the 10 ml sterile contents of wash tubes. Finally the culture is resuspended in the contents of the fourth wash tube and this is used to inoculate the assay.

Alternate methods of storing the organism including deep agar stabs and dried discs are acceptable.

Method

1. Set up 3 150 × 19 mm tubes for each sample.
2. Add 2 ml of serum extract to each of the 3 tubes.
3. Add 3 ml glass-distilled water to each tube.

Note. Where a low B_{12} level is expected, the amount of serum extract can be increased to 3, 4, or 5 ml and a correspondingly lesser quantity of water added.

4. Set up the standard curve (Table 6.2), blank and 4 wash tubes. Cap wash tubes and blank.
5. Add 5 ml assay medium to all tubes.
6. Place lids over the tubes in all racks and autoclave these for 10 minutes at 116°C. Allow to cool.
7. Using a sterile 50 dropper Pasteur pipette add one drop of washed *L. leichmannii* suspension to all tubes except the blank.
8. Incubate the racks at 37°C for 18–20 hours.
9. Resuspend organisms in each tube by vibrating on a vortex mixer.
10. Read the optical density of all tubes on a photometer at 540 nm, zero setting the machine with the blank.
11. Take the mean of the optical density of triplicates in the standard curve provided that they are reasonably close and plot pg B_{12} against optical density on 3-cycle semi-log paper.
12. Take the mean optical density of sample triplicates and read the B_{12} value from the plot.

Calculation

$$B_{12} \text{ level} = B_{12} \frac{\text{reading} \times \text{dilution}}{\text{volume}}$$

$$= \frac{B_{12} \text{ reading} \times 10}{2}$$

$$= B_{12} \text{ reading} \times 5 \text{ pg/ml}$$

Standard and recoveries should read within 10% of expected values.

Comments

— Appropriate use of calibrated and automated pipettes is useful in simplifying additions of serum, diluents and medium. Care must be taken in maintaining cleanliness of such equipment as traces of medium can encourage bacterial contamination.
— Irregular growth suggests unclean glass ware. Disposable tubes, if available, are an advantage.
— Poor growth indicates a declining assay organism.
— Overgrowth is due to contamination, probably of the assay organism.
— Fresh glass-distilled water must be used. Ion-exchange columns can harbour organisms which may release cobalamin.
— Growth of *L. leichmannii* is inhibited by penicillin, ampicillin, erythromycin, co-trimoxazole, folate antagonists, carbenicillin, lincomycin, chloramphenicol, cephalothin and rifampicin.

Reagents

● *0.4 N Acetate buffer, pH 4.5*
   A. sodium acetate $3H_2O$ 27.0 g in 500 ml distilled water.
   B. glacial acetic acid 11.6 ml in 500 ml distilled water. Mix 320 ml of A to 480 ml of B.
● *0.1% Sodium cyanide*
   0.5 g in 500 ml distilled water.
● *0.2 mol K_2HPO_4*
   6.96 g in 200 ml distilled water.

MICROBIOLOGICAL ASSAY FOR VITAMIN B_{12} IN SERUM USING *EUGLENA GRACILIS*

The euglenoid flagellates have an absolute requirement for vitamin B_{12}, without which they become large, with large nuclei and without the condensation of nuclear chromatin observed in replete cells (Ford & Hutner 1955, Bertaux & Valencia 1973, Bre et al 1983). Initially, the bacillaris variety of *Euglena gracilis* was used to assay vitamin B_{12} concentrations in fluids (Ross 1950, Mollin & Ross 1952). A growth response can be detected to as little as 1 ng/litre (0.73 picomolar) of added vitamin B_{12}. The organism synthesises its own folate, and is thus very sensitive to inhibition by sulphonamides. Subsequently, the z strain of *Euglena gracilis* was found to have comparable sensitivity to the bacillaris strain but grew more rapidly. This assay system became the standard assay used for measurement of vitamin B_{12} in human serum.

Assay of vitamin B_{12} with *Euglena gracilis* is inconvenient because of the long incubation period required for growth (6–7 days), special growth conditions including light and carefully controlled temperature, and because the organism is inhibited by very small concentrations of sulphonamides in the medium, other assay techniques have replaced this assay in many laboratories. Numerous studies have demonstrated that vitamin B_{12} concentrations greater than 150–200 pg/ml in serum assayed with *Euglena gracilis* reliably and almost invariably excluded significant clinical deficiency of vitamin B_{12} (Lear & Castle 1954, Anderson 1964, Raven et al 1972, Mollin et al 1976).

Euglena gracilis utilises a variety of corrinoids including all known forms of vitamin B_{12} (forms with biological activity in mammals) and several non-B_{12} corrinoids including pseudo-cobalamin (adenosine as nucleotide), Factor A (2-methyladenine as nucleotide), and certain others (Ford & Hutner 1955, Adams & McEwan 1971, Kolhouse et al 1978, Kondo et al 1982). It will not utilise cobinamide which lacks a nucleotide.

Principle

The amount of growth obtained is proportional to the amount of B_{12} available to the organism.

Release of cobalamin from endogenous ligands. Vitamin B_{12} in serum is bound to transcobalamins. Before vitamin B_{12} in serum can be assayed, it must be released from these binding proteins, since *Euglena gracilis* has little proteolytic activity.

Vitamin B_{12} concentrations which can be assayed by Euglena gracilis. Growth rate of *Euglena gracilis* is maximum in vitamin B_{12} concentrations in excess of about 30 pg/ml (20 picomolar) (Cooper 1959), but its growth rate is proportional to extracellular cobalamin below this. Samples must thus be diluted into this range for assay.

Conditions of growth. Euglena gracilis grows well at acid pH, requiring a source of energy (e.g. carbohydrate), ammonia, CO_2, a tricarboxylic acid cycle intermediate (e.g. succinate), a nitrogen source (e.g. glutamate and glycine) and thiamine. It requires illumination to produce chlorophyll which then satisfies other nutrient requirements. The minimum light required for optimal growth is about 50 foot-candles with growth decreasing at more than 75 foot-candles. The spectrum preferred has not been delineated but white visible light is effective. One would presume that the most effective light would be that with maximum absorption by the green chlorophyll.

Strains of *Euglena* are very sensitive to temperature, losing chlorophyll production at elevated temperatures, and growing poorly at low temperatures. Growth rate increases as temperature increases, with maximum growth of the z strain at 28.5°C. Growth rate at 26 and 31°C was about 80% of that at 28.5°C. At 33°C bleaching occurs, and at higher temperatures, bleaching (loss of chlorophyll) may be permanent.

Growth is slow, and maximum growth is achieved only after 6–8 days at 28.5°C. Shorter incubation times may be used during assay because growth rate is proportional to vitamin B_{12} concentration, but this is not usually done.

Growth in aqueous media is greater and more variable at any concentration of cobalamin than in the presence of serum. Growth decreased progressively with addition of serum until 1 μl of serum was added per 4 ml culture. Growth in 1 μl of serum was 85% of that in aqueous medium. Addition of serum in excess of this did not further decrease growth. Because the serum concentration decreases as the specimen is progressively diluted, inhibition of growth by serum will be most marked in assay tubes containing the lowest serum dilutions (corresponding to vitamin B_{12} content less than 200 pg/ml). Serum samples containing such concentrations of vitamin B_{12} will thus be read as containing smaller concentrations than are actually present.

Cleaning of glass ware. Growth of *Euglena gracilis* is inhibited by traces of ionic detergents. Glass ware cleaned with detergent cannot be used for the assay without meticulous washing (e.g. 15–20 times with water). Glass vessels are preferred over plastic for the assay, and disposable culture tubes and pipettes, vessels and tubes are recommended. Culture tubes must be transparent to permit even illumination of growing cultures. Some laboratories incubate the assay tubes in Erlenmeyer flasks to provide maximum light exposure. Glass test tubes are adequate.

Cultures of *Euglena gracilis* generate a vitamin B_{12} binder which makes some vitamin B_{12} unavailable for assay. Growth of the organism is faster and greater if the stock culture is washed once before use (Kristensen 1956).

Reagents

The organism

Euglena gracilis var z (ATCC no 12716) may be obtained from the American Type Culture Collection, Washington D.C., USA, or from the Culture Collection of Algae, Department of Botany, University of Indiana,

Bloomingdale, Indiana. The organism is subcultured weekly in assay medium containing vitamin B_{12}. *Euglena gracilis* is aerobic.

Glass ware
○ Euglena gracilis cultures are maintained in 150 × 16 mm screw-capped test tubes.
○ Assays utilise 150 × 16 mm screw-capped disposable test tubes (Pyrex Corning).
○ Pipettes are disposable, graduated glass or plastic pipettes in sizes of 10 ml, 5 ml and 1 ml (non-sterile) and 1 ml sterile graduated disposable pipettes.
○ Large flasks and beakers (Pyrex) are cleaned with water, immersed in sulphuric acid-chromate solution for 1 hour and rinsed with 15 changes of tap water and 5 changes of distilled water.

Solutions
● *Water* is glass-distilled followed by filtration through an IWT research ion exchanger to produce deionised water.
● *Medium* is purchased from Difco Corporation (Euglena Vitamin B_{12} Assay Medium) and prepared double strength in deionised water. It is sterilised by autoclaving and stored in 2 litre volumes at 4°C for up to 2 weeks.
● *Vitamin B_{12}* (cyanocobalamin) is purchased from Sigma Corporation and diluted to a concentration of 2000 pg/ml. This solution may be stored at −20°C for up to 6 months. 1:10 dilutions used for assay are stored in aliquots at −20°C.

Pools of 'high B_{12} serum' and 'low B_{12} serum' are collected from samples assayed, and stored at −20°C in 1 ml aliquots. A sample of each is assayed with each assay. Each pool is used for 2–3 months.

Test samples
Serum is separated from blood taken without anticoagulant and is stored as single aliquots at −20°C until assayed. The frozen samples are thawed at room temperature, and refrozen until after the assay is read. The vitamin B_{12} concentration in these is essentially unchanged when re-assayed. Sera are stored in the dark without precautions to exclude light.

Equipment
● *Incubator*. The incubator is a cabinet with vertically-sliding front in which are four 30 inch 15 watt fluorescent light tubes lying horizontally on the bottom and 4 similar fixtures arranged vertically along the sides and back. Two glass shelves are suspended approximately 30 cm above the lights on the bottom, and with the same interval between the shelves. A thermostat is placed against the back wall of the cabinet. If the ambient temperature is consistently less than 25°C, then the thermostat is attached to a heater; if often above 25°C, the thermostat is attached to a fan which evacuates air from the cabinet and permits entry of air from the room. A simple heater can be constructed from a 100 watt incandescent light bulb placed inside a metal can, but many heating arrangements are possible. A thermometer is placed on one of the shelves and temperature is monitored daily so as to maintain incubation temperature between 27 and 31°C.

Assay tubes may be incubated in wire test tube racks. If light is inadequate, the bottoms of the racks may be removed to permit the assay tubes to rest directly on the glass shelves. Racks are moved to different positions within the incubator every 2–3 days.

If assays require only a single shelf, then vertical light fixtures are not required.
● *Racks* Wire or clear plastic racks holding 150 × 16 mm tubes in rows of 4.
● *Colorimeter* with red filter reading at 600 nm.
● *Automatic pipette* delivering 2.0 ml quantities.

Method
1. Four assay tubes are labelled for each sample. 1.75 ml of water is placed in tube 1, and 1 ml into each of the other tubes.

2. 0.25 ml of well-mixed serum is pipetted into tube 1 using a 1 ml graduated pipette, mixed with a fresh 1 ml pipette, and serial dilutions of 1 ml are made into each of the 4 other tubes using the same pipette as used to mix tube 1. 1 ml is discarded from tube 4.

3. Duplicate standard curves are prepared using the 200 pg/ml solution of cyanocobalamin. The serial dilutions are identical to those for serum, viz: 0.25 ml of the cyanocobalamin solution is added to 1.75 ml of water, and 1 ml of this mixture is pipetted into 1 ml of tube 2, mixed, and 1 ml transferred to tube 3, etc. When the serial dilutions have been completed, 1 ml is discarded from tube 4. These tubes contain 50, 25, 12.5 and 6.25 pg B_{12} respectively (Table 6.3).

Table 6.3 Assay procedure using *Euglena gracilis*.

| | Tube number (volumes in ml) | | | |
	1	2	3	4
Water	1.75	1.0	1.0	1.0
B_{12} 200 pg/ml or serum	0.25; serial dilutions of 1.0 ml into tubes 2–4. Discard 1 ml from tube 4.			
Medium (double-strength)	1.0	1.0	1.0	1.0
Blank	1 ml water + 1 ml of medium			

4. Two assay tubes containing only medium and water without added vitamin B_{12} are also inoculated as 'blanks'.

5. 1 ml of double-strength medium is added to each assay tube of the standard curve, pools of control serum and serum samples to be assayed. This utilises an automatic pipette.

6. Samples are autoclaved for 10 minutes at $+1$ atmosphere pressure.

7. Samples are removed from the autoclave and cooled at room temperature for 30–60 minutes until all tubes are cool to the touch.

8. The inoculum is prepared by adding a 4–8 day culture of *Euglena gracilis* drop wise to a sterile test tube containing 5 ml of sterile water and 5 ml of sterile double-strength medium until a definite greenish tinge is visible.

9. Each test tube is inoculated with 1 drop of the inoculum, observing sterile precautions. Inoculation utilises a sterile Pasteur pipette with care not to touch the pipette tip to the solution or tube. The pipette tip is changed after each 4-tube series. Tubes are placed in racks, caps are removed one at a time, they are inoculated and the hand-held cap is replaced. One standard curve is inoculated as the first assay inoculated, and the other as the last.

10. Reading the assay. After 6–7 days of incubation, the assay tubes are removed from the incubator, and the optical density of the standard curve is read. Optical density is read with a red filter to recognise both turbidity and intensity of green colour. A Spectronic 20 grating type colorimeter (Bauch and Lomb) is a convenient apparatus, with the centre of the band width at 600 nm. We have inserted a flow cell into the colorimeter (volume 2 ml) to facilitate reading. The colorimeter is set to 0 optical density using the blank tubes. These should read about 0.04 against water.

Optical density of each series of dilutions is determined beginning with the greatest dilution (tube 4), and rinsing the colorimeter with water only after all 4 tubes of a series are read. If the optical density of the standard curve is not adequate (based on experience), then all tubes are incubated for an additional day.

Calculation

When optical density on an arithmetic scale is plotted against vitamin B_{12} concentration using a logarithmic scale, an S-shaped curve is obtained. The straight portion of the curve (between 50 pg and 3.125 pg of vitamin B_{12} added) is used to calculate the vitamin B_{12} content of samples.

Alternative techniques

Assay medium may be prepared on site as described in Table 6.4. Water may be glass-distilled only, or in some

Table 6.4 Composition of assay medium for *Euglena gracilis*.

Dry mix

Material	Concentration in grams per 100 ml	Grams for 10 litres of double-strength medium
KH_2PO_4	30	3.0
$MgSO_4.7H_2O$	40	4.0
L-glutamic acid	300	30.0
$CaCO_3$	8	.8
Sucrose	1500	150.0
DL-aspartic acid	200	20.0
DL-Malic acid	100	10.0
Glycine	250	25.0
Ammonium succinate	60	6.0
Thiamine HCl*	.06	.6
Metals**	2.2	.22

* Triturate of 1 gm of thiamine HCl + 99 g of sucrose.
** For 1000 litres of final medium mix 14 gm $FeSO_4$, $(NH_4)2SO_4.6H_2O$, 4.4 gm $ZnSO_4.7H_2O$, 1.55 gm $MnSO_4.H_2O$, .31 gm, $CuSO_4.5H_2O$, .48 gm $CoSO_4.7H_2O$ .57 gm, H_3BO_3 64 gm, $(NH_4)6Mo_7O_{24}.4H_2O$, and .093 gm $Na_3VO_4.16H_2O$ and store in a dry place.
The basal medium is made up double-strength by dissolving the ingredients in distilled water by steaming for 15 minutes, pH is adjusted to 3.6 with NaOH or H_2SO_4, medium is filtered and autoclaved at 116°C for 15 minutes.

locations tap water may be deionised before sterilisation.

Vitamin B_{12} should be purchased chemically pure and care exerted in preparation of standards. Many commercial preparations contain considerably more vitamin B_{12} than indicated on the label. The concentration of the stock solution may be verified by measuring optical density at 361 nm using the well-established extinction coefficient of cyanocobalamin (28,100).

Vitamin B_{12} may be added to the standard curve in known concentrations using micro litre pipettes rather than using serial dilutions. The same volumes of serum must then be assayed.

Samples may be boiled for 15 minutes in a water-bath instead of autoclaving.

The organism may be maintained in single-strength assay medium containing 0.2% tryptone and 50 pg/ml of vitamin B_{12}. These are centrifuged in a bench centrifuge, supernatant removed and the cultures resuspended twice in 20 ml of single-strength medium. The inoculum used may be a 1:20 dilution of this. *Euglena gracilis* may be maintained for long periods as stabs in Trypticase 0.2% and 0.25% agar.

Incubation may be in a glass water-bath with illumination from below which will provide better temperature control than the system described above. Details of this water-bath incubator are described by Anderson (1964).

Comments

— Some assay curves may not be parallel to the standard curve. This may occur due to:

a. high serum concentrations with inhibition of growth in low dilutions.

b. presence of medications in the serum (viz sulphonamides, trimethoprim, phenothiazines, tetracycline, or other drugs).

c. very low levels of vitamin B_{12} in serum such that none of the assay tubes contain enough vitamin B_{12} to support growth.

d. very high concentrations of vitamin B_{12} in serum.

e. certain unexplained causes.

For accurate measurement of very high concentrations of vitamin B_{12}, re-assay using 1:20 dilution of the serum is required. We usually are content to report the result as 'greater than 200 pg/ml'.

For others of the above, examination of the curve often will demonstrate a portion of the assay curve which permits approximation of the concentration of vitamin B_{12}. These are reported as 'equal to or greater than ___ pg/ml'

In others, vitamin B_{12} level cannot be calculated. These represent less than 1% of all sera assayed.

— Precipitation of protein may be observed in some assay tubes containing small dilutions of serum due to increase of pH from 3–4 of the assay to above 6 due to growth of the organism. This is uncommon using the dilutions and the growth medium described above. The growth medium is buffered, representing a significant improvement over media used originally.

— Irregular results may be observed. These usually represent contamination of the *Euglena* culture with fungi which will grow at low pH. A new culture or subculture of a culture of *Euglena* organism used in a previous assay may resolve this.

— All results may be elevated because of contamination of solutions with vitamin B_{12}. This may occur if fungi grow in the de-ionizing column.

— Growth may be poor because of inadequate temperature control or occasionally because of an ineffective batch of assay medium.

VITAMIN B_{12} ASSAY BY SOLID PHASE SATURATION ANALYSIS

Principle

Vitamin B_{12} in serum is mixed with a standard amount of isotopically labelled B_{12} and an aliquot taken up by a protein binding B_{12}, namely, gastric intrinsic factor. The more B_{12} present in the serum the greater the dilution of the labelled B_{12}, and hence less isotope is taken up on the B_{12} binder. This is illustrated in Fig. 6.3. This is utilised in a quantitative assay.

Test samples

Sera are assayed and these are stored at $-20°C$ until required.

Preparation for assay

To a glass screw-capped container add:

Serum	1.0 ml
Acetate-cyanide buffer pH 4.65	9.0 ml

Autoclave at 116°C for 10 minutes or place in a boiling water-bath for 30 minutes. Cool, and filter through No 1 Whatman paper. The clear filtrate is retained for assay. It may be stored at 4°C till required.

Reagents

● *Sodium cyanide 10 mg/ml*

Wearing disposable gloves weigh out 1 g of sodium cyanide and dissolve in 100 ml of glass-distilled water. Label and store in poisons cupboard.

● *Cyanocobalamin standard 200 ng/ml*

Add 400 μl of 250 μg/ml cyanocobalamin solution (Glaxo Pharmaceuticals, Cytamen ampoules) to a 500 ml volumetric flask containing 25% ethanol in glass-

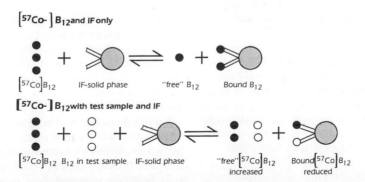

Fig. 6.3 The principle of the solid phase B_{12} assay.

distilled water. Adjust the volume to 500 ml and store at 4°C in an amber glass bottle.

• *Phosphate-buffered saline/azide*

1 g of sodium azide dissolved in 1 litre of sterile phosphate buffered saline (PBS, p. 140).

• *Gastric juice*

Gastric juice is collected, depepsinised and stored at −20° in 10 ml volumes (p. 139). The IF concentration should be greater than 30 ng units/ml and non-IF binding proteins should be as low as possible, but up to 20% of the total binding capacity of the gastric juice is acceptable.

• *Albumin stock solution*

1 g of bovine albumin (Armour Pharmaceuticals, Fraction V) dissolved in 50 ml of glass-distilled water. Store 2 ml volumes at −20°C.

Preparation of solid phase human intrinsic factor

Human intrinsic factor is coupled to polyacrylamide beads (Immunobead reagent, Biorad Laboratories) using 1-ethyl-3(3-dimethylamino propyl) carbodiimide HCl, (EDAC, Sigma Chemicals). At pH 5.3 only IF is coupled and not R-binder.

To prepare 20 mls of reagent:

1. Prepare 2 l of 0.0005 M acetate buffer pH 5.3 and thaw out an aliquot of gastric juice and albumin (p. 140).

2. Dialyse the gastric juice and albumin overnight at 4°C against 500 ml each of acetate buffer pH 5.3.

3. Reconstitute one 20 ml/200 mg bottle of immunobeads with 20 ml of acetate buffer, wash into a glass Universal 25–30 ml container and centrifuge 1000 g/10 min. Wash the beads with two further 20 ml volumes of acetate buffer and discard the supernatant.

4. To the pellet add 1 ml of dialysed albumin, sufficient dialysed gastric juice to contain 200 ng of IF and acetate buffer to bring the volume to 20 ml.

5. Adjust pH to 5.3, leave for 30 minutes at room temperature and re-check pH is pH 5.3.

6. Weigh out 20 mg of EDAC from a fresh previously unopened bottle and add to the coupling reaction mixture. Mix carefully but thoroughly for 10 minutes.

7. Maintain the pH at 5.3 by measuring and adjusting as necessary at 15 minute intervals for 1 hour.

8. The mixture may then be left continuously mixing at room temperature for 2 hours or overnight at 4°C.

9. Centrifuge and wash the pellet with two 20 ml volumes of acetate buffer. Resuspend the pellet in PBS and distribute into two 50 ml plastic centrifuge tubes, make volumes up to 50 ml each with PBS and centrifuge.

10. Suspend the pellets in 50 ml each of cold (4°C) PBS containing 1.4 M NaCl, centrifuge immediately at 4°C. Wash the pellets with cold PBS and stand overnight at 4°C.

11. Wash pellets with PBS containing 1% (w/v) bovine albumin then repeat with two washes with PBS-azide.

12. The two pellets of beads should be pooled and the volume made to 20 mls with PBS-azide. Store at 4°C until titrated.

Titration of solid phase IF

1. Wash 100 μl of IF beads suspension into 10 ml of acetate-cyanide-tween buffer (p. 127), centrifuge at 1000 g for 10 minutes and resuspend pellet with 5 ml acetate-cyanide-tween buffer.

2. Set out 5 pairs of B_{12} assay tubes and place 50 μl, 100 μl, 250 μl, 500 μl and 1000 μl (equivalent to 1 μl to 20 μl of neat reagent per tube) volumes of IF beads into these tubes. Make the volumes to 2.1 ml with acetate-cyanide-tween buffer.

3. Prepare 2 ml of $[^{57}Co]B_{12}$ working solution (p. 140). Pipette 100 μl volumes into each tube and into two additional tubes to be used as counting standards.

4. Mix the tubes containing IF beads by inversion and stand at room temperature for 3 hours. Centrifuge the pellet with 3.8 ml of acetate-cyanide-tween buffer. Centrifuge again, discard the supernatant and count the $[^{57}Co]B_{12}$ bound to the IF beads.

5. Plot the counts in each tube as a percentage of the total $[^{57}Co]B_{12}$ used per tube against the volume of neat reagent per tube.

6. The volume of IF beads that binds 35–45% of the $[^{57}Co]B_{12}$ should be used in the serum B_{12} assay.

7. After titration the IF beads may be stored at −20°C or freeze-dried in suitable volumes each being sufficient for one month's assays.

Equipment

○ Isotope counter $[^{57}Co]$.

○ B_{12} assay tubes, capped polystyrene 4 ml centrifuge tubes.

○ Dispensers to deliver 9 ml, 3.8 ml, 1 ml and 100 μl and convenient for repetitive additions.

○ Pipettes to deliver volumes from 20 μl to 1 ml for preparing standard curve dilutions.

Standards and controls

1. Whole serum. Sera with less than 50 pg/ml, 150–200 pg/ml and 450–650 pg/ml are suitable for low, borderline and high normal controls. Sera should be stored in 1.5 ml volumes at −20°C.

2. Recovery of added B_{12} is assessed as shown on page 121.

Working reagents

● *Buffers.*

Three buffers are used in the assay:

Acetate-cyanide-acetate buffer 0.5 M pH 4.65 containing 25 μg/ml NaCN (ACCN).

Acetate-tween buffer 0.5 M pH 4.65 containing 1% v/v Tween 20 (ACTW).

Acetate-cyanide-tween buffer — equal volumes of ACCN and ACTW.

Prepare buffers fresh each week.

● *B_{12} Standard working solution.*

Dilute stock B_{12} standard solution (p. 140) 1 in 1000 in acetate-cyanide-tween to give a 200 pg/ml working solution.

● *$[^{57}Co]B_{12}$* (Amersham, high specific activity)

This is usually supplied as 1 ml volume containing 10 μCi $[^{57}Co]$ and approximateiy 50 ng B_{12}. Immediately before use dilute a suitable aliquot to give a 750 pg/ml working solution sufficient for 100 μl per assay tube.

● *Solid phase intrinsic factor*

A working suspension is prepared immediately before use. The stock suspension is diluted in acetate-cyanide-tween so that 100 μl binds **35–45%** of the $[^{57}Co]B_{12}$ used per tube. The volume of stock suspension required should be washed once with acetate-cyanide-tween buffer before making up to final volume for use.

Method

1. Number racks and tubes for the assay and for controls. Blank, counting standard, reference and the 6 standard curve tubes are set up in triplicate. Keep counting standard separate from other assay racks. All tests and controls are set up in duplicate.

2. Prepare blank, reference and standard curve tubes (Table 6.5).

Table 6.5 Protocol for serum B_{12} standard curve.

	ACCN buffer (ml)	B_{12} standard working solution (ml)	B_{12} (pg/tube)
Blank	2.1	0	0
Reference	2.0	0	0
Standard 1	1.98	20	4
2	1.95	50	10
3	1.90	100	20
4	1.75	250	50
5	1.625	375	75
6	1.5	500	100

3. Dispense 1 ml of acetate-tween buffer into all test and control tubes.

4. Place 1 ml of each serum extract into test and control tubes.

5. Carefully pipette 100 μl of $[^{57}Co]B_{12}$ working solution into the three tubes as counting standards and place on one side; these should not be inverted.

6. Add 100 μl of $[^{57}Co]B_{12}$ to all other assay tubes.

7. Cap blank tubes.

8. Prepare IF bead suspension and dispense 100 μl into all tubes except counting standards and blanks.

9. Cap tubes and mix by inversion.

10. Incubate at room temperature for 4 hours.

11. Centrifuge all tubes, except counting standard, at 1000 g for 10 minutes, discard supernatant and wash pellet with 3.8 ml acetate-cyanide-tween. Centrifuge and discard supernatant.

12. Count $[^{57}Co]B_{12}$ in all tubes and in counting standards.

Units

Serum B_{12} levels are reported as pg/ml.

Calculation

The method of calculating the results depends on the facilities available. Most modern gamma isotope counters have programmable facilities for standard curve fitting and calculation of the concentrations in test samples. This assay is run routinely with a spline function curve fitting (LKB multigamma 1260). Alternatively a manual plot of $[^{57}Co]$ cpm versus B_{12} in the standard curve can be made on three cycle semi-log paper (Fig. 6.4). Counts in the bound $[^{57}Co]B_{12}$ of the test samples are read off the curve in pg/tube and converted to pg/ml.

B_{12} pg/tube × dilution factor (10) = B_{12} pg/ml.

Comments

— EDAC used for coupling IF does not store well and 'older' samples result in variable coupling. Use a new bottle for each preparation.

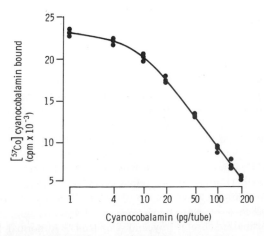

Fig. 6.4 Standard curve in the solid phase B_{12} assay.

— Buffers containing cyanide are at an acid pH which avoids the problems associated with cyanate formation, but it is recommended that buffers are prepared freshly each week.

— $[^{57}Co]B_{12}$ working solution is prepared directly from the material supplied by the manufacturer and the manufacturers storage instructions followed. New batches of reagent should be compared with old batches to guard against inactive impurities.

— Batch to batch variation in the specific activity of the $[^{57}Co]B_{12}$ will produce small shifts in the standard curve. If this is important for quality control procedures then an estimate of the true B_{12} content of the working solution should be made. This is most simply performed by preparing 3 extra reference tubes containing 200 μl rather than 100 μl of $[^{57}Co]B_{12}$ working solution. The counts bound in these tubes are divided by 2 and the pg/tube read off the standard curve. This is the concentration of B_{12} in 100 μl of the $[^{57}Co]B_{12}$ working solution and should be 75 pg.

— The preparation of the IF beads requires the balancing of many factors and the combination described consistently gives a reagent suitable for B_{12} radioassay use.

— The incubation time required for different batches of IF beads to reach equilibrium may vary but has never been above 4 hours. If shorter incubation times are preferred then a comparison with a 4-hour incubation is essential, particularly for sera with low B_{12} content.

— The immunobeads remain in suspension for at least 2 hours and then only sediment slowly. An additional mix after 2 hours of incubation is recommended.

— After centrifugation the IF bead-pellet formed is very stable provided decanting is performed as one smooth inversion, touching the mouth of the tube against adsorbent paper to remove the last drop of liquid.

Interpretation

The normal range for serum B_{12} is 170 to 1000 pg/ml. Reduced levels are normal in pregnancy due to preferential transfer of dietary B_{12} to placenta and fetus. The majority of strict life-long vegetarians have low serum cobalamin levels while remaining normoblastic.

All patients with untreated megaloblastic anaemia due to B_{12} deficiency must have low B_{12} levels. A few patients with chronic myeloid leukaemia complicated by B_{12} deficiency have 'normal' levels. This is due to the presence of very high levels of transcobalamin I in plasma in chronic myeloid leukaemia. A normal B_{12} level in a patient with megaloblastic anaemia (who does not have chronic myeloid leukaemia) excludes B_{12} deficiency as the cause.

Finding a low serum B_{12} level, however, does not necessarily mean B_{12} deficiency, as in pregnancy or in patients with simple atrophic gastritis (Whiteside et al 1964). Such patients are usually normoblastic, absorb B_{12} normally and have normal B_{12} stores on liver biopsy.

Finally, about one-third of patients with megaloblastic anaemia due to primary folate deficiency have a low serum B_{12} level. In these patients treatment with folic acid alone restores the serum B_{12} level to within the normal range within 10 days. All these patients too absorb B_{12} normally (Chanarin 1979).

Thus it is incorrect always to correlate a low B_{12} level with B_{12} deficiency. The circumstances accompanying the low B_{12} level must be considered. In general in those patients in whom B_{12} absorption is normal, or in those patients with a normal blood count and a normoblastic marrow, a low serum B_{12} level does not indicate deficiency.

Elevation of serum B_{12} levels above 1000 pg/ml may occur with liver cell damage (acute hepatitis), and myeloproliferative disorders particularly chronic myeloid leukaemia, polycythaemia rubra vera and chronic myelofibrosis.

FOLATE ASSAY

Assay of the folate levels in serum and red cells is part of the investigation of folate deficiency, usually in patients with megaloblastic anaemia.

Two methods are described:
1. Microbiological assay with *Lactobacillus casei*.
2. Saturation analysis isotope assay.

FOLATE ASSAY WITH *LACTOBACILLUS CASEI*

Principle

L. casei requires preformed folate for growth. The assay medium contains all the ingredients required for growth except folate. The amount of growth is thus determined by the amount of folate supplied either in the standard curve or in the blood sample being assayed.

Test samples

Serum. This must be completely free of haemolysis. Red cells contain 30-fold more folate than serum and even traces of haemolysis will raise the serum folate considerably. If samples are not assayed within a few days, dry ascorbate (up to 5 mg per ml) is added and the serum kept at $-20°C$.

Red cells Whole blood is collected into anticoagulant, usually EDTA but heparin is equally suitable. The haematocrit is measured. One part of whole blood is added to 9 parts 1% ascorbic acid in distilled water (w/v). This is left at room temperature for about an hour and stored at $-20°C$ until assay. Ascorbate not only preserves folate but the resulting pH (4.5) is optimum for the plasma conjugase enzyme which converts methylfolatepolyglutamates in red cells into monoglutamates. Only the monoglutamates produce maximal growth of *L. casei*

Preparation for assay. Add 0.1 ml serum or red cell lysate to 9.9 ml 0.1 M phosphate buffer pH 5.7 (p. 131). Autoclave for 10 minutes at 116°C. Remove precipitate by filtration through Whatman No. 1 filter paper into 25 ml screw-capped containers. The clear filtrate is assayed. Extracts can be prepared a day before the assay and left at 4°C.

Reagents

- *L. casei* may be obtained in the U.K. from the National Collection of Industrial and Marine Bacteria (NCIMB 8081), and in the USA from the American Type Culture Collection (ATCC 7469).
- *Culture and assay media* are most conveniently purchased in dehydrated form, from Difco laboratories or Dano Laboratories and reconstituted as directed. Cultures are grown in Bacto lactobacilli broth AOAC made up in 10 ml aliquots.

  For assay the appropriate amount of dehydrated, double-strength assay medium is weighed out and dissolved in distilled water. It is brought to the boil for 1–2 minutes and then allowed to cool. Ascorbic acid, 2 g/litre is added and the pH of the medium adjusted with 2 M-NaOH to 6.8. When mixed with an equal volume of phosphate buffer pH 5.7 the final pH is about 6.2, which is necessary for the growth response of *L. casei* to methyltetrahydrofolate (in serum and red cells) to equal that of pteroylglutamic acid (in the standard curve).
- *0.1 M phosphate buffer pH 5.7*
- *Pteroylglutamic acid* (Sigma). New batches are dried at 140°C for 2 hours and stored in a dessicator under P_2O_5. Handling of folate should be done well away from the areas where the assay is to be done. 100 mg of pteroylglutamic acid (PteGlu) is made up to 100 ml in 0.01 N NaOH. The folate content is determined by its absorption in 0.1 N NaOH at 365 nm, a 1.0 mg/100 ml solution having an absorbance of 0.199 using a 1 cm light path. Should the absorbance show that only 90% of the solution be pteroylglutamic acid, a corresponding adjustment is made in making up the stock solution. 10 ml of the initial folate solution (10 mg) is made up to 1 litre with 0.01 N NaOH containing 20% ethanol. This stock solution is stored in a dark bottle at 4°C.
- *Fresh glass-distilled water.*

Equipment

○ Pyrex glass test tubes 150 × 19 mm.
○ Metal racks with lids holding 36 × 19 mm tubes.
○ 25 ml capacity screw-cap glass containers.
○ 37°C incubator.
○ Autoclave.
○ Photometer.
○ Pasteur pipettes — 50 drops/ml.
○ Vortex mixer.

Standards and controls

Standard curve

These are folate dilutions containing between zero to 1.0 ng folate per tube. Dilute the stock solution of pteroylglutamic acid (10 µg/ml) as follows in phosphate buffer pH5.7.

Solution A. 25 ml stock to 1000 ml (250 ng/ml).
Solution B. 20 ml solution A to 500 ml (10 ng/ml).
Solution C. 10 ml solution B to 100 ml (1 ng/ml).
Solution D. 20 ml solution C to 100 ml (0.2 ng/ml).

Using dilutions C and D the standard curve is prepared in triplicate in 150 × 19 mm test tubes as set out in Table 6.6. At the same time as setting up the curve it is convenient to prepare a blank tube for zero setting of the photometer, and also solutions to be used for washing the *L. casei* culture prior to inoculating the assay. It is useful to cap the blank tube to ensure that it is not inoculated in error.

Table 6.6 The standard curve for the *L. casei* assay.

Folate content (ng/tube)	Folate solution (ml)		Phosphate buffer (ml)
Zero	Zero	0.25	2.0
0.05	Soln. D	0.5	1.75
0.1	Soln	1.0	1.5
0.2	Soln	1.5	1.0
0.3	Soln	2.0	0.5
0.4	Soln	0.5	Zero
0.5	Soln. C	0.75	1.5
0.75	Soln	1.0	1.25
1.0	Soln		1.0
Blank (1)	Zero		2.0
Washing solution (×4)	Zero		5.0

Controls

Serum. Either a pool of fresh sera or a donation from one individual is prepared, ascorbate 5 mg/ml added and stored at $-20°C$ in 1 ml aliquots. Its value is best determined by several assays, if possible, in more than one laboratory. A sample is included in each assay. Such a pool will retain its folate activity for up to 1 year but not longer. Excess ascorbate must not be added as it may interfere with subsequent protein precipitation.

Haemolysate. A haemolysate is prepared as described for single whole blood samples and stored in 1 ml aliquots at $-20°C$.

Recovery. To 0.5 ml of both serum and haemolysate add 0.5 ml of folate solution B (l0 ng/ml). These are treated and assayed as normal samples.

In general, all controls should assay within 10% of the expected values.

The organism

Using sterile techniques the freeze-dried organism is suspended in 10 ml culture medium and incubated at 37°C overnight. The organism is subcultured into fresh broth morning and evening for 4 days (8 passages). The final overnight culture is distributed in 0.25 ml aliquots into 40 2 ml screw-capped sterile ampoules and stored directly in liquid nitrogen without any further manipulation. The culture should be plated out to check its purity.

For each assay one ampoule is removed from liquid nitrogen, thawed at room temperature and 10 ml broth inoculated with 1 drop from a 50 drop sterile Pasteur pipette. This is incubated for 6 hours at 37°C, and centrifuged at 1500 g for 5 minutes. The supernatant is decanted and the pellet washed three times using 10 ml sterile contents of wash tubes set up with the standard curve. Finally the organisms are resuspended in the contents of the fourth wash tube, which is used to inoculate the assay.

Alternative methods of storing the organism, including deep agar stabs and dried discs, are acceptable.

Method

1. Set up 3 150 × 19 mm tubes for each sample.
2. Add 2 ml serum or haemolysate extract to each set of 3 tubes.
3. Set up the standard curve, blank and wash tubes as set out in Table 6.6.
4. Add 2 ml assay medium to all tubes except the 4 wash tubes.
5. Add 5 ml assay medium + 5 ml 0.1 M phosphate buffer pH 5.7 to the 4 wash tubes.
6. Place lids over the tubes in all racks and autoclave these for 10 minutes at 116°C. Protect the blank with a cap to avoid inadvertent inoculation.

Allow to cool.

7. Using a sterile 50 dropper Pasteur pipette add one drop of washed *L. casei* suspension to all tubes except the blank.
8. Incubate the racks at 37°C for 18–20 hours.
9. Add 5 ml distilled water to all tubes.
10. Mix each tube on a vortex mixer and read the optical density at 625 nm using the blank to zero the photometer.
11. Take the mean of the optical density of triplicates in the standard curve provided they are reasonably close and plot these on squared paper against the folate content.
12. Take the mean optical density of sample triplicates and read the folate content from the plot.

Calculation
Serum folate

$$\frac{\text{ng/folate} \times \text{dilution (100)}}{\text{volume of extract assayed (2 ml)}} = \text{ng/ml}$$

Red cell folate

$$\frac{\text{ng/folate} \times \text{dilution (1000)}}{\text{volume of extract assayed (2 ml)}} \times \frac{100}{\text{PCV}}$$

$$= \text{ng/ml packed red cell}$$

Comments
— Appropriate use of calibrated pipettes is useful in setting up the assay.
— A manual continuous delivery system is useful for adding buffer and assay medium. Care must be taken in cleaning out such equipment as traces of medium will lead to bacterial colonisation of the tubing. The Oxford pipettor (BCL) can be autoclaved.
— Irregular growth suggests unclean glass ware. Disposable tubes, if available, are an advantage.
— Although the assay medium can be made up from simpler ingredients, the difficulty of ensuring that all components are folate-free makes this undesirable in practice. However, on occasion even batches of dehydrated complete assay media may be contaminated with folate.
— Poor growth generally indicates the need to obtain a new assay organism.
— Overgrowth of all tubes is due to contamination, and the likely source is contamination of the assay organism.
— Fresh glass-distilled water must be used. Ion-exchange columns can and do acquire their own bacterial flora which can contribute folate and cobalamin to the water.

Interpretation
The normal range of serum folate is 3–25 ng/ml.

The normal range for red cell folate is 145–600 ng/ml packed red cells. A low serum folate indicates a negative folate balance, that is, less folate is entering plasma from dietary and other sources than is being consumed. This situation can arise after a few days of dietary restriction, for example, after surgery. However it is not a good index of total folate stores which normally last for 3–4 months in the absence of significant folate intake.

In erythropoiesis folate is incorporated by the developing erythroblast, some is lost from the reticulocyte but thereafter the folate is no longer metabolised in the red cell. Change in red cell folate is relatively slow because it depends on release of red cells from the marrow of different folate content. A low red cell folate is unequivocal evidence of folate deficiency.

Reticulocytes have a high folate content, and hence a misleadingly high red cell folate value is obtained in assaying blood with a raised reticulocyte level.

Not only is the red cell folate low in folate deficiency but it is also low in two-thirds of patients with megaloblastic anaemia due to cobalamin deficiency. However in the latter situation the serum folate is usually normal or, in 1 in 10 patients, even elevated.

Composition of solutions
0.1 M phosphate buffer

A.	Sodium dihydrogen orthophosphate	$NaH_2PO_4.2H_2O$	31.2 g to 1000 ml
B.	Disodium hydrogen orthophosphate anhydrous	Na_2HPO_4	28.4 g to 1000 ml

Add 425 ml A and 75 ml B to 500 ml distilled water, add 1.5 g ascorbic acid and re-adjust to pH 5.7.

SATURATION ANALYSIS FOR FOLATE ASSAY

Biochemical basis
The folate in serum is almost entirely in the form of N^5-methyltetrahydrofolate (methyl-H_4PteGlu) monoglutamate which circulates free, or weakly and non-specifically bound to albumin. In erythrocytes, folates are present as polyglutamates of methyl-H_4PteGlu with varying numbers of glutamic acid residues and they are also not bound to any specific binding proteins.

The naturally-occurring folate-binding proteins (FBP) are used as the binding ligands in the radioassays for serum and erythrocyte folate. These FBPs, however, have a higher affinity for the oxidised folate, pteroylglutamic acid (PteGlu), than for the reduced methyl-H_4-PteGlu. Since [^{3}H]PteGlu is used as the radiolabelled tracer, in a competitive assay the FBP will preferentially bind the tracer rather than methyl-H_4PteGlu, thus reducing the sensitivity of the assay. The sensi-tivity of the assay can be increased by using a sequential non-competitive procedure in which the tracer folate is added to the reaction after the methyl-H_4PteGlu standards or test samples are incubated with the FBP (Rothenberg et al 1972). A dose response curve with a sensitivity of 15 pg of methyl-H_4PteGlu can be obtained by this method.

Test samples

Serum Venous blood, preferably a fasting specimen without any anticoagulant, is allowed to clot at room temperature. Separate the serum by centrifugation at 3000 rpm for 10 minutes and store at $-20°C$ after the addition of ascorbic acid, 5 mg/ml. If the serum is assayed on the same day ascorbate can be omitted. Serum folate stored with ascorbate is stable for a month at $-20°C$ and for a week at $4°C$. Folate is measured without deproteinisation. However, if the serum contains a high concentration of unsaturated folate binding protein (vide infra), the folates are extracted by boiling the serum. This is done by pipetting 1 volume of serum into a screw capped Pyrex test tube. Add 4 volumes of Ringer's solution containing ascorbic acid, 500 mg/100 ml, adjusted to pH 4.9 with 1 N NaOH and boil in a water-bath for 5 minutes. Centrifuge at 3000 rpm for 10 minutes and separate the supernatant solution. Assay immediately or store at $-20°C$.

Erythrocytes Collect whole blood into EDTA or heparin. Prepare the haemolysate by centrifuging the blood in a graduated test tube at 3000 rpm for 5 minutes. Remove sufficient plasma to adjust the PCV to 50% and then resuspend the erythrocytes. Pipette 0.1 ml of this suspension into 2.4 ml of distilled water, shake and allow to stand for 5 minutes. Add 2.5 ml of Ringer's solution containing ascorbic acid, 500 mg/100 ml, pH 4.9, and allow to stand at room temperature for an additional 5 minutes. Centrifuge at 3000 rpm for 10 minutes and separate the supernate. Store at $-20°C$ until assayed.

Folate activity is not lost when the haemolysate is stored at $-20°C$ for 2–3 months. Whole blood can be stored at $4°C$ for 5 days without ascorbate and without loss of erythrocyte folate. Haemolysates cannot be stored without ascorbate.

Reagents
- Ringer's solution containing 0.5% ascorbic acid (pH 4.9) for the preparation of erythrocyte haemolysates and the extraction of serum.
- Reaction buffer — borate Ringer's buffer with 0.2% ascorbic acid (pH 8).
- Binder diluent — 1% charcoal-treated ovalbumin.
- Binding protein — β-lactoglobulin (Sigma Chemical Co.).

- 2.5% neutral charcoal suspended in 0.125% bovine haemoglobin.
- D,L-5-methyltetrahydrofolic acid (Sigma Chemical Co.).
- [^{3}H]Pteroylglutamic acid (Amersham).
- Scintillation counting fluid.

Equipment
○ Standard laboratory glassware.
○ 10 × 75 mm borosilicate disposable test tubes.
○ Micropipettes, 0.01–1.0 ml (manual or automatic).
○ Liquid scintillation counting vials.
○ Scintillation counter.

Working solutions
A stock solution of borate-Ringer's buffer is used to prepare all the solutions and diluents. This is prepared as follows:

0.05 M borate-Ringer's solution

Solution A: sodium borate   19.0 g
         sodium chloride   8.5 g
         potassium chloride   0.3 g
   Dissolve in approximately 750 ml distilled water.

Solution B: calcium chloride   0.33 g
  Dissolve in 20 ml of water.

Add solution B to solution A slowly with stirring, and bring the volume to 1 litre with water. Store this buffer at room temperature. If the sodium borate precipitates out of solution, gently warm the solution to resolubilise it before use.

Binder diluent
1% charcoal-treated ovalbumin
Dissolve 10 g of ovalbumin in 100 ml of the stock borate-Ringer's solution adjusted to pH 8 with 2 N HCl. Add Norit A charcoal (15 mg/ml) and stir slowly for 15 minutes. Centrifuge at 30 000 g for 20 minutes to remove charcoal. *Before use dilute the supernate to 1% (v/v) in borate-Ringer's buffer and add Triton X-100 to give a concentration of 0.1% (v/v). The 10% solution is stable at −20°C for 6–9 months.*

Reaction buffer
Add 200 mg of ascorbic acid to 90 ml of stock borate-Ringer's buffer, adjust the pH to 8.0, and bring the volume to 100 ml. Prepare fresh reaction buffer for each assay.

Haemoglobin-coated charcoal suspension
Suspend 2.5 g of neutral Norit A charcoal and 0.125 g of bovine Hb (Sigma) in 100 ml of distilled water. Mix thoroughly before use. The suspension is stable for 2–3 weeks.

N^5methyl-H_4-PteGlu for standards
Methyl-H_4PteGlu acid is purchased as the barium salt from Sigma. Dissolve the powder to a concentration of approximately 1 mg/ml in 0.15 M phosphate buffer, pH 7.2, containing ascorbic acid, 200 mg/100 ml. Adjust the pH to 7.2 with 1 N NaOH. The purity of each batch of the compound must be checked by spectrum analysis. The pure compound has an absorption maximum at 290 nm and minimum at 245 nm with a 290/245 ratio of 3.1:1 at pH 7.2. If this ratio is less than 3:1, the preparation is not sufficiently pure and a fresh sample should be prepared.

The exact concentration of the stock solution is determined spectrophotometrically using $E_{1\ cm}^{1\%}$ at 290 nm as follows: dilute an aliquot of the solution in 0.15 M phosphate buffer, pH 7.2, and read immediately at 290 nm.

The concentration of methyl-H_4PteGlu (mg/ml) in the solution is calculated as follows:

$$\frac{\text{OD of diluted sample} \times \text{dilution} \times 10}{655}$$

After the purity and concentration of this primary solution have been established, prepare a stock solution containing 0.1 mg/ml in the phosphate-ascorbate buffer and store in small aliquots at −70°C. Methyl-H_4PteGlu is labile and is readily denatured in the absence of a reducing agent and with freeze-thawing. Stored at −70°C, this solution is stable for at least 6 months. Its purity and concentration should nevertheless be rechecked once a month.

To prepare the reference standards for the assay, a fresh aliquot of methyl-H_4PteGlu must be used each time. Thaw the stock solution containing 0.1 mg/ml and make the dilutions in the reaction buffer containing ascorbate (Table 6.7)

0.1 ml of solutions C to J contain 300 to 12.5 pg, respectively, of methyl-H_4PteGlu, the concentration range required for the dose response curve. Transfer 0.1 ml from each of these tubes to the appropriately labelled reaction tubes.

Radioactive tracer
Pteroylglutamic acid, labelled with ^{3}H at 3', 5', and 9 positions, ([^{3}H]PteGlu) with a high specific activity (20–54 Ci/mmol) is obtained from Amersham. Dissolve the lyophilised powder, usually 250 μCi, in 5 ml of 20% ethanol and store in aliquots of 0.05 or 0.1 ml at −70°C. To prepare a stock solution, add sufficient 0.05 M borate-Ringer's buffer, pH 8 (without ascorbate), to one of these aliquots to give a concentration of 10 ng/ml, and store at −70°C. Dilute this stock solution five-fold to prepare the working solution as follows: add 1 ml of

Table 6.7 Preparation of standard curve

Solution	Dilution	Methyl-H$_4$PteGlu	Reaction buffer	Concentration of methyl-H$_4$ PteGlu
A	1:100	0.01 ml of stock	0.99 ml	1 μg/ml
B	1:100	0.1 ml of Sol. A	9.90 ml	10 ng/ml
C	1:3.33	1.0 ml of Sol. B	2.33 ml	3 ng/ml
D	1:5	1.0 ml of Sol. B	4.00 ml	2 ng/ml
E	1:2	1.0 ml of Sol. C	1.00 ml	1.5 ng/ml
F	1:2	1.0 ml of Sol. D	1.00 ml	1.0 ng/ml
G	1:2	1.0 ml of Sol. E	1.00 ml	0.75 ng/ml
H	1:2	1.0 ml of Sol. F	1.00 ml	0.50 ng/ml
I	1:2	1.0 ml of Sol. H	1.00 ml	0.25 ng/ml
J	1.2	1:0 ml of Sol. I	1.00 ml	0.125 ng/ml

the stock solution to 4 ml of 0.05 M borate-Ringer (without ascorbate) so that 0.1 ml contains 200 pg of [^{3}H]PteGlu. This is the amount of tracer used in each incubation reaction. Protected from light and stored at -70°C, the [^{3}H]PteGlu is stable for 6–9 months. The purity of the tracer can be checked periodically by determining the percentage of radioactivity which is precipitated with ZnSO$_4$ and an excess of unlabelled PteGlu. The following method is used:

Reaction buffer	0.4 ml
[^{3}H]PteGlu (200 pg)	0.1 ml
PteGlu (10 mg/ml)	0.2 ml
ZnSO$_4$ (5%, anhydrous)	0.2 ml

Vortex the mixture, pellet the precipitate by centrifugation at 3000 rpm for 10 minutes, and add an aliquot of the crystal clear supernatant solution to the scintillation cocktail and determine the radioactivity. The purity of the [^{3}H]PteGlu is computed as a percentage of the total radioactivity as follows:

$$\frac{\text{ct/minute in 0.1 ml of [}^3\text{H]PteGlu} - \text{ct/minute in total supernate}}{\text{ct/minute in 0.1 m of [}^3\text{H]PteGlu}} \times 100$$

The precipitated [^{3}H]PteGlu should be no less than 85% of the total radioactivity.

Scintillation fluid
Dissolve 5 g of 2.5 diphenyloxazole (PPO) and 75 ml of BBS-3 solubiliser (Beckman Instruments Inc.)/L toluene. Alternatively any commercial scintillation cocktail that will solubilise the aqueous reaction mixture can be used.

Stock solution of β-lactoglobulin
Dissolve 100–500 mg of β-lactoglobulin in 4 ml of binder diluent and freeze at -70°C. The folate binding protein in this concentration of β-lactoglobulin remains stable for months.

In order to obtain a sensitive standard reference curve, the amount of binding protein used should bind approximately 50–65% of the [^{3}H]PteGlu in the reaction. This 'working concentration' of binding protein is prepared from the frozen stock solution of β-lactoglobulin as follows:

Binding reaction
Reaction buffer	0.3 ml
[^{3}H]PteGlu (200 pg)	0.1 ml
Serial dilutions of β-lactoglobulin in binder diluent	0.1 ml

Buffer blank
Reaction buffer	0.3 ml
[^{3}H]PteGlu (200 pg)	0.1 ml
Reaction buffer	0.1 ml

Incubate at 4°C for 30 minutes and then add 0.4 ml of cold haemoglobin-coated charcoal suspension. Centrifuge at 3000 rpm for 10 minutes at 4°C and count an aliquot of the supernate in the scintillation solution. Calculate the percentage of [^{3}H]PteGlu bound as in equation 1.

$$\frac{\text{Total ct/minute in supernate} - \text{total ct/minute in buffer blank}}{\text{total ct/minute used in reaction mixture} - \text{total ct/minute of buffer blank}} \times 10 \quad (1)$$

The dilution of β-lactoglobulin required to bind 50–65% of the tracer is used in the assay. This titre remains fairly constant for each batch of stock β-lactoglobulin. β-lactoglobulin loses activity with freeze thawing. A fresh aliquot should be diluted for each assay to be sure that the titre of β-lactoglobulin has not changed. It is simple and convenient to test the diluted binder before setting up the complete assay protocol. The [^{3}H]PteGlu standard, a buffer blank and a binding reaction with the dilution of β-lactoglobulin which is to be used in the assay is incubated for 15 minutes at 4°C and the percentage of the tracer which is bound is quickly determined.

Method

Each assay procedure includes the simultaneous preparation of a reference dose response curve using methyl-$H_4PteGlu$ standards. With each serum to be assayed a 'serum blank reaction' is also prepared to correct for any binding of the $[^3H]PteGlu$ by serum proteins. When whole blood haemolysates and deproteinated serum extracts are to be assayed, these 'sample blanks' can be omitted because haemolysates and deproteinated extracts do not bind $[^3H]PteGlu$. Each reference standard and test sample must be assayed in duplicate.

1. For the dose response standard curve, label 10×75 mm test tubes as follows:

1,2	$[^3H]PteGlu$: This provides the total radioactivity in ct/minute
3,4	Buffer blank
5,6	no methyl-$H_4PteGlu$
7,8	12.5 pg methyl-$H_4PteGlu$
9,10	25 pg methyl-$H_4PteGlu$
11,12	50 pg methyl-$H_4PteGlu$
13,14	75 pg methyl-$H_4PteGlu$
15,16	100 pg methyl-$H_4PteGlu$
17,18	150 pg methyl-$H_4PteGlu$
19,20	200 pg methyl-$H_4PteGlu$
21,22	300 pg methyl-$H_4PteGlu$

From tubes C–J in Table 6.7

Beginning at tube 23, label two tubes for each test sample of whole serum, (or serum extract) and whole blood haemolysate. For each serum assayed label two additional tubes for the 'serum blank'.

Phase I of the assay

2. Add to each tube the appropriate amount of reaction buffer as outlined in Table 6.8.

3. Add 0.1 ml of each concentration of methyl-$H_4PteGlu$ to tubes 7–22 as labelled above and 0.1 ml of the reaction buffer to tubes 5 and 6.

4. Add 0.02 ml of each serum to the appropriately labelled serum sample tube and its serum blank.

5. Add 0.02 ml or 0.04 ml of each whole blood haemolysate to the appropriate tube, making sure to adjust the volume of the reaction buffer when the amount of sample is increased or decreased (see Table 6.8).

6. Starting with tube 5 add 0.1 ml of the diluted binder to all the tubes except the 'serum blank' tubes.

7. Incubate the reaction mixture at room temperature for 30 to 60 minutes and then cool the tubes to 4°C by placing in an ice bath, or in a refrigerator for 30 minutes.

Phase II of the assay

8. Add 0.1 ml of $[^3H]PteGlu$ to each tube and incubate at 4°C for 30 minutes. Add 0.4 ml of the cold haemoglobin-coated charcoal suspension to each tube and vortex vigorously.

9. Centrifuge all the tubes at 3000 rpm for 10 minutes at 4°C to pellet the charcoal.

10. Count an aliquot (usually 0.5 ml) of the supernatant solution from each tube for $[^3H]$ activity.

Calculation

The standard dose-response curve is constructed by plotting the ratio of % $[^3H]PteGlu$ bound (B) to % $[^3H]PteGlu$ free (F) as a function of the amount of methyl-$H_4PteGlu$ in each standard. The calculations are carried out as follows. Average the counts per minute (ct/minute) for each set of duplicate tubes. Subtract the ct/minute in the 'blank' tubes (tubes 3 & 4) from all the other reactions except the whole serum tubes to obtain the *corrected* ct/minute. Subtract the ct/minute of the 'serum blank' tubes, from the ct/minute of the corresponding whole serum tube to obtain the corrected ct/minute. Divide the corrected

Table 6.8 Reaction mixtures for the two-phase ligand-binding assay.

Sample	Phase I				Phase II	
	Reaction buffer (ml)	Methyl-$H_4PteGlu$ (ml)	Test sample (ml)	Diluted binder (ml)	$[^3H]PteGlu$ (ml)	Hb-coated charcoal (ml)
$[^3H]PteGlu$ standard	0.8	—	—	—	0.1	—
Buffer blank	0.4	—	—	—	0.1	0.4
Standard curve	0.2	0.1	—	0.1	0.1	0.4
Serum blank	0.38	—	0.02	—	0.1	0.4
Test serum, or	0.28	—	0.02	0.1	0.1	0.4
Serum extract[a]	0.3	—	0.1	0.1	0.1	0.4
Whole blood haemolysate	0.26–0.28[b]	—	0.02–0.04[b]	0.1	0.1	0.4

a This is only used if the serum contains a substantial amount of an unsaturated folate binding protein. See text for the details.

b Adjust the reaction buffer to give a final incubation volume of 0.5 ml when the volume of test sample assayed is increased or decreased.

average ct/minute of each reaction by the corrected average total ct/minute (tubes 1 & 2) to obtain the % [³H]PteGlu bound (B).

For example, see equation 2.

$$\frac{\text{corrected average ct/minute in tubes 5 and 6 is 3940}}{\text{corrected total ct/minute (tubes 1 \& 2) is 7934}} \times 100 = 49.5\% \qquad (2)$$

This is the % [³H]PteGlu bound (or B) to calculate the first B/F point of the standard curve.

Subtract the value obtained for B from 100 to obtain the % [³H]PteGlu free (or F). Divide the value obtained for B by that obtained for F for each reaction to give the B/F. Calculate the B/F for each point of the standard curve and each test sample. See Table 6.9 for exact examples of the calculation from the ct/minute.

Use arithmetic graph paper to construct the standard curve by plotting the B/F ratio on the Y axis vs. the concentration of methyl-H₄PteGlu on the X axis (Fig. 6.5). Obtain the concentration of methyl-H₄-PteGlu in each test sample by finding the pg of methyl-H₄PteGlu on the X-axis which corresponds to its B/F ratio.

Calculate the concentration of folate per ml of serum as in equation 3.

Equation 3

$$\text{pg methyl-H}_4\text{-PteGlu (obtained by reference to the standard curve)} \times \frac{1}{\text{aliquot of serum (fraction of 1 ml)}} \qquad (3)$$

Calculate the concentration of folate per ml of packed erythrocytes as in equation 4.

Equation 4

$$\text{pg methyl-H}_4\text{PteGlu (obtained by reference to the standard curve)} \times \frac{1}{\text{aliquot of haemolysate assayed}} \times \frac{50}{\text{(dilution factor for whole blood)}} \times \frac{2}{\text{(correction for PCV)}} \qquad (4)$$

An example of the standard curve is shown with a sample calculation in Fig. 6.5.

Results

1. Express the concentration of folate in serum as ng/ml and the concentration of folate in erythrocytes as ng/ml packed erythrocytes.

Table 6.9 Example of calculation of standard curve and sample assays.

	Average ct/min	Corrected[a] ct/min	% Bound(B) $\frac{\text{Corrected ct/min}}{\text{Total Corrected ct/min}} \times 100$	% Free (F) 100−%B	B/F	Folate assayed per aliquot of sample	Folate (ng/ml)
Total [³H]PteGlu	8267	7934					
Buffer blank	333						
Standard curve methyl-H₄PteGlu							
0	4273	3940	49.6	50.4	.98		
12.5	3903	3570	44.9	55.1	.81		
25	3413	3080	38.8	61.2	.63		
50	2633	2300	28.9	71.1	.41		
75	2269	1936	24.4	83.6	.31		
100	1777	1444	18.2	81.8	.23		
150	1412	1079	13.6	86.4	.15		
200	1233	900	11.3	88.7	.12		
300	1043	710	8.9	91.1	.10		
Serum blank	346						
Test serum (0.02 ml)	3426	3080[b]	38.8	61.2	.63	25 pg[c]	1.2[d]
Serum extract (0.1 ml)	3319	2986[e]	37.6	62.4	.60	29 pg[c]	1.4[d]
Haemolysate (0.04 ml))	2833	2500[e]	31.5	68.5	.46	44 pg[c]	110[d]

a. Obtained by subtracting average ct/min of buffer blank from average ct/min.
b. Subtract serum blank.
c. Obtained from standard curve.
d. Calculated from the volume of sample assayed and/or dilution.
e. Subtract buffer blank.

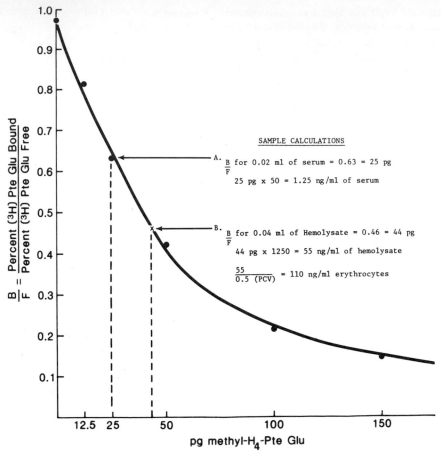

Fig. 6.5 Standard dose response curve obtained with methyl-H₄PteGlu in a two phase sequential non-competitive system. Sample calculations for the determination of serum folate and erythrocyte folate from this dose response curve are shown.

2. The normal range for serum folate is 3.5 ng/ml–20 ng/ml. A folate concentration between 2 and 3.5 ng/ml is indeterminate and a folate concentration below 2 ng/ml usually indicates folate deficiency (Rothenberg et al 1972).

3. The normal range for erythrocyte folate by this method is 200 to 1000 ng/ml of packed erythrocytes (Rothenberg et al 1974). Values below 200 ng/ml indicate folate deficiency. In vitamin B_{12} deficiency the erythrocyte folate concentration may be low but the serum folate concentration in these patients is normal or elevated (Cooper & Lowenstein 1964).

Comments

— A two phase non-competitive sequential system is used to measure methyl-H₄PteGlu in order to increase the sensitivity of the assay. By first reacting the methyl-H₄PteGlu with the binding ligand and then 'titrating' the unoccupied ligand-binding sites

with the [³H]PteGlu the disadvantage of the higher affinity of the binding protein for the tracer than for the competing methyl-H₄PteGlu is minimised.

An important advantage of obtaining a very sensitive radioassay is that it permits the measurement of methyl-H₄PteGlu in 0.01–0.02 ml of serum. Since the serum from some patients with liver disease, folate deficiency, cancer, or from some pregnant women or women who take oral contraceptives, may contain an unsaturated folate binding protein, reducing the volume of serum sample in the assay will reduce the effect of this protein on the radioassay (Rothenberg & da Costa 1976).

— If the [³H]PteGlu bound by the serum blank is substantially greater than the buffer blank, the serum must be extracted by boiling to obtain a correct folate concentration. The high blank is due to an unsaturated folate binding protein in the serum which binds the $[^3H]$PteGlu in the reaction mixture resulting in a higher value for the B/F ratio. This will give a falsely low serum folate concentration.

— It is best to correct the PCV of all the whole blood samples to 50% before haemolysing the erythrocytes to measure erythrocyte folate. The folate concentration measured per ml of packed erythrocytes and the PCV are not linear even after correction for the plasma folate concentration. The erythrocyte folate concentration will be greatly over-estimated in an anaemic patient with a low PCV.

— Phase I of the sequential assay can be incubated overnight at 4°C without loss of sensitivity of dose-response curve.

— For each set of duplicate reactions the ct/min obtained for each reaction should be no greater than ± 15% of the mean value for the two reactions in order to obtain an accurate result. If this value is greater than 15%, this sample should be re-assayed.

INTRINSIC-FACTOR ANTIBODY

Intrinsic-factor (IF) antibodies are present in the serum from over half the patients with pernicious anaemia and hence their detection is useful in diagnosis.

Principle

The normal function of IF is to bind cobalamin (B_{12}) as part of the process of intestinal B_{12} absorption. IF antibody most commonly attaches to that part of the IF molecule that binds B_{12} and hence once IF reacts with antibody, B_{12} is no longer bound.

To detect IF antibodies the amount of $[^{57}Co]B_{12}$ taken up by gastric juice is measured and the uptake repeated after the antibody has reacted with IF. A fall in the B_{12} binding capacity of the gastric juice after the addition of serum is indicative of an IF-antibody in the serum. In the test $[^{57}Co]B_{12}$ is added in excess, and free, unbound $[^{57}Co]B_{12}$ is removed by adsorption onto protein-coated charcoal.

Test samples

Serum is required and stored at −20°C before assay. The patient should not have received an injection of B_{12} in the week prior to the assay since free B_{12} will produce an erroneous result in the assay.

Reagents

As for IF assay (p. 139).

Saliva. Human saliva is collected, the containers being kept on ice. It is filtered through glass wool using a Buchner funnel and stored in 2.0 ml aliquots at −20°C. Determine the B_{12} binding capacity of the saliva (p. 145).

Equipment

As for IF assay (p. 139).

Standards and controls

$[^{57}Co]B_{12}$ standard. As for IF assay (p. 139).

Charcoal control. As for IF assay (p. 139).

Negative serum control. A pool of normal sera, divided into 0.5 ml aliquots and stored at −20°C.

Positive serum control. This is a pool of sera from patients with pernicious anaemia known to have IF antibodies. It is stored in 0.5 ml aliquots at −20°C. It is useful to dilute the pool with negative serum to obtain an IF antibody level of 3–5 ng/ml, which is the lowest level of antibody detectable. A high titre antiserum (100–200 ng/ml) is also useful as a control when titrating high antibody-containing sera.

Preparation of working solutions

Gastric juice IF. The IF content of the gastric juice used in the detection of antibody should be not less than 50 ng units per ml. For use dilute the gastric juice with PBS-albumin so that 5 ng of IF is present in 3.0 ml volume.

Saliva. Dilute saliva in PBS-albumin so that 3.0 ml contains sufficient to bind 5 ng $[^{57}Co]B_{12}$.

PBS-albumin. See IF assay (p. 139).

$[^{57}Co]B_{12}$. See IF assay (p. 139).

Protein-coated charcoal. See IF assay (p. 139).

Method

1. All tests are done in duplicate.

2. Place 4 plastic capped 10 ml centrifuge tubes in a rack for each serum and control to be assayed. Number each with the sample number and label 2 tubes A and 2 tubes B. (Table 6.10).

Table 6.10 Protocol for the detection of antibody to human intrinsic factor. (Volumes in ml)

	$[^{57}Co]B_{12}$ standard	Charcoal control	Serum A	B
PBS-albumin	3.5	3.1	3.0	3.0
Gastric juice	—	—	0.1	0.1
$[^{57}Co]B_{12}$	0.1	0.1	0.1	—
Serum	—	—	—	0.1
Mix, stand 20 min at room temperature				
$[^{57}Co]B_{12}$	—	—	—	0.1
Serum	—	—	0.1	—
Mix, stand 20 min at room temperature				
Charcoal	—	0.5	0.5	0.5
Mix, centrifuge 1000 g, 30 min				

3. Set up 2 centrifuge tubes for the charcoal control and 2 tubes for the $[^{57}Co]B_{12}$ standard.

4. Add reagents in the sequence set out in Table 6.9.

5. After final centrifugation decant supernatants into gamma counting tubes.

6. Count $[^{57}Co]B_{12}$ activity for sufficient time to accumulate a minimum of 10 000 counts for each tube.

Antibody unit

A unit of IF antibody is the amount that blocks the binding of 1 ng B_{12} to IF.

Calculation

A mean of duplicate counts is taken provided they are in reasonable agreement. If they are not the assay should be repeated.

As an example:

$[^{57}Co]B_{12}$ standard		38 700, 38 764/100 sec, mean = 38 732
Charcoal control		578,532/100 sec, mean = 555
Negative serum	tube A	18 868, 18 600/100 sec, mean = 18 734
	tube B	18 430, 18 694/100 sec, mean = 18 562
Positive serum	tube A	18 996, 19 120/100 sec, mean = 19 058
	tube B	17 460, 17 700/100 sec, mean = 17 580
Patient serum	tube A	19 013, 18 895/100 sec, mean = 18 959
	tube B	4537, 4423/100 sec, mean = 4480

1. $[^{57}Co]B_{12}$ standard contains 10.1 ng B_{12}. Thus there are

$$\frac{38\ 732}{10.1} = 3835 \text{ counts/100 s per 1.0 ng } B_{12}$$

2. Charcoal removed 98.6% of $[^{57}Co]B_{12}$ in the charcoal control, that is

$$\frac{38\ 732 - 555}{38\ 732} \times 100 = 98.6\%$$

This confirms the expected activity of charcoal in the removal of free $[^{57}Co]B_{12}$.

3. Serum samples. Tube A measures the $[^{57}Co]B_{12}$ binding to IF in the gastric juice. In tube B the ? antibody has first reacted with IF and produced a corresponding reduction in $[^{57}Co]B_{12}$ binding. Hence subtract the count in tube B from that in tube A:

Tube A–B

negative serum	18 868 − 18 430	=	438 counts/100 s
positive serum	19 058 − 17 580	=	1478 counts/100 s
patient	18 959 − 4480	=	14 479 counts/100 s

Convert counts/100 s (A − B) into ng $[^{57}Co]B_{12}$.

Negative serum. 438 counts is equivalent to 0.11 ng B_{12} and in terms of 1 ml of serum is equal to 1.1 ng units of antibody activity. A difference of less than 2.5 ng B_{12} binding/ml of serum between tubes A and B is a negative result.

Positive serum. 1478 counts is equal to 0.38 ng B_{12} and in terms of 1.0 ml of serum, 3.8 ng of 'antibody activity'.

Patient sample. 14 479 counts is equal to 3.8 ng B_{12} and in terms of 1 ml of serum, 38 ng of 'antibody activity'.

Titration of antibody levels

Positive samples should be titrated (see comments) by preparing dilution in PBS/albumin; 1/5, 1/10 and 1/20 are suitable.

In the patient sample a dilution of 1/10 gave $[^{57}Co]B_{12}$ A−B 2250 counts/100 s.

$$\frac{\text{Counts A–B}}{\text{std count/ng } B_{12}} \times \text{dilution} = \frac{2250}{3835} \times \frac{1000}{10} = 58.7 \text{ ng units}$$

Check for free cobalamin in serum sample

Free B_{12}, i.e. in excess of the serum binding capacity, may occur when the blood is collected after the patient has had a large dose of B_{12} by injection and results in misleading false positive antibody results. This can be checked by using 0.1 ml of salivary R-binder instead of gastric juice in the test. Whereas IF Ab will not affect the $[^{57}Co]B_{12}$ binding to saliva, free B_{12} in serum will compete with $[^{57}Co]B_{12}$ for binding sites and reduce the amount of $[^{57}Co]B_{12}$ bound.

Comments

— *Assay detection limits*

The assay protocol as described can only measure IF antibody concentrations within certain limits. The smallest amount detected depends on the smallest difference between (A) and (B) which can be detected above background counting error and variations due to pipetting/decanting errors etc. —

e.g. the $[^{57}Co]B_{12}$ provides about 40 000 counts/100 s so gastric juice binds about 20 000, of which 16 000 is bound to IF and 4 000 to R (assuming 20% binding was R). The counting error on the 20 000 counts is about $\pm$ 300. A possible pipetting/decanting error of 5% is more than reasonable so that if (B) is 1000 counts less than (A) this could be due to IF-Ab. To illustrate this:

Standard = 40 000 counts = 10 ng B_{12} = 4 000 counts/ng

A − B = 20 000 − 19 000 = 1 000 = 0.25 ng

That is, there is 0.25 ng IF-Ab in 100 μl serum = 2.5 units/ml.

Thus 2.5 mg units is the minimum amount of antibody detectable.

— Antibody binding to intrinsic factor is unlikely to be linear with dilution of the serum because of the polyclonal nature of antibodies. The best estimate of antibody level will be obtained when intrinsic factor is in excess of the amount of antibody so that a large proportion of the antibody is bound. In practice, use for calculation that dilution of serum which inhibits less than 20% of the intrinsic factor present in the gastric juice.

— *False positives*
The main interference is from B_{12} given as therapy or from a flushing dose given with a Schilling test when free B_{12} is present in the circulation for 24–72 hours. Free B_{12} dilutes the radiolabelled B_{12} in the assay, but more importantly the free B_{12} binds to gastric juice and blocks the later addition of $[^{57}Co]B_{12}$, therefore mimicing the effect of antibody.

— *Inactive charcoal*
The commonest cause of a failed assay is inactive charcoal. This is obviated by following the details set out for preparation of charcoal (p. 140) and using charcoal known to be suitable for this type of assay.

Interpretation
IF antibodies are present in the sera of about 57% of patients with pernicious anaemia. Rarely IF antibodies occur in the absence of pernicious anaemia, and the commonest condition is thyrotoxicosis. Such patients usually have a strong personal and family history of auto-immune disorders. IF antibodies in the absence of pernicious anaemia have also been found in a patient with simple atrophic gastritis, in diabetes mellitus, in two relatives of patients with pernicious anaemia and in a patient with nutritional cobalamin deficiency. Such patients usually do not develop pernicious anaemia.

IF antibodies are often present in the gastric secretion of patients with pernicious anaemia.

INTRINSIC FACTOR IN HUMAN GASTRIC JUICE

Intrinsic factor (IF) is a glycoprotein present in gastric juice required for the intestinal absorption of dietary cobalamin. Assay of the amount of IF in gastric juice may be required in the investigation of a patient with megaloblastic anaemia, atrophic gastritis and related disorders.

Principle
IF is assayed by measuring the amount of $[^{57}Co]B_{12}$ that it binds. There are two proteins in gastric juice that bind cobalamin, one is IF, the other is an R-binder present in all body fluids. In order to separate the B_{12} binding due to IF from that of R-binder, an agent that blocks the B_{12} binding site of one of these proteins is added before adding the $[^{57}Co]B_{12}$. This agent can be either an intrinsic-factor antibody that blocks the B_{12} site of IF, or cobinamide, a cobalamin analogue that blocks the R-binder B_{12} binding site.

In both these approaches an excess of $[^{57}Co]B_{12}$ is added. The B_{12} remaining unbound is removed by adsorption on to protein-coated charcoal.

Test sample
Gastric juice is collected from the patient, after an overnight fast, by passing a narrow tube into the stomach via the mouth. Maximum secretion of gastric juice is obtained by giving an injection of pentagastrin or similar substance. Samples may be collected over 30-minute periods before and after the injection.

1. As soon as the gastric juice samples reach the laboratory, measure and record the volume. There should be no delay in processing the samples.

2. Measure the pH with a pH meter. An aliquot may be put aside for titration of the amount of hydrochloric acid present, if required.

3. Add 3 N-NaOH drop-wise until the pH is between 10 and 11. This is to inactivate pepsin, a proteolytic enzyme that will digest IF. Leave for 20 minutes.

4. Add 0.5 N HCl drop-wise to bring the pH back to 7.

5. Particulate debris may be removed by centrifugation.

6. Excessively mucoid samples may be improved by filtration through glass wool using a Buchner filter funnel.

7. Store the neutralised gastric juice at −20°C.

Note. Bile-stained samples cannot be assayed since

bile appears to interfere with the action of charcoal, used in the assay.

Reagents

- *Phosphate buffered saline* (PBS) pH 7.4.
- *Bovine albumin powder* (Fraction V, Armour).
- *Activated charcoal* (Norit GSX, British Drug Houses, or equivalent product). To ensure activity, a small aliquot (enough for 2 weeks' work) is placed in a glass conical flask, tightly capped with metal foil and heated in an oven at 160°C for 2 hours. Fresh charcoal is heated every 2 weeks.
- *Stock cyanocobalamin solution*. 1000 μg of cyanocobalamin (1000 μg/ml pharmaceutical ampoule, Glaxo) is diluted to 100 ml in distilled water. This is divided into 2 ml aliquots and stored at -20°C. The concentration (approximately 10 μg/ml) is determined by assay in a conventional B_{12} assay or preferably determined spectrophotometrically. One mole of cyanocobalamin has an extinction coefficient of 238,057 at 361.5 nm in a 1 cm light path.
- [^{57}Co]-*labelled cyanocobalamin* (Amersham). High specific activity [^{57}Co]-labelled cyanocobalamin should be used and 1.0 ml usually contains about 0.05 μg of B_{12}. Carefully centrifuge the glass bottle of [^{57}Co]B_{12} in its plastic container at the lowest speed setting of a bench centrifuge. Remove the container cap and add 0.5 ml of cyanocobalamin stock solution (10 μg/ml) and 0.5 ml of distilled water. This gives a final volume of 2.0 ml and contains 10 μCi [^{57}Co] and 5.05 μg B_{12}. This is dispensed in 200 aliquots containing 1 μCi and 505 ng B_{12} in 5 ml sterile glass bottles and stored at -20°C.
- *Cobinamide* (Calbiochem). This is stored in an airtight container with silica gel at 4°C. 10 mg is dissolved in 5.0 ml of sterile distilled water and dispensed in 50 μl aliquots (100 μg cobinamide) and kept at -20°C. 100 μg cobinamide is diluted further with sterile distilled water to 25 ml and is stored in 0.5 ml volumes (2 μg cobinamide) at -20°C.
- *Intrinsic-factor antibodies*. About half the patients with pernicious anaemia have a serum antibody against IF. Blood should be obtained from those with higher antibody titres ($>$ 100 ng units/ml). Pooled serum from such patients is stored at -20°C. The antibody titre of the pool is measured (p. 137). Dilute the pool with pooled normal human serum to give a titre of 100 ng units/ml. Store in 2 ml volumes at -20°C.

Equipment

- Disposable, 10 ml, capped, plastic centrifuge tubes (sterilin).
- Capped, disposable isotope counting tubes holding at least 3.5 ml.
- Vortex mixer.

Standards and controls

[^{57}Co]B_{12} standard.

Charcoal control. The charcoal should be capable of adsorbing at least 98% of the free [^{57}Co]B_{12}

Normal human gastric juice. This is treated as described for test samples and stored in 0.5 ml volumes at -20°C. The IF remains stable for several years. An IF content of 25–50 ng units/ml is suitable.

A *specificity control* can be included by assaying human saliva which contains R-binder (and perhaps a trace of transcobalamin II) but no IF.

Working reagents

- *Phosphate buffered saline-albumin.* One gram per litre albumin in PBS is prepared fresh for each assay.
- *Serum-coated charcoal.* Add 0.5 ml of pooled normal human serum to 0.5 g activated charcoal, mix vigorously and leave at room temperature for 10 minutes. Centrifuge at 1000 g for 10 minutes and discard the supernatant. Wash the charcoal once with PBS and resuspend in 5 ml PBS. This suffices for 10 assay tubes and should be used within one hour.
- [^{57}Co]B_{12} Dilute 200 μl (1 μCi and 505 ng B_{12}) of stock [^{57}Co]B_{12} solution to 5.0 ml with PBS-albumin. 100 μl contains 0.02 μCi and 10.1 ng B_{12}
- *Cobinamide.* Dilute 0.5 ml (2 μg) to 5.0 ml with PBS-albumin. 100 μl contains 40 ng cobinamide.
- *IF-antibody.* 100 μl of the stock antibody contains 10 ng units of antibody.

Method

1. All tests are done in duplicate.

2. Place 4 plastic, capped, 10 ml centrifuge tubes in a rack for each gastric juice, including control samples to be assayed. Number all tubes in each set with the sample number and label 2 tubes A and 2 tubes B.

3. Set up 2 centrifuge tubes for the charcoal control and 2 isotope counting tubes for the [^{57}Co]B_{12} standard.

4. Add the reagents in the sequence set out in Table 6.11 if using IF-antibody and Table 6.12 if using cobinamide.

5. After the final centrifugation decant supernatants into isotope counting tubes.

6. Count [^{57}Co]B_{12} activity for sufficient time as to accumulate a minimum of 10 000 counts for each tube.

Unit

One unit of IF is the amount that binds one nanogram of B_{12}.

Calculation

The mean of duplicate counts is taken provided they are

Table 6.11 Protocol for IF assay using IF-antibody. (Volumes in ml)

	$[^{57}Co]B_{12}$ standard	Charcoal control		Gastric juice	
		A	B	A	B
PBS-albumin	3.5	3.1	3.1	3.0	3.0
Gastric juice	—	—	—	0.1	0.1
$[^{57}Co]B_{12}$	0.1	0.1	0.1	0.1	—
IF-antibody	—	—	0.1	—	0.1
Mix, stand 20 min at room temperature					
$[^{57}Co]B_{12}$	—	—	—	—	0.1
IF antibody	—	—	—	0.1	—
Mix, stand 20 min at room tempperature					
Protein-coated charcoal	—	0.5	0.5	0.5	0.5
Mix, centrifuge 1000 g for 30 min					

Table 6.12 Protocol for IF assay using cobinamide. (Volumes in ml)

	$[^{57}Co]B_{12}$ standard	Charcoal control		Gastric juice	
		A	B	A	B
PBS-albumin	3.5	3.1	3.1	3.0	3.0
Gastric juice	—	—	—	0.1	0.1
Cobinamide	—	—	0.1	—	0.1
Mix, stand 30 min at 37°C					
$[^{57}Co]B_{12}$	0.1	0.1	0.1	0.1	0.1
Mix, stand 30 min at 37°C					
Protein-coated charcoal	—	0.5	0.5	0.5	0.5
Mix, centrifuge 1000 g for 30 min					

in reasonable agreement. If not, the test should be repeated. For example:

IF assay using IF-antibody
$[^{57}Co]B_{12}$ counting standard 38 200 and 38 347; mean = 38 274

Charcoal control tubes A 456 and 441; mean = 449
tubes B 739 and 791; mean = 765

Gastric juice   tubes A 18 233 and 18 393
mean = 18 313
tubes B 5413 and 5307
mean = 5360

$[^{57}Co]B_{12}$ counting standard contains 10.1 ng B_{12}.

Thus there are $\dfrac{38\ 274}{10.1}$ = 3790 counts per 1.0 ng B_{12}.

Charcoal control. Charcoal removed

$$\frac{38\ 274 - 449}{38\ 274} \times 100 = 98.6\%$$

of the $[^{57}Co]B_{12}$, confirming that the charcoal could remove in excess of 98% of free $[^{57}Co]B_{12}$.

Gastric juice. The counts in tube A are a measure of the total B_{12} binding capacity of the gastric juice. The counts in tube B represent B_{12} binding after blocking of the IF with antibody. Therefore, the difference between A and B represents B_{12} binding to IF alone. A − B = 18 313 − 5360 = 12 953 counts of B_{12} bound to IF. In order to express the results in terms of ng of B_{12} bound, divide by 3790 counts/ng B_{12}.

$$\frac{12\ 953}{3790} = \begin{array}{l} 3.38 \text{ ng } B_{12} \text{ bound to IF from 100 } \mu l \text{ of} \\ \text{gastric juice.} \end{array}$$

This gastric juice, therefore, had 33.8 ng units of IF per ml.

If the total volume of gastric juice secreted in 1 hour was 200 ml, the total hourly IF output would be 33.8 × 200 = 6760 units.

IF assay using cobinamide

$[^{57}Co]B_{12}$ counting standard	37 941 and 38 821;	mean = 38 381
Charcoal control	tubes A 410 and 431;	mean = 421
	tubes B 463 and 433;	mean = 453
Gastric juice	tubes A 17 667 and 17 553;	mean = 17 610
	tubes B 13 161 and 13 381;	mean = 13 271

$[^{57}Co]B_{12}$ standard contains 10.1 ng B_{12}. Thus there are

$$\frac{38\ 381}{10.1} = 3800 \text{ counts per ng of } B_{12}.$$

Charcoal control. The charcoal has removed

$$\frac{38\ 381 - 421}{38\ 381} \times 100 = 98.9\%$$

confirming that the charcoal can remove in excess of 98% of the free $[^{57}Co]B_{12}$.

Gastric juice. The counts in tubes A are a measure of the total B_{12} binding capacity of the gastric juice. The counts in tube B, which has cobinamide added to block B_{12} binding to R-binder, are due to $[^{57}Co]B_{12}$ binding to IF alone.

Tube B counts − charcoal control (B) = counts bound to IF

$$13\ 271 − 453 = 12\ 818$$

In order to express the results in ng of B_{12}, divide by 3800 counts/ng B_{12}.

$$\frac{12\ 818}{3800} = 3.37\ \text{ng of }[^{57}\text{Co}]B_{12}\ \text{bound to IF from 100 }\mu l\ \text{of gastric juice.}$$

Thus 1 ml of gastric juice contains 33.7 ng units of IF. If the volume of gastric juice secreted over an hour was 120 ml, the hourly output of IF would be $33.7 \times 120 = 4044$ ng units IF.

Comments

— The commonest cause of a failed assay is inactive charcoal which fails to clear all the free B_{12}. This will not occur if all the preparation steps are followed.
— The binding of B_{12} to IF is only linear with concentration up to about 60% saturation. If more than 60% of the $[^{57}\text{Co}]B_{12}$ used in each tube is bound by a particular sample it should be repeated after suitable dilution in PBS-albumin.
— These assays rely on the specific activity of the $[^{57}\text{Co}]B_{12}$ for the calculation of the weight of B_{12} bound. The specific activity provided by the manufacturer is only approximate and an occasion may be up to 30% higher than stated. This can lead to too low results. However, by adding a relatively large amount of unlabelled B_{12} of known concentration, the $[^{57}\text{Co}]B_{12}$ content of B_{12} becomes only a tracer and is insignificant in the calculations — e.g. of the 10.1 ng $[^{57}\text{Co}]B_{12}$ solutions used per assay tube, 10 ng is cold assayable B_{12} and only 0.1 ng is contributed by the original high specific activity $[^{57}\text{Co}]B_{12}$.
— In both methods, the amount of non-IF, i.e. R-binder, can be calculated as follows:
  a. In the IF assay using IF-antibody, counts in tube B minus the charcoal control tube B are due to R-binder.
  b. when using cobinamide, the difference between tubes A and B is due to $[^{57}\text{Co}]B_{12}$ binding to R-binder.

Interpretation

There is considerable variation in the concentration and output of IF, and normal values are shown in Table 6.13. It is useful to note both the concentration and total hourly output both before (resting or basal secretion) and after a stimulant such as gastrin or its

Table 6.13 Values for intrinsic factor content of human gastric juice.

	Concentration ng/units	Output/hour
Basal gastric juice	3–124 mean 36	900–8300 mean 3000
Post-stimulant	14–147 mean 50–60	6000–30 000 mean 16 000

analogue pentagastrin. The concentration is useful because collection of gastric juice after partial gastrectomy will be incomplete. Only about 500 IF units are required in man for normal absorption of a 1 μg dose of B_{12}.

In pernicious anaemia where there is severe atrophy of the gastric mucosa, IF is either absent in half the patients or the concentration is less than 11 ng units/ml, usually less than 5 ng units/ml in the remaining half. Gastric juice volumes are very small and total hourly output is less than 200 units. Patients with simple atrophic gastritis (without pernicious anaemia) have values between the pernicious anaemia and the normal range.

COBALAMIN (VITAMIN B_{12}) ABSORPTION

The absorption of cobalamin may be needed as a test of function of the distal small gut (ileum), as a step in establishing the cause of megaloblastic anaemia, in excluding a possible diagnosis of Addisonian pernicious anaemia, or as a step in investigating a patient who has a low serum cobalamin level.

Principle

Cobalamin in which the cobalt atom has been replaced by an isotope (^{57}Co is preferred) is swallowed by the patient. The amount of dose absorbed from the gut is assessed by measuring
  1. $[^{57}\text{Co}]B_{12}$ in plasma, or
  2. by whole body counting after unabsorbed B_{12} has been excreted in the faeces, or
  3. a large dose of non-radioactive B_{12} (1000 μg cyanocobalamin) may be given intramuscularly (flushing dose) with the oral dose of $[^{57}\text{Co}]B_{12}$ when one-third of absorbed $[^{57}\text{Co}]B_{12}$ will be excreted into urine. The amount of $[^{57}\text{Co}]B_{12}$ in urine is a measure of the amount that has been absorbed.

Biochemical basis

$[^{57}\text{Co}]B_{12}$ given by mouth will bind to intrinsic factor and other B_{12} binding proteins (also called R-binder or transcobalamin I or haptocorrin). In the upper gut proteolytic enzymes will free B_{12} bound to R-binders so that these too will bind to intrinsic factor. The intrinsic factor-B_{12} complex attaches to receptors in the ileum, and B_{12} alone enters the bloodstream, reaching a peak between 8 and 12 hours after the oral dose. All these stages are assessed in the test and malabsorption may follow a defect at any stage.

Combined urinary excretion and plasma level cobalamin absorption

Test samples
20 ml blood in heparin or EDTA is collected between 8 and 10 hours after the oral dose. A complete 24-hour urine collection is made starting at the time of the intramuscular injection of 1000 μg of cyanocobalamin.

Reagents
- $[^{57}Co]B_{12}$ (Amersham).1.0 μg containing not less than 0.1 μCi.
- *Hog intrinsic factor* (Armour, Lederle, Amersham) sufficient to potentiate the absorption of 1 μg B_{12}. With human intrinsic factor (neutralised human gastric juice) 1000 intrinsic factor units is recommended (see 139).
- *Cyanocobalamin* 1000 μg per ml.

Equipment
Gamma counter suitable for counting ^{57}Co.

Standards
If several B_{12} absorption tests are done weekly it is usual to obtain $[^{57}Co]B_{12}$ dose capsules that are swallowed intact by the patient. Under such circumstances the contents of one capsule may be used to serve as a standard for the batch.

The contents of one capsule are dissolved in distilled water and made up to 25 ml in a volumetric flask.

Urine standard. Add 0.2 ml of the standard solution to a 20 ml volumetric flask and make up to 20 ml with distilled water. This is a dilution of 1 in 2500.

Plasma standard. Add 0.4 ml of the standard solution to a 10 ml volumetric flask and make up to 10 ml distilled water. This is a dilution of 1 in 625.

If B_{12} absorption tests are done only occasionally, the dose to be given to the patient is made up 25 ml and 1.0 ml removed to serve as a standard. The 1.0 ml of the dose is diluted with distilled water to 25 ml to serve as a plasma standard (dilution 1 in 625). 5 ml of the plasma standard is further diluted to 20 ml to serve as a urine standard (dilution 1 in 2500).

The removal of 1.0 ml from the dose can be ignored in working out the result.

Method
1. The patient should not eat after midnight before the test, although liquid drinks (tea, water) are permissible.

2. The dose of B_{12} is swallowed accompanied by a drink of water.

3. 1000 μg cyanocobalamin is given i.m. when the dose has been taken.

4. All urine passed in the next 24 hours is collected into an empty container or one containing borate preservative.

5. Eight to ten hours after the oral dose 20 ml venous blood is collected into heparin and the plasma retained for counting.

6. The patient can eat and drink normally 30 minutes after starting the test.

7. Measure the volume of urine passed in 24 hours.

8. Count the $[^{57}Co]B_{12}$ in both the plasma and urine samples, plasma and urine standards and background counts. Equal volumes of all samples must be counted.

Calculation

Urinary excretion

$$= \frac{\text{count/s urine} \times \text{urine volume}}{\text{count/s urine std} \times \text{dilution (2500)}} \times 100$$

$$= \% \text{ of oral dose excreted in urine}$$

Plasma radioactivity

$$= \frac{\text{count/s plasma} \times 1000}{\text{count/s plasma std} \times \text{dilution (625)}} \times 100$$

$$= \% \text{ of oral dose/litre plasma}$$

Example
The gamma counter is set to count either for 1000 seconds or for 10 000 counts.

Urine volume − 2183 ml

	counts (c)	seconds(s)	c/s	c/s − b
Background (b)	558	1000	0.6	−
Urine	7050	1000	7.0	6.4
Urine standard	10 000	374	26.7	26.1
Plasma	1197	1000	1.2	0.6
Plasma standard	10 000	98	102	101.4

Urinary excretion

$$= \frac{6.4 \times 2183}{26.1 \times 2500} \times 100 = 21.4\% \text{ of oral dose}$$

Plasma radioactivity

$$= \frac{0.6 \times 1000}{101.4 \times 625} \times 100 = 0.95\% \text{ of oral dose per litre plasma}$$

Comment

— It should be mandatory to collect both urine and plasma in the test. In a high proportion of cases urine collection is incomplete and a misleadingly low excretion is obtained. If the absorption is normal almost invariably a normal plasma radioactivity level is obtained. It is rare to obtain a complete urine collection in the elderly, and complete reliance can be placed on the result of plasma radioactivity.

— In severe renal failure there will be impaired urinary excretion of the $[^{57}Co]B_{12}$. The plasma radioactivity gives a reliable indication of B_{12} absorption.

— Occasionally batches of $[^{57}Co]B_{12}$ are contaminated with ^{57}Co that is not part of the B_{12} molecule. Such cobalt is excreted into the urine and gives a spurious result in a patient who malabsorbs B_{12}. Such a result can only be suspected when the findings in a patient do not add up. Thus all findings point to pernicious anaemia, yet the absorption of B_{12} is normal. Repeat the test with $[^{57}Co]B_{12}$ from another batch and contact the suppliers in case other complaints have been received.

— With hospital patients in particular other isotopes may have been given such as technetium and these too may be excreted into the urine and give anomalous results. With isotopes having very short half-lives, the samples may be re-counted after the isotopes have been allowed to decay.

— Use cyanocobalamin as the flushing dose. There are little data on the use of hydroxocobalamin in B_{12} absorption tests.

— The test can be repeated with an oral dose of intrinsic factor. This will improve the absorption in pernicious anaemia and after gastrectomy.

— Where an abnormal intestinal bacterial flora is present, the absorption is improved when the test is repeated after 1 week of a wide spectrum antibiotic such as tetracycline.

Interpretation (Table 6.14 and 6.15)

Table 6.14 Percentage of a 1 μg oral dose of $[^{57}Co]B_{12}$ excreted in the urinary excretion tests using a 1000 μg cyanocobalamin flushing injection and a 24-hour urine collection (Chanarin 1979).

	range	mean
Controls	11–32	22
Pernicious anaemia	0–6.8	–
Pernicious anaemia (with intrinsic factor)	3.1–30	10

^{57}Co absorption by whole body counting (Adams et al 1972)

Where an appropriate whole body counter is available, it is very convenient in out-patient work to measure B_{12}

Table 6.15 Percentage of a 1 μg oral dose of $[^{57}Co]B_{12}$ present per litre plasma 8–10 hours after taking the oral dose accompanied by a flushing injection of 1000 μg cyanocobalamin (Coupland 1966).

	range	mean
Controls	0.67–2.19	1.28
Pernicious anaemia	0.02–0.42	0.17
Pernicious anaemia (with intrinsic factor)	0.59–2.0	1.20

absorption by this method. Although it is easier to use $[^{58}Co]B_{12}$ than $[^{57}Co]B_{12}$ for this purpose, both can be used.

The patient is counted before swallowing the dose as a background count. The dose of B_{12} is swallowed and 30 minutes later the count is repeated. The patient then returns about one week later when the count is repeated. The latter represents B_{12} retained by the patient. The result is expressed as a percentage of the oral dose given. As with the urinary excretion test, the test can be repeated with a dose of intrinsic factor.

Normally, not less than 30% of a 1 μg dose of B_{12} is retained, whereas in pernicious anaemia absorption is between 0.3 and 16%. Provided the counter is correctly set at all the counts, all the B_{12} in the gut has been excreted and the dose of labelled B_{12} is all cobalamin, the method should provide a foolproof quantitative measure of B_{12} absorption. But errors do occur. The method is less suited for in-patient work as a week elapses between repeat tests.

TRANSCOBALAMINS

Cobalamin in plasma is bound to two proteins. The bulk of cobalamin in plasma is attached to transcobalamin I (TC I). A relatively small amount (about 10–20%) is attached to transcobalamin II (TC II). The latter, TC II, is the important transport protein carrying cobalamin into cells. The function of TC I is not known. The third cobalamin-binding protein termed transcobalamin III is probably released into plasma from leucocytes after collection of the blood samples. It is immunologically related to TC I.

Congenital absence of TC II, or an abnormal form of TC II, leads to a severe megaloblastic anaemia in the first few months of life. Very high serum B_{12} levels in chronic myeloid leukaemia and myelofibrosis and other myeloproliferative disorders are due to very high levels of TC I. Primary liver cancer may lead to production of an abnormal TC I in large amounts. For these reasons the laboratory may on occasion be called upon to assay these binders.

Principle

In practice the amount of TC is measured by noting the

quantity of $[^{57}Co]B_{12}$ taken up by a unit of plasma or serum. This procedure only assays free binders. TC that is carrying B_{12} will not be measured by this means. This, however, is measured by the B_{12} assay. The total B_{12} binding capacity is the sum of the serum B_{12} level and $[^{57}Co]B_{12}$ uptake.

Total B_{12} unsaturated B_{12} binding may be measured, or TC I and TC II may be separated and quantitated.

Test samples

To prevent release of B_{12} binders from leucocytes blood is collected into a tube containing sodium fluoride 2 mg and disodium EDTA 1 mg for each 1.0 ml of blood. The plasma must be removed as soon as possible and stored frozen. Serum gives higher TC I levels than samples collected into fluoride/EDTA. Heparin produces complexing of TC and should not be used.

Reagents

- $[^{57}Co]B_{12}$ *High specific activity* (Amersham). The vial is handled as described on page 140. To 1.0 ml of the high specific activity $[^{57}Co]B_{12}$ containing 50 ng B_{12} add 0.05 ml cyanocobalamin solution containing 1000 ng cyanocobalamin/ml and 0.95 ml distilled water. The final solution will contain 550 ng B_{12} and 10 μCi radioactivity. This solution is stored in 100 μl aliquots (27.5 ng) at 20°C.
- *Charcoal* (p. 140).
- *Saline*
- *M-glycine*. 75 g glycine in 1 litre distilled water.

Equipment

○ *Chromatography column*, at least 100 cm long and 1.5 to 2.5 cm internal diameter. When in use the column will need to be kept cold at 4°C so that if a cold room or a suitable size refrigerator are not available, a water-jacketed column should be used.
○ *Fraction collector*. Each chromatography run takes 16–24 hours; automatic fraction collection is essential.
○ *Plastic disposable tubes and caps* to hold at least 5 ml and be compatible with fraction collection and gamma counter.
○ *Gamma isotope* counting facility to count ^{57}Co.
○ *Spectrophotomer* to measure absorbance at 280 nm.

UNSATURATED B_{12}-BINDING CAPACITY OF PLASMA

Principle

The amount of $[^{57}Co]B_{12}$ retained by an aliquot of plasma is measured, free B_{12} being adsorbed on to charcoal.

Table 6.16 Measurement of serum unsaturated B_{12} binding capacity. (Volumes in ml)

	$[^{57}Co]B_{12}$ standard	Charcoal control	Plasma
Phosphate-buffered saline	2.5	2.0	1.9
Plasma	0	0	0.1
$[^{57}Co]B_{12}$	0.1	0.1	0.1
Mix, and leave at room temperature for 15 min			
Protein-coated charcoal	0	0.5	0.5
Mix, centrifuge at 1000 g for 30 min			

Standards and controls

Counting standard — see Table 6.16.
Charcoal control — see Table 6.16.
Known plasma sample. This is collected in the same way as the test sample and stored at $-20°C$.

Preparation of working solutions
$[^{57}Co]B_{12}$. Dilute an aliquot containing 27.5 ng B_{12} by adding 4.9 ml saline (0.55 ng/ml).

Protein-coated charcoal (p. 140)

Method

1. All tests are set up in duplicate.
2. Add two 10 ml capacity centrifuge tubes to a rack for each plasma to be tested, two for plasma control, two for charcoal control, and two for $[^{57}Co]B_{12}$ counting standard.
3. Add reagents as shown in Table 6.16.
4. After final centrifugation decant supernatants into isotope counting tubes.
5. Count ^{57}Co to obtain at least 10 000 counts for each tube.

Calculation

Take the mean of duplicate counts provided that they are in reasonable agreement.
$[^{57}Co]B_{12}$ standard 34 060, 34 320   mean, 34 190
Charcoal control   383,401   mean, 392
Plasma   6134,5986   mean, 6060

$[^{57}Co]B_{12}$ standard has 34 190 counts in 0.55 ng B_{12}.

Charcoal control removed $\dfrac{34\ 190 - 392}{34\ 190} \times 100$

$$= 98.8\% \text{ of } B_{12}.$$

Plasma unsaturated B_{12} binding capacity

$$= \frac{\text{plasma counts} \times \text{ng std} \times 10}{\text{std counts}} \text{ ng/ml}$$

$$= \frac{6060 \times 0.55 \times 10}{34\ 190} = 0.97 \text{ ng } B_{12} \text{ bound by 1 ml plasma}$$

MEASUREMENT OF TC I AND TC II (GILBERT'S METHOD)

Principle

B_{12} binding to TC I occurs over a wide range of pH while binding to TC II does not take place at pH 2. This observation is used to measure total B_{12} binding of plasma at pH 7.4 and binding to TC I at pH 2. The difference in B_{12} binding at these two pHs is due to TC II.

Standards and controls

Counting standard (Table 6.17).

Charcoal control (Table 6.17).

Table 6.17 Measurement of TC I and TC II (Gilbert's method). (Volumes in ml)

	$[^{57}Co]B_{12}$ standard	Charcoal control A	Charcoal control B	Plasma or R- binder A	Plasma or R- binder B
Phosphate buffered saline	2.5	2.1	—	1.9	—
Glycine pH 1.85	—	—	2.1	—	1.9
Plasma/R-binder	—	—	—	0.1	0.1
$[^{57}Co]B_{12}$	0.1	0.1	0.1	0.1	0.1

Mix, and leave at room temperature for 15 min

Protein-coated charcoal	0	0.5	0.5	0.5	0.5

Mix, centrifuge at 1000 g for 30 min

R-binder control. Free and virtually pure R-binder is present in saliva. Human saliva is collected, the tube being kept at about 4°C. Debris is removed by either centrifugation or filtration through glass wool. The R-binder content is assayed and aliquots stored at −20°C.

Preparation of working solutions. In addition to those set out on page 145 the following is required.

Glycine 0.1M, pH 1.85. Dilute 100 ml of glycine (75 g/l) and 100 ml N-HCl to 1 litre. Adjust the pH of the solution to 1.85 by careful addition of HCl monitoring pH with a pH meter.

Method

1. All tests are done in duplicate.
2. Set up four 10 ml centrifuge tubes for each plasma to be tested, for the charcoal control, standard plasma and R-binder. Label each pair of tubes A and B.

Two tubes are required for the $[^{57}Co]B_{12}$ counting standard.

3. Set up the tests as shown in Table 6.17.
4. After final centrifugation decant supernatants into isotope counting tube.
5. Count ^{57}Co to obtain at least 10 000 counts for each tube.

Calculation

Take the mean of duplicate counts provided that they are in reasonable agreement.

$[^{57}Co]B_{12}$ Standard		34 060, 34 320,	mean 34 190
Charcoal control	A	383, 401	mean 392
	B	417, 428,	mean 423
R-binder control	A	16 538, 16 488,	mean 16 513
	B	16 248, 16 005,	mean 16 127.
Plasma	A	6134, 5986,	mean 6060
	B	718, 687,	mean 703

$[^{57}Co]B_{12}$ standard has 34 190 counts in 0.53 ng B_{12}

$$or \frac{34\ 190}{0.55} = 62\ 163 \text{ counts per ng } B_{12}$$

Charcoal control removed

$$A \frac{34\ 190 - 392}{34\ 190} \times 100 = 98.8\% \text{ of } B_{12}$$

$$B \frac{34\ 190 - 423}{34\ 190} \times 100 = 98.7\% \text{ of } B_{12}$$

R-binder control. The similarity in counts in A and B indicate that R-binder (in saliva) took up B_{12} at both pH 7 and pH 2 as expected.

Transcobalamin II content of plasma

Counts in tube A = total B_{12} binding (transcobalamin II + R-binder)
Counts in tube B = B_{12} binding by R-binder only.
Counts in tube A − counts in tube B = binding by TC II only.
Total B_{12} binding capacity-R-binder only
= TC II in ng B_{12} bound

$$= \frac{6060 - 703}{62\ 163} = 0.0862 \text{ ng in 0.1 ml plasma}$$

$$= 862 \text{ pg/ml.}$$

Transcobalamin I (R-binder) content of plasma

$$\frac{\text{counts in tube B} - \text{counts in charcoal control B}}{\text{counts in 1 ng } B_{12}}$$

$$= \frac{703 - 423}{62\ 163} = 0.0045 \text{ ng } B_{12}/0.1 \text{ ml plasma}$$

$$= 45 \text{ pg/ml}$$

SEPARATION OF TC I AND TC II BY COLUMN CHROMATOGRAPHY

Principle
The B_{12}-binding proteins are saturated with $[^{57}Co]B_{12}$ and the proteins separated by gel chromatography.

Standards and controls

Preparation of working solutions

Column buffer. Dissolve 58 g of NaCl and 0.2 g of sodium azide in 2 l of PBS (p. 140).

Method

A. *Preparation of chromatography column*
The column is packed with Sephacryl S.200 (Pharmacia) following the manufacturers instructions. Briefly:
1. Prepare a slurry of gel in column buffer with about 75% settled gel.
2. Remove dissolved air by attaching to a vacuum pump.
3. Fix a reservoir on a suitable piece of rigid tube to the top of the column to allow all the gel slurry to be poured in at once.
4. Shut off the bottom of the column and pour in a few ml of buffer, check that air is not trapped under the bottom support net or frit.
5. Carefully pour the gel slurry down the side of the column.
6. Connect a flask of buffer to the top of the column extension and adjust the relative heights of the buffer level in the flask and outlet tubing from the column to obtain a linear flow rate of 40 ml cm^{-2} l^{-1} (see comments). Alternatively use a peristaltic pump.
7. When the gel has settled, remove the extension tube and any excess gel. Allow about 3 cm of buffer above the gel bed and refit the column top. Connect to buffer and adjust the flow rate to 10 ml cm^{-2} l^{-1}. Leave the column to stabilise overnight at this flow rate and at 4°C.

B. *Chromatography of plasma sample*
1. Thaw plasma sample and one vial of $[^{57}Co]B_{12}$ stock solution (p. 140).
2. Pipette 20 μl of $[^{57}Co]B_{12}$ containing 4.5 ng B_{12} into 1 ml of plasma, mix, leave at room temperature 20 minutes.

3. Prepare a $[^{57}Co]B_{12}$ counting standard by adding 20 μl of $[^{57}Co]B_{12}$ solution and 3 ml of column buffer into a gamma counting tube.
4. Disconnect the buffer flask from the column and remove the column top. Allow the buffer to drain until level with the gel surface. Do not let the gel become dry.
5. Layer the labelled plasma sample (usually 1.0 ml) onto the gel carefully avoiding bubbles and splashes. When the sample has soaked into the gel, wash the remaining traces of sample into the column with 1 ml of column buffer layered onto the gel.
6. Refill the column with buffer, replace the top, reconnect buffer flask and start a flow rate of 10 mls cm^{-2} l^{-1}.
7. For a column of 1.5 cm × 100 cm and 1 ml of sample, 100 fraction of 3 ml each should be adequate.
8. Count ^{57}Co in the fractions. If automatic background subtraction is not performed by the counter, an empty tube should be counted to estimate background radioactivity.

Units
Transcobalamins (TC) are measured in the amount of B_{12} bound per unit volume of sample, usually pg/ml or ng/l of plasma. It may be more convenient in some studies to express levels in molar terms. One molecule of B_{12} is bound by one molecule of binding protein so that moles of B_{12} bound represents moles of TC protein.

Calculation
Plot the counts in each fraction against the fraction number (Fig. 6.6) so that the shapes and location of the TC peaks can be visualised. Plot the absorbance (280 nm) of each fraction to outline the three main protein peaks.
Four peaks of $[^{57}Co]B_{12}$ binding are usually apparent:

1. TC O.
2. R-binder
3. Albumin
4. TC II
5. Excess $[^{57}Co]B_{12}$ elutes after the protein bound $[^{57}Co]B_{12}$.

The counts present in the fractions under each peak are added, background subtracted and converted to amount of B_{12} bound — a.

a. $\dfrac{[\text{total count under peak} - (\text{background count} \times \text{number of fractions})]}{\text{counts in counting standard} - \text{background count}} \times 4.5 \times 1000$

= pg/ml of transcobalamin

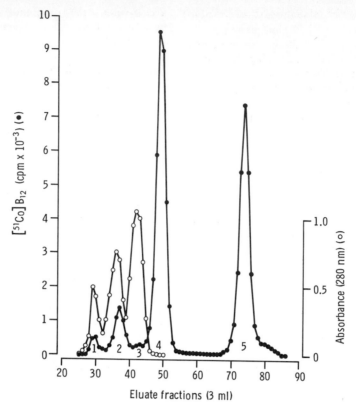

Fig. 6.6 Elution pattern of transcobalamins and protein from Sephacryl S-200 gel filtration column. [^{57}Co]B$_{12}$ containing peaks: 1. TC 0; 2. R-binder; 3. albumin; 4. TC II; 5. free B$_{12}$.

Although only TC II and R-binder levels are reported, the total of [^{57}Co]B$_{12}$ recovered from the column should be calculated from the sum of the counts in all peaks–b.

b. $$\frac{[\text{total counts under peaks} - (\text{background count} \times \text{number of fractions})]}{\text{counts in counting standard} - \text{background count}} \times 100$$

Recovery should be 100% ± 10%

Comments

— Linear flow rate is expressed as the volume of buffer passing through unit cross-sectioned area of the gel bed per unit time, i.e. 40 ml cm^{-2} 1^{-1}, is 40 ml of buffer passing through each square cm of the gel cross-section per hour.

For example: For a 1.5 cm diameter column, the cross sectional area
$$\Pi r^2 = 3.142 \times (0.75)^2 = 1.8 \text{ cm}.$$
A linear flow rate of 40 ml cm^{-2} 1^{-1} indicates that 1.8 × 40 = 72 ml per hour is actually eluting from the column.

A 2.5 cm diameter column at the same linear flow rate gives a $(1.25)^2 \times 40 = 196$ ml per hour.
— After use the column may be stored at 4°C but should not be left at room temperature.
— Peak three probably represents small traces of [^{57}Co]B$_{12}$, present in the [^{57}Co]cyanocobalamin stock solution, which binds to albumin in the plasma sample.
— If the plasma sample binds more than 60% of the added [^{57}Co]B$_{12}$ it should be re-chromatographed using a smaller volume of sample and/or larger volume of [^{57}Co]B$_{12}$.
— Pharmacia produce a very useful free guide 'Gel filtration, theory and practice' which is ideal for first-time users of this technique.

Interpretation

Normal values

Total unsaturated B$_{12}$ capacity   782 ± SD 225 pg/ml
Transcobalamin I   175 ± SD 36
Transcobalamin II   608 ± SD 186

Small variation from these ranges should be disregarded. Indeed, if it is intended to do significant numbers of these tests the laboratory should establish its own normal range.

In TC II deficiency TC II is absent. In myeloproliferative disorders TC I can be considerably elevated. TC II is elevated in Gauchers disease.

Although it is tempting to consider low or absent TC I as a possible cause of an unexplained low serum B_{12} level, this is so rarely the case that it is not recommended as a worthwhile investigation.

FOLATE ABSORPTION

These tests are required occasionally in a research rather than in a clinical context. It is a test of function of the upper small gut, and equally satisfactory results are obtained by measuring absorption of standard substances such as xylose. The test is required in the diagnosis of the rare congenital folate malabsorption disorders.

Principle
After an oral dose of folate the rise in plasma folate levels is measured. With tritium-labelled folate given orally, unabsorbed folate can be measured by counting excreted tritium in faeces.

Test samples
Blood samples without anticoagulant are collected before and at 1, 2 and 3 hours after an oral dose of folate. Sera are stored frozen until assay. Reproducible results are obtained after the patient has been treated with folate to overcome any tissue deficiency. Patients who are folate-deficient clear folate from plasma very rapidly so that misleadingly low blood folate levels after an oral dose are obtained if tissues are not first saturated with folate. An oral dose of 15 mg daily for 2–3 days is adequate, a 36-hour gap being left between the last dose of folate and the absorption test.

In the faecal excretion method, all faeces passed for 4 days after an oral dose (or until a marker substance is excreted) are collected. Only a broad outline of the test is given and details are to be found in the references cited.

Folate absorption by blood levels
After the patient has been saturated with folate an oral dose of 40 μg pteroylglutamic acid per kg body weight is given to the fasting patient. A pre-dose blood sample is collected and 10 ml venous blood at 1, 2 and 3 hours after the oral dose. Serum is separated and assayed by microbiological assay for folate content. Almost all published experience relates to assay using *Streptococcus faecalis* as test organism. A peak blood level of over 40 ng/ml is regarded as normal (Chanarin

and Bennett, 1962). Higher blood levels would be expected with an *L. casei* assay but there are no data on normal levels.

Faecal excretion of tritium-labelled folate
Folic acid or one of its analogues generally labelled with tritium is available and can be used to provide a quantitative measure of the absorption of folate. Between 20 and 50 μCi of tritium and approximately 200 μg folate is given. Faeces is collected for 4 days, weighed, dried and an aliquot combusted in oxygen in a glass chamber. The tritium is thereby oxidised to water, which is trapped by immersing the chamber in dry ice and acetone (Steytler, 1974). At least 80% of pteroylglutamic acid and more than 90% of physiological folate analogues (tetrahydrofolate, methyltetrahydrofolate) are absorbed by normal subjects.

Folate absorption by intestinal perfusion
This is a clinical method in which labelled folate is perfused through a segment of gut via a double lumen tube swallowed by the patient. A non-absorbable marker substance (polyethyleneglycol) is included and variation in its concentration enables one to make allowance for fluxes in volume of carrier fluid. The amount of perfused folate taken up by the gut in unit time is noted. Normally about 50% of a dose of pteroylglutamic acid (2 μmol/litre) is absorbed during 20 minutes perfusion (Halsted et al, 1977).

Tests in congenital folate malabsorption
These children present with a severe megaloblastic anaemia in the first 8–12 weeks of life. Malabsorption of folate is gross. It can be tested by giving an oral dose of 5 mg of pteroylglutamic acid and collecting a blood sample before, and between 1 and 2 hours after, the dose. The sample is prepared and assayed with *L. casei* as described for the serum folate assay. Normally the blood level increases to over 100 ng/ml. In these patients there is virtually no increase at all. The tests would be done after the child has been treated.

URINARY FORMIMINOGLUTAMIC ACID EXCRETION

Increased excretion of formiminoglutamic acid in the urine was proposed as a test for folic acid deficiency because folate is required in its further metabolism. In practice, modestly increased excretion of formiminoglutamic acid occurred in a variety of clinical disorders not related primarily to folate status so that the test lacked specificity. Secondly, some cases of folate deficiency failed to produce significant amounts of formiminoglutamic acid because the breakdown of histidine often stopped following conversion to urocanic acid, a precursor substance of formiminoglutamic acid.

Biochemical basis

Histidine→urocanic acid→formiminoglutamic acid→glutamic acid

$$
\begin{array}{ll}
\text{COOH} & \text{COOH} \\
| & | \\
\text{CH-NH-CH=H} & \text{CH-NH}_2 \\
| & | \\
\text{CH}_2 \quad + \text{H}_4\text{PteGlu} \rightarrow \text{CH}_2 \quad + \text{CH=NH-H}_4\text{PteGlu} \\
| & | \\
\text{CH}_2 & \text{CH}_2 \\
| & | \\
\text{COOH} & \text{COOH} \\
\text{Formiminoglutamic} & \text{Glutamic} \\
\quad \text{acid} & \quad \text{acid}
\end{array}
$$

The enzyme formiminotransferase, transfers the formimino (-CH=NH) group to tetrahydrofolate (H_4PteGlu) to form formiminotetrahydrofolate. At an acid pH this is converted to 5,10 methenyltetrahydrofolate and this is read at 350 nm.

There is a variety of methods for assaying formiminoglutamic acid. In all the patient is given an oral dose of 15 g of L-histidine to stress the pathway and urine passed in the next 8 hours is collected into a container with 2 ml N-HCl.

The only methods recommended are the sensitive enzymic ones which give a quantitative measure of the formiminoglutamic acid excreted. They are not included here but details are to be found in the references.

Interpretation

After 15 g oral histidine the mean urinary excretion is 9 mg with a range of 1–17 mg. A large increase (more than 100 mg) is probably due to folate deficiency, but a smaller increase can be due to B_{12} deficiency because folate function is impaired, or to other disorders including congestive cardiac failure, thyrotoxicosis, liver disease and neoplasia.

URINARY METHYLMALONIC ACID EXCRETION

The further metabolism of methylmalonic acid (MMA) requires vitamin B_{12}. In its absence there is increased urinary excretion of MMA so that it is a specific test for acquired B_{12} deficiency and for congenital impairment of the relevant pathways, the methylmalonylacidurias.

Biochemical basis

$$
\left.
\begin{array}{l}
\text{Valine} \\
\text{Isoleucine} \\
\text{Propionic acid}
\end{array}
\right) \xrightarrow{B_{12}} \text{methylmalonyl-CoA} \rightarrow \text{succinyl-CoA.}
$$

Test samples

24-hour urine is collected into bottles containing 10 ml of 10 N sulphuric acid. 10 g oral valine is given at the start of the collection.

Method

A detailed method is available in the reference papers. A host of colorimetric methods have been described for the measurement of MMA. These are only reliable when large amounts of MMA are excreted, when interference from other weak organic acids is diluted out. These methods are unreliable when there are only small increases in MMA. Gas chromatography after ether extraction of the urine is recommended as a specific assay (see references).

Interpretation

The mean 24-hour urinary excretion of MMA with or without oral valine is 2 mg with a range of 1–15 mg. The majority, but not all patients with B_{12} deficiency have an increased MMA excretion but this remains normal in those with little anaemia and relatively higher (although still low) serum B_{12} levels. The test, however, is specific for B_{12} deficiency provided that a specific assay method is employed.

REFERENCES

Deoxyuridine suppression tests

Chanarin I, Deacon R, Lumb M, Perry J 1980 Vitamin B_{12} regulates folate metabolism by the supply of formate. Lancet ii: 505–508

Das K C, Herbert V 1978 The lymphocyte as a marker of past nutritional status: persistence of abnormal lymphocyte deoxyuridine (dU) suppression test and chromosomes in patients with past deficiency of folate and vitamin B_{12}. British Journal of Haematology 38: 219–233

Deacon R, Chanarin I, Perry J, Lumb M 1980 Marrow cells from patients with untreated pernicious anaemia cannot use tetrahydrofolate normally. British Journal of Haematology 46: 523–528

Ganeshaguru K, Hoffbrand A V 1979 The effect of deoxyuridine, vitamin B_{12}, folate and alcohol on the uptake of thymidine and on the deoxynucleoside triphosphate concentrations in normal and megaloblastic cells. British Journal of Haematology 40: 29–41

Killmann S A 1964 Effect of deoxyuridine on incorporation of tritiated thymidine: Difference between normoblasts and megaloblasts. Acta Medica Scandinavica 175: 483–488

Matthews J H, Wickramasinghe S N 1986b A method for performing deoxyuridine suppression tests on microtitre plates. Clinical and Laboratory Haematology 8: 61–65

Matthews J H, Wickramasinghe S N 1986a Acquired folate deficiency in phytohaemagglutinin-stimulated human lymphocytes. British Journal of Haematology 63: 281–291

Metz J, Kelly A, Sweet V C, Waxman S, Herbert V 1968 Deranged DNA synthesis by bone marrow from vitamin B_{12}-deficient humans. British Journal of Haematology 14: 575–591

Pelliniemi T T, Beck W S 1980 Biochemical mechanisms in the Killmann Experiment. Critique of the deoxyuridine suppression test. Journal of Clinical Investigation 65: 449–460

Wickramasinghe S N 1983 The deoxyuridine suppression test. In: Hall C A (ed) The Cobalamins. Churchill Livingstone, Edinburgh, ch 11, p. 196–208

Wickramasinghe S N, Saunders J E 1977 Results of three years' experience with the deoxyuridine suppression test. Acta Haematologica 58: 193–206

Wickramasinghe S N, Saunders J E 1979 A fault in the design of the deoxyuridine suppression test. Clinical and Laboratory Haematology 1: 69–71

Zittoun J, Marquet J, Zittoun R 1978 Effect of folate and cobalamin compounds on the deoxyuridine suppression test in vitamin B_{12} and folate deficiency. Blood 51: 119–128

Serum cobalamin assay with *Lactobacillus leichmannii*

Beck W S 1983 The assay of serum cobalamin by *Lactobacillus leichmannii* and the interpretation of serum cobalamin levels. In: Hall C A (ed) The Cobalamins. Churchill Livingstone, Edinburgh p 31–50

Microbiological assay for vitamin B_{12} with *Euglena gracilis*

Adam J F, McEwan F 1971 Activities of various cobalamins for Euglena gracilis with reference to vitamin B_{12} assay. Journal of Clinical Pathology 24: 15–17

Anderson B B 1964 Investigations into the Euglena method for the assay of vitamin B_{12} in serum. Journal of Clinical Pathology 17: 14–26

Bertaux O, Valencia R 1973 Blocage de la division cellulaire et malformations induites par carence B_{12} chez les cellules synchrones de Euglena gracilis. Comptes Rendus des Seances de l'Academie des Sciences 276: 753–756

Bre M-H, Pouphile M, Delpech S, Lefort-Tran M 1983 Cytochemical studies of nuclear basic proteins in control and vitamin B_{12} starved Euglena. Journal of Histochemistry and Cytochemistry 31: 1101–1108

Cooper B A 1959 Studies with a more rapid method of vitamin B_{12} assay utilizing Euglena gracilis. Journal of Clinical Pathology 12: 153–156

Ford J E, Hutner S H 1955 Role of vitamin B_{12} in the metabolism of microorganisms. Vitamins and Hormones 13: 101–136

Kolhose J F, Kondo H, Allen N C, Podell E, Allen R H 1978 Cobalamin analogues are present in human plasma and can mask cobalamin deficiency because current radioisotope dilution assays are not specific for true cobalamin. New England Journal of Medicine 299: 785–792

Kondo H, Binder M J, Kolhouse J F, Smythe W R, Podell E, Allen R H 1982 Presence and formation of cobalamin analogues in multivitamin-mineral pills. Journal of Clinical

Investigation 70: 889–898

Kristensen H P O 1956 A vitamin B_{12}-binding factor found in cultures of Euglena gracilis var. bacillaris. Acta Physiologica Scandinavica 37: 8–13

Lear A A, Castle W B 1954 The serum B_{12} concentration in pernicious anemia. Journal of Laboratory and Clinical Medicine 44: 715–722

Mollin D L, Ross G I M 1952 The vitamin B_{12} concentration of serum and urine of normals and of patients with megaloblastic anaemias and other diseases. Journal of Clinical Pathology 5: 129–139

Mollin D L, Anderson B B, Burman J F 1976 The vitamin B_{12} level: its assay and significance. Clinics in Haematology 5: 521–546

Raven J L, Robson M B, Morgan J O, Hoffbrand A V 1972 Comparison of three methods for measuring vitamin B_{12} in serum: radioisotopic, Euglena gracilis, and Lactobacillus leichmannii. British Journal of Haematology 22: 21–31

Ross G I M 1950 Vitamin B_{12} assay in body fluids. Nature 166: 270–271

Vitamin B_{12} assay by solid phase saturation analysis

Chanarin I 1979 The megaloblastic anaemias, 2nd edn. Blackwell, Oxford, 128–141

Muir M, Chanarin I 1983 Solid phase vitamin B_{12} assays using polyacrylamide-bound intrinsic factor and polyacrylamide bound R-binder. British Journal of Haematology 53: 423–435

Whiteside M G, Mollin D L, Coghill N F, Williams A W, Anderson B 1964 The absorption of radioactive vitamin B_{12} and the secretion of hydrochloric acid in patients with atrophic gastritis. Gut 5: 385–399

Folate assay with *Lactobacillus casei*

Chanarin I 1969 The megaloblastic anaemias, 1st edn. Blackwell, Oxford, 308–328

Wright A J A, Phillips D R 1985 The threshold growth response of *Lactobacillus casei* to 5-methyl-tetrahydrofolic acid: implications for folate assays. British Journal of Nutrition 53: 569–573

Saturation analysis for folate assay

Cooper B A, Lowenstein L 1964 Relative folate deficiency of erythrocytes in pernicious anemia and its correction with cyanocobalamin. Blood 24: 502–521

Rothenberg S P, da Costa M 1976 Folate binding proteins and radioassay for folate. In: Hoffbrand A V (ed) Clinics in Hematology: The Megaloblastic Anaemias. W B Saunders, 569–587

Rothenberg S P, da Costa M, Lawson J, Rosenberg Z 1974 The determination of erythrocyte folate concentration using a two-phase ligand binding radioassay. Blood 43: 437–443

Rothenberg S P, da Costa M, Rosenberg Z 1972 Radioassay for serum folate: Use of a sequential incubation ligand binding system. New England Journal of Medicine 286: 1335–1339

Intrinsic-factor antibody

Chanarin I 1979 The megaloblastic anaemias, 2nd edn. Blackwell, Oxford.

Rose M S, Chanarin I, Doniach D, Brostoff J, Ardeman S 1970 Intrinsic factor antibodies in the absence of pernicious anaemiaa, 3–7 year follow-up. Lancet ii: 9–13

Intrinsic factor in human gastric juice

Begley J A, Trachtenberg A 1979 An assay for intrinsic factor based on blocking of the R binder of gastric juice by cobinamide. Blood 53: 788–793

Chanarin I 1979 The megaloblastic anaemias, 2nd edn. Blackwell, Oxford

Cobalamin (vitamin B$_{12}$) absorption

Adams J F, Claw D J, Ross S K, Boddy K, King P, Mahaffy M A 1972 Factors affecting the absorption of vitamin B$_{12}$. Clinical Science 43: 233–250

Chanarin I 1979 The megaloblastic anaemias, 2nd edn. Blackwell, Oxford

Coupland W W 1966 Plasma radioactivity after radioactive vitamin B$_{12}$ given orally. Medical Journal of Australia i: 1020–1023

Siurala M, Erämaa E, Nyberg W 1960 Pernicious anaemia and atrophic gastritis. Acta Medical Scandinavica 166: 213–223

Transcobalamins

Begley J A 1983 The materials and processes of plasma transport. In: Hall C A (ed) The cobalamins. Churchill Livingstone, Edinburgh, p 109–133

Gilbert H S 1977 Inhibition of vitamin B$_{12}$ binding to transcobalamin at low pH: Basis of a procedure for quantitation of circulating TCII and R binders. Journal of Laboratory and Clinical Medicine 89: 13–24

Folate absorption

Chanarin I, Bennett M C 1962 Absorption of folic acid and D-Xylose as tests of small intestinal function. British Medical Journal i: 985–989

Halsted C H, Reisenauer A M, Romero J J, Cantor D S, Ruebner B 1977 Jejunal perfusion of simple and conjugated folates in celiac sprue. Journal of Clinical Investigation 59: 933–940

Steytler J G 1974 The assay of tritium-labelled folate in faeces by the oxygen flask combustion technique followed by liquid scintillation counting. Journal of Clinical Pathology 27: 844–847

Urinary formiminoglutamic acid excretion

Chanarin I, Bennett M G 1962 A spectrophotometric method for estimating formiminoglutamic acid and urocanic acid. British Medical Journal i: 27–29

Tabor H, Wyngarden L 1958 A method for the determination of formiminoglutamic acid in urine. Journal of Clinical Investigation 37: 824–828

Urinary methylmalonic acid excretion

Chanarin I, England J M, Mollin C, Perry J 1973 Methylmalonic acid excretion studies. British Journal of Haematology 25: 45–53

Gompertz D 1968 The measurement of urinary methylmalonic acid by a combination of thin layer and gas chromatography. Clinica Chimica Acta 19: 477–484

7

Malaria and other blood-borne infections

EXAMINATION OF BLOOD FOR PARASITES

WET BLOOD FILM

Principle

This very simple technique can be used to detect motile extracellular parasites in peripheral blood, by allowing direct observation of their movement. It has a sensitivity similar to that of stained thick blood films, however it is not possible to make permanent or stained preparations.

Method

1. A drop of venous or capillary blood, about 5–10 μl in volume, is placed in the centre of a clean 76 × 26 mm slide and covered with a 22 × 22 mm coverslip.
2. The whole area of the coverslip is scanned using × 10 and then × 40 objectives, if possible using phase contrast, but bright field can be used provided the condenser iris is closed to give maximum contrast.

Comments

— Wet films should be checked immediately after preparation to prevent drying of the blood.
— Ideally the sample of blood should be taken straight from the patient without anticoagulant. If anticoagulant is necessary, then heparin is best for wet films.

Interpretation

Diagnosis is made by observation of the vigorous swimming action of the parasites, which set the surrounding red cells into motion. The technique is used for trypanosomes and microfilariae. *Borrelia* (relapsing fever) organisms give a very similar appearance to trypanosomes in this technique. They can be differentiated on Giemsa-stained thin films (see later).

STAINED THIN BLOOD FILM

Principle

Two methods are described. A rapid method, where an urgent diagnosis is required, and a longer method which provides the best staining for the successful identification of species.

Preparation of the smear and the staining is similar to that used for normal haematology, except that ordinary Giemsa stain is used, and dilution is made in alkaline buffer (pH 7.2) instead of the usual slightly acidic buffer used by most laboratories.

Equipment

○ Staining tray, constructed so that the slides may be stained face downwards in a small volume of solution.
○ 20 ml disposable syringe and 5 cm × 19 g needle (point removed).
○ Coplin jars.

Stains and reagents

● Giemsa stain solution (BDH, R66; Product 35086).
● Field's stain solution A (BDH; Product 35056).
● Field's stain solution B (BDH; Product 35057).

As an alternative to commercial stain, the solutions may be made up as follows:

A. Methylene Blue (medicinal) 0.8 g
  Azure I 0.5 g
  Na_2HPO_4 5.0 g
  KH_2PO_4 6.25 g
  Distilled water 500 ml
B. Eosin 1.0 g
  Na_2HPO_4 5.0 g
  KH_2PO_4 6.25 g
  Distilled water 500 ml

The solutions should be filtered after allowing to stand overnight.

● Phosphate-buffered distilled water, pH 7.2.
  KH_2PO_4 0.7 g
  Na_2HPO_4 1.0 g
  Distilled water 1.0 litre
● Absolute methanol (Analar).

Method (Giemsa stain)

1. Prepare thin blood film as for routine haema-

153

tology. Ensure that the film has a good 'tail' and does not reach the edges of the slide laterally.

2. Allow the film to dry in air and fix with methanol for ½ to 1 minute.

3. Tip off excess methanol and place face down on a staining tray.

4. Using the 20 ml syringe and blunt needle, dilute the stock Giemsa 1:10 with buffered distilled water. Mix well and expel air.

5. Infiltrate the stain, using the syringe and needle, under the slide, taking care not to trap large air bubbles. Stain for 40–45 minutes.

6. At end of staining time, rinse slides briefly with tap water and allow to drain dry in a vertical position. Once dry, spread immersion oil thinly over the film, using a finger or swab stick, and examine using the × 10 (for worms) or × 40 objective. Possible parasites should be examined in more detail using the oil immersion lens. A × 50 or × 63 oil immersion objective is invaluable for preliminary examination of blood films.

Comments

— The syringe method for dilution of Giemsa is strongly recommended, as once the stain is diluted with water, precipitation of the stain begins, which is hastened by exposure to air. Staining face-downwards also reduces precipitation, and any that does develop falls away from the smear. Cleanly stained smears are very important when searching for small intracellular parasites.

— The buffered water at pH 7.2 *must* be used for the dilution of stain for blood parasites. It is only at this alkaline pH that proper differentiation of parasite nuclear and cytoplasmic material takes place, as well as the staining of cytoplasmic and membrane changes in infected RBC (e.g. Schuffner's dots in malaria infections). It must be stressed that acidic staining is not suitable for proper diagnosis of blood parasites on thin films.

Method (rapid Field's method)

1. Prepare and fix film as for the Giemsa technique.
2. Dip slide in Field's stain B (in a Coplin jar) for 7–8 seconds.
3. Rinse thoroughly in a beaker of tap water and then drain off excess water onto absorbent paper.
4. Dip slide in Field's stain A for 7–8 seconds.
5. Rinse thoroughly in a beaker of clean tap water and allow to dry in air in a vertical position. Do not blot. When dry examine slide as for Giemsa stain.

Comment

In areas which have a very soft, acidic water supply, it may be necessary to rinse in buffered water, pH 7.2, instead of tap water in steps 3 and 5.

THICK BLOOD FILM

Thick blood films allow a rapid examination of a relatively large volume of blood, enabling the detection of even scanty parasitaemias of all blood parasites. A well-prepared thick blood film gives more than a 10-fold increase in sensitivity over thin films.

As with thin films, two techniques are given; a rapid Field's technique (particularly good for malaria diagnosis) and a slower Giemsa stain method which is more suitable for the extracellular parasites. Two other, more specialised, staining methods are given under the sections on trypanosomes and filarial worms.

Principle

A dried film, about 5–6 RBC thick, is made, and the haemoglobin lysed out either before or during the staining process. The malaria parasites in the film are stained with little interference from the large numbers of RBCs present, and can be seen against a relatively clear background.

Samples

If at all possible, venous or capillary blood should be taken without anticoagulants. Films taken without anticoagulants adhere better to the slides and leave a clearer background after lysis.

Preparation of thick blood film

1. A drop of blood, 3–5 mm in diameter (3–5 μl) is put into the centre of a 76 × 26 mm slide and spread, with the corner of another slide or a swab stick, to cover an oval area of approximately 10–15 mm diameter.
2. The final density of the smear should allow newsprint to be just visible through it.
3. Thoroughly dry the smear, horizontally, in an incubator at 37°C for one hour.

Staining method (Giemsa)

1. Do *not* fix the dry film, but place it in a Coplin jar containing buffered water (pH 7.2) and allow to lyse until no haemoglobin can be seen falling away from the smear (usually 3–5 min).
2. Remove from water, place face-down on staining dish, and stain with Giemsa diluted 1:10 with buffered water, as for thin film method.
3. Stain for 30 minutes; then rinse briefly with tap water and drain dry. Examine film as described for a thin blood film.

Staining method (Field's stain)

1. Do *not* fix the dry film.
2. Dip film for 3 seconds in Field's stain A.
3. Wash thoroughly in tap water and drain off excess water onto absorbent paper.

4. Dip film for 3 seconds into Field's stain B.

5. Wash thoroughly in tap water, and allow to drain dry in a vertical position.

6. When dry, examine as for a thin blood film, paying particular attention to the lower half of the film, where haemoglobin from the lysis stage makes the best colour contrast for detection of the parasites.

Comments
— Films must be absolutely dry before lysis, else the blood smear is likely to detach from the slide.
— In the Field's stain method, the films should be washed, in steps 3 and 5, until no more colour comes away from the film.

BLOOD FILMS FROM SUSPECTED HAEMORRHAGIC FEVERS OR HIV

The recommended technique is as follows:

Thick films
1. Fix the dried smear directly in 10% buffered formalin for 10 minutes.
2. Wash three times (total 3 min) in buffered water and stain with Giemsa as usual.

Thin films
1. Fix in methanol for 5 minutes.
2. Fix in formalin as above, wash and stain in Giemsa.

Comment
Nuclei of malaria parasites stain darker by this technique, and the characteristic RBC stippling is not always satisfactorily stained.

MALARIA

Persons with a history of travel in malarious parts of the world who develop fever within four weeks of return, may be suffering from malignant tertian malaria (*Plasmodium falciparum*). *P. falciparum* infections rarely persist for more than one year untreated, but are often fatal. The other three species of malaria infecting man may, after the initial feverish symptoms have died down, recur after several months to four years in the case of *P. vivax* and *P. ovale* which have dormant liver forms, and up to 40 or more years in the case of *P. malariae*, which can persist in the blood of untreated persons. It should be remembered that malarial infections may be acquired by blood transfusion, syringe-sharing, organ transplants and accidental laboratory inoculation in persons not having travelled to endemic

areas, and a few reports exist of malaria transmission having taken place in the vicinity of airports, owing to the accidental importation of infected vector female *Anopheles* mosquitoes.

Samples and methods
For malaria diagnosis blood should ideally be taken direct from the patient's finger or ear and the smears prepared at the bedside or in the clinic. If it is necessary to use anticoagulants then the films should be made as soon as possible, certainly less than three hours, after the blood was drawn. EDTA is superior to other anticoagulants for this purpose. Parasite and RBC morphology can be seriously affected if the blood has been long in anticoagulant.

Blood should, if possible, be taken during or after pyrexia, and before the administration of antimalarial drugs.

On occasions, bone marrow may contain greater numbers of parasites than the peripheral blood, and bone marrow smears can be used for malaria diagnosis in such cases.

For routine diagnosis of malaria, 4 thin and 4 thick blood films should be prepared. One of the thin films, stained by the method using Giemsa stain should be adequate for detection of normal parasitaemias and for determination of species. To save time, where essential, the rapid Field's technique should be used, but should be backed up by Giemsa-stained thin films. The thick films should be stained using Field's or Giemsa stain. If problems with diagnosis arise the other films are available for further study. In addition, the PHLS Malaria Reference Laboratory would appreciate having unstained films, both thick and thin, for confirmation. If clinical evidence of malaria is strong, yet parasites are not found in the films taken initially, then further films should be taken at 6-hourly intervals.

Interpretation
The presence of intra-erythrocytic bodies, generally consisting of a blue-staining cytoplasmic area closely associated with a small reddish-staining nuclear area, and, in the larger, more mature parasites, the presence within the organism of yellow-brown to black malaria pigment, is diagnostic of malaria infection. As the malaria parasite grows within the erythrocyte, and finally divides to give a maximum of 24 infective merozoites, the host cell may show enlargement (*P. vivax* and *P. ovale*), remain the same size, or shrink (*P. falciparum* and *P. malariae*). The erythrocyte membrane may develop surface markings (Schuffner's and James's dots) which stain pink with Giemsa at pH 7.2 (*P. vivax* and *P. ovale*). All stages of the parasite may be seen in the peripheral blood in the case of *P. vivax*, *ovale* and *malariae*, but generally only the

Table 7.1 Differential diagnosis of *Plasmodium* species of man in Giemsa-stained thin films of peripheral blood.

	Species			
	P. falciparum	*P. vivax*	*P. malariae*	*P. ovale*
Trophozoites (a) Ring forms	0.15 to 0.5 of diameter of RBC; RBC normal size. Cytoplasm — very fine in young rings; thick irregular in old rings. Marginal (accolé) forms, forms with 2 chromatin dots and multiple infections common.	0.3 to 0.5 of diameter of RBC which is unaltered in size. Cytoplasm — circle, thin.	0.3 to 0.5 of diameter of RBC which is unaltered in size. Cytoplasm — circle, thicker.	0.3 diameter of RBC which is unaltered in size. Cytoplasm — circle, thicker.
(b) Growing forms	RBC unaltered in size, sometimes stippled, pale. Parasite compact; pigment dense brown or black mass.	RBC enlarged, stippled. Parasite — amoeboid, vacuolated; pigment fine and scattered, golden brown.	RBC unaltered. Parasite compact, rounded or band-shaped; dark brown or black pigments, often concentrates in a line along one edge of band.	RBC unaltered in size, or slightly enlarged; stippled; may be oval and fimbriated. Parasite — compact, rounded; pigment fine brown grains.
Mature schizonts	RBC unaltered in size, sometimes stippled, pale. Parasites about 0.6 of RBC; nuclei or merozoites 8–24; pigment clumped, black. *Not usually seen in peripheral blood.*	RBC much enlarged, stippled. Parasite large, filling enlarged RBC; nuclei or merozoites 12–24, usually 16; pigment a golden brown central loose mass.	RBC unaltered. Parasite fills RBC completely; nuclei or merozoites 6–12, usually 8, sometimes forming rosette; pigment, brown black central clump.	RBC frequently oval, fimbriated, enlarged, stippled. Parasite as for *P. malariae* but does not entirely fill the slightly enlarged RBC; pigment, brown central clump.
Gametocytes	RBC distorted. Parasite crescentic.	RBC enlarged, stippled. Parasite large, rounded, filling enlarged rbc.	RBC unaltered. Parasite small, round, filling rbc.	RBC slightly enlarged, stippled. Parasite round.
Stippling	Maurer's clefts.	Schuffner's dots.	None. (Fine dots after prolonged staining may be seen).	James' dots.

small ring parasites and (in older infections) the banana-like gametocytes) are found in *P. falciparum*. In infections of *P. falciparum*, a few intra-erythrocytic spots appear, particularly noticeable in erythrocytes inhabited by the thicker ring forms. These are termed Maurer's clefts, and should be distinguished carefully from the finer, much more numerous Schuffner's and James's dots found in *P. vivax* and *ovale*. See Table 7.1 and Plates 1.1–1.6.

Blood which has stood for too long in anticoagulant may manifest several changes.

1. The further development of the sexual stages may occur (even within 20 minutes under the right conditions) and the male gametes released into the plasma may be mistaken for other organisms, such as *Borrelia*. They may be distinguished from *Borrelia* by the central location of the red-staining nucleus, and the absence of marked repetitive sinuous curves.

2. If parasitised blood is left at warm laboratory temperature, re-invasion of released merozoites into red cells may take place, leading, for example, to the occurrence of appreciable numbers of 'accolé' forms, characteristic of *P. falciparum*, in blood parasitised by *P. vivax*.

3. Heavier parasitaemias left for several hours may lead to the build-up of acid in the blood sample, and the serious deterioration of the already delicate parasitised erythrocytes. Those parasitised with early *P. vivax* forms may shrink or become crenated. Later stages of the parasite may become compact, and the erythrocyte membrane may become very delicate so that it stretches when the film is prepared.

Importance of parasitaemia estimation in P. falciparum
An estimate of the percentage of erythrocytes infected is of immediate value to the clinician, especially in the case of *P. falciparum* infections. For example, if parasitaemia exceeds 10%, exchange transfusion may be

indicated in *P. falciparum*. In addition, if late dividing forms of this parasite are seen in the peripheral blood, this should be reported, as it may indicate that the patient is in a critical condition.

BABESIASIS

Like malaria, *Babesia* is an intra-erythrocytic protozoan parasite. Babesias of cattle and rodents are transmitted by ticks, and when the species of tick involved is one that occasionally bites man, the risk of human infection occurs. Cattle babesias, transmitted by *Ixodes ricinus* will infect only splenectomised persons, where they cause a fulminating rapidly fatal disease, with a high parasitaemia. Haemoglobinuria is often seen. *Babesia microti* of rodents will infect normal persons, generally giving rise to chronic disease with intermittent headache, fatigue, fevers and joint pains. Ticks of rodents in Europe rarely bite man, but in North America *Ixodes dammini* will readily do so.

Method
Blood film diagnosis is carried out using thick and thin films stained with Giemsa, as described for malaria. *B. microti* infection can be confirmed by inoculating hamsters or gerbils.

Interpretation
In view of possible confusion with malaria, the history of the patient should be taken with care. In a patient with a fulminating parasitaemia, with non-pigmented parasites in the erythrocytes, who has no recent (1 year) history of travel in malarious areas, lacks a spleen, and has been in contact with infected cattle pastures, babesiasis must be suspected. Presumptive treatment for malaria is often carried out. The intra-erythrocytic parasites of *Babesia* show 'indian club' shaped small forms, which may be arranged as Vs or as Xs.

B. microti generally shows much lower parasitaemias, and animal inoculation may be the best means of diagnosis.

TRYPANOSOMIASIS

Two subspecies of *Trypanosoma brucei*, *T.b. rhodesiense* and *T.b. gambiense*, transmitted to man by the tsetse fly, are responsible for the African trypanosomiases, Rhodesian and Gambian sleeping sickness. Although the South American *Trypanosoma cruzi*, agent of Chagas' disease, may be found in the blood in acute infections, the organism is rarely seen in diagnostic blood specimens taken outside the area of origin.

Principle
Unless the infection is detected during the early acute phase, the number of parasites in the peripheral circulation will be very low, and unlikely to be found without some form of concentration technique. Wet blood films should always be examined in addition to thick blood films, the haematocrit tube method, and if available, the mini-ion-exchange column (MAEC). As the trypanosomes are extracellular and prone to lysis during normal thick film methods, a modified method is given below which helps to protect the parasites during the staining process. (CSF and fluid from enlarged lymphatic glands can also be examined by the following staining techniques.)

Methods
Wet blood films
As previously described.

Modified thick blood film (MacLennan 1957)
1. Prepare standard thick blood films.
2. Dip for 1 second in 0.5% aqueous Methylene Blue (medicinal).
3. Place slide in a Coplin jar containing buffered water pH 7.2 and allow to lyse for 3–5 minutes (change water after 1 minute).
4. Dry slide in air.
5. Fix with methanol for 30 seconds.
6. Stain in Giemsa for 30 minutes.
7. Rinse in tap water and dry in air.
8. Examine under the × 40 objective, having covered the film with oil.

Comments
— Exposure to Methylene Blue appears to stabilise the organisms to lysis.
— The change of buffered water allows the easy observation of dehaemoglobinisation, which is carried out until no further haemoglobin (stained by the Methylene Blue) can be seen leaching out of the smears.
— IMPORTANT. The films must dry thoroughly between lysis and fixation with methanol, otherwise a white precipitate will spoil the result.
N.B. Fixation in this technique improves the result appreciably.

Interpretation
Careful scanning of the film is necessary to pick up the trypanosomes. If stained correctly with Giemsa, the nucleus and kinetoplast (area of DNA associated with the mitochondrial primordium and flagellar basal body) are readily seen as intensely staining pink bodies against the pale blue cytoplasm.

Any suspect organisms should be checked using the

oil immersion lens. Spurious trypanosomes composed of red cell stroma or fragments of leucocyte nuclei will not show any distinction between red and blue areas.

Haematocrit method (Woo 1970)

Principle

This method is a quick and simple adaptation of the standard microhaematocrit method for PCV determination. Like the white blood cells, trypanosomes accumulate during centrifugation with the buffy coat, between the white cells and the plasma. They can then be detected by their characteristic movement when the haematocrit tube is examined under the right conditions. The technique is about 10 times more sensitive than the thick film technique, and will detect very low parasitaemias.

Samples

Capillary blood is taken into a standard heparinised glass capillary tube. Four tubes should be collected at one time from the patient.

Apparatus

○ Microhaematocrit centrifuge.
○ Heparinised capillary tubes.
○ Viewing slide. (This is simply prepared by using strips of Plasticine on a slide, which form a trough in which the sealed capillary can lie in water, and be covered by a coverslip, allowing distortion-free viewing of the contents of the tube.)

Method

1. Fill capillary tubes and heat-seal the contaminated ends.
2. Spin tubes for 4 minutes at 12 000 rpm.
3. Remove a tube and place it on viewing slide under a 22 × 22 mm. coverslip. Flood the space between tube and coverslip.
4. Examine the interface between the 'buffy layer' and the plasma, initially using the × 10 objective. The tube should be gently rolled to ensure all sides are examined.
5. Confirmation of a positive finding may be made by staining a smear of the buffy coat as described above, after cutting the capillary tube.

Comments

— Tubes need to be checked fairly soon after spinning, as the trypanosomes tend to swim away from the interface.
— When viewing the haematocrit tube under the microscope, it is essential that a bright, high-contrast image is obtained. This can be achieved by shutting down the condenser iris or by lowering the condenser.

— It is vitally important to keep focusing up and down through the whole thickness of the capillary tube, or scanty organisms may be missed.

Interpretation

Trypanosomes can be recognised by their active movement at the buffy layer, easily detected using × 10 and confirmed using × 40.

In the case of *T.b. gambiense* infections, very few organisms may be found. It is not unusual to find only two or three trypanosomes in the 4 haematocrit capillaries examined, so all 4 should be examined carefully.

In patients whose clinical history indicates a high likelihood of infection, examinations of further samples may be necessary.

It is not possible to distinguish between *T.b. rhodesiense* and *T.b. gambiense* on blood films. Both are long sinuous flagellated organisms. The former cause a more acute illness, but the latter may often localise in the brain. Distinction follows culture or animal inoculation and electrophoretic studies of enzyme patterns.

Trypanosoma cruzi, when observed in blood, is not sinuous but often takes up a characteristic 'C' shape.

Mini anion exchange method (Lumsden et al 1979)

Principle

This method uses the difference in surface charge between blood cells and trypanosomes to separate the latter. Briefly, heparinised blood diluted with buffer (phosphate-buffered saline, pH 8.0, ionic strength 0.362) is passed through a DEAE cellulose column, which absorbs the blood cells. The trypanosomes are eluted into a finely-drawn Pasteur pipette, which is then centrifuged, and the tip is examined as described for the microhaematocrit technique. Only 80–100 μl of blood or CSF is needed, and the technique is more sensitive than any other. The original reference should be consulted before attempting the technique.

FILARIASIS

Microfilariae found in blood are the larval stages of filarial worms, infective to the dipteran vector. The adults of the genera *Loa*, *Dipetalonema*, *Brugia*, *Wuchereria* and *Mansonella* live in the tissues. *Dipetalonema* and *M. ozzardi*, found in West Africa and South America respectively, rarely cause disease, but may be, like other filarial worms, associated with marked eosinophilia. *L. loa* from Africa, and often found in mixed infections with *D. perstans*, causes a variety of ill effects, one of the most notable being superficial transient oedematous swellings in different parts of the body (Calabar swellings). *L. loa* adults are occasionally seen to move beneath the surface of the conjunctiva.

B. malayi and *W. bancrofti* the former from subtropical and tropical Asia, and the latter found in many tropical countries throughout the world, cause lymphatic filariasis, with elephantiasis occurring in some cases.

Samples

For *Brugia* and *Wuchereria* diagnosis, blood should be collected between 10 p.m. and 2 a.m. since this is when the microfilariae are most abundant in the peripheral blood. In the case of *Loa*, the microfilariae are diurnal, and blood should be collected between 10 a.m. and 2 p.m.

Method

Heavy microfilaraemia can be detected using the wet film technique. Under × 10 the sinuous movements of the microfilariae in fresh blood are readily seen. Fixed and stained thin blood films (Giemsa, long technique) may show the presence of one or two microfilariae in the whole film, but only if scanning of the oiled film is carried out using the × 10 objective.

A haematoxylin technique is valuable for the examination of the nuclei in the tail of the microfilaria. Methanol-fixed films are stained for 20 minutes in Ehrlich's haematoxylin preheated to 60°C (until the stain begins to steam). They are then washed in tap water for 10 minutes. Decolourisation is rapidly carried out by a brief immersion in 1% acid alcohol. A further wash in tap water will blue the stain, and examination under the microscope will verify whether the nuclei are clearly visible.

Thick film examination after staining with Giemsa stain will detect microfilaraemia, but the most sensitive technique is the filtration method.

Filtration method for microfilariae

10 ml of blood is collected in sodium citrate. The blood is filtered through a 'Nuclepore' filter (Sterilin) of 3 μm pore size, using a syringe-mounted filter. After washing through the filter with saline, the membrane is examined under a coverslip using × 10 objective, to detect motile microfilariae. Further examination should be carried out under × 40, for detection of the presence of a sheath. Centrifugal concentration of the blood (700 *g*; 5 min) after lysis with 1% saponin also allows detection of microfilariae on microscopic examination of the sediment (less satisfactory).

Comment

— It is essential to ensure that water for preparation of solutions and for washing the filter is free from free-living nematodes.

Interpretation

Microfilariae of *L. loa* are longer and thicker than those of *D. perstans* (up to 298 μm × 7.5 μm compared with 200 × 4.5 μm), and those of the latter do not possess the characteristic sheath, a transparent envelope covering the whole microfilaria, which in *Loa* stains weakly pink with Giemsa. The microfilariae of *Mansonella* are also small and narrow (173–240 μm × 4–5 μm) and unsheathed. Both *Brugia* and *Wuchereria* microfilariae are sheathed. *Wuchereria* is larger than *Brugia*, (280 μm × 7.5 μm compared with 200–250 μm × 5–6 μm). Distinction between these two species is on the basis of the nuclear arrangement in the tail (*Wuchereria* has no nuclei near the tip, whilst *Brugia* has at least two). In addition, the sheath of *Brugia* stains pink with Giemsa, and that of *Wuchereria* remains colourless.

REFERENCES

Bruce-Chwatt L J 1985 Essential malariology, 2nd edn. Heinemann, London

Lumsden W H, Kimber C D, Evans D A, Doig S J 1979 Trypanosoma brucei: miniature anion-exchange centrifugation technique for detection of low parasitaemias: adaptation for field use. Transactions of the Royal Society of Tropical Medicine & Hygiene 73 (3): 312–317

Maclennan K J R 1957 A staining technique for the identification of trypanosomes in thick blood films. Transactions of the Royal Society of Tropical Medicine & Hygiene 51: 301–302

Manson-Bahr A E C, Apted F I C 1982 Manson's Tropical Diseases, 18th edn. Bailliere Tindall, London

Woo P T K 1970 The haematocrit centrifuge technique for the diagnosis of African trypanosomiasis. Acta Tropica 27: 384–386

8

Pregnancy

KLEIHAUER

This method is used to detect red cells containing fetal haemoglobin in mixtures of cells containing adult haemoglobin. It is of value in two situations:

1. In defining the distribution of fetal haemoglobin in red cells in the inherited conditions characterised by hereditary persistence of fetal haemoglobin (HPFH) (Wood 1983).

2. For detection of fetal erythrocytes in maternal blood following transplacental haemorrhages.

This section describes the use of the method for detection of fetal erythrocytes in maternal circulation and is used in several circumstances.

a. To confirm or refute occult fetal blood loss as a cause of unexplained or unexpected anaemia in the neonate.

b. To semi-quantitate transplacental fetal blood losses in an Rh(D) negative maternal circulation so that appropriate and adequate passive prophylaxis with Anti-D immunoglobulin can be administered.

c. One additional use that is of value is in vascular transfusion to the fetus to check the proportion of fetal cells to transfused adult cells in treatment of anaemia of severe haemolytic disease at early gestation before delivery is feasible.

Principle and biochemical basis

Fetal haemoglobin is chemically more stable in vitro than adult haemoglobin and resists both alkali denaturation and acid elution. The acid elution test of Kleihauer et al (1957) was developed for the detection of fetal erythrocytes in the maternal circulation following transplacental haemorrhages. It is based on the differential elution of fetal and adult haemoglobins at acid pH. It distinguishes between cells containing 90% Hb F (fetal) and those containing virtually none (maternal).

A post-delivery maternal blood film is fixed and then flooded with acid for a short time. On counterstaining the fetal cells which have retained their haemoglobin will stand out in a sea of ghost maternal cells from which the haemoglobin has been eluted. The volume of fetal red cells lost in the maternal circulation can be crudely quantitated (see below).

Test samples

A sample of maternal blood in EDTA should be collected soon after delivery, preferably within 48 hours and kept at 4°C until tested. It is usual to collect a serum sample for checking maternal Rh(D) antibody status at the same time. The delivered baby's blood group is determined and a direct antiglobulin test performed.

Reagents

- Sodium phosphate/citric acid buffer pH 3.3
- Stock solutions:
  1. 0.2 m Na_2HPO_4 anhydrous 28.394 g per litre distilled water
  2. 0.1 m Citric acid 21.0 g/litre distilled water.

Equipment

- Pipettes
- Glass slides
- 37°C Incubator
- 37°C Water-bath
- Staining rack

Preparation of test samples, standards and working reagents

A control is made by adding one drop of compatible cord cells in EDTA to 2.0 ml of adult blood in EDTA. Solutions should be kept at 4°C but working solutions are left at room temperature. Solutions are stable for 3 to 4 weeks.

Solution (1) 0.2 m Na_2HPO_4 sometimes crystallises out at 4°C, therefore warm to 37°C before use. For use, dilute 1 part (1) Na_2HPO_4 and 3 parts (2) citric acid and warm to 37°C.

Method

1. Make thin, uniform blood films on glass slides of maternal specimens and control.

2. These should be air-dried in a 37°C incubator for approximately one hour.

3. Fix in 80% methyl alcohol for 3 minutes.

4. Dry in incubator.

5. Flood slides on staining rack with pH 3.3 buffer for 14–40 seconds. Time depends on each batch of buffer, room temperature, etc. and must be found by trial and error. This step is essential to obtain satisfactory results. Start with control preparation as follows:

1. Flood slides with buffer for 10 seconds.

2. Rock for 10 seconds — total 20 seconds.

3. Wash off with tap water.

Check the unstained preparation under low power to see whether fetal cells stand out in sea of ghost maternal cells. If differentiation is not satisfactory, shorten or lengthen the time of exposure to buffer accordingly. It is more satisfactory to flood and rock the slides for equal lengths of time e.g. 7 seconds flood to 7 seconds rock up to 20 s flood/20 s rock. Always repeat the procedure with the control preparation at the end of a batch. Counterstain with Leishman or any Romanowsky stain. This is far more satisfactory than using Eosin as recommended in some methods. Confusion with small lymphocytes can occur when everything stains pink.

Examine the slides unmounted, under the low power for the presence of fetal red cells.

Interpretation

The aim is to calculate the size of the transplacental haemorrhage in terms of the volume of fetal red cells. Of course this can be assessed most accurately by determining the maternal red cell volume and the ratio of fetal to maternal red cells by counting both types of cells in a large number of microscope fields. This is too tedious and time-consuming for routine purposes.

For practical purposes the important thing is to establish when the transplacental haemorrhage exceeds 4 ml, because the standard dose of 500 IU anti-D immunoglobulin (100 μg) issued will protect the Rh(D) negative mother from sensitisation with up to 4 ml red cells from her Rh(D) positive fetus.

In the vast majority of cases, fetal losses into the maternal circulation are less than 1.0 ml. In devising a convenient screening test it is necessary to consider the numerous sources of error, most of which will be exaggerated by examining only a few microscope fields. The greatest variable of all is in the preparation of blood films. Great care should be taken in spreading. Thin uniform films should be prepared and the aim is to arrive at a density of about 5000 per lower power field. Reference slides for comparison, though frequently referred to in the older literature, do not now seem to be generally available. Fetal red cells tend to concentrate towards the edges of blood films, resulting in lower counts in the central areas. The volume of a fetal red cell is $\simeq$ 22% greater than that of an adult red cell, therefore the number counted under-represents the volume of fetal red cells present. Also, not all fetal red cells stain darkly by the acid elution method. It is assumed that approximately 92% fetal cells retain their haemoglobin. Mollison (1983) has recommended a correction factor of 4/3 to the actual fetal cell count to allow for these sources of error and to give a more accurate estimation of volume of fetal red cells in the maternal circulation.

Assuming that the maternal red cell volume at term is 1800 ml (another possible source of error) then a transplacental haemorrhage of 4 ml will give a ratio of 1:450 by volume. If the correction factor above is applied, the 4 ml will be represented by a count of one fetal cell for every 600 maternal cells. So if the average number of adult cells per low power field is 2400, then a 4 ml fetal bleed would result in an average of 4 fetal cells per lower power field examined. If 5 fields are examined, an average of 20 cells would be seen.

If appropriate tables giving confidence limits for a poisson variable are used, it has been pointed out (Mollison 1983) that 9 at the P=0.1 level would be the maximum number of cells which can be counted in 5 low power fields without arousing suspicion that the actual number is more than 20 and that the fetal blood volume may exceed 4 ml.

As can be seen, this is a very crude quantitation, but is designed to give us a usable method in the laboratory, to detect those fetal bleeds in which the standard dose of anti-D will be insufficient to protect the Rh(D) negative mother from sensitisation.

Procedure is as follows:

1. Inspect thin uniform films prepared and counterstained as described. Use the low power × 10 objective.

2. Count the number of fetal cells in 5 low power fields.

The finding of not more than 9 fetal cells can be regarded as indicating with a high degree of probability that the fetal transplacental haemorrhage does not exceed 4 ml and the standard dose of anti-D (500 IU) may be issued.

In the very few cases in which more than 9 cells are seen in 5 low power fields, the proportion of fetal to adult red cells should be determined by relating the number of fetal to adult cells. The volume of fetal red cells in the maternal circulation can then be derived from the following formula:

$$1800 \quad \times \text{ ratio } \frac{\text{fetal}}{\text{adult}} \text{ red cells} \times \quad \frac{4}{3}$$

Volume of   Correction

maternal red   factor

cells

e.g. if there are 1% fetal cells in the maternal circulation:

$$\text{Volume of fetal cells} = 1800 \times \frac{1}{100} \times \frac{4}{3} = 24 \text{ ml}$$

It is hoped that this simplified, crude semi-quantitative estimate of volume of fetal red cells in the maternal circulation will ensure that no woman will become sensitised because of an inadequate amount of anti-D being administered post-delivery.

AMNIOTIC FLUID BILIRUBIN

Estimation of amniotic fluid bilirubin is important in assessing the severity of haemolytic disease of the newborn during pregnancy.

Principle and biochemical basis
In a normal pregnancy unconjugated bilirubin is present in the amniotic fluid, the concentration decreasing toward term. This is presumed to be due to some leakage of the normal breakdown products of fetal haemoglobin in their transplacental passage to the maternal liver which converts fetal bilirubin to the non-toxic water-soluble form. Since amniotic fluid is, to a large extent, a fetal product, the infant swallowing it and excreting into it, another source of amniotic fluid bilirubin may be tracheal and pulmonary fluid. In a pregnancy complicated by fetal haemolytic disease, the bilirubin concentration in amniotic fluid rises above the known normal level for gestation. This raised concentration of bilirubin is directly related to the severity of haemolysis. By measuring certain parameters in amniotic fluid, viz, total bile pigment, bile pigment/protein ratio and the spectrophotometric curve with quantitations of $\triangle$ 450 nm it is possible to assess the severity of fetal haemolytic disease.

A more accurate picture of the progress of the disease can be obtained if serial measurements are performed. Liley (1961) recommended that the first taps be carried out at between 29 and 32 weeks' gestation, mainly because this was the earliest time that any intra-uterine transfusion could be carried out. However, intraperitoneal transfusions can now be carried out from as early as 22 weeks' gestation and intravascular transfusion from 18 weeks' gestation onwards (Nicolaides et al 1985).

Unfortunately, normal ranges and abnormal amniotic $\triangle$ 450 nm bilirubin values are not widely available or reliably interpretable before 22 to 24 weeks' gestation. After 34–35 weeks' gestation the amniotic fluid becomes increasingly cloudy and it is not possible to obtain reliable spectrophotometric measurements of bile pigment. The bile pigment/protein ratio may be more helpful at earlier gestation.

Amniocenteses for bilirubin content are usually carried out at two-week intervals between 22 and 34 weeks' gestation. By plotting the $\triangle$ 450 nm values on a specially prepared graph relating Liley's zones of severity to gestation (Fig 8.1) it is possible to predict the outcome of the pregnancy and to take the appropriate measures when needed e.g. intra-uterine transfusion or premature delivery of the fetus.

If other parameters (rapidly rising maternal antibody concentration, or previous intra-uterine fetal death) indicate that severe fetal haemolytic disease before 22 weeks' gestation is to be expected, earlier action may have to be taken. This would involve umbilical cord blood sampling at 18 weeks' gestation, when the blood group, haemoglobin, PCV, DAT, etc., can be estimated directly and intravascular transfusion administered if indicated. Normal haematological values have been established for cord blood samples obtained at 18–24 weeks' gestation (Nicolaides et al 1985).

During pregnancy the volume of amniotic fluid increases. If this is not taken into account, it would

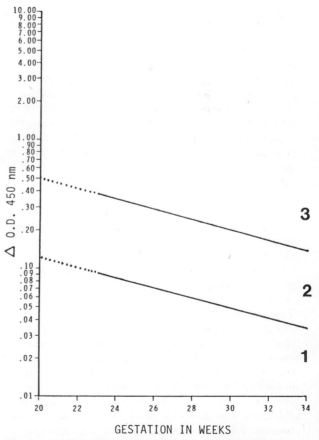

Fig. 8.1 Amniotic fluid spectrophotometry using Liley's three zone concept.

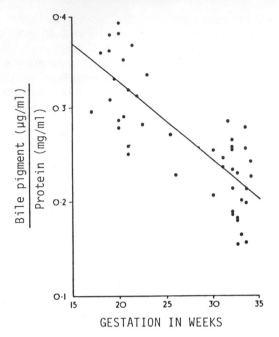

Fig. 8.2 Decrease in liquor bile pigment to protein ratio with increase in gestation in normal pregnancies.

appear that the bile pigment content decreases with increasing gestation. The protein concentration is thought to be inversely related to the total liquor volume and so the ratio of bile pigment to protein is thought by some (Murray et al 1970) to be a better indicator of the severity of haemolytic disease than bile pigment alone. In addition, normal ranges for bile pigment/protein ratio have been established earlier in pregnancy, in a group of mothers between 16 and 26 weeks' gestation (Fig. 8.2).

The method of estimating bile pigment/protein ratio is included here because we have found it valuable additional information in difficult cases and for many years it was the only method of quantifying amniotic fluid bilirubin at Queen Charlotte's Maternity Hospital, which has always had favourable fetal survival rates compared with other referral centres.

Test sample

For all measurements the test sample is treated in the same way. A sample of amniotic fluid is obtained by amniocentesis and put immediately into a sterile container which is protected from light by a black polythene bag. This is important because bilirubin is photolabile. Red cells are removed by centrifugation at 2500 rpm. The hazy supernatant is then clarified in two stages as follows:

1. Millipore pre-filter (cat. no. AP2501300).
2. Filtrate from 1 put through epidural filter of 0.2 μm

cut off (Portex cat. no. 100/385/010).

In both cases a 10 ml plastic syringe is used. At either stage more than one filter may be required because they tend to get blocked with cellular debris. The filtrate from 2 is stored in a sterile container at 4°C and protected from light. The analysis should be performed within 24 hours of taking the test sample.

Estimation of total bile pigment

Reagents

- Diazo A: 1% sulphanilic acid in 0.2 N HCl (245 ml 1% Sulphanilic acid + 5 ml conc HCl).
- Diazo B: 0.5% sodium nitrite (stable 3 weeks at room temperature).
- Diazo blank: 0.25 N HCl.
  Working diazo is made freshly just before use: 5 ml diazo A + 0.15 ml diazo B.
- Methanol.

Equipment

- Double-beam spectrophotometer with scanning facilities between 325 and 700 nm.
- Matched quartz semi-microcuvettes (1 ml volume)

Method

A test and blank are set up for each liquor.

1. 1 ml liquor in test.
2. 1 ml distilled water in blank.
3. 0.5 ml working diazo pipetted into test.
4. 0.5 ml diazo blank pipetted into blank.
5. Pipette 2.5 ml methanol into both tubes and mix well.
6. Incubate at room temperature for 10 minutes.
7. Read absorbances on spectrophotometer at 540 nm.
8. Subtract blank from test absorbance. Value obtained is used to estimate total bile pigment by extrapolation from standard curve (see below).

Preparation of standard curve

The calibration of bilirubin warrants a section in its own right. If there is no established bilirubin assay in the laboratory the reader is referred to Turnell (1985). In order to dispense with the necessity of preparing a standard each time the assay is performed and the expense which this incurs, it is adequate to prepare a calibration curve once and, provided the experimental conditions remain the same, it may be used on all subsequent occasions.

To draw the curve, first prepare a series of bilirubin standards from a stock proprietary standard (several are commercially available).

1. A test and blank are put up for each standard. Both contain 1 ml standard and 1 ml distilled water.
2. 0.5 ml diazo pipetted into blank.

3. 0.5 ml working diazo pipetted into test.

4. Add 2.5 ml methanol into each tube — mix well.

5. Absorbances read at 540 nm after 10 minutes and differences between test and blank plotted against the bilirubin concentration.

Total protein and bile pigment/protein ratio

Reagents

- Saline: NaCl 9g/l.
- Albumin stock standard: 10 g/l (Sigma cat. No. 905–10) Dilute 1 in 40 with saline to give 2.5 mg/ml. This is working standard protein.
- Stock biuret reagent: 45 g sodium potassium tartrate; 15 g copper sulphate (5H$_2$O); 5 g potassium iodide made up to 1 litre with 0.2 M NaOH.
- Working biuret: dilute stock 1:4 with 0.2 M NaOH containing 5 g/l potassium iodide.

Method

1. a. 0.1 ml liquor made up to 1 ml with saline.
   b. 0.25 ml liquor made up to 1 ml with saline.
2. 0.5 ml working standard made up to 1 ml with saline.
3. Blank is 1 ml saline.
4. Add 1 ml working biuret to all 4 tubes.
5. Leave tubes at room temperature for 20 minutes.
6. Read absorbances against the blank at 540 nm.

$$\frac{\text{Value of standard}}{\text{Absorbance of standard}} \times \text{absorbance test}$$

$$\times \text{ dilution factor } \begin{array}{l} ((a) = 5) \\ ((b) = 2) \end{array}$$

Bile pigment/protein ratio

$$= \frac{\text{Total bile pigment } \mu g/ml}{\text{Total protein mg/ml}}$$

The upper limit of normal for the period 16–26 weeks gestation is 0.4. Levels above this, together with other parameters, would be taken to indicate the need for intra-uterine transfusion (Fig. 8.2)

Optical density at 450 nm

Read the absorbance of clarified amniotic fluid at 365, 450 and 550 nm against a water blank.

1. The absorbance at 365 and 550 nm are plotted on semi-log paper and a line drawn between them.

2. The absorbance at 450 nm is read from graph and subtracted from the actual absorbance at 450 nm. This is known as the △ 450 nm value. It corrects for other pigments which may be present in the amniotic fluid. The △ 450 nm is then plotted on a graph against gestational age. The graph is divided into 3 zones — following Liley's concept (Fig. 8.1).

1. Rh(D) negative or mildly affected fetus.

2. Indeterminate — usually moderately severe disease.

3. Severe disease — impending fetal death.

Comment

Contamination of the amniotic fluid with fresh or altered blood diminishes the value of the prognosis. This may be seen directly by eye but sometimes only from the spectral curve. For this reason the amniotic fluid should be scanned in a spectrophotometer from 320 to 700 nm to detect pigments other than bilirubin e.g. methaemoglobin or oxyhaemoglobin. Altered blood classically gives a peak at 405 nm and fresh blood (oxyhaemoglobin) at 413 nm. Later in gestation meconium may interfere with spectrophotometric amniotic fluid examination, but after 34 weeks the bile pigment estimations tend to be unreliable anyway, because of increasing turbidity in the amniotic fluid. One of the main sources of error in assessing severity of haemolytic disease in addition to contamination by pigments other than bile products is incorrect gestational age. It is therefore very important to have the gestational age checked by ultrasound in the early weeks following conception in these high risk pregnancies.

Until skills of safe fetal cord blood sampling have spread to many more obstetric centres, estimation of amniotic fluid bilirubin will continue to play an important part in management of haemolytic disease of the fetus.

REFERENCES

Kleihauer

Mollison P L 1983 Blood Transfusion in Clinical Medicine, 7th edn. Blackwell Scientific Publications, p. 369–370 and Appendix 9 p 792–794

Amniotic fluid bilirubin

Liley A W 1961 Liquor amnii analysis in management of pregnancy complicated by rhesus sensitization. American Journal of Obstetrics and Gynecology 82: 1359–1370

Murray J, Norrie D L, Ruthven C R J 1970 Liquor Bilirubin Levels in Normal Pregnancy: A Reassessment of Early Prediction of Haemolytic Disease. British Medical Journal 4 :387–391

Nicolaides K H, Rodeck C H, Millar D S, Mibashan R S 1985 Fetal haematology in Rhesus Isoimmunisation. British Medical Journal 290 :661–663

Turnell D C 1985 The Calibration of Total Serum Bilirubin Assays. Annals of Clinical Biochemistry 22 :217–221

Leucocytes

9

Morphology and cytochemistry

Among the many cytochemical stains that contribute to the identification of haemic cell lines and maturation stages, the most generally useful are

1. Romanowsky staining
2. the Sudan Black B stain, and
3. the largely equivalent though mostly less informative peroxidase enzyme reactions;
4. the periodic-acid-Schiff (PAS) reaction;
5. esterase enzyme reactions with various substrates, especially butyrate or acetate and chloroacetate esters of α-naphthol, and
6. techniques for acid phosphatase and
7. for alkaline phosphatase.

PREPARATION AND STORAGE OF SLIDES

Haematologists deal chiefly with intact cells in smears and imprints, rather than with sectioned cells. Slides should be grease-free, and thinly spread smears are best made from freshly aspirated material (see Ch. 1). Only a small amount of marrow aspirate containing fragments should be spread. Thick smears, over-rich in particles, are unsatisfactory for cytology and cytochemistry, while smears made from the fluid part of a bone marrow aspirate without particles are commonly too poorly cellular for adequate diagnostic study.

For the preparation of imprints or impressions from lymph node biopsies or similar material it is best to touch the cut surface of the lymph node directly against the slide at two or three sites, and to avoid smearing the resulting impression since this leads to undesirable cell damage.

When fresh material cannot be used immediately or when specimens are poorly cellular and require some form of cell concentration, such as gentle centrifugation, before smears are made, material may be placed in any of the usual anticoagulants such as oxalate, citrate, EDTA or heparin, without detriment to subsequent cytochemical reactivity, provided that slides are made within one or two hours, or within six to eight hours if the specimens are stored in the refrigerator. Heparin has the advantage of giving good morphological pres-

ervation and allowing cells to be used for other purposes, such as surface-marker studies, cytogenetics and in vitro culture.

Unfixed slides may be stored, stacked and wrapped together, with preservation of many cytochemical reactivities, particularly at 4°C or at −20°C. Enzyme reactions, including the commonly used phosphatases, peroxidase and the largely peroxidase-based Sudan Black stain, tend to become progressively weaker with the passage of time, and results cannot be regarded as reliable after much longer than a month at room temperature, 3 months at 4°C or 6 months at −20°C.

Stained slides are generally best preserved unmounted. Azo-dye reaction products are soluble in immersion oil, xylol and many mounting media, but areas of slides not exposed to immersion oil will preserve their positivity for two or three years if stored in the dark. Mounting in glycerine jelly or synthetic media such as DPX is sometimes recommended, the former especially when Fast Garnet GBC is used as coupling agent for the liberated naphthol in phosphatase or esterase reactions, and the latter when hexazotised pararosaniline is used as coupler, since its reaction product is less soluble in xylol. This may be useful when several observers wish to examine the same preparation, but some loss of crispness in disposition of reaction product and a change in colour tend gradually to occur.

FIXATIVE PROCEDURES

For the reactions described in this chapter the fixative procedures chosen are those which provide adequate morphological detail while permitting good cytochemical reactivity. While a single basic fixative procedure, namely, exposure to formalin vapour for four minutes followed by brief washing, will give acceptable results for all the cytochemical methods described here, and is recommended for the esterase and acid phosphatase reactions, a longer fixative exposure is preferable for the Sudan Black reaction to reduce the risk of damage during the long incubation period, while formalin ethanol is preferred for the PAS stain and formalin methanol for alkaline phosphatase because these fixatives give better cell preservation than does formalin vapour alone, yet do not decrease reactivity. To fix slides in formalin vapour it is sufficient to place them in a covered Coplin jar containing a piece of filter paper to which a fresh drop of 40% formalin is added each day.

The tendency for weakly fixed smears to become wrinkled or to be washed off the slide during incubation or washing procedures may be reduced by allowing the smears to dry thoroughly in air for 24 to 48 hours before use, if this is convenient. Such delay is unnecessary when alcohol fixation is to be used, as in Romanowsky staining.

ROMANOWSKY STAINS

Principle

Large numbers of commercially available Romanowsky stains exist. A typical analysis reported by Marshall et al (1975) showed that even the simplest of the Romanowsky stains, Giemsa and Leishman for example, generally contained at least five or six components, although not all appeared to be essential for good staining. After chromatographic separation of dye components of different Romanowsky mixtures in quantities sufficient to carry out detailed staining tests, the characteristic pattern of good Romanowsky staining was found to be achieved by a mixture of pure Azure B and either Eosin Y or a corresponding iodinated fluorescein (Wittekind 1979).

Pure reagents are now available and staining mixtures of consistent quality can now be made up.

Reagents

- Azure B-thiocyanate (Heyl) 1.5 g in 200 ml dimethyl sulphoxide (DMSO) at 37°C.
- Eosin Y (G) (Heyl) 0.5 g in 300 ml methanol.
- Stock stain: mix Azure B and Eosin Y together and store in a dark bottle in a cupboard.
- Buffer: 2.38 g HEPES in 1 litre distilled water (0.01 M). pH adjusted to 6.8 with 1 N sodium hydroxide. Store at +4°C.
- Working stain. Add 3 ml stock stain to 41.5 ml buffer plus 2.5 ml DMSO. Fresh working stain should be made up daily.

Method

1. Fix air-dried smears for 5 minutes using stock stain.
2. Rinse briefly in distilled water.
3. Place slides in Coplin jar with working stain for 25 minutes (blood smears) to 35 minutes (bone marrow smears).
4. Rinse in distilled water for 2 minutes and blot dry.

Comment

Pattern of staining and comparison with older Romanowsky methods

The pattern of staining recognised generally as characteristic of Romanowsky-type stains is illustrated in Plate 2; 1–3, 38–41 Nuclear chromatin stains purple-brown; leucocyte cytoplasm various shades of blue, dark in precursors, lighter in maturing granulocytes, sky-blue in lymphocytes and grey-blue in monocytes; erythroblast cytoplasm again ranges from a deep dark blue in proerythroblasts and early normoblasts, through purple in intermediate normoblasts to light mauve or pink in late normoblasts; 'azurophil' granules of neutrophil promyelocytes are a bright magenta-purple, neutrophil specific granules a darker purple, basophil granules purple-black, and eosinophil granules orange-pink; granules in megakaryocytes and platelets are reddish-purple as are the occasional 'azurophil granules' of large lymphocytes; erythrocytes stain orange-pink and reticulocytes light mauve.

Within this general pattern different stains, different batches of the same stain, and even the same batch at different time intervals after make-up, may show considerable variation in their degree of conformity to the accepted 'best' and most discriminating Romanowsky effect. Using Azure B Eosin Y mixtures, freshly made up each day as described above, a very consistent and reproducible pattern, conforming well to the optimum standard, can be achieved.

Many laboratories use Leishman, Wright or Giemsa stains for rapidity. The difference between such a Leishman-stained preparation and comparable Heyl-stained ones is illustrated in Plate 2; 1–3.

SUDAN BLACK B

Principle

A buffered solution of the diazo-dye Sudan Black B stains neutral fats, phospholipids, and lipoproteins in some cells and tissues by simple physical solubility partition. However, the stable sudanophilia of leucocytes and most other haemic cells appears to be enzymatically linked, perhaps with peroxidase, and also to have a chemical basis resulting from the acidophilia of amino groups in the dye.

Reagents

- *Sudan Black B* (Gurr). 0.3 g in 100 ml absolute ethanol. Store at 4°C, discard after 12 months.
- *Buffer*. Dissolve crystalline phenol 16 g in 30 ml absolute ethanol; add to 100 ml distilled water in which 0.3 g hydrated disodium hydrogen phosphate ($Na_2HPO_4 + 12H_2O$) has been dissolved.
- *Working stain*. Add 40 ml buffer to 60 ml Sudan

Black B solution and filter; store in refrigerator; discard when staining effectiveness weakens. This depends on frequency of use, but will usually be after two to three months.

Method

1. Fix air-dried smears in formalin vapour 10 minutes.
2. Wash briefly in distilled water and blot dry.
3. Immerse in working stain in a Coplin jar for one hour. After use return stain to stock bottle and replace in refrigerator.
4. Wash off with 70% ethanol.
5. Counterstain with Leishman's or MGG.

Comment

Distribution of positivity
Early granulocyte precursors show weak localised granular black cytoplasmic reactions, becoming stronger and more generalised with increasing cell maturity. Both primary (Plate 2; 16) and specific (Plate 2; 4) neutrophil granules are positive, eosinophil granules stain positively but with hollow centres (Plate 2; 39), while basophil granules may show normal black positivity but often show a reddish metachromasia. Monocytes may be negative but some show a characteristic pattern of discrete scattered granules (Plate 2; 4). Normal lymphoid and erythroid cells are invariably negative. In leukaemias the reaction is generally more helpful than peroxidase, though similar. Blasts of acute myeloid leukaemias frequently show positivity, with weak or strong localised reactions in myeloblastic cases (Plate 2; 8), overall dense reactions in acute promyelocytic cases (Plate 2; 16), scattered granules in monocytic cases (Plate 2; 12, 17) and a mixture of the granulocytic and monocytic patterns in mixed myelomonocytic cases (Plate 2; 18). Especially strong localised reactions occur in myeloblastic cases showing the 8;21 translocation. Auer rods are positive, sometimes staining solidly and sometimes showing hollow centres, this latter feature being often seen in t(8;21) and in promyelocytic cases.

Lymphoblasts are almost invariably negative although occasional isolated examples of sudanophilia in leukaemic blast cells having antigenic characteristics of lymphoblasts have been reported (Tricot et al 1982), and one retrospective survey showed 1.6% of 350 cases of ALL in childhood to manifest sudanophilia in 5% or more of the blast cells (Staso et al 1984).

Such positivity is sufficiently uncommon not to interfere seriously with the differential value of the Sudan Black reaction between lymphoid and myeloid elements, but must be borne in mind in apparently anomalous cases, where further investigations are called for.

Sudanophilia is also found in the lipid-storing macro-phages in Gaucher's disease and more conspicuously in Niemann-Pick disease, but the lipid inclusions in marrow macrophages seen in some myeloid leukaemias and dyserythropoietic states and in occasional thrombocytopenic purpuras, and the inclusions of 'sea-blue histiocytosis' show only scanty and weak positivity with Sudan Black.

PEROXIDASE

Principle

Several methods are available for the demonstration of myeloperoxidases which catalyse the oxidation of the respective substrates in the presence of hydrogen peroxide. The methods are essentially similar, but differ in the substrates used.

The standard peroxidase procedure used in haematology since the early years of the century was based on benzidine as substrate. Later modifications followed the demonstration that benzidine was carcinogenic, but some substitutions such as o-tolidine proved equally carcinogenic and others such as diaminobenzidine and 3-aminocarbazole provide a possible hazard. Yet another cytochemical method for peroxidase uses 4-chloro-1-naphthol as substrate. The patterns of positivity found with these various reactions are not identical, nor is the stability of the reaction products. In making a choice between these methods it seemed to us sensible to use the benzidine or o-tolidine-based procedure as a standard of comparison because of its long history of usage, but to accept that this method should itself not be recommended since the manufacture, distribution and handling of benzidine base have been prohibited in some countries, in view of the known carcinogenic risk.

Reactions for myeloperoxidase have close similarities in positivity to Sudan Black B reactions and many laboratories use them as alternatives. In comparing different peroxidase reactions we have taken the opportunity to add comparable Sudan Black reactions to the comparison. Plate 2; 4–15 illustrate typical findings with Sudan Black (Plate 2; 4, 8, 12), benzidine peroxidase (Plate 2; 5, 9, 13), diaminobenzidine (DAB) peroxidase (Plate 2; 6, 10, 14), and 3-aminocarbazole (3AC) peroxidase (Plate 2; 7, 11, 15).

The first column (Plate 2; 4–7), shows the reaction in a buffy coat preparation of normal peripheral blood leucocytes; the Sudan Black (4) gives strong granular positivity in neutrophils, clearly positive eosinophil granules with negative centres, discrete scattered granular reaction in monocytes and entirely negative lymphocytes; the benzidine peroxidase (5) shows equally strong positivity in neutrophils but with a less granular and more blurred and imprecise localisation, a clear positive reaction with a suggestion of hollow centres in eosinophils, a reaction in monocytes which is much less granular and precise than with Sudan Black and is sometimes negative, and again negative lymphocytes; the DAB reaction (6) shows a pattern in neutrophils which is almost as strong as with benzidine but more sharply granular, like Sudan Black reactivity, a strong reaction in eosinophil granules with less suggestion of hollow centres, but perceptibly weaker reactions in monocytes, many of which, as in this field, are virtually negative like lymphocytes; the 3AC reaction (7) gives a bright red reaction product with strong positivity in neutrophils and eosinophils but with a less precise localisation than Sudan Black or DAB peroxidase and some tendency to diffusion as found with the benzidine peroxidase reaction product, a tendency which in this stain may also affect monocytes. A particular drawback of the 3AC reaction is the occasional diffuse peripheral positivity found in lymphocytes and at the edge of platelet clumps in some areas of the smear, as shown in 7.

The second column (Plate 2; 8–11) shows reactions with the same set of stains in a case of AML with strong localised sudanophilia. All the peroxidase reactions show good positivity of generally similar disposition, but a little less strong than with Sudan Black, notably in the case of the DAB reaction (10). Auer rods, concealed amid the heavy positivity in 8 and perhaps in 9 are manifest in both 10 and 11.

The third column (Plate 2; 12–15) shows reactions in a case of AMML with numerous monoblasts. These cells all react with Sudan Black to show discrete scattered granules as well as some localised accumulations of positivity (12). In the peroxidase stains the reaction is weaker in every case, with all monoblasts negative in the benzidine reaction (13) and most negative in both DAB and 3AC reactions (14 and 15). When there is positivity in peroxidase reactions it tends to be a weak localised reaction without scattered granules. In each peroxidase stain the single granulocyte precursor, like the early eosinophil in 12, is strongly positive.

This group of illustrations typifies the findings in many comparative staining trials; Sudan Black is superior to all these peroxidase reactions in sensitivity, as shown especially in monocytes and their precursors and also in weakly reacting myeloblasts; DAB gives more precisely localised and also more stable reaction product than either benzidine or 3AC. We accordingly recommend that, if Sudan Black and peroxidase are regarded as alternatives, Sudan Black should be preferred, but that if both reactions are to be used — and this may have advantages in the demonstration of Auer rods, for example, in cases of t(8;21) AML — then DAB is the substrate of choice.

Another recent substrate, 4-chloronaphthol, used in some automated differential analysers, gives a strong black reaction product in neutrophils, but this does not appear superior to DAB in localisation or stability.

The diaminobenzidine (DAB) method for peroxidase

Reagents
- *Fixative*. Buffered formol acetone: anhydrous Na_2HPO_4 40 mg, KH_2PO_4 200 mg, acetone 90 ml, concentrated formalin 50 ml; distilled water 60 ml. Store at 4°C and use cold for fixation.
- *Stock phosphate buffer*. Dulbecco A, pH 7.3. NaCl 40 g. KCl 1.0 g. Na_2HPO_4 anhydrous 5.75 g, KH_2PO_4 1.0 g. Distilled water 1 l.
- *Working buffer*. Dilute stock buffer 1 l with 4 l distilled water.
- Substrate: 3,3′ diaminobenzidine tetrachloride (Sigma).
- H_2O_2 (100 vol).
- *Working incubation solution*. Dissolve 30 mg DAB in 60 ml working buffer and add 120 μl of 100 vol H_2O_2: use immediately.

Method
1. Fix air-dried smears in buffered formol acetone for 45 seconds.
2. Rinse with distilled water and drain dry.
3. Incubate in working substrate solution for 10 minutes.
4. Rinse with distilled water.
5. Counterstain with Carazzi's (or other water-soluble) haematoxylin (see PAS method) 1 minute.
6. Rinse with distilled water and air dry.

Comment

Distribution of positivity
As discussed already, the general pattern of distribution is essentially similar to that of sudanophilia, with granulocytes of neutrophil and eosinophil lines showing weak to strong localised or heavy overall granular reactions, from early promyelocyte stage onwards. Basophils are negative. Monocytes may show fine granules or a faint diffuse or localised positivity but are more often negative to peroxidase than to Sudan Black. Lymphocytes, erythroid cells, megakaryocytes and platelets are negative to DAB using the standard techniques such as that listed above; some positivity in lymphocytes, megakaryocytes and platelets may occur in very weakly fixed preparations or with the 3AC technique. In leukaemias the reactions parallel those of Sudan Black but are usually weaker and less discriminatory, although the DAB reaction is very effective in the demonstration of Auer rods. Polymorphs in AML may be negative and in CML may be exceptionally strongly positive.

PERIODIC-ACID SCHIFF (PAS) REACTION

Principle

Periodic acid oxidises the 1-2 glycol group of various compounds — chiefly glycogen — in blood and marrow cells to produce a di-aldehyde, which then gives the Schiff's spot reaction with basic leuco-fuchsin to release the strongly magenta-coloured fuchsin. The reactivity of glycogen can be removed by pretreatment of the cells with salivary amylase.

Reagents

- *Periodic-acid solution.* Dissolve 5 g periodic-acid crystals in 500 ml distilled water; store in dark bottle at 20°C. Keeps for three months.
- *Basic fuchsin.* Bring 500 ml distilled water to boil in a litre flask. After cooling for 2 to 3 minutes take it to a fume cupboard, add 5 g basic fuchsin (Gurr), and mix for 2 to 3 minutes. Allow to cool to room temperature (overnight). Filter through Whatman no. 1 or similar paper. Bubble sulphur dioxide (SO_2) gas slowly through a Pasteur pipette to the bottom of the flask until saturated, when bubbles rise more slowly, or until liquid is dark brown colour (usually 30 min). (A 500 g canister of SO_2 with tap (from BDH Ltd.) will last 2 to 3 years). Remove the Pasteur pipette from the flask before turning off the SO_2 tap; this avoids corrosion of the metal by the solution. Add activated charcoal gradually, 2 g or so at a time, shaking flask each time for a few seconds, until nearly all of the brown colour has been removed, leaving a slight straw tinge only. Basic fuchsin strength seems to vary considerably and so does the amount of charcoal required. Usually between 2 g and 7 g suffice for 500 ml of solution. After adding charcoal and shaking, a little of the solution must be filtered off from time to time to check colour. Finally, filter into a brown glass bottle with ground stopper; store in fume cupboard if possible (exposure to daylight is acceptable). The prepared solution keeps for 3 to 6 months depending on how often it is used. Discard when staining appears less than optimal.
- *Carazzi's aqueous Haematoxylin.* Dissolve 75 g potassium aluminium sulphate in 1200 ml warm distilled water. Add 1.5 g Haematoxylin powder (Gurr) dissolved in 300 ml glycerol by grinding with pestle and mortar. Dissolve 0.3 g sodium iodate in a little water and add gradually. The stain is conveniently made up in this large quantity because it is used for several reactions and discarded each time.

Method

1. Fix air-dried smears for 10 minutes in a solution of 10 ml 40% formalin and 90 ml absolute ethanol.
2. Wash briefly in tap water.
3. Treat with periodic-acid solution for 10 minutes.
4. Wash and blot dry.
5. Immerse in Schiff's basic fuchsin in a Coplin jar for 30 minutes. (The fuchsin solution is returned to the stock bottle immediately after use.)
6. Wash in tap water 5–10 minutes.
7. Counterstain with Carazzi's aqueous Haematoxylin 10–15 minutes.

All steps except 5 may conveniently be carried out on a staining rack and the reagents discarded.

Comment

Distribution of positivity

Very full practical details on the preparation of leuco-basic fuchsin solution are given because the quality of this reagent appears of the greatest importance in achieving really bright PAS reactions. Commercially available prepared reagents are not reliable substitutes.

Early granulocyte precursors are negative or show weak diffuse staining, but positivity increases with increasing cell maturity in the neutrophil series and mature polymorphs show very strong granular positivity (Plate 2; 20). Eosinophil granules remain unstained against a positive cytoplasmic background and coarse intergranular positivity may also be seen in basophils. Monocytes and their precursors range from negative to coarsely granular positive, but usually with a diffuse background tinge. Lymphocytes are often negative, but some 10–20% normally show one or two rings of perinuclear granules in a clear background. Platelets are positive and megakaryocytes show strong positive granularity. Leukaemic precursors reflect these patterns in the variants of AML as illustrated in Plate 2; 21–27. Coarse granules or blocks of positivity against a negative background are often conspicuous in leukaemic lymphoblasts (Plate 2; 44 and 45). Erythroblasts are normally negative but may show coarse granular positivity or strong diffuse staining in erythroleukaemia and erythraemic myelosis (Plate 2; 28). Plasma cells, normally and in myeloma, are usually negative or show weak diffuse positivity. Hairy cells usually show moderately strong diffuse and finely granular positivity as illustrated in Plate 2; 46.

ESTERASES

Principle

Leucocytic esterases include many isoenzymes with differing electrophoretic mobilities and substrate affinities, but two important groups may be separated that have a degree of substrate specificity respectively for simple acyl or for chloroacyl esters of α-naphthol (or naphthol AS-D).

The first group occurs chiefly in monocytes and macrophages and to some extent in megakaryocytes, platelets, and certain lymphocytes. It is demonstrated by exposing the slides to α-naphthyl butyrate (or acetate) as substrate with either Fast Garnet GBC or Fast Blue BB as diazonium salt capture agent.

The second group occurs predominantly in granulocytes and their precursors and is demonstrated by the use of α-naphthol AS-D chloroacetate as substrate and one of the same pair of diazonium salts as capture agent. Both reactions can conveniently be demonstrated in the same preparation by the method described here.

Dual esterase reaction with double incubation

Reagents

- *Chloroacetate substrate solution.* 0.1 M phosphate buffer (pH 8.0) 10 ml; α-naphthol AS-D chloroacetate (0.7×10^{-4} M) 0.25 mg in 0.1 ml acetone; Fast Blue BB salt (5×10^{-3} M) 15 mg. Use at once.
- *Butyrate substrate solution.* 0.1 M phosphate buffer (pH 8.0) 10 ml; α-naphthyl butyrate (2.33×10^{-4} M) 0.5 mg; Fast Garnet GBC salt (9×10^{-4} M) 3 mg. Use at once. For testing fluoride inhibition add NaF 1.5 mg/ml to buffer.
- *Carazzi's aqueous Haematoxylin.* See PAS method.

Method

1. Fix air-dried smears in formalin vapour for 4 minutes.
2. Wash briefly in distilled water and blot dry.
3. Incubate in freshly prepared chloroacetate substrate solution for 5 to 15 minutes at room temperature.
4. Wash briefly in distilled water and blot dry.
5. Incubate in freshly prepared butyrate substrate solution for 15 to 30 minutes at room temperature and away from light.
6. Wash briefly in distilled water.
7. Counterstain in aqueous Haematoxylin for 5 minutes.
8. Wash in distilled water, blot dry, and examine.

Comments

The following additional technical details may be helpful:

— The naphthol AS-D chloroacetate reaction presents no trouble and slides can be stained on a rack over the sink or in a Coplin jar for larger numbers of slides. The α-naphthyl butyrate reaction is best carried out in a Coplin jar and probably better in the dark — for example, in a drawer.
— Solutions should be made up quickly — for example, place 10 ml buffer in a measuring cylinder first, dilute the AS-D chloroacetate in a small jar with acetone, quickly mix, then add Fast Blue BB to buffer, again quickly mix (ignore what does not go rapidly into solution), add the acetone solution to measuring cylinder, quickly mix, and pour on to slides.
— The same applies to the butyrate substrate. Place 10 ml buffer in a measuring cylinder; remove α-naphthyl butyrate from deep freeze to thaw and, using a micro-syringe to pierce the suba-seal of vial, take 0.01 ml (= 10 mg) of the anhydrous liquid into 0.5 ml of acetone; then use 0.025 ml of this solution which contains 0.5 mg butyrate. Discard the remainder. Add Fast Garnet GBC to the buffer, quickly mix, add 0.025 ml of the butyrate solution, quickly mix, and place in a Coplin jar for the 30 minutes incubation period.
— Control smears should always be used: stored normal buffy coat smears serve well for this purpose. The neutrophils show good chloroacetate esterase positivity, while the monocytes and T lymphocytes present give butyrate esterase positivity. RE cells are always butyrate-esterase positive for marrow smears and provide a built-in control.

Dual esterase reaction with single incubation (after Swirsky 1984)

Reagents

- Buffered formalin/acetone (20 mg Na_2HPO_4, 100 mg KH_2PO_4, 30 ml distilled water, 45 ml acetone, 25 ml concentrated formalin).
- 50 ml 0.1 mol/l phosphate buffer pH 8.0.
- 2.5 mg naphthol AS-D chloroacetate (Sigma no. N-0758) in 1 ml acetone.
- 4 mg (4 μl) α-naphthyl butyrate (Sigma no. N-8000) in 1 ml acetone.
- 80 mg Fast Blue BB salt (Gurr/BDH no. 34177).

Method

1. Fix air-dried smears in buffered formalin/acetone for 30 seconds.
2. Wash briefly in distilled water and air dry.
3. Mix the Fast Blue BB vigorously with the buffer.
4. Add 1 ml of acetone to the naphthol AS-D chloroacetate, agitate until dissolved, and mix with the buffer/Fast Blue BB.
5. Add the α-naphthyl butyrate to 1 ml of acetone, agitate until dispersed, and mix with the buffer/Fast Blue BB/naphthol AS-D chloroacetate.
6. Pour substrate solution into a Coplin jar in which the fixed slides have been placed and allow to incubate at room temperature for 15–30 minutes.
7. Wash in distilled water.
8. Counterstain with aqueous Haematoxylin for 2–5 minutes.
9. Rinse in distilled water, air dry, and coverslip using aqueous mounting medium.

Steps 4 and 5 should be carried out as rapidly as possible. Step 7 should be carried out by running distilled water into the Coplin jar until the substrate solution (deep violet) has been cleared. The dark brown reaction product with α-naphthyl butyrate is soluble in organic solvents.

Comment

Distribution of positivity (Plate 2; 29–37, 48, 51)

Butyrate esterase (BE). Shows positivity as red-brown granules in most normal monocytes (29) and in leukaemic monoblasts (32–34), but some 20% have weak reactions. Unlike other BE-positive cells, monocytes have fluoride-sensitive enzyme. Granulocytes are usually negative and megakaryocytes and platelets usually react weakly as do their leukaemic counterparts or precursors (36) (though stronger acyl esterase reactions occur with acetate instead of butyrate as substrate (37)). Lymphocytes vary in BE-positivity. Normal B cells are negative; T cells (especially the T helper subset) have localised coarse, dot-like paranuclear positivity; while null cells and some T cells have scattered fine granules. These patterns may be reflected in pathological states (51), but some B-cell CLL cases have scattered granules or resemble hairy cells of hairy-cell leukaemia (48) in having a crescentic granular positivity. Erythroblasts are normally negative or only weakly positive, but megaloblasts and erythraemic erythroblasts are often strongly positive (35).

Chloroacetate esterase (CE). Shows strong positivity as bright blue granules in both the normal (29) and leukaemic granulocyte series. Auer rods are strongly CE-positive (30 and 31) and sometimes appear hollow or with BE-positive cores in acute promyelocytic leukaemia. Occasional CE-positive granules occur in monocytes.

With the single incubation dual esterase method the colour discrimination is very similar, with granulocytes and their normal and leukaemic precursors staining a bright blue and with monocytes and some T cells having butyrate positivity staining a brown or even black colour, sometimes with a greenish tinge. Examples of this staining reaction are shown in Plate 2; 34 and 41.

ACID PHOSPHATASE

Principle

At acid pH this phosphatase will hydrolyse phosphates of naphthol or of naphthol derivatives to release insoluble naphthols which couple with appropriate diazonium salts to produce a coloured precipitate. L(+)-tartaric acid inhibits most acid phosphatase isoenzymes but not isoenzyme 5, which occurs most characteristically in the neoplastic cells of hairy-cell leukaemia.

Reagents

- *Substrate solution*. Dissolve 10 mg naphthol AS-BI phosphoric acid and 10 mg Fast Garnet GBC salt in 60 ml acetate buffer, 0.1 mol/l, pH 5.0. Mix well. Filtration is not required.
- *Acetate buffer*. Stock solution A: 60 ml glacial acetic acid in 1 litre distilled water. Stock solution B: 82.04 g sodium acetate in 1 litre distilled water.

  Working buffer should be made up freshly before use by diluting the stock buffer solutions 1 in 10 and, for pH 5.0, mixing 59 parts of A to 141 parts of B — for example, for one Coplin jar (60 ml) take 3 ml A and dilute to 30 ml with distilled water, and take 5 ml B and dilute to 50 ml with distilled water, then add 18.0 ml diluted A to 43.0 ml diluted B.
- *Carazzi's aqueous Haematoxylin*.

Method

1. Fix air-dried smears in formalin vapour for 4 minutes.
2. Wash briefly in tap water.
3. Incubate in substrate solution for 60–90 minutes at 37°C.
4. Wash briefly in tap water.
5. Counterstain with Carazzi's aqueous Haematoxylin for 10 minutes.

To assess tartrate resistance of acid phosphatase add 120 mg L(+)-tartaric acid to 60 ml substrate and incubate slides in this medium in parallel with tartrate-free medium at step 3.

Comment

Distribution of positivity

This method, using naphthol AS-BI phosphoric acid as substrate and Fast Garnet GBC as capture agent, gives chiefly granular positivity in all reacting cells and appears more specific, precise, and sensitive than other methods, notably those using hexazotised pararosaniline as naphthol receptor which commonly give diffuse positivity in both granulocytes and monocytes.

A reddish-brown granular deposit occurs in most nucleated blood and marrow cells, with plasma cells, osteoclasts, eosinophils, monocytes, megakaryocytes, platelets, and some macrophages showing the strongest reactions. Neutrophil granulocytes show much weaker positivity, though stronger in immature cells rich in primary granules than in later cells. Lymphocytes generally show a few localised paranuclear granules, more conspicuous in T cells than in B cells and certainly more so in leukaemic T-cell precursors (Plate 2; 50 and 52) than in the lymphoblasts of common ALL. Among AML variants, cases with a marked monocytic component generally show stronger positivity than do more purely myeloblastic cases. Tartrate-resistant acid phosphatase positivity is almost always found in at least a proportion of the abnormal lymphocytes of hairy-cell leukaemia (Plate 2; 47).

ALKALINE PHOSPHATASE

Principle

Several azo-dye methods using phosphates of naphthol or of naphthol derivatives as substrates and various diazonium salts as capture agents give satisfactory results. Users are advised to keep to a single method for routine use to facilitate scoring the extent of positivity in peripheral blood neutrophils in comparison with an established normal range.

Reagents

- *Stock propanediol buffer solution (0.2 M)*. Dissolve 10.5 g 2-amino-2-methyl propane-(1:3)-diol in 500 ml distilled water. Store at 4°C, discard after 3 months.
- *Working buffer (0.05 M)*. Prepare by mixing 25 ml stock buffer with 5 ml 0.1 N HCl and make up to 100 ml with distilled water.
- *Methyl Green*. Make a 2% solution in distilled water and free from contamination with Methyl Violet by extraction with one-half of its volume of chloroform for 48 hours. The dye solution is stored at 20°C in contact with the chloroform to allow continuous extraction of newly produced Methyl Violet. We usually make up 2 litres and store in large medical flats or similar container through which the chloroform level can be seen. This quantity lasts about a year and need not be discarded sooner.

Method

1. Fix air-dried smears in 10% formalin in absolute methanol for 30 seconds (use stopwatch) at 0–5°C.
2. Prepare substrate solution as follows:

Sodium α-naphthyl phosphate (Gurr)	35 mg
Fast Garnet GBC salt (Gurr)	35 mg
Working 0.05 M propanediol buffer	35 ml

3. As soon as the substrate has been mixed pour it directly on to the slides and allow to incubate at room temperature for 5 to 10 minutes. The substrate must be used within 5 minutes of preparation.

4. Rinse slides in tap water for 10 seconds.
5. Counterstain with Methyl Green for 10 to 15 seconds.

Controls. Slides from polycythaemia, infection, hairy-cell leukaemia, or Hodgkin's disease provide good positive controls.

Comment

Distribution of positivity

The intensity of staining and number of positive reddish-brown granules in each of 100 neutrophils may be scored as follows:

0 = negative or colourless.
1 = faint diffuse positivity or occasional granules.
2 = diffuse positivity with moderate numbers of granules.
3 = strong positivity with numerous granules.
4 = very strong reaction with very numerous coarse granules, often obscuring the nucleus.

The sum of a 100 cell ratings gives a 'leucocyte alkaline phosphatase (LAP)' score with a possible range from nil to 400. The normal range with this method is 14 to 100 (mean 46). Higher scores, up to twice the normal adult level, may be found in childhood and during pregnancy.

In normal blood and marrow cells positivity is confined to macrophages (Plate 2; 57), osteoblasts, and to a proportion of the later neutrophils from metamyelocyte onwards. Very occasionally, normal lymphocytes in the peripheral blood may show a weak cytoplasmic reaction, but neoplastic lymphocytes, especially of B-cell lineage and moderate differentiation, may sometimes be clearly positive, more often in node imprints than in blood smears. The isoenzyme involved in these cases seems likely to be the lymphoid APase. The LAP score in neutrophils is generally raised in polycythaemia vera; myelofibrosis; inflammatory leucocytosis; leukaemoid reactions; Hodgkin's disease in relapse; carcinomatosis; myeloma; aplastic anaemia; hairy-cell leukaemia (Plate 2; 49); and, less markedly, in CLL. Low scores are usual in CML, in some AML cases with myeloblastic preponderance, in paroxysmal nocturnal haemoglobinuria (PNH), and in infectious mononucleosis.

REFERENCES

Marshall P N, Bentley S A, Lewis S M 1975 An evaluation of some commercial Romanowsky stains. Journal of Clinical Pathology 28: 680–685
Staso S A, Pui C-H, Melvin S, Rovigatti O, Williams D, Motroni T, Kalwinsky D, Dahl G V 1984 Sudan black B positive acute lymphoblastic leukaemia. British Journal of Haematology 57: 413–21
Swirsky D M 1984 Single incubation double esterase cytochemical reaction using a single coupling reagent.

Journal of Clinical Pathology 37: 1187–1190
Tricot G, Broeckart-von Orshoven A, van Hoof A, Verwilghen R L 1982 Sudan black B positivity in acute lymphoblastic leukaemia. British Journal of Haematology 51: 615–621
Wittekind D 1979 On the nature of Romanowsky dyes and the Romanowsky-Giemsa effect. Clinical and Laboratory Haematology 1: 247–262

10

Leucocyte preparation and separation

Separation techniques may be required for the study of lymphocytes and lymphocyte subsets, neutrophils and monocytes, but rarely for other cell types such as eosinophils and basophils. For surface marker studies these separation procedures need not be performed aseptically, but since sterile techniques are required for functional studies it is sensible policy to use sterile technique routinely.

PREPARATION OF STERILE LYMPHOCYTES

Principle
Lymphocytes and monocytes are separated from granulocytes and erythrocytes by buoyant density centrifugation over a layer of Ficoll-hypaque. After centrifugation, the agglutinated red cells and granulocytes sediment to form a pellet whereas lymphocytes and monocytes remain on the interface between the Ficoll-hypaque and plasma layers; platelets remain suspended in the plasma. The method is also suitable for separating bone marrow cells since blast cells and immature myeloid cells are also retained at the interface.

Test Samples
Venous blood or bone marrow collected into heparin. Note that some heparin tubes contain plastic beads; these should be tipped out before the blood is collected since they interfere with the cell separation. 20 ml of blood is adequate for most tests.

Reagents
- Ficoll-hypaque purchased commercially under such names as Lymphoprep. Store in the dark.
- Physiological saline ('normal' saline), autoclaved.
- Fetal calf serum or — depending on the tests to follow — human AB serum, both inactivated by heating for 30 minutes at 56°C.
- Standard tissue culture medium such as RPMI 1640.

Equipment
○ Test tube rack.
○ Sterile 10 ml capped plastic tubes such as Falcon.
○ Bench centrifuge.
○ Laminar flow hood.
○ Sterile glass conical flask.

Method
1. Collect blood into sterile container with sterile heparin. Perform subsequent steps in Laminar flow hood.
2. Dilute blood 1:2 with sterile normal saline. Use a sterile conical flask.
3. Aliquot blood in 9 ml lots in sterile 10 ml Falcon tubes (no mouth pipetting). Simply pour the diluted blood from the flask into the tubes.
4. Underlay aseptically with sterile Ficoll-hypaque using a pasteur pipette. Take 2 ml of Ficoll-hypaque into the pipette and push to the bottom of the tube before gently expelling contents.
5. Spin 25 minutes at 1200 rpm (200 g), room temperature.
6. Aseptically remove layer of mononuclear cells from the interface. Use a Pasteur pipette in a vacuuming motion.
7. Wash cells × 2 with RPMI + 10% human AB serum. Count and adjust concentration to 2×10^6/ml.

Comment
One ml of blood should yield approximately 10^6 mononuclear cells (lymphocytes and monocytes).

SEPARATION OF GRANULOCYTES

Principle
Leucocytes are separated from red cells on the basis of their differential velocity of sedimentation. Polymorphonuclear cells are separated from the mononuclear cells and platelets by virtue of their greater density. Contaminating red cells are eliminated by hypotonic lysis.

The resulting cell preparation contains about 97% neutrophilic and about 3% eosinophilic granulocytes, with generally less than 1% contaminating lymphocytes, monocytes or basophils. The yield is about $1-3 \times 10^6$ cells/ml of blood.

Test sample
Blood or marrow taken into heparin (10 u/ml).

Reagents
- Dextran (MW 150 000–500 000), 10% (w/v) in normal saline.
- Ficoll-sodium metrizoate (density = 1.077 g/ml, e.g. Lymphoprep, Nyegaard, or Ficoll-Paque, Pharmacia).
- Sodium chloride, 1.8% (w/v), containing heparin (5 u/ml).
- Saline or PBS, containing heparin (5 u/ml).
- RPMI 1640 medium (or PBS containing 10 mM glucose) with heparin (5 u/ml).

Equipment
- Syringes (5, 20, 50 ml).
- Needles (19 G×2).
- Conical plastic tubes (50 ml).
- Centrifuge with a swing-out rotor with buckets for 50 ml tubes.

Method
All procedures are at room temperature.

1. Sedimentation. Dextran solution (10% by volume) is aspirated into the heparinised blood (20–50 ml) while still in the syringe into which it has been drawn. The syringe is fixed in an upright position for 45 minutes with the needle end on top.

2. Density centrifugation. The leucocyte-rich layer of plasma is gently expressed through a bent needle onto 10–15 ml Ficoll-sodium metrizoate in a 50 ml conical tube, taking care to minimise mixing of the phases. The tube is centrifuged in a swing-out rotor at 800 g for 15 minutes. The mononuclear cells and platelets remain at the interphase and the pellet consists of granulocytes and contaminating red cells.

3. Hypotonic lysis of red cells. Everything above the pellet is aspirated. The pellet is resuspended in 25 ml distilled water, vigorously pipetting up and down for 30 seconds. Tonicity is restored by the immediate addition of 25 ml 1.8% sodium chloride containing heparin.

4. The cell suspension is centrifuged at 220 g for 5 minutes and the pellet resuspended in 10–20 ml saline or PBS containing heparin.

5. The purified polymorphonuclear leucocytes are centrifuged at 220 g for 5 minutes and resuspended in either RPMI 1640 medium or PBS containing 10 mM glucose (both with heparin) at a final concentration of 10^7-10^8 per ml.

Comments
— Freshly drawn blood should be used. If this is not possible, it may be stored for up to 24 hours at room temperature. Blood samples should not be cooled to 4°C as this induces the granulocytes to clump.

— If hypotonic lysis (step 3) is incomplete, as evidenced by a ring or layer of erythrocytes on the surface of the neutrophil pellet after centrifugation, a second cycle of hypotonic lysis may be performed although this increases the risk of cell damage.

— It is best to use the cells immediately, although they may be kept for 2–3 hours at room temperature with little deterioration in function. Clumping can usually be reversed by vigorous agitation. Mucoid clumps that do not resuspend well are a clear indication of the release of DNA and irreversible cell damage.

— Concentrated cell suspensions may appear to lose function with time. This is commonly due to acidification of the medium and may be corrected by pelleting the cells and resuspending them in fresh medium.

SEPARATION OF MONOCYTES

Principle
The property of monocytes to adhere to glass or plastic surfaces is used to separate them from the other mononuclear cells.

Test samples
Blood taken into heparin (10 u/ml)

Reagents
As for isolation of granulocytes, plus:
- RPMI 1640 medium containing HEPES (25 mM), glutamine (2 mM), sodium bicarbonate (0.2%, w/v); penicillin (50 U/ml), streptomycin (50 μg/ml) and amphotericin B (2.5 μg/ml).
- Fetal calf serum.
- EDTA (sodium salt), 200 mM (pH 7.4).
- PBS containing 2 mM EDTA.
- PBS containing 2 mM EDTA and 10 mM glucose.

Equipment
As for isolation of granulocytes, plus:
- Tissue culture dishes (3–10 cm diameter).
- Conical plastic tubes (10–15 ml).
- Slides.
- Cytocentrifuge.
- Sterile cabinet.
- 5% CO_2 incubator.
- Microscope.

Method

All the procedures are carried out at room temperature and, if monocytes are to be cultured, sterile conditions should be used. The latter involve the use of sterile solutions and materials and a laminar flow cabinet.

1. Mix heparinised blood with dextran, sediment and centrifuge as described for granulocytes (p. 177).

2. The supernatant plasma is discarded and the interface cells are then aspirated and transferred to a 50 ml conical tube, diluted 2–3 fold with saline, and centrifuged at 220 g for 5 minutes.

3. Platelets are removed from the cell pellet by repeated washing in saline. At least 3 cycles of resuspension and centrifugation at 170 g for 3 minutes are required to eliminate most platelets.

4. After removal of the platelets, the mononuclear cells are resuspended at a concentration of approximately 10^7 per ml in RPMI 1640 medium prewarmed to 37°C and plated onto the tissue culture dishes at a concentration of about $0.5–1.0\times10^6$ cells per cm^2. The dishes are placed in a 5% CO_2 incubator for 1–2 hours at 37°C.

5. The non-adherent cells are then removed by gently shaking the plates and aspirating the supernatant. The adherent cells are washed twice with saline or PBS, after which they consist of about 80–90% monocytes and 10–20% lymphocytes. If the plates were adequately rinsed, there should be less than 0.5% of contaminating neutrophils which will detach within 2 days if kept in culture.

6. Freshly adherent cells are harvested by adding EDTA to a final concentration of 2 mM and gently scraping the surface of the plate with a latex rubber stopper or transecter rubber tubing. The detached cells are transferred to conical centrifuge tubes and the plates are again scraped after the addition of a small volume of PBS containing EDTA.

7. The combined cell suspension is centrifuged at 250 g for 5 minutes and the pellet washed once with PBS with EDTA.

8. The cells are resuspended in PBS with EDTA and glucose to a concentration of about $1–2\times10^7$ cells/ml. The yield of monocytes is $0.5–1.5\times10^5$ per cm^2 of plate.

Comments

— It is important to eliminate as many platelets as possible from the mononuclear cell suspension before plating.
— Contaminating neutrophils also adhere to the plates. They detach readily on shaking, forming clumps that can be aspirated and discarded.
— The monocyte/macrophage cell suspension should be used for functional assays within 1–2 hours.

CYTOCENTRIFUGATION

Principle

This technique is a means of transferring cells in suspension to a circumscribed area on a glass slide. The method greatly concentrates the cell suspension and minimises cell damage.

The cytocentrifuge (Shandon; Runcorn)

The plastic block, together with slide and filter paper, are spring-loaded onto the centrifuge as indicated in Fig. 10.1. The centrifugal force causes the cells to be deposited in a circular area on the slide and the filter paper absorbs the suspension fluid. A balance slide and block must be used.

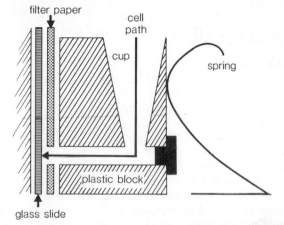

Fig. 10.1 Cross-section of cytocentrifuge block with attached slide.

Method

1. Put one drop of H/HBSS or RMPI-1640 medium into the cup and add 30 μl of a 1×10^6 cells/ml suspension, followed by a further drop of medium.

For rosette preparations, after completing counting, remove all but 20 μl of test suspension, add 700 μl of medium (i.e. fill to the top of the LPL rosette tube) and finally centrifuge 50 μl of this diluted suspension in the usual way.

2. Centrifuge for 10 minutes at 700 rpm (setting 50 on cytocentrifuge).

3. Remove slides, air dry and stain in the same way as blood films.

4. Wash and dry centrifuge blocks for re-use.

Notes on technique

1. The initial drop of medium prevents damage by any water persisting after washing. Also, together with the subsequent drop of medium, this gives a more uniform spread of cells on the slide.

2. Centrifugation at substantially greater than

700 rpm causes disruption of rosettes and damages leucocyte morphology.

Comment

Cytocentrifugation is ideal for establishing the content of a given cell suspension and for determining the nature of rosetting cells. It is less good, however, for scoring rosettes which, for accurate results, should be done in cell suspensions. Examination of rosettes should be confined to the central area of the preparation since non-rosetting erythrocytes tend to accumulate at the edge where they may appear to form pseudorosettes.

The method is equally useful in concentrating cells from CSF, for example, in a patient with possible meningeal leukaemia.

CRYOPRESERVATION

Principle

Storage of viable cells for long periods of time requires that they be in a frozen state at the lowest feasible temperature. Liquid nitrogen has. evolved as the environment of choice.

When stored in purpose-designed liquid nitrogen refrigerators, material is maintained at $-196°C$ when stored below the liquid level or at $-190°C$ when held in the vapour phase. Three methods of freezing are given; the preparation and reconstitution of cells is common to all these methods.

Reagents/equipment

Liquid nitrogen (BOC Ltd.).
Liquid nitrogen refrigerator.
Freezing ampoules.
Dimethyl sulphoxide (DMSO; Sigma).
RPMl Medium and calf serum.
Crushed ice.

Method

1. Leucocytes to be frozen should be separated from red cells.
2. After washing, resuspend cells at 5×10^6 to 1×10^7 cells/ml in RPMI 1640 medium containing 40% inactivated calf serum. Accurately measure the volume added and place cell suspension on ice for 30 minutes.
3. Prepare 20% DMSO in RPMI 1640 (exactly the same final volume as in step 2) and place on ice for 30 minutes.

4. Label freezing ampoules.
5. With constant mixing, slowly add the DMSO solution to the cell suspension keeping both solutions on ice. This results in a freezing mixture of 10% DMSO, 20% calf serum in RPMI 1640.
6. Transfer cell suspension/ freezing mixture (approx 1.5 ml) into ampoules and freeze by steps 7, 8 or 9 below.
7. Programmable freezing machine: A programme which has proved satisfactory involves reducing the temperature by $5°C$ each minute to $4°C$ and then proceed as below:

> hold for 5 minutes at $+4°C$
> then $-1°C/min$ to $-30°C$
> and then $-2°C/min$ to $-60°C$

8. Storage tank freezer: small numbers of ampoules may be frozen in the 'neck' of certain nitrogen storage containers. Follow manufacturers instructions for setting rate of cooling to $-1°C/min$.
9. Polystyrene Igloo freezing: place ampoules in a rack in an 'Igloo' ice container with a lid. Immediately place assembly in $-70°C$ freezer and leave overnight.
10. When freezing has been completed, ampoules should be transferred to the nitrogen storage container as quickly as possible, using a pre-cooled transfer flask if necessary.

Cell retrieval
1. Heat water-bath to $37°C$.
2. Remove ampoule(s) from storage and rapidly thaw in water-bath with manual agitation.
3. As soon as thawing is complete, centrifuge at 1000 rpm for 2 minutes and remove 50% of the supernatant.
4. Resuspend cells and add RPMI 1640 + 20% calf serum to original volume. Centrifuge as before.
5. Repeat this washing procedure three times and finally remove all supernatant and resuspend cells in RPMI 1640/10% calf serum. Check cell yield and viability.

Comments

— If sterile disposable syringes are used for measuring volumes, care must be taken to leave an air gap between the plunger and the surface of the DMSO. Some syringe lubricants will dissolve in DMSO only to form a precipitate when added to RPMI.
— The overall procedure for good recoveries requires a controlled and steady freezing of cells and rapid thawing.

11

Immunological markers

Immunological marker techniques, particularly since the introduction of monoclonal antibodies, have had a profound impact on immunobiology and thereby on haematology. Initially, these methods added a new dimension to the earlier morphological/cytochemical approach to identifying haematological cells, and consolidated the concept that leukaemic/lymphomatous proliferations are clonal expansions of a normal counterpart 'frozen' at a given stage of differentiation. More recently, by providing a means of identifying and influencing functionally important surface molecules, monoclonal antibodies have yielded increasingly important information concerning the biology of haemic cells. These new data will be increasingly applied to haematology in the next few years; for example, monoclonal antibodies are already being used to 'purge' bone marrow of specific cell types.

Hitherto, however, the clinical use of monoclonal antibodies and immunological marker methods has largely related to the refinement of diagnosis based on morphological/cytochemical criteria. For example, such techniques have been used to classify acute leukaemia, to investigate the nature of lymphocytoses, and to distinguish chronic lymphocytic leukaemia from other chronic lymphoproliferative disorders affecting the blood.

In the small proportion (less than 10%) of cases of acute leukaemia remaining unclassified after careful morphological and cytochemical analysis, appropriate immunological markers allow the majority of cases to be identified as a particular type of ALL or as AML including erythroid or megakaryocytic variants.

Regarding lymphocytoses, markers readily allow recognition of B versus T proliferations. Most B proliferations are neoplastic and this is confirmed by the demonstration of light-chain-restricted surface immunoglobulin. T proliferations can be neoplastic or reactive. Although aberrant marker expression suggests neoplasia, markers will usually provide no definitive information concerning the clonality of T proliferations and the demonstration of clonal rearrangement of T-cell-receptor genes is required.

The detection of haematologically relevant cellular antigens has been done in three main ways — immunofluorescence, rosetting and immunocytochemistry — considered in turn below. Each of these methods has advantages and disadvantages, and which technique is used will depend on the circumstances of a given laboratory. For straightforward diagnostic work in departments with little previous experience, it is likely that the immunocytochemical (e.g. by APAAP) staining of air-dried smears will prove the method of choice.

For all three methodologies, positive and negative control samples should be periodically included and spurious positivity minimised. The two major causes of such spurious reactivity are non-specific reagent and extrinsic antigen binding. Reagent Fc binding can be eliminated by using Fab fragments of the test antibodies or minimised in various ways such as avoiding rabbit antisera which have a high affinity for human Fc receptors, by including high-speed centrifugation to remove Ig aggregates (spin at 100 000 g for 30 minutes and freeze as small aliquots), and by incorporating normal calf serum in the test medium. Lyophilised monoclonal antibodies frequently contain aggregates, whereas culture supernatants usually avoid this problem. Inclusion of irrelevant antibodies of the same class provides a control for non-specific reagent binding. Extrinsic antigen can be removed by, for example, pre-incubation of leucocytes in serum-free medium or by an acetate wash (see below), but definitive demonstration of the intrinsic nature of antigen may require that it be re-expressed after removal by enzyme treatment or by capping and shedding with the relevant antibody.

MONOCLONAL ANTIBODIES (MAb)

Most antibodies in use in the haematology laboratory for phenotyping are now monoclonal and derive from the hybridoma technology introduced by Kohler & Milstein in the late 1970s. Such MAb have identified numerous previously unrecognised antigens, but have also replaced many polyvalent reagents against well-characterised antigens. Most MAb are murine in origin, but rat and human MAb are also available.

A great many MAb have been developed and new reagents are constantly being produced. In order to inter-relate different MAb, clusters of MAb with very similar reactivity within cells of a given lineage and therefore against the same differentiation antigen have been identified; these have been designated as Clusters of Differentiation (CD) (see below). Rather than attempt to list all haematologically useful MAb, the CDs so far established are given below, where well-known examples within each CD group are included. Haematologically useful MAb are considered further in Table 11.1 and in the relevant text.

Clusters of Differentiation (CD)

The Clusters of Differentiation defining human leucocyte differentiation antigens were established initially at the First International Workshop on Human Leucocyte Differentiation Antigens in Paris in 1982. The protocol used for delineation of Clusters of Differentiation was defined by the following criteria: distribution of reactive cells in blood, lymphoid tissues and leukaemias/lymphomas, as well as the molecular weights of the antigens. After the First Workshop, 15 clusters were defined and the list was expanded to 25 at the Second Workshop in 1984 and to 45 at The Third in 1986 (Table 11.1; McMichael, 1987).

Table 11.1 Leucocyte differentiation antigens; clusters of differentiation (CD) identified by 1986

Antigen	M.Wt. (kd)	Distribution	Function	Value in diagnosis
CD1	49	Thymocytes	Unknown, but member of Ig gene superfamily	Identifies thymic proliferations, (e.g. NA1/34, T6) but expression too limited for routine diagnosis of T lineage
CD2	50	Immature and mature T cells	Sheep erythrocyte (E) receptor; involved in T-cell activation	Good marker of T and NK lineage (e.g. T11), but occasional very early T-cell proliferations may be CD2$^-$
CD3	19,25	Mature T cells	T-cell antigen receptor	Membrane marker of mature T-cells (e.g. T3 & Leu 4) and cytoplasmic marker (cCD3 for thymocytes and T-ALL)
CD4	60	T subset	Interacts with class II MHC molecules in T-cell help	Useful for diagnosis (e.g. T4, Leu 3a) of cutaneous T-cell lymphomas/leukaemias. In conjunction with CD8 is useful in monitoring AIDS
CD5	67	Mature T cells + subset of B cells	Involved in T-cell activation.	Typical CLL is CD5$^+$(Leu 1$^+$).
CD6	120	Mature T cells + subset of B cells	As for CD5	Probably none
CD7	40	Immature and mature T cells	Receptor of the Fc of IgM?	Best marker for T-ALL (e.g. 3Al) apart from cCD3
CD8	32	T subset	Interacts with Class I MHC in T-cell suppression/cytotoxicity	Identifies (e.g. OKT8, Leu 2) certain proliferations of granular lymphocytes associated with peripheral cytopenias
CD9	24	Not lineage specific	Unknown	Probably none
CD10	100	pre-pre B cells, granulocytes and some plasma cells.	Unknown	Identifies common ALL (e.g. J5) and some follicular-centre-cell proliferations
CD11a	180	Leucocytes	α chain of LFA-1;	Absent in rare immunodeficiency disease
11b	160	Monocytes, granulocytes	α chain of MAC-1(also Mo1, OKM1) C3bi receptor	Immunodeficiency disease

Table 11.1 (*cont'd*)

Antigen	M.Wt. (kd)	Distribution	Function	Value in diagnosis
11c	150	Monocytes	α chains of p150.	Useful marker of monocytes and hairy cells
CDW12	—	Myeloid cells	Group not well defined	None
CD13	150	Monocytes, granulocytes and myeloid precursors	Not known	In conjunction with CD33 (My 9) a useful marker (e.g. My7 and MCS2) of AML
CD14	50–55	Monocytes	Not known	Of some value in the identification of monocytic proliferations
CD15	—	Antibodies from subgroups and some are macrophage and granulocyte restricted	Sugar sequence in lacto-N-fucopentose	One antibody in this group (Leu M1) detects Reed-Sternberg cells
CD16	50–60	Large granular lymphocytes, granulocytes	Low affinity receptors for the Fc of IgG	Useful (e.g. Leu 11) for detecting NK cells among mononuclear populations
CD17	—	Granulocytes and some monocytes	Lactosyl ceramide	None
CD18	95	Leucocytes	β chain associated with CD11 α chains	Absent in rare immunodeficiency diseases
CD19	95	Immature and mature B cells	Unknown	Good marker (e.g. Leu 12, B4) of B lineage
CD20	35	B cells	A few of these Abs are involved in B-cell activation	Good marker (e.g. B1) of peripheral B lineage, but less reliable for pre-B-cells
CD21	140	B cells and dendritic reticulum cells	C3d receptor	Limited
CD22	135	Mature B cells	Augments anti-Ig-induced B-cell proliferation	Cytoplasmic in cALL and 'null' ALL and membrane expression in peripheral B cells and malignancies. Typical CLL shows low expression.
CD23	45	Activated B cells	Involved in B-cell activation	None at present
CD24	45	Earlier B cells, lost with maturation. Granulocytes (intracellular)	Unknown	A marker for cALL and some AML
CD25	55	Activated T and B cells. Monocytes, come early myeloid cells	IL-2 receptor	Strongly expressed (e.g. Tac) in Japanese acute T-cell leukaemia and in hairy-cell leukaemias
CDW26	120	Activated T cells	?T200 (CD45)-associated antigen on T cells	Not yet clear
CD27	120	T cells, plasma cells	Unclear	Not yet clear
CD28	44	T subset	Antibody maintains growth of activated T cells	Not yet clear
CDW29	135	T subset	Identifies a CD4 subset which induces help	Probably none (4B4)
CD30	110–130	Activated T and B cells	Unknown	Good, but not specific, marker of Reed Sternberg cells (e.g. Ki 1)

Table 11.1 (*cont'd*)

Antigen	M.Wt. (kd)	Distribution	Function	Value in diagnosis
CD31	130–140	Myeloid cells, platelets and some T cells	May be glycoprotein IIa	Not yet clear, but probably limited
CDW32	40	Myeloid cells, platelets, B cells	A second type of γFc receptor (c.f. CD16)	Not yet clear but probably limited
CD33	67	Early myeloid cells	Unknown	One of the marker of AML cells, (e.g. My 9), used in combination with CD13
CD34	115	Primitive myeloid and lymphoid progenitors	Unknown	Useful in distinguishing acute leukaemias from more mature proliferations (e.g. My 10, BI-3c5)
CD35	220	Widely distributed	CR1	Probably none
CD36	85	Monocytes and platelets	Glycoprotein IV	Not yet clear
CD37	40–45	Mature B cells	Unknown	Not yet clear
CD38	45	preB, germinal centre B cells and plasma cells. Weakly expressed by certain T-cells	Unknown	Not yet clear
CD39	80	Most B cells, but not B-cell specific	Involved in B-cell activation	Not yet clear
CDW40	50	B cells, carcinomas	Involved in B-cell mitogenesis	Not yet clear
CDW41	115–130	Platelets and neutrophils	gp IIb/IIIa fibrinogen, receptor	Useful marker of primitive megakaryocytes
CDW42		Platelets	gp Ib	Useful marker of primitive megakaryocytes
CD43	95	Widely distributed	Unknown	Not yet clear
CDW44	65–68	Widely distributed	Unknown	Not yet clear
CD45	$\simeq$ 200	Leucocyte	Leucocyte common antigen; function largely unknown but involved in lymphoid cell killing	Important in distinguishing haemic from non-haemic cell tumours
CD45R	220,205	Subsets of T and B cells and monocytes	Largely unknown	Not yet clear(2H4)

IMMUNOFLUORESCENCE

Modern microscopes use incident-light illumination (epi-illumination) instead of transmitted light excitation, with the following advantages. First, the exciting light passes through the specimen downwards and is lost without interfering with the fluorescence image, while the elicited fluorescent light passes from the sample upwards through a chromatic beam splitter into the eyepieces. Secondly, the design of reflector housing is compact, and the switch between fluorescein filters and rhodamine filters is rapid. A further advantage is that the compact epifluorescence condenser is easily fitted to a standard microscope and converts it into a fluor-escence microscope. The small epifluorescence condensers which use HBO 50 small mercury lamps give higher total energy yield (and brighter image) in the specimen plane than most of the larger and more expensive photomicroscopes. Narrow band filters to examine the excitation of fluorescein-isothiocyanate (FITC) and tetramethyl-rhodamine-isothiocyanate (TRITC) are available as standard sets. There are differences in the quality of filters supplied by the different manufacturers.

The brightest lenses are the Planapochromatic 63 Ph3 oil objectives with numerical aperture (NA) 1.4. Membrane marker studies are difficult to perform with cheaper 100 Ph3 lenses (NA: 1.25–1.3). It is important that fluorescence studies should always be combined with morphological analysis using phase contrast. Distinct populations such as granulocytes, promyelocytes, myeloblasts with nucleoli, normoblasts, lymphocytoid and lymphoblastic cells of different sizes, etc. can be readily observed with precision — and their phenotypic features recorded. These observations are as valuable as the quantitative analysis performed by fluorescence activated cell analysers (FACA-s).

In the late 70s and early 80s conventional antisera that were deemed to be important were:

a. anti-ALL antiserum reacting with common acute lymphoblastic leukaemia antigen (cALL antigen; M.Wt 100 kd);

b. antisera to HLA-DR (p 28,33, HLA Class II) molecules,

c. anti-T cell reagents (anti-HuTLA), and

d. anti-Ig.

An antiserum made against a nuclear enzyme terminal deoxynucleotidyl transferase (rabbit-anti-TdT) complemented these reagents and helped to elucidate the 'normal equivalent cells' in the common form of ALL (an early lymphoid precursor in the bone marrow; Janossy et al 1979) and in T-ALL (immature thymic blasts). These markers are not leukaemia specific and react with rare precursor cells from which the leukaemia cells originate (Greaves & Janossy 1978).

Recent developments have extended these observations. Diagnostic precision has been refined by the use of fluorochromes in addition to FITC and TRITC. Some of these, like phycoerythrin (PE), are suitable for double colour analysis with a single laser on FACA-s. The greatest impact has been made by the introduction of monoclonal antibodies (MAb), and these antibody clusters are set out in Table 11.1 (Bernard et al 1984, Reinherz et al 1986 McMichael, 1987).

With experience there has been a simplification of diagnostic panels. A few crucial reagents with clearly established reactivity patterns are now recognised. These antibodies are available from commercial sources.

The investigation of lymphoid subsets, most important in the study of immunoregulatory disorders, are based on the development of pan-T reagents (reacting with thymocytes and most T cells; e.g. CD2 antibodies), pan-peripheral T reagents (reacting with mature T lymphocytes; e.g. CD3) as well as from the discovery of a dichotomy between T cells of helper function (identified by CD4) and suppressor/cytotoxic function (identified by CD8; Reinherz & Schlossman 1980). The correlation of phenotype and function is nevertheless not absolute. For this reason phenotypic and functional studies remain complementary. Immunofluorescence (IF) methods have the following advantages:

1. The speed of the technique. Staining of cells in suspension with directly-labelled antibodies takes 10–15 minutes, and in an indirect IF assay 20–30 minutes. Large numbers of samples can be assessed rapidly in a microplate assay.

2. The economy of tests. Only small amounts of reagents are required when a microplate assay is used.

3. Analytical precision of studying the expression of two different antigens with antibodies labelled with different fluorochromes such as FITC (green) and TRITC (red) or, more recently PE (orange). Only two colour IF, viewed by separate filters, is capable of revealing small amounts of antigen-1 in the presence of larger quantities of antigen-2. Alternatively, two colour histochemistry might be applied, but this procedure takes longer to perform and the colours may interfere on doubly-labelled cells: the stronger colour masks the tint of the weakly-expressed antigen.

4. The ease of concomitant morphological assessment with phase contrast. It is also possible to stain the IF labelled slides with haematoxylin without quenching fluorescence.

5. The extension of the technique to flow cytometry for quantitative analysis. The microplates are directly applicable to flow cytometry. In these studies two separate antibodies, labelled with FITC and PE, can be investigated with one single laser (see p. 198).

6. The two-colour investigations are essential for defining asynchronous expressions of markers, as characteristic aberrations of leukaemic cells can be exploited for defining minimal residual disease (see conclusions on p. 205).

Control of immunofluorescent techniques

Great care is necessary to avoid spurious results due to a number of potential artefacts. Binding of aggregated immunoglobulin (Ig) to cell membranes is mediated by Fc receptors which are present on many cell types including lymphocytes, myeloid and monocytic elements. When blood is taken from patients with circulating immune complexes, cells with Fc receptors carry passively absorbed Ig. This can be eluted from the cells by a wash in acetate buffer. Aggregates can also bind to receptors on viable cells during the IF test. Rabbit Ig has particularly high affinity for human Fc receptors and rabbit antisera should be avoided unless one wishes to use F(ab)$_2$ fragments. Goat Ig does not bind efficiently to human Fc receptor and goat antisera give clean results. After purchase the reagents are centrifuged (100 000 g 30 min) to remove aggregates, and these are stored as aggregate-free reagents frozen at −30°C in small aliquots. These small aliquots are then spun again at 1000 g for 5 minutes before use. MAb may also contain aggregates when stored in lyophilised form and reconstituted. These aggregates should also be removed by high speed centrifugation.

MAb culture supernatants containing 10% fetal calf serum store particularly well at $-30°C$ and can be relatively free of aggregates. Finally, if a reagent still gives strong binding to Fc receptors, e.g. on subsets of monocytes and acute monocytic leukaemias, the sample should be pre-incubated with rabbit serum in an attempt to block the 'non-specific' binding of MAb to Fc receptors.

ACETATE WASHING OF CELLS (TO REMOVE CYTOPHILIC PROTEINS)

Principle
Serum immunoglobulin and other proteins attach to leucocytes and interfere with the analysis of surface membrane Ig (SIg). The bulk of passively absorbed protein can be eluted with a gentle acetate wash method which allows the demonstration of monoclonality in malignant B-cell disorders.

Reagents
- Acetate buffer: solution 1 — glacial acetic acid 12.0 ml/l
  solution 2 — anhydrous sodium acetate 16.4 g/l.
  Mix 8.8 ml of solution 1 to 41.2 ml of solution 2 and make up to 200 ml with distilled water. To each 200 ml add 1.8 g NaCl and 0.2 g anhydrous $CaCl_2$. Store 10 ml aliquots at $-20°C$.
- Medium (TC-199, or Dulbecco modified MEM or RPM1 with 10% FCS).
- Water-bath, 37°C.
- Cell suspension (1 to 2×10^7/ml).

Equipment
Bench centrifuge.

Method
1. After Ficoll-Triosil separation (see Ch. 10), resuspend cells in acetate buffer (pH 5.5) and incubate at 37°C for 10 minutes with occasional shaking.
2. Wash cells twice and resuspend in medium. Put cells into water-bath at 37°C and incubate for 2 hours with occasional mixing.
3. Wash cells twice and resuspend in medium.

Comment
After the acetate wash, minimal dot-like polyclonal Ig staining on myeloid cells is still observed. The staining of malignant B-lymphocytes seems to be stronger than before wash and shows genuine monoclonality.

MEMBRANE IMMUNOFLUORESCENCE STAINING IN TUBES

Principle
Antibodies react with membrane marker determinants of viable cells in suspension. In order to prevent extensive movement of the membrane protein-antibody complexes (which can lead to 'cap-formation' and shedding of caps), 0.2% sodium azide, a metabolic inhibitor, is added. Antibodies are either directly labelled with fluorochromes (direct IF test) or the cells are incubated with unlabelled antibody (first layer), washed and re-incubated with labelled antibodies (second layer) directed against the first layer (indirect IF test). The indirect test is more sensitive than the direct test. Afterwards, washed cells are viewed with a fluorescence microscope either in suspension under a sealed coverslip or in freshly prepared fixed smears.

Reagents
- Antisera (of known specificity and strength) and normal control serum (from the same species). Goat anti-mouse Ig labelled with FITC (e.g. Sigma cat.no. F1010. Seralab cat.no. FAES-084, or Kallestad cat.no. 147).
- PBS containing 0.2% bovine serum albumin and 0.2% azide (PBSA). PBS is prepared as follows: sodium chloride 8.00 g/l; potassium chloride 0.20 g/l; di-sodium hydrogen phosphate (Na_2HPO_4) (0.008 M) 1.15 g/l; potassium di-hydrogen phosphate 0.20 g/l in 1000 ml of distilled water.
- Plastic tubes (volume: 2 ml, LP3, Sterilin Ltd).
- Automatic pipette (50 μl) and tips.
- Glass micropipettes (1,2 and 5 μl volume).
- Microscope slides and coverslips.
- Fine Pasteur pipettes.
- Bucket with chips of ice.
- 8% formalin.
- Capillary tubes.

Test samples
Cells (1 to 2×10^7/ml in PBSA + 0.2% bovine serum albumin + 0.2% azide) separated from the sample with the Ficoll-Triosil method.

Equipment
○ Bench centrifuge.
○ Microscope with epifluorescence attachment.

Method
1. Dispense 50 μl of cell suspension (0.5 to 1×10^6 cells/tube) with automatic pipette into LP3 tubes according to the number of antisera tested. Include controls for staining with normal serum.

2. Add antibody with glass pipettes, mix well by tapping and incubate for 10 minutes at room temperature. Agitate samples once or twice during incubation.

3. Top up tube with PBSA, spin (3 min, 400 g) and discard supernatant and wash resuspended cells twice.

4. If indirect test is used, leave approximately 50 μl fluid on the cells after the last wash. Add second antibody with glass pipettes. Repeat incubation and washing as above.

5. Keep the tubes on ice while slide preparations are made. Collect cells directly from the pellet with a capillary tube, place on slide, cover with coverslip and press gently. Finally seal with nail varnish.

6. Study cells immediately. If cells cannot be analysed within 30 minutes add one drop of 8% formalin (approximately 2% final concentration) in order to fix cells as soon as possible (before preparing the slides).

Comments

— Sodium azide under acid conditions yields hydrazoic acid which is extremely toxic. Azide compounds should be diluted with running water before being discarded to avoid deposits in the piping where explosive conditions may develop.
— It is important to wash samples well. Residual traces of the first antibody in the supernatant can form soluble complexes with the second antibody and bind to Fc receptors on irrelevant cells.

Interpretation

The fine morphology of membrane staining is informative. If azide is omitted and the samples are left on the bench for a long period, the binding of antibodies (i.e. the crosslinking of membrane antigens) will result in active membrane movement. This leads to 'cap-formation' and to shedding and/or endocytosis of membrane receptors (Fig. 11.1). Obviously this must be prevented and the tests are therefore performed in the presence of azide, and the tubes are kept on ice 10 minutes after adding the final antibody. Nevertheless minimal membrane movement (patch formation) does occur even in the presence of azide, and in fact helps to identify genuine membrane staining. This staining pattern is distinct from the binding of Ig-aggregates or complexes to cells that express strong Fc receptors. In the latter case little 'lumps' seem to be lifted out from the plane of the membrane, and do not tend to show a linear apposition. Also, rarely, viable cells can show a weak but perfect ring-staining (Fig. 11.1) which is an artefact. Some overconjugated commercial reagents can give this non-specific staining pattern. Dead cells in the suspension may stain homogeneously with labelled antibodies. Some investigators prefer to read the results of membrane staining in viable (or formalin-fixed) suspensions of cells, using phase-contrast microscopy. Others resuspend cells in a droplet of buffered glycerol. An important point is to avoid an excessive amount of fluid on the slides under the coverslip. This results in a 'halo' effect around the cells when viewed under phase. Apply a gentle pressure on the coverslip. This slightly flattens the cells and facilitates photography by preventing their movement. Other investigators prefer to spread droplets of cells on slides, let them dry on the bench, fix for 5 minutes in ethanol, wash in PBS and mount in glycerol. Interestingly, the intensity of fluorescence staining increases when the stained cells are smeared, but cells can shrink as they dry out. Finally, one can prepare

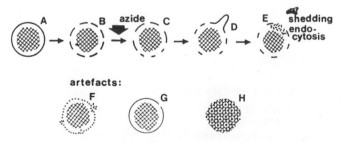

Fig. 11.1 *Morphology of membrane staining.* Normally, antigens are evenly distributed on the cell surface, as demonstrated by labelling cells prefixed in formalin (A). If viable cells are incubated with Abs the crosslinking of antigens leads to formation of patches (B,C) and caps (D). Finally, antigens are shed and endocytosed (E). This energy dependent process is inhibited by cold (4°C) and azide (0.2%) and only patch formation occurs (B). *Artefacts.* Soluble Ig aggregates bind to Fc receptors (F). Perfect ring-staining on viable cells is an artefact of reagents over-conjugated to FITC. Sometimes dead cells show homogeneous staining all over the cell (H). The aim of good IF labelling is to observe cells of B and C morphology (see also Fig. 11.6).

fixed preparations of pre-stained cells on a cytocentrifuge (p. 179).

A RAPID MICROPLATE METHOD FOR MEMBRANE IMMUNOFLUORESCENCE

Principle

Four elements contribute to the economy of this test:

a. microplates with U-wells are used to provide a
vehicle for simultaneously staining and washing 96
samples,

b. antibody panels are constructed as multiples of
six tests, and Titertek multipipettes are employed to
handle six reagents and six samples simultaneously.
These samples are transferred onto slides, for viewing,
in a pre-arranged pattern of 2 × 6;

c. 12-well multitest slides receive the 12 droplets of
cells and are fixed in formalin and viewed on a standard microscope under coverslip. Bright 63 × Phaco
objectives with numerical apertures 1.4 are used and
there is no compromise on optical quality;

d. depending on the results, it is possible

(i) to re-stain the residual cells left in the microplate
wells (e.g. by using directly labelled second Ab);

(ii) to prepare cytospins from selected microwells
and stain these with anti-TdT, etc.,

(iii) to analyse cells from selected microwells on the
cell sorter.

Reagents

- Monoclonal antibodies for diagnosing acute leukaemia

(Table 11.2) and for investigating immune disorders
and chronic leukaemias (Table 11.3).

- Microplates with U-bottom wells (Sterilin; cat.no.
M24A).
- Adhesive microplate cover (Flow Labs; cat.no.
77–400–05).;
- Plastic stoppers for individual wells (e.g. from
Pierce & Warriner Ltd).
- Microplates with V-bottomed wells (in order to keep
the panel of reagents in a pre-established order).
- PTFE coated multispot slides with 12 wells (cat.no.
PH001, Headley, Essex, U.K.).
- Formalin vapour (40% formaldehyde in a tight moist
chamber).
- Permanent mountant: 20 g poly-vinylalcohol in
80 ml PBS + 40 ml glycerol containing 3 g diaza-
bicyclooctane (DABCO), pH 8.6 or semipermanent
mountant: PBS and glycerol in 1:1 ratio.

Equipment

○ Beckman TJ-6 centrifuge with plate carriers (cat.no.
340509).
○ Microscope with epi-illumination, filter sets for FITC
and TRITC, phase contrast condenser and objective
63 Phaco N.A. 1.3–1.4.
○ Plate shaker (Dynatech; cat.no. AM69).
○ Titertek 8-fold multipipettes: 5–50 μl (cat.
no.77–858–00); 50–200 μl (cat.no.77–969–00;
both from Flow Labs), together with trays for
solutions; also tips in unlimited quantity, changed
after each operation. Note that only 6 of the 8 channels of the Titertek pipettes are used.

Table 11.2 Diagnostic reagents in leukaemia ('acute leukaemia' panel)[a,b].

	Ab	M.Wt. of antigen(kd)
(a)	T associated	40
	1. CD7 (3A1,	50
	2. CD2 (T11,	
(b)	myeloid	150
	3. CD13 (My9)	67
	4. CD33 (My7, MCS2)	50–55 or 150
	5. CD14 (UCHM1) or CD11c	
(c)	common-ALL and B	94
	6. CD19 (B4)	100
	7. CD10 (J5, common ALL)	35
	8. CD20 (B1)	135
	9. CD22 (RFB4, T015)	
	10. K/λ double labelling	
(d)	stem cell associated	120
	11. CD34 (BI-C35)	28,33
	12. Class II anti-HLA-DR	

[a] For further details about the CD groups see Table 11.1
[b] For reactivity on common ALL, T-ALL and AML see Fig. 11.2. and Table 11.7. After
the completion of the microplate assay with the 12 reagents, the intracellular staining for
TdT, cytoplasmic IgM, CD3 and CD22 is recommended (Fig. 11.9, 11.10, Table 11.7)

Table 11.3 Diagnostic reagents in lymphoid disorders ('lymphocyte' panel)[a,b]

		M.Wt. of antigen(kd)	Comments
(a)	T-cell associated		
	1. CD7 (3A1)	40	
	2. CD2 (T11)	50	
	3. CD3 (T3)	19,29	
	4. CD5 (T1) + anti-IgM	65 + 7S membrane IgM	double labelling for CLL
	5. CD4	55	
	6. CD8	32	
(b)	B-cell associated		
	7. Class II, HLA-DR	28,33	
	8. CD20 (B1, RFB7)	35	
	9. CD22 (RFB4, To15)	135	
	10. CD21 (RFB6, B2)	140 (C3d receptor)	
	11. anti-κ + anti-λ	light chains	double labelling for monoclonality
	12. CD10 (RFAL-1) or normal mouse serum	100	used as negative controls

[a] For further details about CD groups see Table 11.1.
[b] For reactivity in normal blood, AIDS and CLL see Fig. 11.3.

○ Repette repeating dispensers, 2 ml total volume with Teflon piston (Jencons Scientific; cat.no. H9/255/22) for rapid repeated delivery of 50 μl cell suspensions.

Microplate method

1. 50 μl aliquots of 2–4 × 10^6/ml suspension (1–2 × 10^5/well) are placed into 12 microwells in a U-bottomed microplate with a repeating dispenser.

2. 12 (2 × 6) MAb (Table 11.2 or 11.3), kept in an adjacent plate as a row of concentrated stock solution and diluted with PBSA prior to use, are transferred in 50 μl volumes onto the cells with a Titertek multipipette (using 6 of the 8 available channels).

3. The individual wells on the whole plate are covered with an adhesive sheet and gently shaken while incubating for 10 minutes at 20°C.

4. The wells are topped up with 100 μl PBSA, spun in a centrifuge for 30 seconds at 1500 rpm, and the supernatant is removed by forcefully inverting the plate.

5. The cells are suspended on a plate shaker, and washed with cold PBSA 4 times.

6. Cells are then incubated again for 10 minutes with diluted goat-anti-mouse-Ig-FITC (50 μl), and washed 4 times.

7. After the last wash, 5–6 μl PBSA (with azide) is added to each of the small cell pellets using a smaller Titertek multipipette and 2 μl of resuspended cells are transferred, as two rows of 6 samples, onto a PTFE coated multispot slide.

8. One slide (12 samples) for each patient is placed into formalin vapour for 15 minutes, dried and covered with glycerol: PBS (1:1) and a coverslip.

Comments

— The antibodies for the acute leukaemia panel (Table 11.2) are classified as (a) T lineage associated, (b) myeloid, (c) B lineage associated and (d) precursor cell associated. These terms are merely convenient phrases to describe the most obvious activity of the antibodies.

a. In the field of acute leukaemia diagnosis one of the most prominent groups of reagents is the CD7 group detecting an antigen of 40 kd. This group includes 3A1, WT1, RFT2, Leu-9, all strongly reactive with T blasts and positive in virtually all cases of T-ALL including those which are negative with sheep erythrocyte rosetting and the corresponding T11-like CD2 antibodies. On the other hand, virtually all cases of common ALL are CD7-. It is interesting to note that CD7 Abs show reactivity with some cases of AML (see below).

b. Three types of myeloid antibodies which are included in the first screening range. The first two react with most myeloid leukaemias. These are CD13 including My-9 and CD33 including My-7 or MCS-2. The highest percentage of AML reactivity has been recorded with CD33 although the staining intensity in some AML can be low and the proportion of positive blasts is variable (Drexier, 1987). The third MAb is to detect malignancies with monocytic component such as AMMoL and AMoL. As yet there is no general agreement which CD group is the best for the latter aim, and the two best candidates are the CD14 group (such as UCHM1) and the CD11c group (also referred to as p 150/95; Table 11.6) CD11c reagents are also strongly positive with hairy cell leukaemia.

c. There are five groups of antibodies within the common ALL-B cell associated category. The widest 'cover' from early precursors to B-lymphocytes is provided by the CD19 cluster of antibodies (e.g. B4 and Leu-12). These Abs, available from Coulter, Becton-Dickinson and Seralab, are reactive with an antigen of 95 kd which is expressed even on 'null' ALL cases which do not carry the cALL (p 100, CD10) antigen, but are negative with T-ALL or AML blasts. A few cases of AMMoL might be CD19 positive (but see Fig. 11.5). A further important group of antibodies is the CD10 cluster. These reagents are Abs to the common ALL Ag (cALL; 100 kd). The next reagent, CD20 (to 35 kd antigen; e.g. B1) shows strong anti-B cell reactivity without reacting with most cases of cALL+ cells. (The RFB7, an unclustered new MAb, is used as an alternative). The CD22 cluster of MAbs also show positivity with the membrane of mature B cells and include RFB4 or TO15 antibodies. Finally, the most conventional B-cell markers, a mixture of anti-κ and anti-λ antibodies labelled with different fluorochromes (Fig. 11.6), complete the range by providing a rapid test for membrane Ig expression and monoclonality. (See p. 196.)

d. The stem-cell related Abs such as CD34 (BI-3C5 or My-10) and anti-HLA-DR are found on immature cells without discriminating between acute myeloid (AML) and the common form of acute lymphoid leukaemias (cALL). Large numbers of positive cells in a sample immediately indicate a preponderance of 'immature' leukaemic cells. In addition, anti-HLA-DR is reactive with B-cell disorders. The characteristics of pluripotent stem cells, in man, are unknown and in this respect the reactivities of CD34 and anti-HLA-DR (just as any other reagents) are still unclear (see below).

— As the reactivity pattern with the first antibodies emerges, further tests might be required. These are largely dependent upon the location of the laboratory (i.e. leukaemia centre, general hospital or pediatric oncology group, etc.). An immediate task is double staining for TdT (p. 202). The 'second round' reagents include additional monocytic, erythroid (glycophorin C) and megakaryocytic (gpIIIa) reagents as well as anti-Ig heavy chain antibodies (anti-IgM, IgG, -IgA; heavy chain specific) for B cell malignancies. For further useful antibodies and their CD numbers see Table 11.1.

— The 'lymphocyte panel' of MAbs in the microplate assay for immunoregulatory disorders and chronic lymphoid leukaemias (Table 11.3) are classified as (a) T cell associated, and (b) B cell associated. The T cell associated markers are CD7, CD2, CD3 and CD5, together with the subset markers for T cells of predominantly helper function (CD4) and suppressor/cytotoxic function (CD8). The CD5 marker is used in two-fluorochrome combination with anti-IgM in order to detect B-CLL (Fig. 11.3). The B cell associated group includes anti-Class II reagents, which in normal conditions, are dominantly B lymphoid (strong) and monocytic marker (weak) as well as antibodies of the CD20, CD22 and CD21 groups. Finally, the assay for monoclonality and Ig expression using two-fluorochrome combination of anti-κ and anti-λ completes the range (Fig. 11.3 and 11.6).

— The microplate assay can be assessed on the microscope or measured quantitatively on fluorescence activated cell analysers. This and two-fluorochrome methodology is described below.

QUANTITATIVE ASSESSMENT OF FLUORESCEIN ISOTHIOCYANATE (FITC) STAINING

Principle

The advantages of flow cytometers over microscopy are the speed of analysis (>500 cells/sec) and the accurate quantitative assessment of at least two independent parameters of the same cell: the light scatter and the fluorescence intensity of label. These parameters are obtained as the light emitted from a laser source intersects the path of the cells while they are travelling with the speed of 10 m/sec in the middle of a fluid stream. The light scatter detector is sensitive to light at the unchanged wavelength of the laser beam, while the fluorescence detector, set at 90° to the laser beam, picks up the light of a longer wavelength which is emitted by the fluorochrome bound to the cell. The modern cytometers are capable of routinely analysing two types of light scatters:

1. The detector of forward angle light scatter (FALS) looks into the laser beam. The direct entry of laser light into the sensor is blocked by a 'beam-stop', but the light scattered by cells is recorded. FALS is roughly proportional to cell size.

2. The second light scatter detector is situated at 90° to both the laser beam and the fluid stream, and the observations are recorded as '90° light scatter' (90°LS). These values are proportional to the 'granularity' of cells: irregularities of the nuclear and surface membrane, and the abundance of granules and organelles inside the

cytoplasm. When the FALS and 90°LS are used together the discrimination of viable red cells, lymphoid cells, monocytes and granulocytes is excellent, and dead cells are also separately recorded. Populations of chronic lymphocytic leukaemia are observed in the lymphoid peak, and acute leukaemias are positioned amongst larger lymphocytes and monocytes. It is common practice that the flow cytometers are gated to demonstrate IF labelling within these populations only, while the maturing myeloid and granulocytic forms are usually excluded from routine analysis.

The fluorescence of cells, within the gates set on FALS and/or 90°LS, is collected, analysed and displayed in a form of histogram. The relative fluorescence from each individual cell is stored in an analyser, and the number of cells with any given fluorescence intensity is plotted as a function of increasing fluorescence (Fig. 11.2). Other displays, such as the correlative data between two parameters (light scatter versus fluorescence), are also frequently used but not described here. These are referred to as 'dot plots' or 'scattergrams'.

Reagents
Same as in the microplate method. In addition: 2% formalin or 1% paraformaldehyde in 0.85% saline (adjusted to pH 7.4 with 0.1 M NaOH or 0.1 M HCl).

Equipment
○ Several instruments are available for flow cytometry. The most popular models are manufactured by Becton Dickinson (FACS systems), Coulter Electronics (EPICS systems) and Ortho Diagnostics (Cytofluorographs).
○ Vortex mixer (Jencons Ltd; cat.no. H79/7)

Method
1. Following the third wash of the cell suspensions in tubes (p. 186) or the fourth wash in the microplate method (p. 188), 100 μl formalin or paraformaldehyde solution is added to the cell pellets. The cell suspension is immediately but gently mixed with the Vortex. The cells can be stored for months in the dark at 4°C.

2. FITC is excited mostly by monochromatic laser light of 488 nm wavelength. The required population is gated on FALS and/or 90°LS. FITC fluorescence above 515 nm is collected, reflected 488 nm laser light being blocked out with filters; 10 000 cells are studied and the results are displayed in a histogram form.

3. Most analysers have computer programs to calculate the percentages of fluorescence positivity and mean fluorescence of the studied population. Graphic programs are available to produce comparative displays of results, such as the data obtained with a range of MAb in a microplate assay. One of these, referred to

as 'COMPOS', lines up histograms in horizontal rows (Fig. 11.2, 11.3). Subtraction of control from test histograms is facilitated by programs such as IMMUNO, available on EPICS (Coulter) analysers (Fig. 11.4). The IMMUNO program is useful for analysing samples where the positive cell distribution overlaps with the negative (or control) distribution. The program provides statistics for both the positive and negative (control) populations.

Comments
In Figure 11.2 the 'acute leukaemia' microplate is demonstrated. In Figure 11.3 the 'lymphocyte' microplate is shown as applied to the analysis of chronic lymphocytic leukaemia, and immunoregulatory disorders, such as AIDS.

As demonstrated in the case of common ALL, this diagnosis is established by the strong reactivity with anti-Class II and CD10 (cALL antigen) and the weaker but still clear reactivity with CD19. This particular patient's leukaemic cells show some peculiarities which can also be observed in 20–30% of cases with common ALL. The blast cells are virtually negative with CD34 a stem-cell marker but show some pre-B features: e.g. weak reactivity with CD20, a B-cell marker. The few CD7+, CD2+ cells are residual T lymphocytes.

The selected case of T-ALL shows typically strong reactivity with CD7. The staining intensity of T-ALL blast cells is frequently higher than observed on the majority of normal peripheral T lymphocytes (e.g. in Fig. 11.3). Note the lack of Class II labelling and the CD2 positivity on T-ALL blast cells. These T-ALL blasts also show weak expression of CD10 (cALL antigen) and other thymic features, such as the co-expression of CD1, CD4 and CD8, but no membrane CD3. The CD3 expression by T-ALL will be reinvestigated in cytospin smears, and the labelling of nuclear TdT, particularly in cases of early relapse, will also be important to avoid the confusion of T-ALL blast cells with normal reactive T lymphocytes (see below).

In the case of AML shown, the background labelling with goat anti-mouse Ig (negative control) is higher than the negative controls seen in ALL and T-ALL. Clearly, the labelling with a whole range of anti-lymphoid MAb does not exceed the level of staining detected in the negative control, and these are regarded as negative. Positive labelling is, however, depicted with the anti-Class II, CD13 and CD33 reagents, but not with the anti-monocytic CD14 (but see Fig. 11.5). Very few cells (2.1%) strongly react with glycophorin; these are residual normal normoblasts.

In Fig. 11.3 the findings for mononuclear cells taken from normal blood are compared with those seen in CLL of B-cell type. Amongst the B-cell reagents CD20 appears to give the highest intensity on both the normal

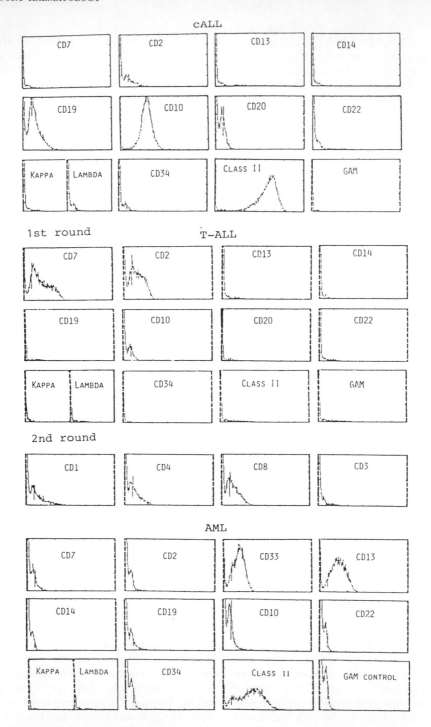

Fig. 11.2 cALL TALL and AML analysed by flow cytometry. The typical reactivity of MAb panels used in the microplate assay on malignant cells in acute leukaemia as demonstrated by the COMPOS program on a fluorescence activated cell analyser, EPICS V. cALL: common acute lymphoid leukaemia (Class II[+], CD19[+],CD10[+] mostly CD24[+] and CD9[-]). T-All: thymic ALL (Class II[+], CD7[+],CD2[+]). The study with additional markers confirms the thymic phenotype (CD1[+], CD4[+], CD8[+]) although some of these Abs show weak or variable staining on T-ALL AML: acute myeloid leukaemia (Class II mostly positive, My9[+],MCS-2[+],My7[+]). This particular case of AML shows no monocytic (UCHM1[+]), erythroid (glycophorin) or megakaryocytic (J15[-]) differentiation, but in other cases these Abs further differentiate between variants of non-lymphoid leukaemia.

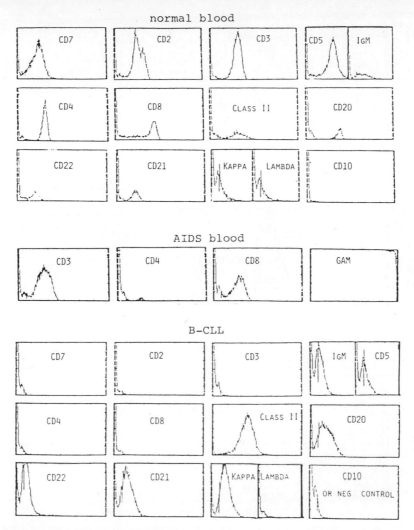

Fig. 11.3 Normal, AIDS and B-CLL blood analysed by flow cytometry. The typical reactivity of a MAb panel used in a microplate assay are shown. Normal blood contains 10–15% B cells (Class II$^+$,CD20$^+$,CD22$^+$,CD21$^+$,IgM$^+$), some of which are κ^+ and others are λ^+ in a normal 2:1 ratio. T cells are the majority cell type (CD7$^+$,CD2$^+$,CD3$^+$,CD5$^+$). Most T cells are CD4$^+$, while the others are CD8$^+$ in 2:1 ratio. In acquired immune deficiency, CD4$^+$ cells are absent. In B-CLL, malignant B cells, predominate and co-express CD5 and IgM. In this particular example, the B-CLL population is κ^+ and λ^- (monoclonal).

and malignant B cells, but these CD20+ cells are in a minority in the normal sample (10%), while they predominate in B-CLL. The CD2, CD3 and CD5 antibodies strongly mark normal T cells including the small residual T-cell population in B-CLL. The weak positivity of malignant B-CLL with CD5 is a well known phenomenon, a characteristic feature both of this disease and centrocytic lymphoma. Finally, in the normal blood, a few B cells are κ+ and λ+. Double colour IF will be required to prove that the κ+ and λ+ cells are different cells with no sign of monoclonality (see below). By contrast, in the example of B-CLL shown in Fig. 11.3 only κ light chain is detected, as

seen in two-thirds of cases. One-third of cases are λ positive.

From the data presented in Figures 11.2 and 11.3 the reactivity of lymphocytes with CD4 (T4) antibodies against T cells of helper phenotype were selected for statistical analysis using the IMMUNO program on the EPICS flow cytometers (Fig. 11.4). Two samples, in this case CD4 Ab and its negative control are compared in Figures 11.4a and c. Then the control values are subtracted in order to show genuine positivity with CD4 (Figs. 11.4b and d). The results demonstrate that 47% of mononuclear cells are strongly positive. These are normal T lymphocytes representing the 'positive range'

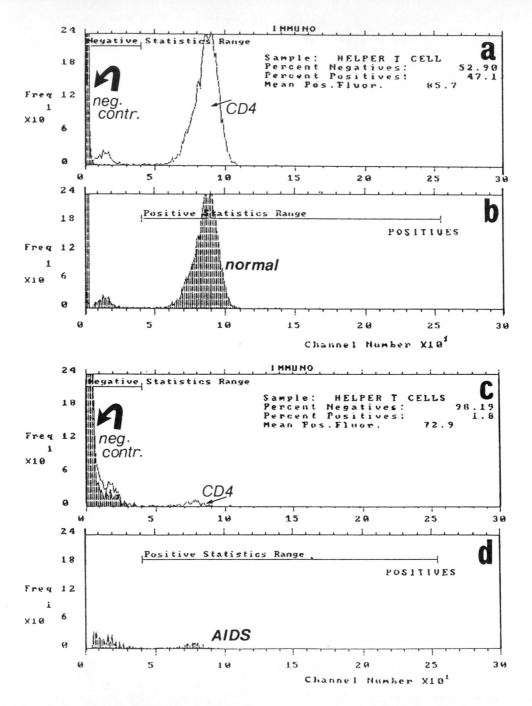

Fig. 11.4 Quantitation of IF with fluorescence activated cell analysers. As an example, the IMMUNO program on an EPICS V analyser is shown. The staining of CD4+ cells is compared to irrelevant mouse Ab plus goat anti-mouse-Ig-FITC (negative control in a and c; see large arrows). The positive results are expressed following the subtraction of negative controls (b,d). Figures a and b are from normal blood; c and d are CD4 deficient samples from AIDS with very low numbers (1.8%) of residual T4+ cells from Klaus, G.G.B., (ed). Lymphocytes, The Practical Approach; ICR Press, p. 82 With the permission of the publishers.

(channel 4–25). Cells in the other peak express CD4 very weakly (channel 1–3). In the blood of a patient with HIV infection (Fig. 11.4d) only 1.8% positive CD4+ cells are present, indicating severe depletion of CD4+ T cells. The low number of CD4+ lymphocytes together with the clinical symptoms of opportunistic infections indicate that this HIV antibody-positive patient has AIDS.

The quantitative resolution of programs such as the IMMUNO is so sensitive that the exact comparability of samples becomes important. It is therefore advisable to use, instead of murine serum (negative control, first layer), murine myeloma proteins with the same isotype applied in the same concentration as the MAb used in the test. The demonstration of the problems which are caused by binding of Abs to Fc receptors will be discussed below.

Interpretation

The microplate assays above include the most informative reagents used in many laboratories. In spite of their reliability, these reagents show some 'idiosyncratic behaviour' and none of them can be regarded, when used on its own, to be the sole feature of any given leukaemic type. CD19, a very good marker for common ALL, is also present on normal B cells and on B-CLL. CD10 is present on both common ALL, and on 15–20% of T-ALL, as demonstrated above, and shows many extra activities, e.g. on granulocytes. CD7 is a good T-ALL marker which is negative on common ALL but is recorded on 20% of cases with AML. The reactivity patterns of MAb in the CD9 (BA2) and CD24 (BA1) groups are virtually impossible to interpret when they are used on their own. These Abs might be included in the panel because they may have some prognostic significance (Kersey et al 1982). In addition, there are 'idiosyncratic cases' of leukaemias with peculiar phenotypes where some strange combination of antibody reactivity is accompanied by multiple chromosomal aberrations. For these reasons, the use of a rapid method with a panel of markers, such as the microplate assay, is important to avoid misinterpretation of data. Furthermore, specialised laboratories establish 'second panels' of reagents to investigate further the most cumbersome cases of leukaemias with additional markers (as shown in the case of AML in Fig. 11.2).

The methods shown are rapid and informative in leukaemias presenting with high WBC counts. Nevertheless, samples sent for immunological analysis may contain only low proportions of malignant cells. In these cases single colour IF may not be sufficient to reach a diagnosis, and double labelling techniques are helpful (p. 196).

BLOCKING OF THE BINDING OF MONOCLONAL ANTIBODIES TO FC RECEPTORS

Principle

Certain leukaemias of myelo-monocytic origin and subpopulations of monocytes may express Fcγ receptors in exceptionally high density. In these cases mouse MAb of IgG type give disconcertingly high levels of binding even when used with goat-anti-mouse-Ig-F(ab)$_2$ second layers. This phenomenon is identified by the high level of false positivity in the 'normal mouse serum' negative control, and can be proven by the efficient blocking of Fc binding by normal rabbit serum. Aggregated rabbit Ig has particularly high affinity to human Fc receptor, and incubation with rabbit serum saturates Fc receptors without interfering with the binding of MAb to other membrane antigens.

Reagents

See microplate method. In addition:
○ Normal rabbit serum stored for >1 month or frozen-thawed a few times to ensure that it is full of Ig aggregates. Use in 1:10 dilution without previous centrifugation.
○ Goat anti-mouse-Ig-FITC, free of anti-rabbit Ig activity (negative on cells incubated with rabbit serum alone).

Method

1. When, in the microplate assay, the négative control (mouse serum) yields high positivity (Fig. 11.5d), the test is repeated by adding 50 μl rabbit serum (prediluted 1:10) to the cells in microplate wells.
2. Incubate cells for 10 minutes at 20°C, top up well with 100 μl PBSA and wash samples twice.
3. Compare results with the previous observations (Fig. 11.5).

Interpretation and comment

In Figure 11.5 observations are shown in a case of acute monocytic leukaemia (AMoL). The first superficial impression may indicate B-cell malignancy because the blast cells are strongly Class II positive (Fig. 11.5a) and react with a 'B-cell-specific' reagent, CD19 antibody (Fig. 11.5b). There are, however, other disturbing 'irregularities' in the reactivity of other Abs, and both the UCHMI (anti-monocytic; Fig. 11.5c) and negative controls (normal mouse serum; Fig. 11.5d) are strongly positive. Following the incubation with rabbit serum, there is a dramatic decrease in the binding of CD19 (anti-B cell; Fig. 11.5f) and negative control (normal mouse serum; Fig. 11.5h) but the staining intensity of both the anti-Class II (Fig. 11.5e) and UCHMI (Fig. 11.5g) remains high. The diagnosis is AMoL.

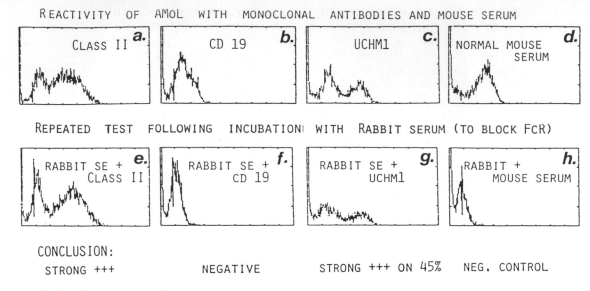

Fig. 11.5 The efficient blocking of binding of mouse Ig molecules to the Fcγ receptor expressed by blast cells of acute monocytic leukaemia. Samples are incubated with mouse Ig and MAb as shown, followed by goat-anti-mouse-Ig-FITC; in e–h similar samples were pre-incubated with rabbit serum prior to mouse Ig and second layers. For conclusions and interpretation see text.

DIRECT TWO-COLOUR FLUORESCEIN ISOTHIOCYANATE-TETRAETHYL RHODAMINE ISOTHIOCYANATE (FITC-TRITC) IMMUNOFLUORESCENCE (IF) IN SUSPENSION

Principle
This is a rapid, simple and sensitive method. Abs are directly labelled with fluorochromes FITC or TRITC, applied in combination and viewed with selective filters. The basic features of this method are;

1. its speed;
2. good performance with antigens which are abundantly expressed: for example surface Ig, HLA-DR, some B-cell antigens such as CD20 and some T-cell antigens such as CD3, CD8 and CD4;
3. relative wastefulness and high costs, when compared to indirect IF, due to the use of large amounts of first layer Ab without second layer amplification.

This method is highly recommended when one wishes to investigate the absolute amounts of antigens expressed on the cells; in this type of experiment single-layer MAb are used at saturation conditions with the IMMUNO, or an equivalent, program (Fig. 11.4). A number of companies market MAb of high quality directly conjugated to FITC or TRITC. The reagents shown below are used to perform three separate tests, all of which are linked with leukaemia diagnosis in the microplate assay but demonstrate different aspects of the same method.

Reagents
See microplate method. In addition:
- Goat anti-human κ-TRITC (cat.no. 2060–03, Southern Biotechnology Associates; referred to as SBA) and goat anti-human λ-FITC (cat. no. 2070–02, SBA) or equivalent reagents, both light-chain specific.
- Goat anti-human IgM-TRITC, μ-heavy-chain specific (cat.no. 2020–03, SBA) or rabbit anti-human IgM-FITC F(ab)₂ (Kallestad, cat.no. 140).
- TRITC conjugated MAb to Class II antigen (e.g. anti-HLA-DR, cat.no. 7364. Becton Dickinson).
- Mouse serum used at 1:10 dilution.

Method
1. When the 'lymphocyte' microplate is performed (Table 11.3; Fig. 11.3) a mixture of goat-anti-Hu-κ-TRITC and goat-anti-Hu-λ-FITC is placed into the 11th well. After washing four times, FITC- and TRITC-positive cells are counted on the microscope with separate filters (Fig. 11.6)
2. The 8th well of the same microplate has been incubated with MAb of CD5 (T1-type) and to this well, in addition to goat-anti-mouse-Ig-FITC, goat-anti-Hu-IgM-TRITC is also given. After washing four times, it is determined whether the CD5+ (T) cells and IgM+ (B) cells represent separate populations, as in normal blood or, alternatively, whether malignant IgM+ (B) cells co-express CD5, as seen in B-CLL.

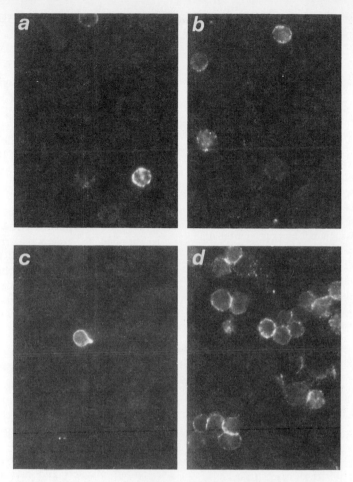

Fig. 11.6 Two-colour direct IF investigation in cell suspension of normal blood (a,b) and B cell lymphoma with circulating monoclonal B cells (c,d). Cells in a microplate were incubated with anti-λ light chain directly labelled with TRITC (in a and c) and with anti-κ directly labelled with FITC (in b and d). In normal blood the labelled B cells are a minority, present in 2:1 κ/λ ratio (a,b). In this case of B lymphoma most cells are k⁺ (d) with one residual λ⁺ (normal) B lymphocyte. Note the typical 'patch' formation of membrane antigens.

3. The first reading of the microplate assay frequently reveals that the cell populations detected with the various reagents are heterogeneous, and may contain variable proportions of leukaemic cells admixed with normal myelo-/erythro-poietic populations and T lymphocytes. As some pre-stained cells are still left in the individual microplate wells, add 20 μl mouse serum for 5 minutes in order to block goat-anti-mouse-Ig activity and wash once.

4. Now MAb anti-Class-II-TRITC is added to these wells. The plate is incubated for 10 minutes, washed four times, and the minority, potentially leukaemic, population is assessed by HLA-DR positivity (TRITC filter) in combination with any other

selected marker (CD10, anti-T or anti-myeloid in separate wells: FITC filter).

Comment and interpretation

In samples labelled for κ and λ, the microscopic analysis of normal blood rapidly reveals that, amongst the total numbers of lymphocytes, 10–15% of cells show characteristic patch and cap-formation (Fig. 11.1B,C), and these B cells show a 2:1 ratio of κ/λ positivity on separate cells (Figs. 11.6a,b). Occasionally, some cells are doubly stained with both reagents, in spite of acetate washing, but the staining pattern on these cells indicates the presence of Ig aggregates (Fig. 11.1F). In leukaemia/lymphoma the diagnosis of malignant involvement can be made if the κ/λ ratio is >10:1 or <1:5 (Figs. 11.6c,d). When the sample is not heavily involved (e.g. when B lymphoma is studied in the bone marrow), a two-colour combination may be necessary for accurate diagnosis. It is important to emphasise that the percentage positivity with anti-Ig reagents has to be interpreted in the light of positivity with other B-cell markers such as CD19, CD20 and anti-Class II, because some B-cell malignancies express low or undetectable amounts of SIg, and still show 'monoclonal' rearrangements of their Ig genes.

The CD5/IgM combination, in normal blood with separately stained cells, is a convenient two-colour method to count T cells (CD5+) and B cells (IgM+) in the suspension, but in leukaemia this double staining is a virtually tumour associated marker combination. These doubly-labelled cells are present in the normal primary nodules of the fetal lymph nodes and spleen but such cells are rapidly diluted out with CD5-negative B cells so that in normal adult lymphoid tissue, blood and bone marrow the CD5/IgM-positive cells are very rare (Caligaris-Cappio & Janossy 1985).

The combination staining with anti-HLA-DR can also be very useful in leukaemia/lymphoma with low numbers of infiltrating cells, particularly peripheral blood samples of low count common ALL, where large numbers of Class II negative T lymphocytes are present and the study has to be focused on SIg-negative, Class II+ blast cells.

DIRECT TWO-COLOUR (FLUORESCEIN ISOTHIOCYANATE-PHYCOERYTHRIN) IMMUNOFLUORESCENCE IN SUSPENSION

Principle

See FITC-TRITC method with modifications which follow from the features of phycoerythrin (PE). Both FITC and PE absorb 488 nm (blue) light emitted by the laser tube. FITC emits at a 520 nm peak (green), and PE emits with a maximum at 575 nm (orange). Thus both FITC labelled cells (apple green; arrows in Fig. 11.7b) and PE labelled cells (orange; asterisks in Fig. 11.7b) can be viewed simultaneously on the microscope without switching filters. Furthermore, these double-labelled preparations can be studied on flow cytometers equipped with a single laser (Fig. 11.7c), because argon lasers efficiently emit light in the 488 nm range (but not in the 530 nm range required for TRITC). As a result, the samples from cells studied on the microscope can be re-investigated and quantitatively documented on the flow cytometer. The advantages of this method are demonstrated by the example set out below in which double labelling CD4 (T4) and CD8

(T8) positive cells with directly labelled MAb is performed.

Reagents

The same as the previous assay, except that PE label is used instead of TRITC. In addition: FITC conjugated MAb to T cells of suppressor/cytotoxic type (CD8; Leu2a-FITC, cat.no. 7313) used together with PE conjugated reagent to T cells of helper type (CD4; Leu-3a-PE, cat.no. 7327; from Becton Dickinson).

Equipment

○ Microscope with epi-illumination. In most epifluorescence attachments a narrow band FITC filter set is supplied in order to carry out FITC analysis without interference from TRITC or PE, as demonstrated in Figure 11.7a. From this filter set one of the selective barrier filters has to be removed, and then both orange (PE) and green (FITC) cells become visible (Fig. 11.7b).
○ Flow cytometer.

Method

1. Incubate mononuclear cells with mixtures of CD8-FITC and CD4-PE for 10 minutes as described in the microplate method and wash cells three or four times.

2. Add 2% formalin or 1% paraformaldehyde to the cell pellet and mix.

3. Count 100–200 lymphocytes on the microscope and ignore platelets and monocytes. The latter may exhibit weak CD4 labelling. Calculate the percentage of CD4 (orange)- and CD8 (green)-positive cells within the total lymphoid population.

4. Gate the flow cytometer on cells with the scatter characteristics of lymphocytes. Count 10 000 cells and express the results, on the basis of two-colour histogram (Fig. 11.7c, d), as percentage positive cells in the CD4-PE (orange; Y) channel, percentage positive cells in the CD8-FITC (green; X) channel.

Comment

— The technique described here has wide applications. Figures 11.7c and d demonstrates the CD4 T cells of helper type in the normal blood and their deficiency in a patient with AIDS. The method is simple and precise. It is important in terms of establishing T cell subset (CD4) deficiency in HIV infections, and in the over production of T cells of suppressor-cytotoxic type in viral infections. Other combinations of reagents are equally important. MAb of CD4 or CD8 type can be used in combina-

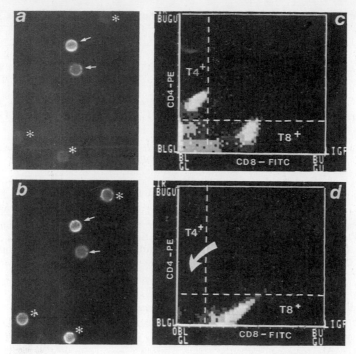

Fig. 11.7 Features of double staining with phycoerythrin (PE) and fluorescein (FITC). The sample contains T4⁺ (CD4-PE) and T8⁺ (CD8-FITC) cells. When photographed with FITC filters (a) using a selective barrier filter, only T8⁺ (green) cells are visible (arrows). Using the same FITC filters without the selective barrier filter (b), both the T8⁺ (green; arrows) and T4⁺ (orange; asterisks) cells are seen. Under this condition PE fades slowly. PE is also visible with TRITC filters but fades rapidly (not shown). The fluorescence activated cell analysers (c) use a single laser to visualise both orange (PE: CD4) and green cells (FITC: CD8). These are shown as separate groups of cells along the X and Y axes, respectively. In this sample there is a normal ratio of T4/T8 cells (2:1). In d a sample from a patient with AIDS is shown and the CD4⁺ peak is virtually missing (arrow) (1.8% CD4⁺ cells) but many CD8⁺ cells are present.

tions with pan-T reagents (CD3), activation markers (e.g. Tac, CD25) and further functionally related markers such as 4F2, TQ1, Leu-8, CD45R (2H4) and CDW29 (4B4). This trend leads from phenotyping on the microscope to cell sorting and the analysis of cell function (Lanier et al 1986).

Interpretation
Although this method is eminently suitable to give an exact T4/T8 ratio in samples with even low numbers of T cells such as the bone marrow or blood of patients during the regeneration of immune system following bone marrow transplantation, it is also essential to express the values in terms of absolute numbers within the circulating T-cell populations. Each laboratory should establish the normal ranges for the various lymphocyte subsets. In the authors' Department these are:

T cells $1.0–3.2 \times 10^9/l$; T4 $0.6–1.7 \times 10^9/l$; T8 $0.2–0.8 \times 10^9/l$; T4/T8 ratio $1.2–3.5$

INDIRECT TWO-COLOUR IMMUNOFLUORESCENCE IN SUSPENSION

Principle
The advantages of indirect IF are three-fold:

1. the second layer amplifies the intensity of labelling, and gives good results even if the given antigen is expressed in low density;

Table 11.4 Examples of antibodies recognising the same CD clusters but showing different isotypes.

	IgM		IgG$_2$		IgG$_1$	
T-cell antibodies						
CD2 (T11) pan-T	9–2	(1)*	OKT11a	(2)	RFT11	(3)
CD3 (T3) periph. T (mitogenic)	T10B9	(4)	OKT3	(2)	UCHT1	(5)
CD4 (T4) helper	66.1	(6)	OKT4	(2)	Leu 3a	(7)
CD8 (T8) suppressor/cytotoxic	RFT8μ	(3)	OKT8	(2)	RFT8γ	(3)
Precursor cell associated						
CD10 common ALL antigen	RFAL3	(3)	RFAL2	(3)	RFAL1	(3)
Class II non-polymorphic	RFDR1	(3)	RFDR2	(3)		
B-cell antibodies						
CD19 pre-B + B	SB4	(8)			B4	(9)
CD20 pan-B	RFB7	(3) 10)	B1	(9)		

* The numbers in brackets refer to the Laboratories where the reagents are made or distributed from. (1) Naito and Dupont, Sloan Kettering, New York;(2) ORTHO, Raritan, New Jersey; (3) Royal Free Hospital, London; (4) Thompson, Kentucky; (5) Beverley, University College Hospital, London; (6) Hansen, Seattle; (7) Becton-Dickinson, Mountain View, California; (8) Sanofi, Montpellier; (9) Coulter, Hialeah, Florida. (10) CD20-like reactivity but not identical to the known CD20 MAbs.

2. it is an economical test for the first-layer Ab, and

3. the same fluorochrome-labelled second Ab can be used with a wide variety of first layers. With the establishment of numerous MAb reacting with the same membrane antigen (CD groups), there is an increasing chance that within the same CD group MAb of different isotypes (Ig classes) are available. Two MAb, one of mouse IgG and another of IgM class, reacting with any two separate antigens can then be grouped in informative pairs, providing that the corresponding fluorochrome-conjugated anti-mouse IgM and anti-mouse IgG second layers are powerful reagents and class specific. Such reagents are now commercially available.

Reagents

• A short list of MAb of different classes which react with the most commonly used leukaemia/lymphocyte markers is shown in Table 11.4. In the test described below an Ab of CD19 group (B4 of IgG class, cat.no. 660 2683; Coulter) was used in combination with MAb of CD10 group (RFAL-3 of IgM class, made at Royal Free Hospital, London).

• Affinity-purified goat antibodies to mouse Ig are available from Southern Biotechnological Associates (SBA) or Seralab. U.K. One pair of the following four reagents can be selected: goat-anti-mouse-IgM-FITC (cat.no. 1020–02), goat-anti-mouse-IgM-TRITC (cat.no. 1020–03), goat-anti-mouse-IgG-FITC (cat.no. 1030–02) and goat-anti-mouse-IgG-TRITC (cat.no. 1030–03).

• 10% mouse serum or irrelevant myeloma proteins of IgM class (MOPC 104e) and IgG class (5563) used at a 1 mg/ml concentration (referred to as negative controls of IgM and IgG class).

Method

1. The standardisation of the two-colour indirect IF assay is as follows. Prepare cell suspension (50 μl each into 4 tubes) from a high count leukaemia of common ALL type (as described on p. 177).

2. Add MAb CD19 (IgG) into Tubes 1 and 2, and the negative IgG control into tubes 3 and 4. Add MAb CD10 (IgM) into tubes 1 and 3, and the negative IgM control into tubes 2 and 4. Incubate for 10 minutes in the presence of 0.2% azide, and wash tubes three times.

3. Add a mixture of appropriately diluted goat-anti-mouse-IgG-FITC and goat-anti-mouse-IgM-TRITC to all tubes, and incubate for 10 minutes and wash again three times.

4. Prepare slides and examine cells under sealed coverslips. The expected results are as follows. Both CD19 and CD10 Abs label large proportions of ALL blast cells, and most of the blast cells are double labelled in tube 1 (Figs. 11.8b,c). Nevertheless, the membrane molecules labelled with CD19 (FITC) do not fully overlap with those labelled with CD10 (TRITC), and occasional blast cells are positive with one or other Ab (see arrow in Fig. 11.8). This indicates that the antigens recognised by the two Abs are different, and that the second layers do not cross-react with the irrelevant mouse Ig class or with each other. This is confirmed in tube 2 where only FITC-labelled blast cells can be detected, and in tube 3 where only TRITC-stained blasts are seen. If the reagents are well standardized, tube 4 is negative.

Comment

— This standardisation experiment for the two fluorochrome labelled anti-mouse Ig class specific

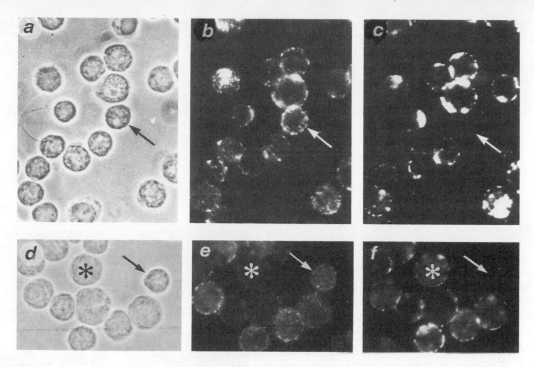

Fig. 11.8 Two-colour indirect IF investigation in suspension. Cells of a patient with common ALL (phase contrast: a and d) were incubated with two MAb of different Ig class: CD19 of IgG_1 (b,e) and CD10 of IgM class (c,f). Cells in b were labelled with class specific goat anti-mouse IgG (FITC) and in c with goat anti-mouse IgM (TRITC). The method is very sensitive for detecting unusual cells ($CD19^+$, $CD10^-$, see arrow) amidst the majority of $CD19^+,CD10^+$ (>99%) leukaemic blast cells. In d–f the cells were stained with CD19 and goat-anti-mouse-Ig-FITC (first (e) followed by mouse serum and reincubated with CD10-biotin, and avidin-TRITC (f). Note that there is no cross-reaction between the two channels, and some cells are $CD19^+,CD10^-$ (arrow) or $CD10^+,CD19^-$ (asterisk).

reagents indicates that these particular second layers can be used with any of the dozens of IgG-IgM combinations for which MAb are potentially available (Table 11.4). This assay is a powerful analytical tool in finding even minute proportions of leukaemic blasts of unusual phenotype (Fig. 11.8) and has many clinical applications.

IMMUNOFLUORESCENCE STUDIES USING BIOTIN-AVIDIN

Principle

Conjugaton of MAb with biotin is simple, and Ab-biotin conjugates can be powerfully visualised by commercially-available fluorochrome-labelled avidin or streptavidin. The principle of biotin conjugation is that biotin succinimide ester (BSE) dissolved in dimethylsulphoxide (DMSO) binds to Abs at pH 8.6.

Reagents

- MAb (purified antibody, 1 mg/ml) in 0.1 M $NaHCO_3$ (pH 8.6) without azide or preservative.

- BSE (stored in dessicator), dissolved prior to use in DMSO: 1 g/ml.
- PBS (pH 7) with 0.2% azide.
- Avidin (Sigma, cat.no. A-3275), labelled with TRITC, FITC or PE in the laboratory. Alternatively: streptavidin-Texas Red (RPN 1233) or -FITC (RPN 1232, both from Amersham Biochemicals).

Method

1. Take 3×1 ml samples of MAb solution and add 30, 60 and 120 μl BSE in DMSO, respectively. Leave at 20°C for 4 hours.

2. Dialyse against PBS overnight at 4°C.

3. Investigate which one of the three samples is the optimal conjugate with bright staining using (strept) avidin fluorochrome, without non-specific IF or loss of Ab activity.

4. Incubate cells with Abs followed by washes in the following sequence:

    a. MAb-1

    b. goat-anti-mouse-Ig-TRITC

    c. mouse serum to block binding to goat-anti-mouse-Ig-TRITC

d. MAb-2, biotinated, and

e. avidin- or streptavidin-FITC (Figs 11.8d–f).

Comment
— This technique (Figs 11.8d–f) is an alternative to the class specific double combinations (Figs. 11.8a–c), although it takes longer to perform.

INVESTIGATION OF CELLS IN CYTOCENTRIFUGE PREPARATIONS AND SMEARS

Principle
The analysis of IF in cytospins has several advantages.

Readily stored slides
Once the membrane antigens on viable cells are labelled in cell suspension, it is convenient to view these cells on a slide, and store them, if needed, in the dark at 4°C without loss of fluorescence for longer than 1 month. Many of the photographs above were made with this simple modified method (e.g. Figs. 11.7, 11.9).

Detection of cytoplasmic antigens
Slides are prepared from unstained cells and labelled with Abs after fixation. Under these conditions the labelling of cytoplasmic and nuclear antigens predominates, and the specificity of many MAb is different from that seen in suspension. Strongly expressed membrane antigens are also stained but the morphology of labelling is different from that seen in suspension. Typical examples of this method are the analysis of normal and malignant pre-B cells (Fig. 11.10), and that of benign and malignant plasma cell disorders (Caligaris-Cappio et al 1985).

Combined surface and intracytoplasmic staining
Finally, following membrane staining of cells in suspension with FITC-labelled MAb, cytospins are made and restained for cytoplasmic or nuclear antigens with MAb labelled with TRITC. A typical example of this method is the further analysis for nuclear TdT of cells stained for surface antigen by the microplate method (Fig. 11.11; see also Janossy et al 1980).

Reagents
- Fixatives:
  - (i) pure methanol to fix cells for nuclear staining with anti-TdT reagents
  - (ii) 5% glacial acetic acid in 95% ethanol to fix plasma cells for labelling with anti-Ig reagents
  - (iii) in addition, acetone and formalin vapour might be tried for staining with various MAb which

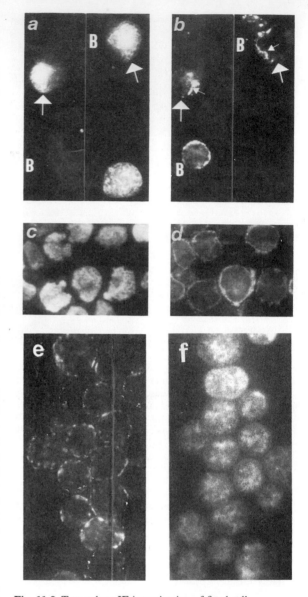

Fig. 11.9 Two-colour IF investigation of fixed cell populations on cytocentrifuged preparations. Cells of normal bone marrow (a,b) ALL with pre-B features (c,d) and AML with TdT expression (e,f) were labelled for nuclear TdT (FITC; a,c,e), cytoplasmic IgM (TRITC; b,d) and membrane CD33 (TRITC;f). In the normal bone marrow most TdT$^+$ cells and Ig$^+$ cells are separate but rarely some TdT$^+$,cIgM$^+$ pre-B cells are seen (arrows). Ig labelling is perinuclear (small arrows). In pre-B ALL (c,d) TdT$^+$ cells are cIgM$^+$. In this case of AML (CD33$^+$;f) the blasts are TdT$^+$ (e). No normal equivalent of this TdT$^+$, CD33$^+$ population is detectable in normal and regenerating bone marrow (not shown).

may give weak staining following methanol fixation.

- Microscope slides, absorbent cytospin paper, coverslips and mounting media for permanent storage.

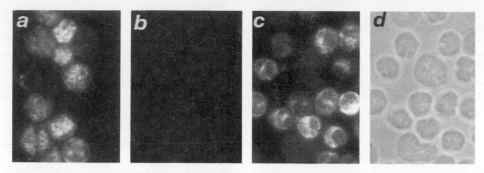

Fig. 11.10 Comparative study of cytoplasmic and membrane antigen expression with two-colour IF. This sample of T-ALL contained TdT$^+$ blast cells (a). When labelled for membrane antigens with anti-CD3, this leukaemia was CD3$^-$ (b). The same cells smeared and restained for cytoplasmic CD3 showed strong positivity (c). Phase appearance for b and c is as shown in d. Similar findings (cytoplasm positive, membrane negative) have been reported for the CD22 antigen in the common form of ALL (Campana et al 1985).

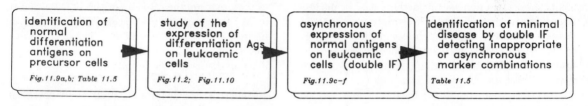

Fig. 11.11 Stages of investigation with two-colour immunofluorescent studies. These methods are ideal for identifying minimal disease in a substantial number of patients with leukaemia.

- Glass micropipettes (2, 5 and 10 μl volume) for adding Abs to smeared cells.
- Antibodies:
  (i) Rabbit antibody to calf terminal deoxynucleotidyl transferase (rabbit-anti-TdT, affinity purified; cat.no. 004, Supertech or Seralab), and swine anti-rabbit Ig-TRITC second layer (Dakopatt, cat.no. R156). Alternatively, goat anti-rabbit Ig-FITC second layer (Supertech or Seralab, cat.no. 008).
  (ii) Goat anti-human IgM-TRITC (cat.no. 2020–03, SBA).
  (iii) Goat-anti-mouse-Ig-FITC or TRITC from reliable commercial source (such as SBA, Seralab, Kallestad, Tago, Meloy, Nordic, etc.) or locally produced.
  (iv) Goat antisera to mouse IgG and IgM as described in indirect two-colour IF method (p. 199).
  (v) directly conjugated goat antisera to human light chains κ and λ, and to human isotypes μ, γ, and α from reliable commercial sources (see in iii), or mouse-anti-Hu Ig MAb used with second layers.
- 10% Mouse serum.

Equipment
○ Bench centrifuge for Ficoll-Triosil separation (p. 177).
○ Cytocentrifuge (Cytospin-2; Shandon, cat.no. 59900101)
○ Moisture chamber, to prevent the evaporation of reagents from cytospins.

Method
1. Place microscope slides with absorbent paper into the cytocentrifuge.
2. Adjust cell concentration of unfixed viable cells to $5–7 \times 10^5$/ml. You may choose to use unstained fresh cell populations. Alternatively, you may wish to use unfixed cells from selected microwells of a microplate, already labelled for membrane antigen and FITC-second layer (see above). Add 1–2 drops (100 μl) into the plastic well of the cytocentrifuge and spin at 800 rpm for 5 minutes. Let the deposits dry rapidly, and check for optimal cell density (40–50 cells per high power field).
3. Fix slides for 30 minutes in cold methanol at 4°C for TdT staining, and for 15 minutes in ethanol with 5% acetic acid for cytoplasmic Ig staining in plasma cells. Use other fixatives, if required, after careful standardisation with individual MAb. Wash slides in PBS.

4. If necessary, draw a circle with a diamond around the cytospin. While leaving the cytospin fully covered with PBS (approximately 20 μl), wipe the moisture off the rest of the slide. Add reagent diluted in 10 μl PBS to the droplet covering the cells and mix fluid gently with the micropipette.

5. Incubate at 20°C for 30 minutes, wash in three successive batches of PBS. If indirect IF is performed, leave 20 μl fluid on the smear and add 10 μl pre-tested second layer Ab. After incubation (30 min), wash three times and mount the preparations.

Controls

1. Cytospins from known cases of acute lymphoblastic (TdT+) and acute myeloid leukaemia (TdT−).

2. Cytospins of normal lymphoid cells from blood as well as from suspension of tonsil lymphocytes.

3. Some poorly standardized commercial anti-TdT reagents show extra non-specific activity against nuclear antigens in normal (activated?) lymphocytes. These reagents can lead to the dangerously misleading diagnosis of 'ALL' rather than to the correct diagnosis of lymphocytosis. Thus tonsil cells need to be tested with each new batch of anti-TdT. The anti-TdT reagents from supertech and seralab are devoid of non specific activities and are well standardized.

Comment and interpretation

— The method for labelling cytoplasmic and nuclear antigens plays an important part in investigating normal and malignant lympho-haemopoietic cells. There are three areas where the study of various intracellular antigens is essential.

— It has been recently emphasised that at the end-stage of B lymphoid differentiation both normal and malignant plasma cells lack the vast majority of B-cell-associated membrane antigens such as CD19, CD20, CD21, CD22 and SIg, and express only cytoplasmic Ig (Caligaris-Cappio et al 1985). When a plasma cell disorder is suspected on the basis of haematological findings, membrane marker studies for B cell antigens or for surface Ig are not sufficient. The analysis of monoclonality of cytoplasmic Ig (with antibodies to κ and λ, and to various heavy chains) within the plasmacytoid population is required in cytospin smears. Plasma cell associated markers, such as MAb PC1 also have to be studied.

— In the diagnosis of the common form of acute lymphoblastic leukaemia, nuclear TdT is one of the most characteristic markers. When the microplate assay is performed, samples with membrane-labelled unfixed cells are taken from the relevant wells (e.g. CD10+, or HLA-DR+), spun in a cytocentrifuge and restained for nuclear TdT with TRITC-labelled second layers (Janossy et al 1980; Fig. 11.10).

— Here we also emphasise that the detection of lineage specific cytoplasmic antigens within TdT+ blast cells can also help both the diagnosis and the clarification of the origin of acute lymphoid leukaemia. In the normal bone marrow 'early' forms of the B-lymphoid lineage are TdT positive without detectable cytoplasmic Ig expression, but a very small proportion of TdT+ cells (Fig. 11.10a) express detectable cytoplasmic (but not membrane) IgM (Fig. 11.10b, Table 11.5). In common ALL, the accumulating TdT+ blast cells reflect the phenotypic features of the normal TdT+ bone marrow precursors (Greaves & Janossy 1978): most cases of common ALL are TdT+ and cytoplasmic Ig negative. In approximately 25–30% of common ALL cases, however, the malignant cells carry cytoplasmic, but no surface, IgM (Fig. 11.10c,d): these cases are referred to as pre-B ALL. It is interesting to note that another B-cell antigen (CD22; detected by MAb To15 and RFB4) is also first exhibited, like Ig, in the cytoplasm of TdT+ precursors, and in the corresponding common ALL. This cCD22 positivity is detected by staining in cytospins using IF or immunocytochemistry. This antigen is then exhibited in the membrane of B lymphocytes at a later stage of development (Campana et al 1985).

— Nuclear TdT is also an 'early' marker for immature cortical thymocytes in the normal thymus, and in their corresponding leukaemia — T-ALL. Normally, cells with thymocyte features are restricted to the thymus. In blood and lymph nodes all T cells (CD2+, CD7+) are TdT- when tested in double marker combinations. In the bone marrow TdT+, CD7+ cells are also virtually absent. Thus outside the thymus CD7+, TdT+ blast cells are likely to be leukaemic if they represent >20% of the TdT+ population (Table 11.5). An additional recently established finding is that these immature normal thymocytes and cases of T-ALL do not express CD3 (T3-like) antigens on their surface (Figs. 11.2, 11.10b), but accumulate CD3 in their cytoplasm (Fig. 11.10c). The TdT+, surface CD3-, cytoplasmic CD3+ (cCD3+) phenotype is therefore characteristic of immature thymocytes and T-ALL. (Campana et al. 1986).

— From the results above, it is clear that at least three antigens are expressed in the cytoplasm first, and in the membrane later: immunoglobulin and CD22 during B lineage maturation, and CD3 during T lineage development. The most recent observations reveal that cCD22/TdT and cCD3/TdT are the most reliable marker combinations with two important applications: (a) precise immunodiagnosis of common ALL, T-ALL and AML in >98% of acute leukaemias; and (b) the exquisite sensitivity in single cell

Table 11.5 TdT$^+$ cells in human haemopoietic tissues[a].

	cCD22$^+$ HLA-DR$^+$, CD10$^+$, CD7$^-$	cCD3$^+$ CD7$^+$, HLA-DR$^-$, CD10$^+$
Bone marrow	0.01–2.0	<0.001[b]
Blood	0.01[c]	<0.001
Thymus	<0.05	>60
Cerebrospinal fluid	<0.1[d]	<0.1

a TdT$^+$HLA-DR$^+$ cells in bone marrow are normal components and are present in high numbers during fetal development. Ig gene rearrangement studies are required to distinguish between normal and malignant TdT$^+$ cells.

b 0.01% CD7$^+$,TdT$^+$ cells seen in patients on maintenance therapy (<20% of all TdT$^+$ cells) but cCD3$^+$, TdT$^+$ cells include only thymocytes and T-ALL (Fig. 10.10).

c >0.05% TdT$^+$ cells in blood indicate residual or relapsing ALL.

d Single TdT$^+$ cell has been detected in non-leukaemic conditions.

Table 11.6 Antibodies for the immunocytochemical typing of haematological samples.

Antigen	Specificity	Source
T-cell markers		
CD1 (T6)	Cortical thymocytes	Dako
CD2 (T11)	Pan T	Dako
CD3 (T3)	Pan T	Dako
CD4 (T4)	T helper cells	Dako
CD5 (T1)	Pan T	Dako
CD7	Pan T	Dako
CD8 (T8)	T suppressor cells	Dako
B-cell markers		
CD19 (B4)	Pan B	Dako
CD20 (B1)	Peripheral B	Coulter
CD22	Pan B	Dako
Miscellaneous		
HLA-DR	B cell, monocytes, macrophages	Dako
CD10 (CALLA)	Common ALL antigen	Dako
CD33	Early myeloid cells	Coulter
Platelet glycoproteins (Ib, IIb/IIIa and IIIa)	Platelets megakaryocytes	Dako
CD11c	Monocytes/macroph ages, myeloid cells	Dako
Myeloperoxidase	Myeloid cells	Dako
Terminal transferase (TdT)*	Haemopoietic precursors	Supertechs or Seralab
Immunoglobulin	B cells	Dako

* Polyclonal reagent

assays, facilitating the delection of minimal disease (Table 11.6).

Conclusions

The investigation of leukaemia by immunological methods has had a shifting aim during the last 15 years (Fig. 11.11). Normal differentiation antigens such as cALL antigen, Class II molecules and T lineage markers have been defined and used for classifying leukaemias according to their origin (Greaves & Janossy, 1978). These studies have been concluded by

establishing both the differentiation schemes and the origin of leukaemias (Table 11.7). With the use of double immunofluorescence techniques a new phase is opening up in the analysis of minimal disease. It has been known for a long time that leukaemic cells show an asynchronous nuclear and cytoplasmic development. This asynchrony can be defined by demonstrating aberrant combinations of normal differentiation antigens on leukaemia. The essential difference between the earlier stages of investigations and these new developments is that these special features are characteristic for individual leukaemic samples, and need to be investigated at presentation in order to find the minor deviation from normalcy.

Such features are, for example, the regular double expression of cytoplasmic IgM and TdT in pre-B ALL, a phenomenon exquisitely rarely seen in normal and regenerating bone marrow (Fig. 11.9cd), or the double expression of TdT and myeloid antigens in some cases of AML (Fig. 11.9ef), etc. We cannot find normal TdT$^+$ cells with myeloid antigen expression. These unusual features can then be exploited to detect minimal residual disease. These studies might be useful to define the speed of remission induction, to demonstrate the absence of residual leukaemia in true remission as well as to diagnose early relapse. Two colour immunofluorescence represents a natural technique for investigating such questions. Finally, it is important to emphasize that in cases of T-ALL the presence of single cCD3$^+$, TdT$^+$ cells represents residual leukaemia in the blood, lymph nodes and bone marrow (Fig. 11.10) because normal cells of this type are restricted to the thymus (Campana et al. 1986).

ROSETTE TECHNIQUES

Rosette techniques involve the detection of surface structures by means of indicator particles which are usually erythrocytes; cells possessing the test structure

Table 11.7 Reactivity of leukaemias with monoclonal antibodies.

	CD2 (T11)	CD7[a]	CD13	CD33	CD14 or CD11c	CD10 (CALL)	CD19	CD20	CD22[b]	κ or λ	Class II	CD34	TdT[c]	cIgM[d]
Acute lymphoblastic T-ALL	+	+	–	–	–	–/+	–	–	–	–	–	–	+	–
Acute myeloid leukaemia	–	–/+	+	+	–	–	–	–	–	–	+/–	+/–	+/–	–
Acute (myelo)-monocytic leukaemia	–	–	–/+	–/+	+	–	–/+	–	–	–	+	+/–	–/+	–
Acute lymphoblastic common ALL	–	–	–	–	–	+	+	–	c	–	+	+	+	–
Acute lymphoblastic 'null' ALL	–	–	–	–	–	–	+	–	c	–	+	+/–	+	–
pre-B ALL	–	–	–	–	–	+/–	+	–/+	c/+	–	+	–	+	+
Chronic lymphocytic (B type)	–	–	–	–	–	–	+	+	+	+	+	–	–	m
Chronic lymphocytic (rare T-type)	+	+	–	–	–	–	–	–	–	–	–/+	–	–	–
rare leukaemias:														
hairy cell (HcL)	–	–	–	–	+	–	+	+	+	+	+	–	–	m
erythroleukaemia[e]	–	–	–	–	–	–	–	–	–	–	–/+	–	–	–
acute megakaryocytic[f] leukaemia	–	–	–	–	–	–	–	–	–	–	–	–	–	–

Key: + All (or the great majority of) cases positive.
+/– More than 50% of cases positive.
–/+ More than 50% of cases negative.
– All (or the great majority of) cases negative.
a cytoplasmic CD3 positive (Fig. 11.10)
b CD22 is cytoplasmic in common ALL, 'null' ALL and pre-B ALL and expressed on the membrane in B cell malignancies
c detecting nuclear TdT with polyclonal or monoclonal anti-TdT antibodies (Fig. 11.9 and 11.10)
d detecting cytoplasmic IgM in pre-B ALL (Fig. 11.10) B cell malignancies show membrane IgM (m).
e additional reagent such as anti-glycophorin is required.
f additional reagent is anti-gp IIIc

form a rosette consisting of a central leucocyte surrounded by adherent erythrocytes.

Rosetting erythrocytes can be used either for the detection of leucocyte surface structures interacting directly with an integral component of the red cell membrane (e.g. sheep and mouse erythrocyte rosettes), or as indicator particles to which various antibodies have been coupled. In the latter type of use, the reagent can be employed in a direct or indirect technique. For direct rosetting, the test anti-human antibody is coupled to indicator erythrocytes, whereas the indirect method employs red cells coupled to anti-first-layer antibody (usually goat or sheep anti-mouse Ig). Previously, erythrocytes specifically bound to IgG or IgM ($\pm$ complement) polyclonal anti-erythrocyte antibody were used to detect Fc and complement receptors. Such methods are now rarely used because there is little current interest in receptors for IgM and because monoclonal antibodies are now available for the detection of IgG Fc and complement receptors.

Rosette techniques have the disadvantage that they require considerable attention to technical detail, and direct rosetting with monoclonal antibodies requires more reagent than is usually available from commercial sources. Rosette techniques, however, are more sensitive than immunofluorescent and immunocytochemical methods are easier to score than immunofluorescent preparations, and in cytocentrifuge preparations allow detailed morphological examination. Furthermore, rosetting has the considerable advantage of allowing positive and negative enrichment of cells (by centrifugation over Ficoll-hypaque) without highly expensive cell-sorting equipment.

General comments
— Rosette assays can be performed in tubes of various sizes or in microtitre plates. We have most experience with LP2 plastic tubes (Luckham's) and have found them entirely satisfactory.
— As with fluorescent methods, reacting cells should be kept on ice to avoid capping.
— Many authors regard three adherent erythrocytes as the minimum number required to form a rosette, but we recommend that at least five be present.
— Scoring rosettes is greatly facilitated by adding a fluorescent reagent and it is usual to count 200 viable cells.
— A reagent incorporating two fluorescent dyes makes it possible to identify both viable and non-viable leucocytes. Acridine Orange selectively enters dead cells which then fluoresce an orange-red colour, while ethidium bromide is taken up by viable cells which as a result appear a light-green colour under UV light. The combined fluorescent reagent is prepared as follows: 0.1 g Acridine Orange (Sigma,

cat.no. A6014) is dissolved in 100 ml distilled water and stored at $-20°C$ in 4 ml aliquots; 0.2 g ethidium bromide is dissolved in 50 ml distilled water and stored at $-20°C$ in 2 ml aliquots; the working solution is provided by adding 4 ml of the Acridine Orange, together with 2 ml of ethidium bromide to 494 ml 0.9% saline; the working solution can be stored at 4°C for at least 6 months, but aliquots should be used at room temperature for the actual addition to cell suspensions.

SHEEP ERYTHROCYTE ROSETTING

Principle
Unsensitised sheep erythrocytes (E) detect a 50 kd glycoprotein present on most immature and all mature T cells. The glycoprotein structure, which can now be detected by a range of monoclonal antibodies (designated CD2, e.g. OKT11 and Leu5), is probably involved in non-antigen-specific T-cell activation and proliferation.

Although largely specific for cells of T lineage, the E receptor is present on some non-B, non-T cells with natural killer activity and may also very occasionally be found on a range of pathological cell types.

Treatment of the indicator red cells with AET (E-AET) (AET = aminoethylisothiouronium bromide hydrobromide), neuraminidase or papain, enhances the sensitivity of the test and increases the stability of the rosettes. E rosetting is now usually performed with E-AET or E-neuraminidase, and the preparation of both reagents is described here.

Reagents
● *Sheep red cells.* Sheep blood is available from a number of sources and is usually collected into Alsever's solution.

Indicator sheep red cells are obtained by washing the sheep blood five times in 0.9% NaCl solution (e.g. 5 ml of blood mixed with 20 ml saline). After each wash, blood is centrifuged for 5 minutes at 300 g and supernatant, together with any white cells at the red-cell interface, carefully removed.
● *AET solution.* 0.403 g AET (Sigma, cat.no. A5879) is dissolved in 10 ml distilled water and adjusted to pH 9.0 with 4 N NaOH. Since the E-AET may be used for upto 10 days, the AET solution is usually filter sterilised.
● *AET-treated sheep erythrocytes.* E-AET are prepared by mixing 1 volume (e.g. 2 ml) of pelleted washed red cells with 4 volumes of freshly prepared AET solution. The mixture is then incubated at 37°C for 30 minutes with repeated mixing. The red cells are then washed four times; to avoid lysis, this should

be done by gentle centrifugation for 10 minutes at 80 g and inversion resuspension in phosphate-buffered saline (PBS), before finally diluting an aliquot to 1% v/v in HEPES-buffered Hanks balanced salt solution (H/HBSS) containing 0.2% bovine serum albumin. The stock E-AET is kept at 4°C as 50% v/v in RPMI-1640 supplemented with 10% calf serum.

- *E-neuraminidase*. E-neuraminidase are obtained by mixing 0.5 ml pelleted washed red cells with 0.2 ml neuraminidase (1 unit/ml, Sigma, Type V purified) in 5 ml PBS and incubating at 37°C for 30 minutes with intermittent mixing. The E-neuraminidase are then washed three times in PBS before final suspension at 1% v/v in H/HBSS containing 0.2% bovine serum albumin.

Method

1. Add 100μl of 1% sheep erythrocyte suspension to 50 μl of test mononuclear cell (1×10^6/ml).
2. Mix either by flicking or on a vortex mixer and incubate at 37°C for 15 minutes (incubation unnecessary for E-AET and E-neuraminidase).
3. Centrifuge 200 g for 1 minute at room temperature.
4. Place on ice for 60 minutes.
5. Remove overlying medium from cell pellet, replace with 100 μl fluorescent reagent and gently suspend with a pasteur pipette.
6. Transfer 1 drop of mixture to glass microscope slide, add coverslip, and score under combined UV/white light illumination.

Comments

— Fresh stock sheep blood in Alsever's should be obtained weekly.

— AET- or neuraminidase-treated red cells have a shelf life of 3–4 days at 4°C but, if the treatment is performed aseptically with sterile reagents and the cells stored in RPM1 + 10% heat-inactivated calf serum, they may be used for up to 10 days.

— The washed indicator sheep erythrocytes should be checked for contamination by sheep leucocytes since a significant number may sometimes remain after repeated washing.

— Omission of the incubation of the leucocyte/red cell pellet on ice markedly reduces the percentage of E cells, and detects 'active' E rosettes.

— A reactive (non-neoplastic) T-cell population is present in many leukaemias/lymphoproliferative disorders, so care must be exercised in interpretation. To diagnose a T-cell lymphoproliferative disorder, the E receptor must be demonstrably present on the malignant cells. It also should be noted that E rosetting gives no indication of monoclonality.

— On pathological cells, some disparity between E positivity and CD2 monoclonal antibody staining may occur.

— Although cells expressing E receptor in general also express T-cell antigens, exceptions may be observed in haematological malignancies.

Interpretation

Normal peripheral blood mononuclear cells consist of approximately 70% E^+ cells, and in terms of numbers E^+ cells are $1863 \pm 388/\mu$l.

ROSETTE METHODS EMPLOYING INDICATOR ERYTHROCYTES COUPLED TO ANTIBODY

Principle

For direct rosetting, first-layer antibody is coupled to indicator cells which are then directly exposed to the test leucocytes.

For indirect rosetting, second-layer antibody is coupled to indicator erythrocytes which are then used to detect bound first-layer antibody (Mills et al 1983). Since so much current work involves mouse monoclonal antibodies, the appropriate second-layer reagent will usually be heterologous anti-mouse Ig, although in some instances protein A can be substituted. Polyclonal sheep or goat anti-mouse Ig are very suitable reagents, since, when coupled to indicator erythrocytes, they display minimal non-specific reagent binding and are widely available, well characterised, and relatively cheap.

Ox erythrocytes have been most used as indicator cells and are therefore recommended. Sheep erythrocytes are probably best avoided since they potentially react directly with the CD2 structure. Rabbit erythrocytes, although they may enchance the sensitivity of rosetting, have been little used and are probably therefore best avoided for the present.

Reagents

- *Preparation of antibody*. All antibodies used for coupling should be affinity purified, dialysed for 4 days against 0.9%NaCL (4 changes of 1l), and employed at approximately 5 mg/ml protein. Since most commercial monoclonal antibodies are supplied at much lower concentrations, the direct method is only suitable for polyclonal or home-produced monoclonal antibodies. When protein A is to be coupled it can be used directly from a commercial source.
- *Ox erythrocytes*. These are available commercially from Tissue Culture Services, and are washed in exactly the same way as sheep erythrocytes (see above) except that the saline must be either freshly

prepared or filter (not autoclave) sterilised if sterile work is being performed.

- *Chromic chloride coupling.* Aged chromic chloride (1 mg/ml in 100 ml normal saline, adjusted to pH 5.0 with N NaOH, and at least 4 weeks old) is used. Immediately before use an aliquot of the aged chromic chloride is diluted 1 in 10 with normal saline.

The actual coupling is performed in glass bijous containing 100 μl of packed ox cells and 0.3 mg antibody protein or protein A (e.g. 60 μl of 5 mg/ml antibody). While continually mixing on a vortex, 500 μl of diluted chromic chloride is added drop-wise. Approximately 1 ml of saline is then carefully layered on top of the cells by running down the side of the bijou. The indicator cells are left overnight at 4°C and then washed three times in H/HBSS and made up to 4 ml (i.e. 2.5% v/v of erythrocytes) in RMPI-1640 containing 5% calf serum.

Method

1. 50 μl of test leucocytes (1 × ;10^6/ml) are placed in an LP2 plastic tube, 500 μl of H/HBSS added, and the mixture centrifuged for 1 minute at 300 g. The supernatant is discarded.

2. For indirect rosetting, 50 μl of appropriately diluted first-layer antibody is added to cell pellet, mixed on a vortex and incubated on ice for 30 minutes, with occasional mixing. Leucocytes are then washed three times with ice-cold H/HBSS and finally resuspended in 50 μl RPMI-1140 containing 5% calf serum.

3. 100 μl of 2.5% second-layer-antibody-coupled indicator cells are added, vortex mixed, centrifuged (1 min, 200 g), and placed on ice for 30 minutes before reading.

4. For direct labelling, 100 μl of indicator cells are added to 50 μl of test leucocytes (1 × 10^6/ml) and processed as in step 3.

5. For both indirect and direct rosetting, remove overlying medium, replace with 100 μl of fluorescent reagent and gently suspend with a Pasteur pipette.

6. Transfer 1 drop of mixture to glass microscope slide, add coverslip, and score under combined UV/white light illumination.

Comments

— The washed ox cells should be checked for contamination by ox leucocytes.

— The precise technical details of the chromic chloride coupling are important. For example, the chromic chloride must be aged, the glass ware must be scrupulously clean, and the system must be totally free of phosphate. Even the type of glass used in the reaction vessel is important and the method is not reproducible in certain types of glass ware. We have not made a systematic study of this phenomenon but find the method completely reproducible in clean bijous.

— Aseptically prepared indicator cells in RPMI-1640 + 5% calf serum have a shelf life up to 1 month at 4°C.

— Because the indirect rosette method is more sensitive than indirect immunofluorescence, it is often possible to use much less first-layer monoclonal antibody.

— The incubation times quoted are probably not critical, and various authors use 15 minutes to 2 hours.

— The advantages and disadvantages of direct and indirect rosetting have been discussed on page 207 and the preparative use of the method is considered below.

MOUSE ERYTHROCYTE ROSETTING

Principle

Some B cells, but not other cell types, possess a surface receptor for unsensitised mouse erythrocytes. The nature of this receptor and its physiological function are largely unknown. However, there is some evidence to suggest that receptor expression may be related to cell maturity, mature B cells lacking receptor.

Reagents

Mouse erythrocytes: mouse blood is obtained by bleeding from the ophthalmic venous plexus; 0.5–1 ml of blood is collected into a tube containing Alsever's solution. The erythrocytes are then washed four times in H/HBSS supplemented with 1% BSA and finally resuspended to 1% v/v.

Method

1. Add 50 μl of test mononuclear cells (1 × 10^6/ml) to 100 μl of 1% mouse erythrocyte suspension.

2. Mix on a vortex and centrifuge (200 g for 1 minute at room temperature).

3. Place on ice for a minimum of 1 hour.

4. Remove overlying medium from cell pellet, replace with 100 μl fluorescent reagent and gently suspend with a pasteur pipette.

5. Transfer 1 drop of mixture to glass microscope slide, add coverslip, and score under combine UV/white light illumination.

Comments

Mouse rosetting is greatly affected by technique, but such affects are probably quantitative rather than qualitative. The techniques described above consistently demonstrate the mouse receptor, but the percentage of positive cells detected will be influenced by the precise technique employed (Irving et al 1984).

— The species of mouse used does not seem to be critical. BALB/C mice are certainly satisfactory and are widely available.
— The bench life of mouse cells is relatively short. Although we have not formally established their usable life, we use the indicator cells within 48 hours of collection.
— Various mainly enzyme modifications of indicator cells have been employed. These in general enhance rosette formation, but the significance of this enhancement is not clear since a second receptor may be involved (Forbes et al 1982).
— Pretreatment of test leucocytes with neuraminidase may enhance rosette formation, but this manipulation is not essential for consistent demonstration of receptor.
— Serum protein must be present in the lymphocyte-erythrocyte mixture for optimal formation of rosettes. The mechanism of this dependence on the presence of protein is poorly understood and the type of protein and its concentration may influence the precise percentage positivity observed.
— Different temperatures and durations of incubation have been employed. These do not seem to be especially critical, but short incubations (< 1 hour) at higher temperatures (e.g. 37°C) are probably best avoided.

Current haematological use of mouse rosetting is largely related to its potential value in distinguishing chronic lymphocytic leukaemia (CLL) from related chronic lymphoproliferative disorders. The diagnosis of CLL is no longer straightforward and it is clear that the term may encompass several chronic B-cell disorders including, for example, centrocytic-cell (CCL) and lymphoplasma-cell (LPL) leukaemia. Most cases of CLL are mouse rosette positive, whereas some other CLL-like disorders (e.g. CCL and LPL) lack mouse receptors. Some disorders clearly distinguishable from CLL (e.g. centroblastic-centrocytic lymphoma) display mouse rosetting.

ROSETTING AS A PREPARATIVE TECHNIQUE

Principle
Rosetting leucocytes, by virtue of their attached erythrocytes, are more dense than their non-rosetted counterparts. When subjected to Ficoll-hypaque centrifugation, rosetting leucocytes enter the pellet, leaving the non-rosetting mononuclear cells at the interface. The indicator erythrocytes are then removed from the pellet by some form of lysis. Because of the forces to which they are subjected during centrifugation, only stable rosettes are suitable. For this reason mouse rosetting has been little used as a preparative technique.

Reagents
Indicator erythrocytes are prepared in exactly the same way as for the corresponding assay technique.

Standard Ficoll-hypaque is used (see p. 177).

Method
The manipulations are carried out in conical-tipped universals.

For separation of E+ cells

1. 300 μl of 50% AET-treated sheep erythrocytes are added to 2×10^7 mononuclear cells in H/HBSS.
2. The cells are mixed on a vortex, centrifuged (200 g for 5 min) and placed on ice for 1 hour.
3. Approximately 10 ml of chilled H/HBSS is then added to the contents mixed by repeated inversion.
4. The cell suspension is now underlayed with 7 ml of Ficoll-hypaque and centrifuged at 4°C (600 g for 30 min).
5. Non-rosetted (E−) leucocytes are harvested from the interface (and washed three times before use) and the remaining supernatant (including Ficoll-hypaque) is removed by pipetting.
6. To lyse the indicator sheep erythrocytes, 5 drops of autologous plasma are added to the rosette pellet and the resuspended cells transferred to a clean universal.
7. A further 2 ml of plasma are added and the mixture left for 10 minutes at 37°C.
8. The E+ lymphocytes are then washed three times before use.

For separation of leucocytes rosetting with antibody-coated ox erythrocytes.

1. For indirectly labelled cells, 300 μl of appropriately diluted first-layer antibody is added to a cell pellet containing 1.5×10^7 mononuclears. The cells are suspended by mixing on a vortex, incubated for 30 minutes on ice with occasional mixing and then washed three times with chilled H/HBSS.

Subsequent processing is identical for both indirect and direct methods, except that for the former the ox erythrocytes are coupled to second-layer antibody whereas for the latter they are, of course, coupled to test first-layer antibody.

2. 1 ml of 1.5×10^7 leucocytes are mixed with 1 ml of 2.5% ox erythrocytes, centrifuged (200 g, 5 min) and then incubated on ice for 30 minutes.
3. Cells are then resuspended and centrifuged through Ficoll-hypaque in exactly the same way as described above for E+ separations.
4. The ox erythrocytes in the rosette pellet are lysed in the same way as sheep erythrocytes except that Geys solution (5 ml and 10 min incubation) is substituted for autologous plasma.
5. Rosette-positive and -negative cells are then

washed before further use. Care will be necessary in further surface-marker analysis of the positive fraction (see comments).

Comments

— The erythrocyte:leucocyte ratio for preparative methods is lower than that for analytical tests. This reduces costs and, in the case of E+ separation, minimises the red-cell clumping which may trap non-rosetting lymphocytes which then appear in the E+ fraction.

— Some methods employ more dense Ficoll-hypaque (sg 1.082) but usually the standard lymphocyte separation reagent (sg 1.077) is satisfactory.

— Autologous plasma lyses sheep erythrocytes without damaging the E+ leucocytes. Lysis depends on the presence of naturally occurring heterophile antibodies and, being complement-dependent, requires fresh plasma. We employ the plasma supernatant from the initial mononuclear-cell separation; it is therefore diluted approximately 1:1 (see p. 177). This technique is not applicable to ox erythrocytes or to certain disease states such as chronic lymphocytic leukaemia and some other form of lysis must be employed. We have found Geys solution less damaging to leucocytes than hypotonic lysis with distilled water.

— Antigen detected by rosetting with monoclonal antibodies does not readily cap and shed at 37°C, and antibody may persist at the cell surface for a prolonged period. Therefore, if cells positively enriched by rosetting are to be retested with monoclonal antibodies, potentially persisting antibody must be removed by capping and shedding with polyclonal reagent against the original first-layer antibody.

— Rosetting is highly effective as a method of negatively enriching a given population; the negative population contains very few contaminating positive cells and is not subject to possible functional alteration resulting from exposure to antibody and/or erythrocyte lysing agent. The positive fraction tends to be somewhat less pure and has potentially been modified by exposure to antibody.

Composition of solutions

Geys solution
Solution A

NH$_4$Cl	35.0 g
KCl	1.85 g
Na$_2$HPO$_4$.12H$_2$O	1.5 g
KH$_2$PO$_4$	0.119 g
Glucose	5.0 g
Phenol Red	0.05 g
Gelatin	25.0 g

Make up to 1 litre with distilled water and autoclave to sterilise.

Solution B

MgCl$_2$.6H$_2$O	4.2 g
MgSO$_4$.7H$_2$O	1.4 g
CaCl$_2$	3.4 g

Make up to 1 litre with distilled water and filter sterilise.

Solution C

NaHCO$_3$	22.5 g

Make up to 1 litre with distilled water and filter sterilise.

Working solution: 7 ml of distilled H$_2$O + 2 ml solution A + 0.5 ml solution B + 0.5 ml solution C. Work and stock solutions are stable for many months when stored at +4°C.

IMMUNOENZYMATIC LABELLING OF HAEMATOLOGICAL SAMPLES

Until recently the usual approach to labelling cellular antigens in haematological samples has involved incubating living cells in suspension with a monoclonal antibody, followed by a second incubation with FITC-labelled anti-mouse Ig. The cells are then analysed either by flow cytometry or by fluorescence microscopy.

The technique described here represents a departure from this traditional technology. Its origin lies in two shortcomings of the immunofluorescent procedure which (whilst being of little importance for immunological research laboratories) are particularly evident to the diagnostic haematologist. The first of these is that the haematologist cannot assess immunofluorescently-labelled preparations by conventional light microscopy; and secondly, that immunofluorescent labelling of cell samples has to be performed without delay after their receipt.

The development of immunoenzymatic techniques for staining antigens in cell smears (rather than in cell suspension) preceded the advent of monoclonal antibodies. However, the availability of monoclonal antibodies removed a major obstacle to the wider application of the cell smear staining technique by greatly increasing the number of antigens detectable.

In the technique described here alkaline phosphatase is used to tag the primary monoclonal antibody. It should be noted that staining of cell smears with monoclonal antibodies can also be performed using immunoperoxidase procedures (e.g. the PAP technique), and indeed peroxidase was the label used in the initial stages of developing the cell smear labelling procedure. However, immuno-alkaline phosphatase methods are preferable when staining haematological samples: problems due to endogenous enzyme activity in haemopoietic cells (e.g. myeloperoxidase and eosinophil peroxidase) are avoided; and the red reaction product produced by alkaline phosphatase (see Plate 3) is more easily visualised than the brown product of the immunoperoxidase reaction.

The important characteristics of the APAAP immuno-alkaline phosphatase procedure as described in this chapter are listed below.

Compatibility with conventional microscopy
APAAP-stained cell smears are permanent and are viewed by conventional light microscopy, allowing antigen labelling and cell morphology to be visualised simultaneously. Haematological samples stained by this procedure thus take their place as one further special stain, to be examined by the haematologist alongside conventional Romanowsky stained smears.

Storage of samples
Antigens present in air-dried cell smears survive for long periods (provided the smears are kept frozen). In consequence labelling can be performed at the convenience of the laboratory.

Visualisation of surface and intracellular antigens
When cells are stained in suspension by immunofluorescent techniques, the only antigens which can be detected are those on the cell surface. In contrast, when staining cell smears, antigens within the cell are demonstrated. These include antigenic constituents in both the cell cytoplasm, (such as mu chains in ALL blasts and neutrophil granule proteins and the nucleus, (e.g. terminal transferase).

Number of cells needed
The cell smear technique is particularly suitable for staining small specimens (e.g. heel prick samples) or samples which contain very few cells (e.g. cerebrospinal fluid), from which it may be difficult or impossible to obtain sufficient cells for conventional immunofluorescent labelling.

Detection of rare cells
APAAP training, because of the vivid red labelling of antigen-positive cells and the absence of non-specific background staining, allows cells present at very low frequency (eg less than one in a thousand) to be visualised. This is of potential value in a variety of settings, including the detection of carcinoma cells in bone marrow smears and the demonstration of low numbers of circulating micromegakaryocytes in acute leukaemia and myelodysplasia.

APAAP TECHNIQUE

Principle
The sandwich of reagents used for APAAP immuno-alkaline phosphatase labelling (see Fig. 11.12) comprises a three layer sequence. The primary monoclonal antibody (the reagent responsible for recognising the cellular antigen) is itself recognised by the anti-mouse Ig in the second stage. This latter antibody is added in excess so that only one antigen binding site on the anti-mouse Ig is occupied, leaving a free site available for binding the complexes of alkaline phosphatase and monoclonal anti-alkaline phosphatase (APAAP complexes) which comprise the third stage in the sequence.

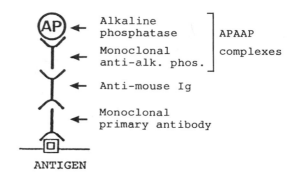

Fig. 11.12 Schematic illustration of the APAAP immuno-alkaline phosphatase labelling technique.

By repeating the linking second stage of the method and the APAAP complex stage, considerable enhancement in the intensity of the reaction can be obtained (see below for details). The result of such additional incubations is shown schematically in Fig. 11.13.

The alkaline phosphatase enzyme reaction is developed using a conventional cytochemical substrate. A variety of colour reactions may be generated by using different diazonium salts, but Fast Red provides an optimal reagent since the vivid red reaction contrasts well with haematoxylin counterstaining and is easily seen in the light microscope.

The APAAP technique is used primarily for detecting antigens which are recognised by monoclonal antibodies (e.g T and B lymphocyte markers, common ALL antigen, etc.) but, by a simple modification, it can also be used to detect antigens recognised by rabbit antisera (e.g. terminal transferase). This is shown schematically in Fig. 11.14.

Test samples

Type of sample to be labelled. APAAP labelling can be performed equally well on either routinely prepared

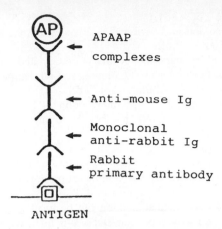

APAAP
complexes

Anti-mouse Ig

Monoclonal
anti-rabbit Ig

Rabbit
primary antibody

ANTIGEN

Fig. 11.13 Schematic representation of the way in which APAAP labelling may be enhanced by repeating two of the incubation steps in the technique. The amount of additional enzyme which binds as a result of this modification of the basic procedure has not been experimentally determined, but in practice the intensity of labelling is strikingly increased and this diagram gives an idea of how the creation of a network of antibodies and enzyme molecules can produce this result.

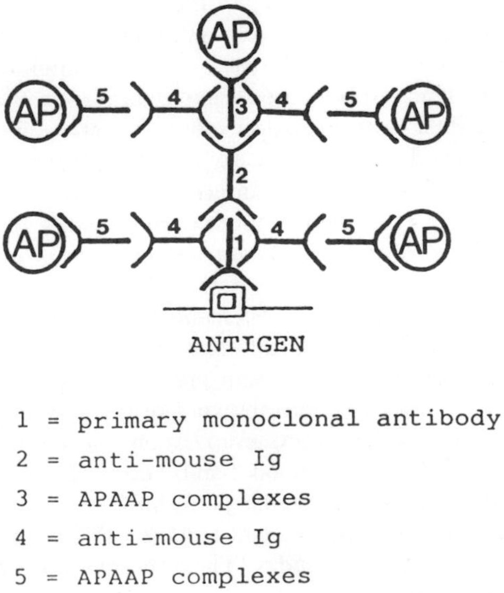

ANTIGEN

1 = primary monoclonal antibody

2 = anti-mouse Ig

3 = APAAP complexes

4 = anti-mouse Ig

5 = APAAP complexes

Fig. 11.14 Schematic illustration of how the APAAP technique may be used to label rabbit antibodies. This modification of the basic procedure (see Fig. 11.12) involves using a monoclonal antibody against rabbit Ig as a second stage reagent.

smears of blood and bone marrow or on cytocentrifuged mononuclear cell preparations. Staining of blood and marrow smears has the advantage that minimal sample preparation is required and cellular morphological detail is optimally preserved. Cytocentrifuged preparations should be used when staining for immunoglobulins and when the blood sample to be studied is leucopenic (or the marrow hypocellular). However the preparation of cytocentrifuged samples is time-consuming and cellular morphology may show some distortion.

Preparation of cell smears. Air-dried smears of blood or bone marrow are prepared by conventional methods, using routine microscope slides. Smears should be thoroughly dried by leaving them on the bench for at least one hour (although drying for longer periods — e.g. up to 48 hours at room temperature — will also give optimal results).

Cytocentrifuged cells (e.g. from cerebrospinal fluid, serous effusions, gradient-isolated mononuclear cells). These should be handled in the same way as blood and bone marrow smears. When staining for surface immunoglobulin (e.g. to show light-chain restriction) cytocentrifuged cells should be used (since they are free of serum immunoglobulin).

Storage. If it is necessary to keep smears for long periods before staining, they should be stored wrapped in aluminium foil at −20°C (although in practice smears kept unfixed at room temperature for as long as a week are satisfactory). When stored frozen, smears are stable for long periods (e.g. at least one year). In order to prevent condensation forming on cold slides, the foil wrapping should be removed only after the slides have been out of the freezer for a few minutes (and have hence warmed to room temperature).

Reagents

Antibodies

Monoclonal antibodies. Antibodies for immunocytochemical typing of haematological samples are obtainable from a variety of sources. Table 11.6 lists commercial reagents which are known to be suitable for typing by the APAAP technique.

Rabbit anti-mouse immunoglobulin, APAAP immune complexes and monoclonal anti-rabbit Ig. These are obtainable from Dakopatts (cat. nos. Z259, D651 and M737 respectively).

Buffers

Tris-buffered saline (TBS). Prepare a stock solution of 0.5 M Tris HCl, pH 7.6. Prepare the working buffer by dilution of the stock solution 1/10 in 0.15 M isotonic saline.

Tris buffer for alkaline phosphatase substrate. Prepare a stock solution of 0.01 M Tris, pH 8.2.

Fixatives

Acetone:methanol

Acetone	1 part
Methanol	1 part

Acetone:methanol:formalin

Acetone	19 parts
Methanol	19 parts
Formaldehyde (40%)	2 parts

Substrate

Naphthol AS-MX phosphate (Sigma, cat. no. N4875)	2 mg
Dimethylformamide	0.2 ml
Tris buffer (pH 8.2)	9.8 ml
Levamisole (1 M)	10 μl
Fast Red TR salt (Sigma, cat. no. F1500)	10 mg

Prepare this solution by dissolving the naphthol AS-MX phosphate in dimethylformamide in a glass tube. Dilute to 10 ml with the pH 8.2 Tris buffer and add levamisole (which blocks endogenous alkaline phosphatase activity). This solution can be stored if necessary at 4°C for several weeks (and for longer at −20°C). Immediately before applying the substrate (i.e. at the completion of the APAAP sandwich — see below) dissolve the Fast Red salt in the substrate solution and filter directly onto the slides.

Equipment

○ Chamber for incubating slides (see Comments section below).
○ Eppendorf (or similar) pipette and disposable pipette tips.
○ Test tubes (for diluting antibodies).
○ Slide racks and tanks (for washing slides).

Method

Fixation

1. Fix smears in acetone:methanol or acetone:methanol:formalin for 90 seconds. When staining cells for common ALL antigen, fixation in acetone (10 min) alone will usually give better results (see Comments section below). Fixation for terminal transferase detection should be for 15 minutes at 4°C in methanol.
2. Transfer directly to TBS. (Do not allow the slides to dry at any stage after fixation.)
3. Leave for 1–5 minutes.

Staining

After fixation and washing, take slides from TBS and remove excess buffer.

1. Add primary monoclonal antibody and incubate in a moist chamber for 30 minutes at room temperature.
2. Wash for 1–2 minutes in TBS.
3. Add anti-mouse immunoglobulin (at 1/25 dilution) and incubate in a moist chamber for 30 minutes at room temperature.
4. Wash for 1–2 minutes in TBS.
5. Add APAAP complex (1/25 dilution) and incubate in a moist chamber for 30 minutes at room temperature.
6. Wash for 1–2 minutes in TBS.

The intensity of final staining can be greatly enhanced at this point by repeating steps 3–6 inclusive. When carrying out this repeat cycle the incubation time for steps 3 and 5 can be reduced to 10 minutes.

7. Add alkaline phosphatase substrate (see above) and incubate for 15–20 minutes at room temperature.
8. Wash in TBS and then tap water. Counterstain with haematoxylin and mount in a suitable aqueous mounting medium (e.g. Apathy's medium).

Comments

Fixation. Fixation of cell smears represents a compromise between, on the one hand, the need to fix sufficiently to preserve cell morphology and, on the other, the necessity to avoid antigen denaturation through excessive fixation. The two acetone:methanol mixtures provide a satisfactory compromise, and the addition of a small amount of formalin improves morphological preservation. However, one antigen (common ALL antigen) tends to be more sensitive to fixation than are other cellular antigens, and fixation in acetone alone for 10 minutes (followed by air drying) yields better results. When staining for cALL antigen, cytocentrifuge preparations are preferable to routine smears since red cells (which tend to lyse in acetone) are only present in small numbers.

Incubation conditions. The chamber in which the slides are incubated with the different immunocytochemical reagents can be of any design provided it supports the slides in a level position (to avoid reagents running off the smear), and prevents evaporation. A suitable tray is available from Raymond Lamb. For small numbers of slides incubation can be performed in Petri dishes containing lengths of orange sticks (or suitable alternatives) to support the slides. The atmosphere should be kept moist by putting a few drops of water or wet filter paper in the chamber.

Dilutions of antibodies. No recommendations are given in this text concerning the optimal dilution at which individual monoclonal antibodies should be used, since this varies from one reagent to another. Laboratories should follow suppliers' recommendations, but also perform preliminary staining with a limited range of dilutions to be certain that staining is of optimal intensity. Note that antibodies supplied in the form of ascitic fluid or purified immunoglobulin can usually be diluted by a greater factor than can supernatant (and are hence usually distributed in smaller volumes). However, it is preferable to perform staining with supernatants (if there is a choice) since this minimises the risk of unwanted staining due to the presence of non-specific mouse immunoglobulin.

Staining with rabbit antisera. This may be performed by first applying the rabbit antiserum (appropriately diluted) in step 1 above. Slides are then washed in TBS (step 2) and incubated with monoclonal anti-rabbit Ig. The APAAP sequence is then completed by performing steps 2 to 8.

Interpretation

Antigen-positive cells are distinguishable by their red reaction product, whereas antigen-negative cells should be completely unstained. Typical examples of the type of labelling which should be obtained on leukaemic samples are shown in Plate 3, and the reactivity in different leukaemias is shown in Table 11.7.

It is advisable, particularly when first establishing the technique in the laboratory, to run positive controls, the labelling reactions of which are already known. It is convenient to make a large batch of smears from one sample and store these frozen for use as positive controls over a period of time. The following samples provide convenient positive controls, although with time additional material (e.g. from cases of leukaemia) is likely to accumulate and may prove valuable.

Normal blood smears. Anti-HLA-DR will label a minor proportion (approximately 15%) of normal lymphocytes (representing B cells) and the majority of blood monocytes. Anti-T-cell reagents will label 75–90% of blood lymphocytes, and antibodies to helper and suppressor T-cells (anti-CD4 and CD8) will label approximately 55 and 30% of blood lymphocytes respectively. Anti-B cell reagents will label approximately 10–25% of normal blood lymphoid cells.

Chronic lymphocytic leukamia. Anti-HLA-DR will label the neoplastic small lymphocytes in the majority of CLL samples since they are usually of B-cell type. B-cell monoclonal antibodies will also usually label CLL smears (although the reaction may be relatively weak). T-cell antibodies, in contrast, will label only occasional cells (representing normal lymphocytes), with the important exception that T1 (CD5) monoclonal antibodies will label the neoplastic lymphoid cells (as well as normal T cells), although this reaction may be weak.

REFERENCES

Immunofluorescence techniques

Bernard A, Boumsell L, Dansset J, Milstein C, Schlossman S F 1984 Leucocyte typing I.Springer-Verlag, Berlin

Caligaris-Cappio F, Janossy G 1985 Surface markers in chronic lymphoid leukaemias of B cell type. Seminars in Hematology 22: 1–12

Caligaris-Cappio F, Bergui L, Tesio L et al 1985 Identification of malignant plasma cell precursors in the bone marrow of multiple myeloma. Journal of Clinical Investigation 76: 1243–1251

Campana D, Janossy G, Bofill M et al 1985 Human B cell development. I. Phenotypic differences of B lymphocytes in the bone marrow and peripheral lymphoid tissue. Journal of Immunology 134: 1524–1530

Campana D, Thompson J S, Amlot P, Brown S, Janossy G. The cytoplasmic expression of CD3 antigens in normal and malignant cells of the T lymphoid lineage. Journal of Immunology 1987; 138: 648–655

Drexler H G Classification of acute myeloid leukaemias — a comparison of FAB and immunophenotyping Leukemia 1987; 697–705

Greaves M F, Janossy G 1978 Patterns of gene expression and the celullar origins of human leukaemias. Biochimica et Biophysica Acta 516:193–230

Greaves M F, Chan L C, Furley A J W, Watt S M, Molgaard H V 1986 Lineage promiscuity in hemopoietic differentiation and leukaemia. Blood 67: 1–11

Janossy G, Bollum F J, Bradstock K F, McMichael A, Rapson N, Greaves M F 1979 Terminal transferase positive human bone marrow cells exhibit the antigenic phenotype of common acute lymphoblastic leukemia. Journal of Immunology 123: 1525–1529

Janossy G, Bollum F J, Bradstock K F, Ashley J 1980 Cellular phenotypes of normal and leukemic hemopoietic cells determined by analysis with selected antibody combinations. Blood 56: 430–441

Kersey J H, Goldman A, Abramson C, Nesbit M, Perry G, Gajl-Peczalska K, LeBien T 1982. Clinical usefulness of monoclonal antibody phenotyping in childhood acute lymphoblastic leukaemia. Lancet ii: 1419–1421

Kohler G, Milstein C 1976 Derivation of specific antibody-producing tissue culture and tumour cell lines by cell fusion. European Journal of Immunology 6: 511–519

Lanier L L, Phillips J H, Warner N L 1986 Monoclonal antibodies to human lymphocytes. In: Beverley P C L (ed) Methods in Hematology. 13. Monoclonal antibodies. Churchill Livingstone, Edinburgh, p 207–221

McMichael A J Ed. Leucocyte Typing III. 1987, Oxford, Oxford University Press.

Reinherz E L, Schlossman S F 1980 Regulation of the immune response. Inducer and suppressor T lymphocyte subsets. New England Journal of Medicine 303: 370–373

Reinherz E L, Haynes B F, Nadler L M, Bernstein I D 1986 Leucocyte typing II. Springer-Verlag, New York

Rosetting techniques

Forbes I J, Zalewski P D, Valente L, Gee D 1982 Two maturation-associated mouse erythrocyte receptors of

human B cells. 1. Identification of four human B-cell
subsets. Clinical and Experimental Immunology
47: 396–404

Irving W L, Youinou P Y, Walker P R, Lydyard P M 1984
Receptors for mouse erythrocytes on human lymphocytes:
technical aspects. Journal of Immunological Methods
69: 137–147

Mills K, Armitage R, Worman C 1983 An indirect rosette
technique for the identification and separation of human
lymphocyte populations by monoclonal antibodies: a
comparison with immunofluorescent methods. Immunology
Letters 6: 241–246

Immunoenzymatic labelling of haematological samples

Cordell J L, Falini B, Erber W N et al 1984
Immunoenzymatic labelling of monoclonal antibodies using
immune complexes of alkaline phosphatase and monoclonal
anti-alkaline phosphatase (APAAP complexes). Journal of
Histochemistry and Cytochemistry 32: 219–229

Erber W N, Mynheer L C, Mason D Y 1986 APAAP
labelling of blood and bone marrow samples for
phenotyping leukaemia. Lancet i: 761–765.

12

Diagnosis of infectious mononucleosis

Infectious mononucleosis is a disease largely of teenagers, presenting with fever, sore throat, swollen tender glands, a skin rash and other features. It can be due to infection with the Epstein-Barr virus (infectious mononucleosis) but the identical clinical picture can be due to the cytomegalovirus or to toxoplasma.

The clinical presentation gives rise to a request for a blood count and for a Paul-Bunnell test. The blood shows a raised lymphocyte count with very characteristic morphology. These aberrant lymphocytes are T cells reacting against virus-containing B lymphocytes.

DETECTION OF THE HETEROPHILE ANTIBODY OF INFECTIOUS MONONUCLEOSIS

Principle
Heterophile antibodies are antibodies that have the ability to react with antigens that are apparently entirely unrelated to those that stimulated antibody production.

Infectious mononucleosis (IM) is characterised by the presence of an IgM heterophile antibody which is distinguished from naturally occurring and other heterophile antibodies by its specific pattern of reactivity: it agglutinates horse and sheep erythrocytes; is absorbed by ox erythrocytes but does not cause their agglutination and it does not react with guinea-pig kidney cells.

IM antibody is now universally detected by various commercial slide tests which either incorporate absorption of other heterophile antibodies with guinea-pig kidney antigen or employ aldehyde-treated horse erythrocytes considered to be specific for the IM antibody (Hoff & Bauer 1965).

Screening test

Test samples
Non-haemolysed serum or plasma free from cells or debris should be used. Samples may be stored at 2° to 8°C for up to three days but must be frozen if prolonged storage is required. Some kits are designed to be used with whole test blood.

Method
Detailed instructions are provided with the various commercial kits and these should be followed. A positive result is indicated by agglutination of the test red cells. It is usual to proceed to confirm a positive screen by carrying out a standard Paul-Bunnell test.

PAUL-BUNNELL TEST

This test confirms a diagnosis of infectious mononucleosis (glandular fever) due to the EB virus and is usually done when a positive screening test for this disorder is obtained.

Principle
Patients with infectious mononucleosis develop a heterophile antibody that agglutinates sheep red blood cells. The antibody is not removed by absorption of the serum with guinea pig kidney but is removed by absorption with ox red blood cells. These steps differentiate the glandular fever antibody from the common Forssman heterophile antibody present in many normal sera and from the antibody that may appear in serum sickness.

Test samples
Serum is used.

Reagents
- *Sheep cells*. 0.4% in isotonic saline. Wash sheep cells in isotonic saline and add 0.04 ml packed cells to 10 ml saline.
- *Guinea pig kidney*. Strip the capsules and perirenal fat from at least two pairs of guinea pig kidneys. Wash the kidneys well in running tap water and macerate them through a fine wire sieve using a pestle. Mix the sieved kidneys with 0.9% saline and autoclave at 15 lb pressure for 20 minutes. Process the autoclaved material through the wire sieve to prepare a fine suspension. Centrifuge to deposit the suspension, discard the supernatant and wash twice

more with normal saline. Add 4 volumes of 0.5% phenol in 0.9% saline to 1 volume of the kidney deposit, centrifuge in a haematocrit tube and estimate the additional amount of 0.5% phenol required to produce a 1 in 6 suspension. Dilute the kidney suspension accordingly. This is used undiluted. It is stored at 4°C and will keep at least a year.

• *Ox red cell suspension.* Ox red blood cells are washed three times in normal saline and a 30% suspension is made. This is autoclaved at 15 lb pressure for 30 minutes. After cooling the autoclaved preparation is strained through muslin and the solid material present estimated by centrifugation in a haematocrit tube. A 20% suspension in normal saline is made. An equal volume of 1% phenol in normal saline is added to give a 10% suspension. This is diluted 5-fold (2% suspension) for use. It is stored at 4°C and will keep for at least a year.

Sheep red blood cells, guinea pig kidney and ox red cell preparations may all be purchased ready for use (for example, from Diagnostic Reagents Ltd).

Equipment
○ 75 × 9 mm glass tubes.
○ 37°C incubator.

Method
1. Inactivate sera at 56°C for 3 minutes.
2. Set out 3 tubes (A, B and C) for each serum being tested.
3. Add 0.25 ml inactivated serum into tubes A, B and C.
4. To tube A add 1.0 ml 0.9% saline.
5. To tube B add 0.75 ml of 0.9% saline and 0.3 ml guinea pig kidney preparation.
6. To tube C add 0.75 ml of 0.9% of saline and 0.25 ml of ox red cell preparation.
7. Leave tubes A, B and C at 4°C overnight, centrifuge at 3000 rpm for 10 minutes and take off supernatant. (= 1 in 5 dilution of original serum).
8. Set out 3 rows of 9 75 × 9 mm tubes, that is, one row for tubes A, B and C. Make serial dilutions in saline using 0.2 ml volumes and discarding 0.2 ml from tube 9. This gives a range of dilution from 1 in 5 in tube 1 to 1 in 1280 in tube 9.
9. Add 0.2 ml of 0.4% sheep cells to all tubes and gently mix. The final dilutions of serum are now from 1 in 10 to 1 in 2560.
10. Incubate at 37°C for 2 hours and read for agglutination macroscopically.

Interpretation
A positive result shows an agglutinin titre greater than 1 in 10 after the serum has been absorbed by guinea pig kidney. A positive screening test may just give agglutination at 1 in 10 but not at a higher titre and is reported as a negative test. A positive result also shows a significant fall in titre in the samples absorbed by ox red cells. The naturally occuring (Forssman) heterophile antibody against sheep cells is removed by adsorption with guinea pig kidney but not by ox cells. By contrast, the antibody that may appear after treatment with serum (serum sickness) is absorbed by both reagents.

The Paul-Bunnell becomes positive during the course of glandular fever and persists in diminishing titre for a few months after the infection. When the Paul-Bunnell test is negative in a patient with a blood picture of 'glandular fever' either cytomegalovirus or toxoplasma is the likely causative agent.

REFERENCES

Barratt A M 1941 The serological diagnosis of glandular fever (infectious mononucleosis). Journal of Hygiene 41: 330–343
Davidsohn I, Stern K, Kashiwagi C 1951 The differential test for infectious mononucleosis. American Journal of Clinical Pathology 21: 1101–1113
Hoff G, Bauer S 1965 A new rapid slide test for infectious mononucleosis. Journal of the American Medical Association 194: 351–353

13

Investigation of paraproteinaemia

Paraproteins, or monoclonal immunoglobulins (Ig), provide the best available serum marker for tumours of the lymphoid system such as myeloma or macroglobulinaemia. They are recognisable in serum as electrophoretically homogeneous Ig, often accompanied by an increase in the concentration of the paraprotein Ig class and depletion of the normal Ig components. More than 75% of patients with myeloma, 100% of patients with macroglobulinaemia and a small number of patients with non-Hodgkin's lymphoma and chronic lymphocytic leukaemia have paraprotein in their serum, arising from a single clone of lymphoid or plasma cells. Occasionally two paraproteins can be found and this occurs in 0.3% of patients with myeloma. Where two paraproteins arise, they may be either the products of the same clone or of two different clones. Abnormal Ig heavy chains without attached light chains are found in serum and urine of the rare patients with μ, γ or α heavy chain disease.

In the majority of cases paraproteins are the products of malignant clonal proliferations, but occasionally patients with a paraprotein may demonstrate a benign state with little or no evidence for disease. Such states have been designated as monoclonal gammopathy of undetermined significance (MGUS) or benign paraproteinaemia. The occurrence of this benign condition is more common among the elderly and in such cases reassessment of the patient at six-month intervals is recommended. An increase in the monoclonal component with depletion of the normal Ig levels is suggestive of malignancy.

In myeloma, macroglobulinaemia and other lymphoid tumours, serial quantitation of the monoclonal Ig can be used to monitor disease progress or response to therapy. In this regard, the use of antibodies to idiotypic determinants on the paraprotein molecule for the specific detection of tumour derived Ig can provide a sensitive monitor of disease (Stevenson et al 1983). The demonstration of idiotypic determinants is the definitive method of establishing the monoclonality of a homogeneous Ig product; however as this approach involves the raising of antiserum for each patient it tends at present to be restricted to the research laboratory.

In normal individuals, Ig production is accompanied by synthesis of an excess of free light chain which can be detected in small amounts in urine from all individuals. These light chains are polyclonal and therefore electrophoretically heterogeneous. In patients with lymphoid tumours the neoplastic clone is also capable of producing either κ or λ free light chain, which is detectable in urine as Bence-Jones (BJ) protein by the classical heat test (where concentrations exceed 4 g/l), or more conventionally by electrophoresis, where it appears as a homogeneous monoclonal band. Monoclonal light chains can be found in 80% of patients with myeloma and 30% of patients with macroglobulinaemia by simple electrophoresis of concentrated urine. In approximately 25% of patients with myeloma, BJ protein may be the only detectable tumour product, while in a small percentage of patients (<2%) a paraprotein or BJ protein may be undetectable. In heavy chain diseases, monoclonal free light chains are sometimes found in the urine from patients with μ chain disease.

Approximately 10% of patients with B-cell chronic lymphocytic leukaemia and non-Hodgkin's lymphoma have monoclonal light chains detectable in concentrated urine by electrophoresis, but this detection rate can be increased to 50% by the application of isoelectric focusing. It is therefore useful to apply this technique where other diagnostic criteria are equivocal.

The appearance of a homogeneous band on electrophoresis (EP) and confirmation by immunoelectrophoresis (IEP) are usually sufficient to identify a monoclonal Ig in serum or urine. Isoelectric focusing (IEF) should be used where these techniques are not sufficiently discriminating or sensitive.

ELECTROPHORESIS

Principle
This is the first step in the examination of serum for the presence of abnormal immunoglobulins. The technique

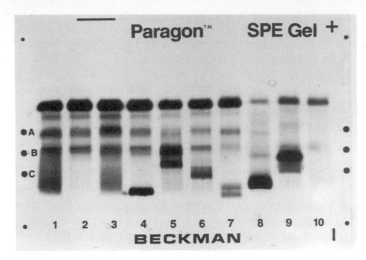

Fig. 13.1 Electrophoresis of serum or urine from patients with various immunological disorders. Serum (lanes 1–7) or concentrated urine (lanes 8–10) was applied at B, and staining was with Paragon Blue. The top anodic band in serum is albumin. The bands of interest extend from B towards the cathode. The disorders illustrated are as follows:
1. Hypergammaglobulinaemia
2. Hypogammaglobulinaemia
3. Normal
4. Myeloma: IgG paraprotein
5. Myeloma: IgM and IgA paraproteins
6. Macroglobulinaemia: IgM paraprotein
7. Myeloma: IgGκ + κ light chains in serum
8. Urinary Bence-Jones protein
9. Urinary Bence-Jones protein + and IgG paraprotein leakage
10. Normal urine

involves the separation of proteins according to their charge. Serum proteins are separated into their constituent entities with the immunoglobulins diffusely located at the cathodal end of the electrophoresis strip (Fig. 13.1).

There are a variety of electrophoresis units employing either cellulose acetate or agarose support media, available commercially such as the Beckman Paragon system. The method adopted by a particular laboratory will ultimately depend on the system available and for this reason the method given is intended as a guide. For those who wish to prepare their own agar support media, the reader is referred to Thompson (1981).

Test samples

1. Serum rather than plasma is preferred, because of the confusing band caused by fibrinogen. Serum should be examined for the presence of a cryoprecipitate and, if present, electrophoresis should be carried out at 37°C. Cryoglobulins are Ig or immune complexes which precipitate at temperatures below 37°C and can be detected by the formation of a precipitate in serum left

for 72 hours at 4°C. Before electrophoresis, serum samples are diluted 1:5 with electrophoresis buffer.

2. CSF and effusions with less than 7 g/l of total protein are not diluted. Specimens must be centrifuged at 720 g for 10 minutes to remove cells before investigation.

3. Urine is filtered before concentrating (× 100) using immersible CX-10 ultrafiltration units (Millipore). A random 20 ml sample or preferably an aliquot of a 24-hour collection is suitable.

Reagents
- Agarose gels (Beckman) or cellulose acetate (Millipore) strips, depending on the system adopted.
- Electrophoresis buffer: buffer pH 8.6 is supplied with the Beckman system. Alternatively barbiturate buffer can be prepared by addition of 15.4 g sodium barbitone and 2.76 g diethylbarbituric acid to 1 l of distilled water.
- Staining solutions:
  Paragon Blue 5 g (Beckman) made up in 1 l 5% acetic acid.

Ponceau S: 2 g Ponceau S, (Gelman Sciences, Inc.,), 30 g trichloroacetic acid made up to 1 l with distilled water.

Coomassie Brilliant Blue R (Sigma) 0.5% in methanol: distilled water: glacial acetic acid (4:4:1).

Silver stain: solution A, 5 g anhydrous sodium carbonate in 100 ml distilled water. Solution B, 0.3 g ammonium nitrate, 0.3 g silver nitrate, 1.5 g tungstosilicic acid, 2.1 ml 37% (w/v) formaldehyde, 150 ml distilled water. 13.5 parts of solution B is added to 6.5 parts of solution A immediately before use.

Method

The Beckman system is used according to the manufacturers' instructions. Basically, the technique of electrophoresis incorporates the following steps:

1. Fill each compartment of the electrophoresis cell with equal volumes of electrophoresis buffer.

2. Load 3–5 μl sample onto the gel with the aid of a template. Ensure that the electrophoresis tracks are correctly numbered on the underside of the gel base.

3. Place gel in electrophoresis cell, connect power supply and electrophorese for 25 minutes at 100 volts.

4. At completion of electrophoresis remove gel and stain. The choice of stain will depend on the sensitivity required (see comments). Paragon Blue staining should be carried out as instructed (Beckman). Alternatively gels can be stained in Ponceau S for 5 seconds and destained in 3 changes of 5% glacial acetic acid, or with Coomassie Brilliant Blue R for 5 minutes followed by destaining in methanol:distilled water:glacial acetic acid (4:4:1). Silver staining must be carried out in thoroughly clean containers; the gels are allowed to stain for 10–15 minutes, transferred to 1% acetic acid for 5 minutes and finally rinsed in distilled water.

5. Dry stained gels in a drying oven at 40°C.

Comments

— All the stains are suitable with agarose gels. Ponceau S and Coomassie Brilliant Blue R are suitable for staining cellulose acetate membranes. Ponceau S and Paragon Blue are satisfactory at detecting homogeneous bands in serum at a concentration of 1 g/l. Sensitivity with Coomassie Blue can be as low as 0.1 g/l and is suitable for staining electrophoretic strips of urine. Bands at a concentration of 0.01 g/l can be detected by the silver stain; this method is suitable for electrophoretograms of urine or CSF.

— Scanning the EP strips with a densitometer will give a semi-quantitative estimate of the serum proteins present.

Interpretation

Figure 13.1 illustrates some examples of electrophoretic patterns found in the laboratory. They include sera and urine from patients with myeloma (lanes 4–9) and sera from patients with immunological disorders giving rise to raised or depleted levels of normal polyclonal Ig (lanes 1 and 2). In normal serum (lane 3), albumin comprises 50–70% of the total protein, while the immunoglobulins comprise 10–18%. Often the position of the paraprotein on the electrophoretic strip is a guide to its Ig type: IgG bands tend to be located towards the cathode while IgM and IgA tend to be more anodic (lanes 4–6). The presence of a paraprotein band in serum from a patient with myeloma is often accompanied by immunoparesis or a reduced level of the normal Ig comparable to that seen in patients with hypogammaglobulinaemia (lanes 4–7 c.f. lane 2).

Misinterpretation of Ig bands on urinary EP strips from patients with myeloma can arise when there is also renal impairment, leading to the leakage of paraprotein into the urine (Fig. 13.1, lane 9): this shows a major anodic band of BJ protein with an IgGk paraprotein located more towards the cathode. Failure of the kidney to clear tumour-derived light chains will occasionally give rise to their detection in serum as well as in urine; this finding is unexpected but will occur where there are high levels of production, possibly combined with renal damage (lane 7). This lane shows two bands, the more anodic being a light chain and the other an IgG paraprotein. These illustrations demonstrate the necessity of further analysis for the identification of bands on EP strips by immunoelectrophoresis or isoelectric focusing.

IMMUNOFIXATION

Principle

The technique of immunofixation applied to agarose or cellulose acetate electrophoresis strips allows rapid identification of a paraprotein and is comparable to immunoelectrophoresis. However problems can be encountered with sera containing immune complexes, which can be misinterpreted as a paraprotein, as there is often an apparent κ light chain predominance on immunofixation.

Reagents

- Cellulose acetate (Celagram, Shandon Southern Instruments).
- Antibodies to Ig heavy and light chains (Dako Immunoglobulins).
- Stains: Ponceau S, Coomassie Brilliant Blue R.

Method

1. Carry out electrophoresis of samples in agarose or cellulose acetate and overlay tracks with strips of cellulose acetate (50 × 20 mm) moistened with the appropriate Ig antiserum.

2. Leave the strip with overlay in a humid chamber for 30 minutes.

3. Remove overlay strip and wash acetate strip in saline with three changes for 1 hour to remove antiserum and unfixed proteins. Agarose strips require the more vigorous washing procedure described for immunoelectrophoresis.

4. Stain and dry.

Comment

Antiserum should be diluted to give optimal immunofixation.

IMMUNOELECTROPHORESIS

Principle

This technique is used for demonstrating monoclonality of Ig components in serum and urine. In principle, it depends on the formation of antibody:antigen precipitates in agarose gel following the separation of serum proteins by electrophoresis, giving rise to lines or 'arcs' of immunoprecipitation characteristic of each serum protein component. Monoclonal Ig components give rise to thickening and distortion of the normal immunoprecipitation arc. In urine monoclonal light chains may give a single arc in the absence of detectable normal Ig components. The method described is for use with agarose gels and the Beckman electrophoresis system.

Test samples

Serum or urine, which on electrophoresis exhibit abnormal banding, should be prepared in a similar manner to that for electrophoresis, with the exception that serum is not diluted.

Reagents

- Agarose M (LKB Instruments).
- Gel bond (FMC Corporation, Marine Colloids Division) and templates (Millipore).
- Barbiturate buffer pH 8.6 as used for electrophoresis.
- Antibodies to Ig heavy and light chains (Dako Immunoglobulins).
- Coomassie Blue stain.

Method

1. Preparation of agarose gels: swell 0.5 g gel in 50 ml of barbiturate buffer for 1 hour and dissolve by gently stirring on a heated magnetic stirrer. Cool to 75°C and pour into moulded templates supplied with preformed agarose gels by Millipore. Cover with a square of gel bond, being careful to eliminate air bubbles and leave to set in a humid chamber at 4°C.

2. Add equal volumes of barbiturate buffer to each compartment of the Beckman electrophoresis cell.

3. Remove gel from template, label appropriately by marking the underside of the gel support and load 1.2 μl of sample into the respective well. Place gel in electrophoresis cell.

4. Connect power supply and electrophorese for 25 minutes at 100 volts.

5. Remove gel and add 45 μl of appropriate antiserum to each trough. Leave the gel in a humid chamber overnight at 4°C.

6. Remove unprecipitated protein by immersing the gel in saline for 4 hours at room temperature. Rinse three times with distilled water and dry between layers of paper towel before staining with Coomassie Brilliant Blue R as described for electrophoresis.

7. Dry the stained gels at 40°C for 15 minutes.

Comments

— Discard damaged or dehydrated plates.
— Do not overload sample well or troughs as this will cause smearing and spurious or multiple precipitation arcs with specific antisera.
— Electrophoretic separation must be adequate otherwise immunoprecipitation arcs will be difficult to interpret.
— Antiserum should be diluted to give immunoprecipitin arcs that are easily interpretable.

Interpretation

This technique is suitable for establishing the identity of a clear band on the electrophoretic strip. By using antibodies to the various heavy and light chains, identification and some estimate of the proportion of abnormal Ig can be made (Fig. 13.2). With serum monoclonal Ig comprising less than 20% of the normal Ig of the same isotype and with urine concentrations of monoclonal light chains less than 0.5 mg/ml, IEP arcs can be very difficult to interpret. In particular, IgM and polymeric IgA paraproteins, which do not diffuse well, can give ambiguous precipitin arcs.

ISOELECTRIC FOCUSING

Principle

Isoelectric focusing (IEF) is more sensitive and discriminating than EP or IEP and should be used where these techniques provide an equivocal result. A pH gradient is established in a polyacrylamide-agarose gel and the protein is allowed to move under the influence of an electric field until it reaches the pH of its isoelectric point where it then carries no net charge and stops moving. By this procedure, normal Ig or light chains, because of their charge heterogeneity, form multiple bands. However, monoclonal Ig form discrete bands at their isoelectric points and can be distinguished readily

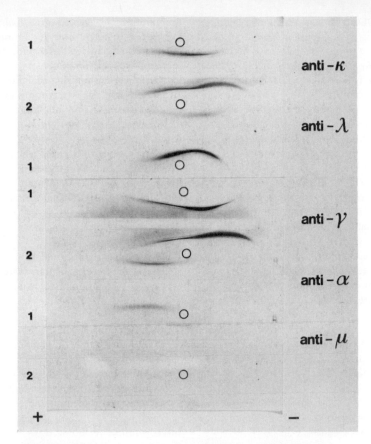

Fig. 13.2 Immunoelectrophoresis of sera from two patients with myeloma. Serum was electophoresed in agarose and the separated components were allowed to interact with antisera as indicated.

Sample 1: an IgGλ paraprotein reacting with anti-λ and anti-γ to give strongly curved arcs; residual normal Ig gives a small reaction with anti-κ anti-α and anti-μ.

Sample 2: an IgGκ paraprotein reacting with anti-κ and anti-γ to give strongly curved arcs; residual normal Ig gives a small reaction with anti-λ and anti-α.

from the background of normal components. A suitable power supply and dedicated electrophoresis bed are essential; many are available commercially such as the Pharmacia FBE-3000 Flatbed unit.

Test samples

Isoelectric focusing can be useful under the following circumstances.

1. Sera containing IgM or IgA paraproteins at concentrations <20% of the same normal Ig isotype.

2. Sera containing high levels of immune complexes which may mask an underlying paraprotein.

3. Sera giving several bands on electrophoresis that are not readily identifiable as monoclonal Ig.

4. Urines which have suspicious faint bands on electrophoresis, often with accompanying proteinuria.

5. CSF for monoclonal or oligoclonal Ig components.

Reagents

- Tris-EDTA buffer 0.02 M, pH 8.0 prepared from 0.2 M stock (2 g sodium azide, 58.4 g sodium chloride, 24.2 g Tris, 3.7 g disodium ethylenediamine-tetra acetic acid, 20 ml 5 N hydrochloric acid made to 1 l with distilled water).
- DTT, Dithiothreitol (British Drug Houses), 6.15 mg/ml in Tris-EDTA buffer.
- IAM, Iodoacetamide (purified for biochemical work, British Drug Houses) 18.3 mg/ml in tris EDTA buffer.
- TEMED, N, N; N^1, N^1-tetraethylmethylenediamine (British Drug Houses).
- Agarose, IEF grade (Pharmacia).
- Ampholines, 40% carrier ampholytes pH 3.5–9.5 (LKB Instruments).
- Gel Bond.

- Acrylamide (British Drug Houses) monomer solution: 20% solution in Tris-EDTA buffer containing 0.2% (v/v) TEMED.
- Ammonium persulphate (Analar, British Drug Houses). Dissolve 0.14% (w/v) in Tris EDTA buffer immediately before use.
- Fixative and Stains: 5% trichloroacetic acid, 3.5% sulphosalicylic acid in methanol:distilled water (1:2). Coomassie Brilliant Blue R or silver stain.

Preparation of test samples

In some circumstances it is necessary to expose serum to reducing agents in order that polymeric IgM and IgA can enter the gel. This is not necessary for urine or CSF samples as these usually contain light chain or IgG respectively. Serum is treated with DTT, a disulphide bond reducing agent and, after reduction, the sulphydryl bonds are alkylated with IAM so that they cannot reoxidise. The method is as follows:

1. 270 μl serum is treated with 30 μl DTT for 1 hour at room temperature.

2. To this solution add 30 μl IAM and incubate at room temperature for 30 minutes.

3. Treated serum can be stored at $-20°C$ if IEF cannot be done immediately.

Method

1. Gel preparation: prepare the polyacrylamide polymer before addition of agarose.

a. Prepare the linear polyacrylamide polymer by mixing equal volumes of acrylamide monomer solution containing TEMED with freshly prepared ammonium persulphate solution. After mixing, the solution is immediately transferred to dialysis tubing and left for 2 hours at room temperature. The viscous solution obtained is then dialysed against 8 changes of distilled water for 48 hours and stored in a dark bottle at room temperature.

b. Add 4 g polyacrylamide preparation and 0.7 g agarose to 76 ml distilled water and place on a heated stirrer until dissolved.

c. Add 4 ml ampholines, mix and pour gel into templates (those made for IEP analysis by Corning are suitable), overlay with Gel Bond and store overnight at 4°C before use.

2. Apply sample (1–8 μl) to the gel and place on a Pharmacia FBE-3000 Flatbed unit (or equivalent), usually with sample wells towards the anode, but reversed for the more acidic IgM and IgA.

3. Apply electrode strips soaked in 0.5 M sodium hydroxide for the cathode or 0.5 M acetic acid for the anode.

4. Gels are run at 10°C for 35 minutes at a constant 7 mA per gel followed by 15 minutes at 1000 v.

5. At completion of focusing, gels can be either immunofixed or treated with fixative and stained with Coomassie Brilliant Blue R. Immunofixation is carried out as described previously with cellulose acetate strips soaked in specific antibody. Antiserum should be tested for the most economical use (most of the antisera can be diluted 1 in 5). After immunofixation for 1 hour in a humid chamber the gels are thoroughly washed with 0.9% saline overnight. Next day, the gels are washed with distilled water (10 min) and squashed between sheets of ashless filter paper using a glass plate with 1 kg weight for 2 minutes; this procedure is repeated twice before drying at 70°C and staining with Coomassie Brilliant Blue R or silver stain, as described for electrophoresis.

Comments

— A standard monoclonal protein is normally run on each gel to check the system. Haemoglobin or protein standards of known isoelectric points obtained from Pharmacia can also be used for this purpose.

— Cryoglobulins usually lose their cold precipitability after reduction with DTT and can be analysed by IEF.

— Immunofixation of gels gives increased sensitivity and discrimination compared with TCA fixation.

— Silver stain is recommended for CSF samples.

Interpretation

Illustrations of the application of this technique are given in Figures 13.3–13.5. In Figure 13.3a the identification of an IgGλ paraprotein is shown. Several bands can be seen with both anti-γ and anti-λ antisera; this is thought to be due to either single charge differences between individual components arising from deaminidation of some glutamine or asparagine residues, or to heterogeneity in the number of sialic acid residues attached to the carbohydrate chains of the IgG. The pattern should be compared with Figure 13.3b which shows the result obtained from normal serum. Many bands and diffuse areas can be seen and there is staining with both anti-κ and anti-λ antisera. Figure 13.3c shows a less clearly defined paraprotein which formed about 30% of the total IgG. The monoclonal IgGκ can be clearly seen. Figure 13.3d shows an interesting serum which contained two paraproteins, both IgGλ of different isoelectric point. Figure 13.4 shows the results of IEF on a serum with a suspected IgM paraprotein. The gel has been run in the opposite direction and there is clear definition of an IgMκ paraprotein. An illustration of the application of IEF to urinary light chain analysis is shown in Figure 13.5 where a κ light chain in the absence of λ or IgG has been demonstrated.

The sensitivity of IEF is high and we can detect as

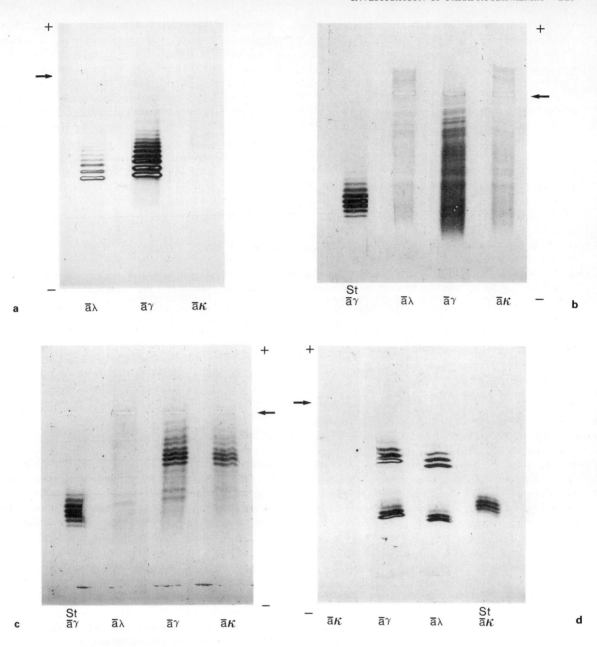

Fig. 13.3 Isoelectric focusing patterns immunofixed and anti-γ, anti-λ and anti-k antibodies as indicated.
a. Isoelectric focusing of serum from a patient with myeloma: identification of an IgGλ paraprotein. Serum
(1 μl), diluted 0.5 mg/ml of IgG, was applied at the arrow to agarose gel and focused. **b.** Isoelectric
focusing of normal human serum. Serum (1 μl), diluted to 0.5 mg/ml of IgG, was applied at the arrow to
agarose gel and focused. A standard IgG (St) paraprotein has been run for comparison. **c.** isoelectric
focusing of serum from a patient with a minor IgGκ paraprotein band. A standard IgG paraprotein was run
for comparison. **d.** Isoelectric focusing of serum from a patient with two paraprotein bands, both IgGλ. A
standard IgGκ paraprotein was run for comparison, and immunofixed with anti-κ.

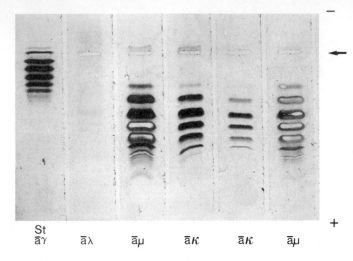

St
āγ   āλ   āμ   āκ   āκ   āμ

Fig. 13.4 Isoelectric focusing of serum from a patient with an IgMκ paraprotein. Serum was reduced and alkylated and diluted to 1 mg/ml of IgM. 1 μl (two central lanes) or 0.5 μl (two right hand lanes) was applied at the arrow. The electric field was applied in the opposite direction to that used for IgG. Detection was by immunofixation using anti-μ, anti-λ and anti-κ. A standard IgG paraprotein was run for comparison.

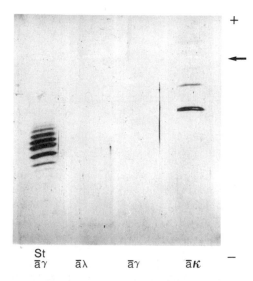

St
āγ   āλ   āγ   āκ

Fig. 13.5 Isoelectric focusing of concentrated (× 100) urine from a patient with a κ Bence-Jones protein. Urine (1 μl) was applied at the arrow, focused and detected by immunofixation using anti-λ, anti-γ and anti-κ. A standard IgG paraprotein was run for comparison.

QUANTITATION OF IMMUNOGLOBULINS

Various procedures exist for quantitation of the major Ig classes (IgG, IgA and IgM) and the choice of method is usually dictated by the degree of automation required in the laboratory. Single radial immunodiffusion (SRID) introduced in 1965 by Mancini, is still popular and is particularly useful for patients with suspected infections such as acquired immunodeficiency syndrome or hepatitis, since it can be carried out in contained facilities. For laboratories handling large numbers of specimens there are a number of automated systems available commercially.

In recent years, immunoassays have become increasingly important for the detection and quantitation of proteins. The use of enzymes rather than radioisotopes has enabled the application of the enzyme-linked immunosorbent assay (ELISA) to the quantitation of proteins at ng levels and can be used for IgD, IgE and light chain determinations.

It is usually not necessary to identify the subclass of a paraprotein except to provide standards for assaying sera of patients with suspected deficiency of a subclass of IgG or IgA. So far, the monoclonal antibodies specific for the individual subclasses of IgG 1 to 4 do not seem to have sufficient affinity for an ELISA technique and they are used in an SRID method.

little as 3 μg/ml of light chain or 10–20 μg/ml of monoclonal Ig against a background of normal Ig. Its main disadvantage is that it is more expensive than IEP (~ 4 times) but in our view this is outweighed by its unique discriminating power. It should of course be reserved for difficult cases such as those described under test samples.

SINGLE RADIAL IMMUNODIFFUSION

Principle

This technique involves the radial diffusion of antigen from sample wells into surrounding agar gel impregnated with antibody. Quantitation is based on the fact that at equivalence point, the square of the diameter of the precipitin ring plotted against known antigen concentrations is a straight line. Measurement of unknown antigen concentration can therefore be determined by reference to this standard relationship.

Test samples

Serum for quantitation of IgG, IgA or IgM, and CSF for quantitation of IgG; the method can be adapted to measure serum IgD or urinary light chains, but the ELISA method is recommended for this purpose.

Reagents

- Barbiturate buffer pH 8.6 as for electrophoresis.
- Agarose (Miles Laboratories).
- Antibodies to IgG, A, M.
- Plastic petri dishes, 9 cm diameter (Nunc).
- Antigen standards which comprise sera containing known concentrations of IgG, A and M.
- Tannic acid (British Drug Houses) 2% in distilled water.

Method

1. Preparation of agar plates: Dissolve 0.5 g agarose in 50 ml of barbiturate buffer by boiling. Cool to 56°C, and to 10 ml of the gel in a universal add appropriate antisera usually of the order 10–50 μl/ml of gel, depending on the antibody titre. After mixing, pour into flat bottomed petri dishes placed on a levelling table. Allow to set, cover and store at 4°C until ready to use. Immediately prior to use, cut 2 mm diameter holes with a gel punch at 1 cm intervals in the gel.

2. Prepare standards by doubling dilution of a commercial serum or normal serum previously assayed for Ig content. Add 3 μl of neat and diluted standards to 4 wells in the appropriate plate.

3. Fill remaining wells on the gel plate with 3 μl of sera to be tested.

4. Place agar gels in a humid chamber at room temperature. IgG and A gels are left for 24 hours. IgM gels are left for 48 hours.

5. Stain gels with 2% tannic acid for 5 minutes, rinse with distilled water.

6. Read the diameter of the precipitin rings over a light box with an eye-piece fitted with a graticule marked in millimetres.

7. Plot the standard curve and read off the unknown sample concentrations.

Comments

— Sample spillages cause irregular precipitin rings.
— Dilutions of test sera with 0.9% saline may be necessary to achieve optimal precipitin rings.

Interpretation

The method is suitable for the assessment of IgG, A and M in serum and IgG in CSF. We do not recommend it for the assessment of IgD or IgE or for the assessment of urinary light chains.

Automated immunoprecipitation

Methods used for automated quantitation include the centrifugal analyser (Anderson 1969) nephelometry (Cloppet et al 1982) or turbidimetry (Ritzmann et al 1981). Several units are available commercially such as the Hyland Disc 120 nephelometer based on the principle of forward light scatter and end point titration. Results with this instrument are comparable with other methods within the National Quality Control Scheme. The disadvantage of the end point method compared with rate nephelometry is that high levels of Ig, which cause antigen excess, may give a false low value resulting from dissolution of the antigen-antibody lattice. If the laboratory carried out serum electrophoresis before quantitation this problem can be avoided by dilution of sera with high levels of monoclonal or polyclonal Ig. The Hyland system is suitable for quantitating IgG, A and M in serum and other body fluids including CSF.

ENZYME-LINKED IMMUNOSORBENT ASSAY

Principle

The method is suitable for measuring proteins in the 0–100 ng/ml range. It is applicable to any antigen for which a specific antibody and its enzyme-linked derivative can be prepared or purchased including serum IgD or IgE with mean values of 30 μg/ml and 0.05 μg/ml respectively, and for urinary κ or λ light chains. It can also be used to measure tumour derived idiotypic Ig.

The general principle is to bind antibody to the wells of a microtitre plate, expose it to antigen which is then 'captured' by the antibody, and detect captured antigen by using either the same antibody (single determinant assay) or an antibody reactive to a different epitope of the antigen (double-determinant assay), each of these detecting antibodies being coupled to an enzyme such as horse radish peroxidase. Bound enzyme is then detected by placing substrate in the wells and developing a chromogenic product. Colour can be read either by eye or by spectrophotometry. If suitable standards are used, the procedure can be made quantitative, and in our hands compares in specificity and sensitivity with radioimmunoassay.

Test samples

Serum, CSF and 24-hour unconcentrated urine specimens.

Reagents

- Coating buffer pH 9.6: 1.59 g sodium carbonate, 2.93 g sodium bicarbonate and 0.2 g sodium azide made up to 1 l with distilled water. Store at 4°C for up to 3 weeks.
- *Wash solution.* Phosphate-buffered saline (PBS), pH 7.3: 7.0 g sodium chloride, 0.79 g potassium dihydrogen phosphate, 3.44 g disodium hydrogen phosphate dissolved in 1 l distilled water with either 1% bovine serum albumin (PBS-BSA) or 0.1% Tween 20 (PBS-Tween) added.
- *Substrate.* Immediately before use dissolve 10 mg ortho-phenylenediamine in 50 ml phosphate-citrate buffer (pH 5.0), (4.68 citric acid, 7.30 g disodium hydrogen phosphate made up to 1 l with distilled water) and add 20 μl of 30% hydrogen peroxide. Stock phosphate-citrate buffer can be stored at 4°C for up to 2 weeks.
- Coating antibodies and horse radish peroxidase-labelled antibodies are available from Dako Immunoglobulins or Serotec.

Preparation of standards and working reagents

Immunoglobulin D. Coating antibody and horse radish peroxidase-labelled antibody can be purchased from Dako Immunoglobulins. Standard IgD should be prepared from an IgD myeloma. IgD in serum is stable at −70°C but should not be stored diluted. Add the plasmin inhibitor 6-amino-n-hexanoic acid (British Drug Houses) at 0.13% to the diluent and wash solution (PBS-Tween) for IgD analysis.

Immunoglobulin E. A good coating antibody is a mouse monoclonal anti-human IgE (MCA 24, Serotec). Horse radish peroxidase-coupled rabbit anti-human IgE is available (Serotec). Results with this assay compared well with the commercially available kits.

Urinary light chains. Rabbit antibody to free light-chain determinants is used as coating antibody, and horse radish peroxidase-labelled rabbit antibody to free and bound light-chain determinants is used for detection (Dako Immunoglobulins). Standards in this laboratory consist of pooled preparations of Bence-Jones proteins of known concentration as measured by the Lowry technique.

Idiotypic Ig. Idiotypic Ig is a tumour specific marker for myeloma, macroglobulinaemia or lymphoma. Polyclonal anti-idiotypic antibody is particularly useful as a capture antibody (Tutt et al 1983). Enzyme-labelled antibody against the heavy chain constant region of the idiotypic Ig (IgG, IgM or IgA) is suitable for detection.

Method

1. The capturing antibody is suitably diluted (1 in 1000 for most commercial antibodies) in coating buffer and 200 μl aliquots are placed in a 96-well microtitre plate (Nunc). A lid is placed over the wells and the plate is incubated for 1 hour at 37°C and overnight at 4°C.

2. Antibody solution is shaken out of the wells and 200 μl aliquots of PBS-BSA are added. After incubating for 1 hour at 37°C, this is shaken out and wells are washed three times with PBS-Tween at room temperature using a Handiwash 110 (Titertek, Flow Laboratories).

3. Antigen is diluted in PBS-Tween to cover the assay range (usually 0–50 ng/ml) and 200 μl aliquots placed in the wells, normally triplicates for each doubling dilution point. Standards and unknown solutions are diluted similarly. After incubation for 1½ hours at 37°C the solutions are shaken off and the wells are washed four times with PBS-Tween.

4. Horse radish peroxidase-labelled antibody is suitably diluted in PBS-Tween (1 in 1000 for most commercial conjugates) and 200 μl aliquots placed in the wells. Incubation is for 1 hour at 37°C, after which the wells are shaken out and washed four times with PBS-Tween.

5. Substrate is freshly prepared and 200 μl aliquots placed in the wells. Incubate in the dark for 30 minutes, visually scanning the wells at intervals. The reaction is stopped by addition of 80 μl aliquots of 2.5 M sulphuric acid, and the colour reaction is read by a spectrophotometer such as the MicroElisa reader MR 580 (Dynatech) at 492 nm.

Comments

- In establishing new ELISA procedures, it is necessary to assess optimal dilutions of the antibody reagents and to work within an assay range which does not exceed an optical density of ~ 1.2 for the most concentrated solutions. Specificity checks should also be included to ensure the accuracy of the claims of the manufacturers.
- The substrate for development of the colour reaction is light sensitive and development must be carried out in the dark.
- Heterophile antibody or rheumatoid factor in serum can recognise the capturing antibody and either bind enzyme-labelled antibody or be recognised by it, leading to spurious results. Tests of patients' sera with high levels of rheumatoid factor should be checked by carrying out the ELISA with control plates coated with normal IgG of the same species and at the same concentration as the capture antibody and substracting any colour developed from the test value.

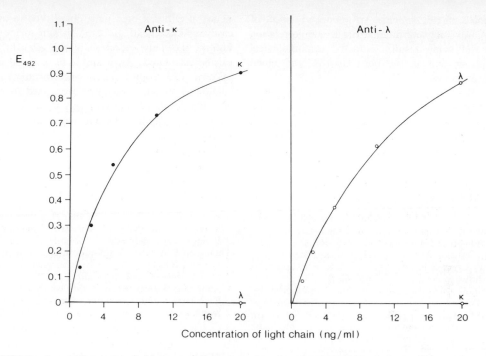

Fig. 13.6 ELISA for the measurement of either κ or λ light chains in urine of patients with myeloma. The coating antibody is anti-free κ or λ which binds κ or λ light chains respectively; detection is with the appropriate horse radish peroxidase-labelled anti-light chain antibody. The clear specificity of the assay is indicated, and urine samples can be assayed without concentration.

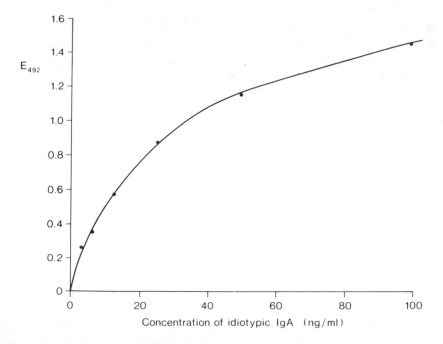

Fig. 13.7 ELISA for the measurement of idiotypic IgA in serum from a patient with an IgA myeloma undergoing intensive chemotherapy. The coating antibody is anti-idiotype which binds the idiotypic IgA; the latter is then detected by horse radish peroxidase labelled anti-α. The response curve with isolated idiotypic IgA is shown and levels in sera can be read off this.

Correlation with cell analysis. An important aspect of the investigation of paraproteinaemia is the correlation of serum and urine results with the immunological investigation of cells in the bone marrow and blood (Stevenson et al 1983).

Interpretation

Examples of response curves obtained for the assay of κ or λ light chains are shown in Figure 13.6. Predomi-nance of either κ or λ light chain type in urine can be easily assessed and, if the 24-hour urine volume is known, the daily excretion of the relevant light chain can be calculated. An example of a response curve for idiotypic IgA from a patient with myeloma is shown in Figure 13.7. This assay has been used to monitor the very low levels of idiotypic IgA which can result after high-dose chemotherapy and which cannot be detected by conventional assays.

REFERENCES

Anderson N G 1969 Analytical techniques for cell fractions XII. A multiple-cuvet rotor for a new microanalytical system. Analytical Biochemistry 28: 545–562

Cloppet H, Francina A, Coquelin H, Bourcard-Maitre Y, Hutinel P, Creyssel R 1982 Laser nephelometry and radial immunodiffusion compared for immunoglobulin quantification in pathological sera. Clinical Chemistry 28: 180–182

Ritzmann S E, Aguanno J J, Ash K O, Wenk R E 1981 An evaluation of the immunoglobulin G, A and M. Methods and calibrators for the duPont ACA. Wilmington: duPont de Nemours

Stevenson G T, Smith J L, Hamblin T J 1983 Immunological investigation of lymphoid neoplasms. Churchill Livingstone, London

Thompson R A 1981 Techniques in clinical immunology, 2nd edn. Blackwell Scientific Publications, London

Tutt A L, Stevenson F K, Smith J L, Stevenson G T 1983 Antibodies against urinary light chain idiotypes as agents for detection and destruction of human neoplastic B lymphocytes. Journal of Immunology, 131: 3058–3063

14

Lymphocyte function

In some immunodeficiency diseases the number of lymphocytes and the relative proportions of the major subsets appear normal. Yet cells from these patients fail to respond normally to a variety of stimuli resulting in an increased susceptibility to infection. This failure of lymphocyte response can be detected in the laboratory and, in addition, such tests of lymphocyte function can point to an underlying disease which may have been unsuspected.

Upon encountering their specific antigen, the relevant T and B cells become stimulated to express a series of so-called activation antigens; these include receptors for growth factors, transferrin, and insulin to enable rapid cell division when the appropriate signals are received. The appropriate signals are provided by factors secreted by T helper (TH) cells: these include T-cell growth factor (interleukin 2; 1L2) and B-cell growth (BCGF) and differentiation (BCDF) factors. Thus after stimulation the relevant populations of cells are prompted to undergo blast transformation followed by division and differentiation, the T cells to develop into mature TH or to cytotoxic or suppressor cells and the B cells into antibody-secreting plasma cells.

Each step in the cascade of events which occurs with antigen stimulation can be measured: factor release, expression of activation antigens, blast transformation, proliferation, helper function, plasma cell numbers, antibody secretion, e.t.c. — and all are relatively simple assays. However, since the cells which respond to a given antigen are in relatively low numbers — for example only about 1 T cell among 10 000 peripheral blood cells responds to influenza virus — less specific forms of stimulation are generally used for clinical studies. For this, polyclonal mitogens are of value. Such mitogens, usually of plant origin such as phytohaemagglutinin (PHA) or pokeweed mitogen (PWM), non-specifically stimulate a large number of clones regardless of their specificity for particular antigens, thus providing a convenient assay for gross deficiencies in lymphocyte responsiveness; with the use of these mitogens and purified subpopulations of lymphocytes, simple assays measuring proliferation or immunoglobulin synthesis and secretion can reveal defects in TH cells or B cells.

The mixed lymphocyte reaction is the proliferative response which takes place when T lymphocytes encounter foreign major histocompatibility antigens (HLA-DR) presented on allogeneic lymphocytes. The mixed lymphocyte cultures (MLC) used to generate the reaction usually employ stimulator cells which are irradiated or treated with mitomycin C to prevent them from proliferating, and responder cells which are able to proliferate: hence these reactions are described as one-way MLC. Because of the nature of the reaction, the MLC causes proliferation of a large number of clones and thus the magnitude of the response is almost equivalent to that induced by non-specific mitogens. Nevertheless the reaction is specifically in response to foreign MHC antigens and the MLC is also used for tissue typing to detect differences in the DR region of potential tissue donors. In addition to the proliferative response, MLC causes the generation of cytotoxic T lymphocytes (CTL) which are specific for class I MHC antigens on the stimulating cells, and this effect also provides a valuable measurement of function.

These responses represent the specific or non-specific activation and differentiation of T or lymphocytes. In addition to these lymphocytes which mediate specific immune responsiveness, about 1 in 50 of circulating blood lymphocytes belongs to the subset known as natural killer (NK) cells. NK cells are essentially defined by the assay which describes their function, that is their ability to kill certain tumour cell targets without prior sensitisation or MHC restriction. Nevertheless these cells can be recognised morphologically as large granular lymphocytes, and they express distinct surface antigens recognised by monoclonal antibodies such as HNK1. It is becoming increasingly recognised that NK cells play a major role in vivo in regulating haematopoiesis and in graft-versus-host reactions, therefore functional assays for NK cells will continue to be of importance in the haematology laboratory.

MIXED LYMPHOCYTE CULTURE (MLC) REACTIONS

Principle

Lymphocytes are induced to proliferate in response to foreign HLA-DR antigens and this response also gives rise to cytotoxic T lymphocytes (see below). The *stimulating* lymphocytes from a pool of normal donors (or from B lymphocytes stimulated with Epstein-Barr virus (EBV) and grown as continuous B lymphoblastoid cell lines) are first irradiated or treated with mitomycin C to prevent them from proliferating. Proliferation of the *responder* lymphocytes is measured by the incorporation of ^{3}H-thymidine (tritiated thymidine; ^{3}H-TdR) into newly-synthesised DNA.

Test samples

Lymphocytes are prepared from 20 ml heparinised peripheral blood (p. 177). Lymphocyte preparations from 10 normal individuals are also required; these can be reconstituted from pooled lymphocytes stored above liquid nitrogen. All lymphocytes are resuspended to 2×10^6 cell/ml in tissue culture medium.

Reagents

- Tissue culture medium: any standard tissue culture medium such as RPMI 1640 or DME can be used. The medium should be supplemented with antibiotics (penicillin and streptomycin) and 10% (v/v) of pooled human AB serum or fetal calf serum inactivated at 56°C, and 2-mercaptoethanol 5×10^{-5} M. The RPMI medium should also be buffered with 20 mM HEPES.
- Tritiated thymidine (^{3}H-TdR): this is normally supplied sterile as 1000 μCi/ml. A stock solution of 100 μCi/ml is prepared by diluting in culture medium and stored at 4°C. Immediately before use dilute 1/2.5 (40 μCi/ml) in medium (this provides 1 μCi/25 μl).
- Scintillation fluid.

Equipment

- Round-bottomed 96-well microtitre tissue culture plates (such as Linbro).
- Sterile plastic 2 ml or 10 ml tubes.
- An automated cell harvester.
- A CO_2 incubator.
- A beta counter.
- Preferably, a laminar flow hood.
- Source of gamma irradiation.

Method

Preparation

Lymphocytes from the test subject and from 10 normal donors are prepared as described under lymphocyte preparation and resuspended to 2×10^6 cells/ml. Equal numbers of cells from each of the normal donors are pooled and the majority frozen down in aliquots for future use (see p. 180).

1. One-half of the pooled normal lymphocytes and one-half of each of the lymphocytes from test subjects are placed in sterile tubes and irradiated with 1500 rad or treated with mitomycin C (25 μg/ml at 37°C for 30 min). After treatment these stimulator cells are washed three times in tissue culture medium and resuspended to 2×10^6 cells/ml.

2. All assays are carried out in triplicate because of variation in the harvesting system. It is also better to avoid the outside wells of the microtitre plates because these are subject to evaporation and fluctuations in pH. Use sterile pipette tips throughout.

3. Into wells B2, B3 and B4 of the microtitre plate add 100 μl of pooled stimulator cells. (These serve as stimulator-alone control.) Depending on the number of subjects under test, add 50 μl of pooled stimulator cells to wells 2, 3 and 4 in rows C, D, E etc. To these wells add 50 μl of test responder lymphocytes, that is test 1 to row C, test 2 to D, test 3 to row E etc.

4. Wells, 5, 6 and 7 serve as responder controls. Thus into B5, B6 and B7 add 100 μl of responder cells from test subject 1, into C5–7 responder cells from subject 2 etc.

5. As a positive control the reverse procedure is carried out, that is, using the non-irradiated (or non mitomycin C-treated) pooled normal lymphocytes as responder cells and the irradiated test subjects lymphocytes as stimulator cells. These are set up in wells 8, 9 and 10 of the appropriate rows.

6. Replace the lid and culture the cells for 6 days in 5% CO_2 in a water-saturated atmosphere.

7. To all the wells of the plate add 25 μl of ^{3}H-TdR.

8. Incubate the plate for a further 4 hours at 37°C.

9. Harvest the assay using multi-harvest apparatus. (^{3}H labelled DNA — will stick to nitrocellulose paper).

To use harvester:

a   Check water level and turn on suction pump.

b. Place nitrocellulose paper, shiny side up, in harvester and harvest each row according to the instructions on the harvester.

c. Before harvesting sample, a blank run should be done to clean harvester and avoid contaminated results from a previous harvest.

10 Place nitrocellulose paper(s) to dry at 50°C overnight.

11. Place dried sample from each well in separate scintillation vials and add 3–4 ml of scintillation fluid.

12. Count samples on beta counter, usually 1 minute per vial.

Interpretation

Results can be expressed as stimulation index (SI): mean cpm in test/mean cpm in unstimulated controls. The SI varies considerably from individual to individual and from day to day, therefore a normal range of values should be established. An SI of <10 should be suspected as being abnormally low.

A positive MLC response provides useful evidence of the ability to recognise and respond to immunological stimuli, and negative responses (against a panel of MHC antigens) indicate gross defects of T-cell function such as in severe combined immunodeficiency disease. In milder defects of immune function such as those found in Hodgkin's disease there may be dissociation between the MLC and PHA responses.

B-CELL FUNCTION

B cells differentiate with T-cell help into immunoglobulin-secreting plasma cells. There are a number of immunodeficiency diseases, from infantile X-linked agammaglobulinaemia without B lymphocytes, through hypogammaglobulinaemia, to deficiencies only in the B cells secreting IgM or IgA. The underlying defect can be among the T helper cells, the B cells themselves, or both. Laboratory tests can readily differentiate the major defective cell type. Two assays are presented in this section. The first detects circulating antibody-secreting B cells by a reverse haemolytic plaque assay: this detects the 30% or so of blood B cells which are presumably activated in vivo and which spontaneously secrete small amounts of immunoglobulin without requiring in vitro stimulation. The second assay depends on the ability of pokeweed mitogen (PWM) to cause resting B cells to differentiate into immunoglobulin-secreting plasma cells in the presence of T helper cells. This latter assay when used with purified T and B cells enables discrimination by TH-cell defects and B-cell maturation defects.

REVERSE HAEMOLYTIC PLAQUE ASSAY

Principle

Ox (or sheep) erythrocytes are coated with protein A and these indicator cells are mixed with lymphocytes. Rabbit antibody against human immunoglobulin is added together with a source of complement. The red cells and lymphocytes form a monolayer in the chamber (or microtitre well) and, upon incubation, some of the B lymphocytes spontaneously secrete (human) immunoglobulin. The secreted immunoglobulin is bound by the rabbit anti-human immunoglobulin, these complexes are then bound by the protein A on the erythrocytes and the complex-bound erythrocytes are lysed by complement. In this way clear areas of lysis (plaques) are formed around the immunoglobulin-secreting B cells.

Test samples

10 ml of peripheral blood. The lymphocytes are separated as described under Lymphocyte Separation.

Reagents

- HEPES-buffered Eagles Medium containing 0.2% bovine serum albumin (HEM/BSA).
- Protein A-coupled erythrocytes prepared as described under Rosetting (p. 208).
- Commercial rabbit anti-human immunoglobulin antibodies. Affinity purified antibodies are best and, if desired, the test can be adapted to identify cells secreting IgM, IgG, IgA etc. by employing the appropriate antiserum.
- Fresh guinea pig serum (as a source of complement): this should be absorbed with sheep erythrocyte and stored in aliquots at −70°C until use. Thaw only once.
- Molten wax.
- Cunningham chambers: these are prepared by thoroughly washing glass slides in detergent and then absolute alcohol. Two slides are then stuck together with double-sided tape as illustrated in Figure 14.1.

Note. If a large number of samples are being tested, the Cunningham chamber technique should be replaced by flat-bottomed microtitre plates: the method is almost the same but the monolayer of erythrocytes and lymphocytes is obtained by centrifuging the cells to the bottom of the wells of the plate rather than between two glass slides. The microtitre plate method is rapid and sensitive but slightly more technically demanding. For further details of this method see Librach & Burns 1983.

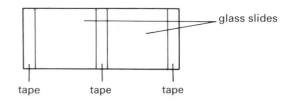

Fig. 14.1 A Cunningham chamber.

Method

1. In preliminary experiments the batches of antibody and guinea pig complement must be titrated to yield the optimum number of plaques. Thereafter these dilutions are used for each assay.

2. Reaction mixture: the following reagents should be mixed together in a small tube.

10 μl of HEM/BSA

100 μl of mononuclear cells (at 1×10^6/ml in HEM/BSA).

20 μl of protein A-RBC (at 25%).

20 μl of rabbit antiserum (at $\log_2$ dilutions 1–20 until tested, then over a narrower, appropriate dilution range).

60 μl of guinea-pig complement (at dilutions 1/5, 1/8, 1/8, 1/10, 1/20 until tested, then at optimal concentration, usually 1/7 or 1/8).

3. Prepare molten wax by heating in a wide-necked container (a convenient wax contains a 1:1 mixture of paraffin wax and petroleum jelly). Do not overheat.

4. Mix the tube containing the reaction mixture then, using a Pasteur pipette, further mix the contents and transfer completely into both sides of a Cunningham chamber. Seal the filled chambers with wax by gently dipping the long edges of the chamber into the wax to a depth of about 2 mm. Incubate the chambers overnight on a flat surface at 37°C.

5. In the morning, count the plaques on both sides of the chamber. This can be done roughly by eye but more accurate results are obtained by using a dissection microscope with the mirror rotated to give a dark background. Express the results as plaques per 10^6 mononuclear cells (i.e. per whole chamber).

Comment

— The main problems which occur with this technique (which is very simple to perform after one or two trials) are:

1. protein-A coupling to the RBC.

2. the wrong concentration of antibody and/or complement.

Interpretation

Normal subjects yield plaque numbers varying between 200 and 700 per 10^6 mononuclear cells. Increased numbers may be seen in some patients with auto-immune diseases such as systemic lupus erythematosus. Very few or no plaques are seen in patients with B-cell immunodeficiencies.

POKEWEED MITOGEN (PWM) STIMULATION

Principle

PWM stimulates both B and T cells. The TH cells provide factors which enable the B cells to differentiate into antibody-secreting plasma cells. This B-cell function can be measured by enumerating the numbers of plasma cells which are generated and by measuring the amount of immunoglobulin secreted. By using separated populations of B and T cells, TH function can also be assessed.

Test samples

For simple B-cell function, 20 ml heparinised peripheral blood; for assessing B- and T-cell function, at least 50 ml of blood from the test subject and from one normal donor is required.

Reagents

● Pokeweed mitogen: depending on the commercial source this is normally used at a final dilution of 1/200 (Gibco) or 10 μg/ml (Grand Island Biological Co.)

● Tissue culture medium: as described above under MLC.

● Reagents for intracytoplasmic staining (see Immunofluorescence Techniques, p. 202).

● Reagents for immunoglobulin quantitation (RIA or ELISA, see p. 227).

Equipment

○ Sterile pipettes and tips.

○ 96-well round-bottomed tissue culture microtitre plates.

Method

If a simple functional assay is required, whole mononuclear-cell populations from the patient are used (p. 177). For this assay ignore steps 1–3 and pass straight to step 4. A slightly more complex assay requires separation of B and T cells.

1 Using the method given in Leucocyte Separation p. 210, isolate separate populations of B and T cells from the test patient and from the normal control subject. Resuspend the B cells to 1×10^6 cells/ml in tissue culture medium and the T cells to 5×10^5, 1×10^6 and 5×10^6 cells/ml in the same medium.

2. Set up assays in duplicate and do not use the outside wells of the microtitre plate. Replace tips between each procedure. Into rows B2 to B7 inclusive and C2 to C7 add 50 μl of patients' B cells. To rows D2 to D7 inclusive and E2 to E7 add 50 μl of normal B cells. In duplicate add 50 μl of patient T cells to the patient B cells in row B as: 5×10^5 into wells 2 and 3; 1×10^6 into wells 3 and 4; and 5×10^6 into wells 6 and 7. Repeat exactly in row E but this time note that the patient's T cells are being added to B cells from the normal subject. Reverse the procedure by adding the normal subject's T cells to the patient's B cells in row C. Add normal T cells to autologous B cells in row D.

3. Set up the controls in rows 8 to 11 as: Row B, wells 8 and 9, 100 μl of patient B cells.

Row B, wells 10 and 11, 100 μl of patient T cells at 5×10^6/ml.

Row D, wells 8 and 9, 100 μl of normal B cells.

Row D, wells 10 and 11, 100 μl of normal T cells at 5×10^6/ml.

4. If separated populations of B and T cells are not being tested; simply plate out, in duplicate, 3 dilutions of patient and normal mononuclear cells at 5×10^5, 1×10^6, 5×10^6 cells/ml as 100 μl per well.

5. To all wells add 100 μl of PWM diluted 1/50 in tissue culture medium.

6. Incubate for 6 days at 37°C in a water-saturated atmosphere of 10% CO_2.

7. Carefully harvest the supernatants from each well and measure the immunoglobulin concentration by RIA or ELISA.

8. Pool the cells from each duplicate culture, check the viability and total cell count with Trypan Blue, then prepare smears or cytocentrifuge preparations.

9. Stain the cell preparations for intracytoplasmic Ig and count the total number of plasma cells for each culture.

Comments

— It is as well particularly if more than one subject is being tested, to draw a plan of the microtitre plate on a sheet of paper (this can then be photocopied to produce multiple copies) then write in the contents of each well before beginning the assay.

— If plasma cells are generated in any of the control cultures, the B- and T-cell separation was not adequate. Monocytes are required in the assay but very few are necessary and unless these have been extensively depleted they need not be reconstituted.

Interpretation

In cases of severe immunodeficiency, no plasma cells and very little immunoglobulin secretion will be seen from the patient's B cells. Among normal subjects the number of plasma cells generated per 10^5 B cells varies considerably. In selective B-cell deficiencies, the patient's B cells will not develop to antibody-producing plasma cells even in the presence of normal T cells; conversely if the patient has a TH defect, no plasma cells will be generated among the normal B cells.

T-CELL FUNCTION

T-cell deficiencies are frequently combined with B-cell deficiencies, but selective inherited T-cell deficiency syndromes occur and there are several forms of (acquired) late-onset deficiencies of T cells. The laboratory tests for T-cell function include proliferative assays in response to MLC and mitogens (and specific antigens), and measurements of mature T-cell function such as the help and suppression of B cells and cytotoxic reactions. The PWM assay for TH cells was given in the preceding section. In this section assays for PHA stimulation and for cytotoxic T lymphocytes (CTL) will be presented.

MITOGENIC RESPONSE TO PHA

Principle

At optimal concentrations PHA can non-specifically activate the great majority of circulating blood T cells, causing their proliferation. As with the MLC, proliferation is conveniently measured by the incorporation of tritiated thymidine (^{3}H-TdR) into the DNA of dividing cells.

Test samples

10 ml heparinised peripheral blood.

Reagents

- Phytohaemagglutinin (PHA): various commercial sources. Reconstitute in distilled water and dilute in medium.
- Tissue culture medium as in the preceding tests.
- ^{3}H-TdR, see under MLC (p. 232).
- 96-well, round-bottomed tissue culture microtitre plates.
- Scintillation fluid.

Equipment

○ 37°C, CO_2 incubator.
○ Laminar flow hood.
○ Automated cell harvester.
○ Beta counter.

Method

Preparation

Prepare mononuclear cells as described in Leucocyte Preparation (p. 177). Resuspend cells to 1×10^6 cells/ml.

Prepare dilutions of PHA in tissue culture medium to 0.25, 0.5, 1 and 2.5%.

1. For each assay, use triplicate cultures in the microtitre wells. One row per test subject.

Add 100 μl cells to each well of the first row (if the whole plate is not being used, i.e. <12 samples it is better to avoid the outer wells, therefore start in row B).

2. To the first 3 wells add 25 μl of medium.

3. To the next 3 wells add 25 μl of 0.25% of PHA.

4. Repeat, in triplicate, for PHA concentrations to 2.5%.

5. Incubate plate for 3 days at 37°C in 10% CO_2 in a water-saturated atmosphere.

6. Harvest the plates on the automated harvester, dry the paper, and count the samples in scintillation fluid as described under MLC above.

Comments

— Different individuals respond better to slightly different concentrations of PHA. Some batches of

PHA may require testing over a wider concentration range but, after testing, each assay should still incorporate 2–3 different concentrations of PHA.

— Some individuals are late responders. If the response is very low the assay should be repeated with a wider range of PHA concentrations and harvested after 3, 4, 5 and 6 days.

Interpretation

If the stimulation index (see MLC) is <10 a T-cell defect should be suspected.

CYTOTOXIC T LYMPHOCYTES

Principle

Cytotoxic T-cell precursors can be sensitised to foreign MHC antigens in MLC. During this response the precursor T cells develop into mature functional cytotoxic T lymphocytes (CTL) with the ability to kill the sensitising cell but not other cells bearing different MHC antigens. The killing assay is most conveniently performed by loading the target cells with ^{51}chromium and then measuring ^{51}Cr released when these target cells are mixed with the sensitised CTL effector cells.

The assay can be divided into four parts. Preparing the effector CTL — essentially a one-way MLC; preparing the target cells — involves a PHA response; labelling the target cells; the final killing assay.

Test samples

10 ml heparinised peripheral blood from the test subject and from one normal donor.

Reagents

As for MLC.
- PHA.
- Tissue culture flasks (small).
- V-bottomed microtitre plates.
- Saponin or other cell lysis reagent such as Zap-Oglobin.
- 100 μCi ^{51}Cr.
- Pipettes and sterile tips.
- Serology tubes.

Equipment

- 37°C incubator.
- Gamma-irradiation source.
- Plate holders to centrifuge microtitre plates.

Preparation

Separate the mononuclear cells from blood over Ficoll-Triosil.

Method

Preparation of CTL effectors

1. Resuspend mononuclear cells from both donors in tissue culture medium to 10×10^6 cells per ml.

2. Set aside an aliquot (about 10^6 cells) of the mononuclear cells from the normal donor (these will be cultured separately). Treat the remaining mononuclear cells from this donor (stimulator cells) with 1500 rad (or with mitomycin C) as described under MLC.

3. Into a sterile flask add 1 ml of cells from the test subject together with 1 ml of irradiated cells from the normal subject and add 8 ml medium (final cell concentration 2×10^6/ml).

4. Incubate the flask for 7 days at 37°C in 10% CO_2. This will generate the CTL effector cells (EC).

5. After 7 days, collect the EC and wash in medium by centrifuging at 1200 rpm. Resuspend vigorously (using vortex mixer) in medium, count the viable cells using Trypan Blue and adjust the viable cell concentration to 2×10^6 cells/ml. (If there are sufficient cells at this stage these cells can be separated over Ficoll-isopaque to remove dead cells).

Preparation of target cells

1. The aliquot of cells set aside in step 2 above is placed in tissue culture in a flask with 10 ml of medium (approximately 1×10^5 cells/ml) and maintained at 37°C for 3 days.

2. To this flask add 0.5% (or 10 μg/ml) of PHA on day 4.

3. On day 7 (when the EC are being harvested) these PHA blasts, or *target* cells (TC) are also collected and washed.

4. The TC are counted, and if the viability is less than 90% these must be centrifuged over Ficoll-Triosil to remove dead cells (which sediment to the bottom).

Labelling of target cells

1. Targets from various flasks are removed and counted.

2. Suspend TC at 2×10^6 cells/ml in tissue culture medium.

3. Add 500 μl of medium containing 100 μCi ^{51}Cr + 500 μl target cells (i.e. 1×10^6 cells).

4. Incubate 90 minutes at 37°C, shaking every 30 minutes.

5. Wash the cells with tissue culture medium by centrifuging for 5 minutes at 1000 rpm. Tip first washing down radioactive sink.

6. Resuspend/wash (×2) at 1000 rpm for 10 minutes with RPMI + 10% FCS, (tipping supernatant down sink). Note: Do not vortex labelled target cells to resuspend. Tap tube lightly between washes. (Targets must be resuspended using Pasteur pipette).

7. Make to 10 ml (i.e. 1×10^5/ml) in tissue culture medium.

Killing assay

1. All assays are performed in triplicate and the killing is measured at different EC:TC ratios.

Add 100 μl of TC into the first 15 wells of a V-bottomed microtitre plate. Note: If several assays are being performed it is advisable to prepare a written template, as for the PWM assay, such as:

	1 2 3	4 5 6	7 8 9	10 11 12
A	Patient 1 E: T = 20:1	Patient 1 E: T = 10:1	Patient 1 E: T = 5:1	Maximum release
B	Minimum release			
C				

2. The effector cells are at 2×10^6 cells/ml. Prepare two doubling dilutions to yield 1×10^6/ml and 5×10^5/ml.

3. To the first 3 wells containing target cells add 100 μl of effector cells at 2×10^6/ml (EC:TC = 20:1).

4. To the next 3 wells of TC add 100 μl of EC at 1×10^6/ml (10:1) and to the next 3 add 100 μl of EC at 5×10^5 (5:1).

5. The next 3 wells are the maximum release, that is the amount of ^{51}Cr available for counting. To these wells add 100 μl of Zap-Oglobin.

6. For the minimum, or spontaneous, release control add 100 μl of tissue culture medium.

7. Prepare a balance plate (which can be re-used many times) by weighing the test plate and then bringing another V-bottomed plate to the same weight by adding water to the wells.

8. Centrifuge the plates at 1000 rpm for 1 minute.

9. Incubate the plates for 3–4 hours at 37°C.

10. Re-centrifuge the plates for 1 minute at 1000 rpm.

11. With a change of pipette tip for each sample, remove 100 μl of medium from each well into a serology tube (or whichever tube fits your gamma counter) taking care not to disturb the pellet.

12. Count each tube for 1 minute on the gamma counter.

Calculation of results

The resulting count from each set of 3 values is meaned. From this is obtained the mean specific lysis (msl) or percentage cytotoxicity from the formula:

$$msl = \frac{\text{Experiment count} - \text{minimum count}}{\text{Maximum count} - \text{minimum count}} \times 100$$

Where the experimental count is the mean count obtained with the patient's effector cells (hence 3 different values, with one for each of the 3 ratios used). the maximum count is the mean count from the Zap-Oglobin-treated target cells, and the minimum count is the mean from the target cells and medium-alone wells.

Comment

— The relationship between the values of percentage cytotoxicity for the 3 different ratios should be approximately linear.

Interpretation

No killing indicates severe T-cell immunodeficiency.

NATURAL KILLER (NK) CELL FUNCTION

There are certain conditions such as Chediak-Higashi syndrome where the patients have a selective defect in NK-cell function, and this function is also reduced in patients with X-linked lymphoproliferative disease and in kidney allograft recipients. However, the variation in NK-cell function among normal subjects means that a single testing is generally of little value. For a given individual the level of NK-cell activity is relatively consistent, and valuable information can be gained by monitoring changes in NK-cell function over a period of time: this may be of particular value in bone marrow recipients where it is thought that NK cells may play a role in graft versus host disease.

Principle

NK cells circulate in the peripheral blood as large granular lymphocytes. These can be isolated separately from T cells and B cells but for simple functional assessment this is unnecessary since whole mononuclear cell preparations contain sufficient numbers of NK cells to kill certain target cells without prior sensitisation, and this is the basis of the test. But the range of target cells susceptable to NK cell-mediated lysis is quite limited, with cells from the erythroleukaemic cell line K562 and from the T-cell line MOLT4 being the most sensitive.

Test samples

10 ml heparinised peripheral blood from the test patient and from the regular standard donor (see below).

Reagent

As for the killing assay for CTL above.
- K562 cells.

Equipment

○ 37°C incubator.

Standard

Blood from a normal healthy subject whose NK-cell level has been frequently tested should be included in every assay.

Method

Preparation of sample

Separate the mononuclear cells from blood over Ficoll-Isopaque.

1. Label the K562 target cells with ^{51}Cr exactly as described for target cell labelling in the CTL section above.

2. Resuspend to 1×10^5 cells/ml.

3. Adjust the washed mononuclear cells to 4×10^6 cells/and prepare a series of doubling dilutions in medium to provide 2×10^6, 1×10^6 and 5×10^5 cells/ml. (These will provide E:T ratios of 40, 20, 10 and 5:1.)

4. Add the labelled target cells to the wells of the V-bottomed plate followed by the effector mononuclear cells and proceed exactly as described for the CTL killing assay described above. Remember the maximum and minimum controls for ^{51}Cr release.

Calculation of results

Calculate the msl values as described above for CTL.

Plot the values of percentage cytotoxicity versus E:T ratio on a linear scale. Keep an individual record for each patient.

Comments

— The assay does vary according to the health of the K562 cells. These should be subcultured regularly to maintain the cells in logarithmic growth and should be free of mycoplasma contamination which can affect the results.

— The blood from the normal subject will serve as control for variations in the assay since individual values remain relatively constant: Donors with high or low activities are useful. Any changes in the patient's NK-cell function are only valid if no changes have taken place in cells from the control subjects. Note, however, that NK-cell activity does increase with colds or influenza.

REFERENCE

Librach C L, Burns G F 1983
Scandinavian Journal of Immunology 17: 171–181

15

Granulocyte function

Neutrophils and monocytes are the 'professional' phagocytic cells of the body's defence system. Reduced numbers or malfunction of these cells are associated with increased susceptibility to infection. If severe enough it manifests itself by frequent, protracted or severe infections, commonly with bacteria or fungi that are often not pathogenic in normal subjects. Unfortunately, seemingly normal individuals also become infected, and thus infection does not necessarily signify a primary neutrophil or monocyte abnormality. It is therefore not always clear which patients to subject to detailed investigation. Generally, anyone whose life is being seriously interfered with by pyogenic infection should be investigated. All such patients should have measurements of serum immunoglobulins and complement, as abnormalities of these systems are at least as common as phagocytic cell dysfunction.

It is obviously unnecessary to perform all the studies described here on each patient. An in-depth investigation is determined by initial screening tests such as serum immunoglobulin concentrations, serum complement (CH50), full blood count, differential leucocyte count and cellular morphology, skin window test (for cell movement), whole blood phagocytosis and killing of *Candida*, and nitroblue tetrazolium slide test (for chronic granulomatous disease).

LOCOMOTION

A mechanism for ensuring the rapid accumulation of phagocytes in vivo at sites of injury and pathogen entry in time to prevent lodgement and multiplication of pathogens, is essential for effective host defence. To arrive at sites of injury and infection, neutrophils must leave blood vessels and traverse extravascular tissues. In vivo, cells are attracted by a mixture of factors, including complement components, other inflammatory mediators and microbiological products. Skin windows offer a convenient and acceptable, and probably the only, means of assessing this complex in vivo response,

and should therefore form part of any comprehensive testing of phagocyte function.

There are many methods of measuring cell movement in vitro, which allow the influence of added factors to be measured. These factors can influence movement in two main ways, by changing the speed of movement independent of direction — chemokinesis — and by changing movement in relation to a concentration gradient of a factor — chemotaxis. Most factors alter both these parameters and most methods fail to distinguish between these functions. It is thus more accurate to refer to stimulated locomotion in relation to these tests than to specify chemotaxis unless this has been measured specifically.

NEUTROPHIL LOCOMOTION IN VITRO: RAFT TECHNIQUE

Principle
Neutrophils are stimulated to move into micropore membranes and the penetration and/or density of infiltration assessed microscopically. The cell suspension is contained in plastic cups which are inverted on strips of membrane resting on a moist pad which can be saturated with chemo-attractant solutions. Plasma is used as the stimulant in routine studies.

Reagents
● Phosphate-buffered saline pH 7.2 (Mercia Brocades).
● Cedarwood oil.

Equipment
○ Filter paper (e.g. Whatman, hardened type).
○ Micropore membranes, 3 μ pore-size (Sartorius).
○ Flat-ended forceps (Millipore).
○ Plastic petri dishes, 9 cm diameter.
○ Plastic caps (LP35, Luckhams).
○ Coverslip mounting fluid (Ralmount, Raymond A. Lamb).

Method

1. Blood is taken into heparin (5 U/ml, preservative-free or standard lithium heparin bottle). It is centrifuged at 250 g for 5 minutes to separate the plasma which is retained for use later. The cells are made back to volume with medium and then neutrophils separated as described on page 177. Cells are made up to a concentration of 2×10^6 per ml and plasma added to a final concentration of 30%.

2. Two layers of filter paper are placed in a petri dish and moistened with medium, pouring off excess fluid.

3. Strips of micropore membrane are placed on the filter paper, taking care to ensure that they moisten evenly. Underlying air bubbles must be stroked away.

4. The plastic caps are filled to the brim with cell suspension (0.25 to 0.3 ml) and inverted onto the membrane and gently tapped to raise any air trapped between the cell suspension and the membrane. Three test and one control sample can be placed on one strip.

5. The petri dish is placed in a moist chamber (e.g. a sandwich box lined with wet tissues) at 37°C for 25 minutes.

6. The caps are removed and the membranes processed as follows:

Rinse with medium;
Fix in 10% formal saline for 2 minutes;
Rinse in tap water;
Stain in Harris Haematoxylin for 5 minutes;
Wash in tap water for 5 minutes and then twice in propanol for 10 minutes;
Soak in xylene until the membrane is glass clear. Propanol treatment should be repeated if clarification is not complete in a few minutes.

7. The stained membranes are then mounted. Xylene or cedarwood oil are used for immediate observation. They enable the coverslip to be removed and examined from the other side. However, these agents evaporate and mounting fluids must be used for permanent preparations.

Interpretation

The distance travelled by the furthest cells is determined — this is known as the leading front method. The microscope is used at a magnification of × 200–400. It is initially focused on the starting surface, which is identified by a layer of well-spread cells, and the micrometer reading of the focusing screw recorded. The field of focus is then moved down through the cell-filled area in the membrane until the furthest two to five cells are in focus. The micrometer reading is again recorded and the distance travelled by the leading front calculated. Three fields are examined in each cell patch (avoiding the edges) and the mean from the three patches calculated. The test results are compared with those from a simultaneously tested control preparation.

Comments

— Placing sets of test and control samples on one strip of membrane facilitates handling and ensures the homogeneity of test conditions.

— Movement in the membranes can be assessed in several ways.

a. The leading front has been described above.

b. The number of cells in focus at 10 μ steps through the membrane can be counted. This gives a better overall picture of movement by the population as a whole but is more laborious.

c. The number of cells passing beyond a given depth of filter may be counted. In essence this resembles the original method of counting numbers of cells on the far surface.

— Unseparated blood can be used. This is particularly useful when the volume of the blood sample must be restricted, for example when testing infants. The technique is as described above, with the following modifications:

Blood is diluted with an equal volume of medium.
The incubation time is increased to 2 hours.
The membranes must be washed extensively to remove erythrocytes.

— The above method uses plasma to stimulate movement. This can be replaced by any solution under investigation.

— The absolute results of cell function studies vary from day to day, irrespective of the expertise and care with which the tests are performed. Therefore, the function of the patient's cells is assessed in comparison with that of a normal control tested simultaneously as well as of a set of normal values.

The conditions described give leading fronts of 50–100 μ. Although standard statistical tests can be used to compare patient and control, a clinically significant abnormality is unlikely if the difference between patient and control is less than 30%.

— The same technique can be used to measure monocyte locomotion by means of the following modifications:

a. A suspension of monocytes is purified as described on page 178 and adjusted to a density of 5×10^6 per ml in 33% plasma.

b. The pore size of the membrane is 8 μ or more.

c. The incubation time is increased to 90 minutes.

d. Staining: monocytes are identified by staining for non-specific esterase.

NEUTROPHIL LOCOMOTION IN VIVO: SKIN WINDOW TECHNIQUE

Principle
The skin is abraded down to the dermis without causing bleeding. A micropore membrane is applied to this abrasion and the inflammatory mediators released by the trauma induce neutrophils and monocytes to emigrate from dermal capillaries into the membrane. Examination of a series of membranes applied for different times over 5 to 6 hours demonstrates the types, numbers and locomotory activity of emigrant cells.

Equipment
In addition to those items listed in the previous section:
○ Dental stone, pear-shaped, maximum cross-section 50 mm (e.g. Meisinger type 677, Cottrells Dental Supplies).
○ Electric drill — variable speed, slow running, hand held.
○ Micropore membranes — 8 μ pore size (Sartorius). Large sheets can be cut to size.
○ Dialysis membrane.
○ Moisture-proof film. (e.g. Nescofilm, Clingfilm, etc.).
○ Micropore surgical tape (Medical Products Division. (3M).
○ Tubular support bandage — Tubigrip.
○ Diff-Quick haematological stain (Merz Dade).

Method
1. The subject's arm is held so as to tighten the skin on the flexor surface which is gently wiped with spirit and then with sterile saline (vigorous rubbing will affect the subsequent response).
2. The rounded surface of a pear-shaped dental stone, mounted in a variable speed drill, is applied to an area about 5 to 7 mm in diameter of the skin for periods of a few seconds at a time until red specks can be seen through a magnifying glass. This state is reached before any bleeding is visible, though glistening at the surface may be seen.
3. The abrasion is covered in succession with:
A piece of membrane moistened with sterile saline.
Dialysis membrane pre-wetted with saline.
A pad of saline-moistened filter paper.
A square of moisture-proof film, overlapping the above. These are secured with adhesive plaster and a sleeve of tubular support bandage.
4. Successive filters and dialysis membranes are left on for 4 hours and 20 and 60 minutes.
5. At the end of the test, the abrasions are left uncovered, except in some severely immunodeficient patients in whom antimicrobial powder and a dressing may be used.
6. The micropore membranes are fixed in 10% formol saline for 2 minutes and then kept in water until stained. The 4-hour and 60-minute micropore membranes are treated by the non-specific esterase technique and the 20-minute micropore membrane is stained with Haematoxylin. The dialysis membranes are stained by Diff-Quick (10 seconds in the fixative, 10 seconds in solution 1, and 20 seconds in solution 2). The membranes are cleared and mounted as described above. Dialysis membranes are mounted in water.

Interpretation

4-hour membranes
These are in place while the response is getting going. In normals the micropore membrane should be fully infiltrated with neutrophils, which may have travelled right through to form a carpet of cells on the distal dialysis membrane. Monocytes (NSE-positive cells) should be scattered throughout the micropore membrane, and a few may be morphologically detectable on the dialysis membrane.

20-minute membranes
These are used to test the rate of neutrophil migration which is assessed by the leading front method. Normal values are 50–90 μ and there will be an even infiltration of membrane overlying areas of emigration.

60-minute membranes
These are to measure the monocyte response. This is never as florid as that of neutrophils, hence leading cell distances rather than leading fronts may be measured. Normal values are 25–50 μ.

Comments
— This is a painless and reproducible technique.
— All materials except the moisture-proof film can be autoclaved and the latter can be sterilised with propanol.
— Cells which have adhered to dialysis membrane can be tested further:
   a. For reduction of NBT (see below).
   b. For phagocytosis and killing of opsonised *Candida* (see below, p. 242), but staining has to be performed with Diff-Quick, since May Grunwald-Giemsa does not seem to give a clear result with dialysis membrane.
   c. Fixed in acetone and stained for phenotypic markers by the APAAP method (p. 212).

PHAGOCYTOSIS AND KILLING

Neutrophils ingest particles or aggregates provided they are coated with IgG, complement components, fibronectin, etc. — generally referred to as opsonins. Receptors on the plasma membrane of neutrophils interact with the coated particles and phagocytosis takes place. Live organisms such as yeasts or bacteria are then killed and digested. The opsonising capacity of plasma and the different cellular functions (phagocytosis, killing and digestion) can be impaired independently, and the various tests assess one or more of these processes.

PHAGOCYTOSIS AND KILLING USING UNSEPARATED BLOOD

Principle

Live yeast cells are added to diluted whole blood and incubated while being mixed. Slide preparations are stained and examined by light microscopy for particles that have become associated with leucocytes and for intracellular particles demonstrating alterations in staining indicative of killing. Autologous plasma supplies the required opsonin, as *Candida* fixes complement by the alternative pathway. Blood may be washed and resuspended in another plasma to differentiate cellular and humoral defects.

Reagents

- Yeast-maltose broth (Difco): dissolve 21 g in 1000 ml of distilled water. Autoclave at 15 lb/in² for 15 minutes and aliquot 10 ml volumes aseptically.
- *Candida guilliermondiae* culture.
- Medium — e.g. Hanks balanced salt solution, HEPES-buffered (avoid bicarbonate-buffered medium as it changes pH rapidly on exposure to air).

Equipment

○ LP3 tubes and LP/35 caps (Luckham Ltd.).
○ Rotating (end-over-end) blood mixer (Matburn or similar style, Gallenkamp).
○ Cytocentrifuge (Cytospin, Shandon Ltd.).

Method

1. Yeast-maltose broth (10 ml) is inoculated with *Candida guillermondiae*, incubated overnight at 37°C, centrifuged, and resuspended in medium.
2. Blood is taken into heparin (5 U/ml or lithium heparin tube). Total and differential WBC counts are performed. Blood is diluted with an equal volume of medium.
3. The diluted blood (0.25 ml) is placed in duplicate tubes and the *Candida* added (in 50 μl of medium, diluted to give 2 *Candida*/neutrophil).

4. Tubes are incubated on an end-over-end blood mixer for 60 minutes at 37°C.
5. The tubes are mixed with a vortex mixer and 15 μl added to 1 ml of medium. Cytocentrifuge preparations are made of these mixtures using 0.1 ml per cup and spinning at 60 rpm for 10 minutes.
6. Slides are stained with May-Grunwald-Giemsa and observed by light microscopy (at × 1000).

Interpretation

Live *Candida* appear as homogeneously stained cigars. The appearance of dead *Candida* varies considerably from swollen, balloon-like objects to small shrivelled structures, which stain irregularly or poorly.

The following parameters can be determined:
1. Mean number of *Candida* associated with each neutrophil.
2. Full frequency distribution of association of *Candida* and cells, i.e. numbers of cells with 0, 1, 2, 3, 4, etc. associated particles.
3. Proportion of cells containing one or more *Candida*.
4. Proportion of cell-associated *Candida* staining as dead.
5. Mean number of dead *Candida* per cell.
6. Number of dead *Candida* per cell as a function of the total number in a cell (i.e. is the proportion of ingested *Candida* which a cell kills affected by the total number it has ingested?).

1, 3 and 4 are used for most routine testing.
  Sample normal values for these parameters are:
  1. 1.5
  3. 80%
  4. 50 to 70%
Every laboratory must establish its own range of expected results. Results are usually expressed in comparison with those of simultaneously tested normal controls.

Comment

Candida guilliermondiae is used because it is non-pathogenic, manifests post-killing degradation by particularly clear alterations in staining, and remains in the convenient yeast form when incubated with plasma (El-Maalem & Fletcher 1976). However, other species can be used, including the clinically significant *C. albicans*.

PHAGOCYTOSIS AND KILLING USING PURIFIED GRANULOCYTES

All phagocytosis and killing experiments are performed in a chamber that is rapidly stirred (to provide the greatest possible frequency of collisions between cells and particles) and maintained at a temperature of 37°C. By using the chamber of an oxygen electrode, oxygen consumption and phagocytosis by the cells can be measured simultaneously. After 2–3 minutes in the chamber for temperature equilibration, an aliquot of the test particles (latex, oil droplets, heat-killed or live *S. aureus*) is added. Aliquots of the mixture are then removed at timed intervals for analysis.

PHAGOCYTOSIS OF LATEX PARTICLES

Principle (Segal & Jones 1979)
This technique involves the microscopic examination of neutrophils to visualise the ingestion of opsonised polystyrene particles. It gives no indication of killing, and does not clearly differentiate engulfed from adherent particles.

Reagents
- A suspension of granulocytes, prepared as described earlier, p. 177.
- Polystyrene beads, 0.8 μ diameter (Difco).
- Tricine-NaOH buffer, 100 mM (pH 8.5).
- Human immunoglobulin (150 mg protein/ml, Blood Products Laboratory).
- Saline.
- Saline containing N-ethylmaleimide (1 mM).

Equipment
- Microcentrifuge.
- Microcentrifuge tubes (1.5 ml).
- Oxygen electrode (Clark type, Rank Bros.), provided with a thermostat-controlled chamber.
- Microscope.

Method

Opsonisation of latex particles.
1. Resuspend 10^{10} polystyrene beads (1 ml of the Difco suspension) in 2 ml of the tricine-NaOH buffer containing human immunoglobulin (50 mg).
2. Incubate at 37°C for 15 minutes.
3. Dilute with 1 ml of saline and centrifuge for 5 minutes at 10 000 g, in a microcentrifuge.
4. Wash the pellet twice by resuspension in 2 ml saline and centrifugation.
5. Resuspend the opsonised latex particles in 1 ml of saline and store at 4°C.

Phagocytosis
1. Place an aliquot of the granulocyte suspension (1 ml, containing 0.1–1.0 $\times$ 10^8 cells) in the chamber at 37°C, with rapid stirring.
2. Add opsonised latex in a particle/phagocyte ratio of 20:1.

3. Take samples (0.1 ml) at variable times between 30 seconds and 5 minutes, pour into 0.1 ml of saline containing N-ethylmaleimide and count the number of cell-associated particles by direct microscopy ($\times$ 1000, with condenser depressed).

Interpretation
Compare, as a function of time, the number of particles ingested by a range of normal (control) and test cells. It is more important to assess the rate of ingestion than the total number of particles ingested after a long period.

PHAGOCYTOSIS OF OIL DROPLETS

Principle
The ingestion of paraffin oil particles containing Red O is measured by extraction of the associated dye, which is quantitated spectroscopically.

Reagents
- Oil Red O dye.
- Paraffin oil (heavy, colourless, 0.86–0.89 g/ml, BDH).
- RPMI 1640 medium.
- Human immunoglobulin (150 mg protein/ml, Blood Products Laboratory).
- Saline containing N-ethylmaleimide (1 mM) and heparin (5 U/ml).
- Dioxan.

Equipment
- Mortar and pestle.
- Bench centrifuge.
- Medium speed centrifuge (20 000 rpm).
- Sonicator.
- Glass conical tubes (10–15 ml).
- Spectrophotometer.
- Oxygen electrode (Clark type, Rank Bros.), provided with a thermostat-controlled chamber.

Method
Preparation of Red O-oil particles:
1. Homogenise Red-O (2 g) and paraffin oil (50 ml) with a mortar and pestle.
2. Centrifuge at 20 000 g for 15 minutes, at room temperature.
3. Decant the red oil supernatant (Red O-paraffin) and store (it can be stored indefinitely).
4. Mix 1 ml of Red O-paraffin with 3 ml of RPMI 1640 medium containing 80 mg human immunoglobulin and sonicate for 90 seconds. This is the particle suspension to use for ingestion.

Phagocytosis

1. Add Red O-paraffin particle suspension (0.4 ml) to 5 ml of the cell suspension (0.5–1.0 × 10^8 per ml) in the chamber, with rapid stirring.

2. Take aliquots (1 ml) immediately (time 0) and at 30, 60, 120 and 240 seconds into ice-cold saline (9 ml) containing N-ethylmaleimide and heparin, to stop phago-cytosis, and leave on ice until step 3.

3. Centrifuge at 250 g for 5 minutes, at 4°C, and discard the red oil phase at the top of the tube together with the rest of the supernatant.

4. Wash the pellets twice by centrifugation as in 3 and resuspension in 5 ml of cold saline containing N-ethylmaleimide and heparin.

5. Resuspend the pellets in 2 ml of dioxan and leave 1 hour at room temperature.

6. Centrifuge at 250 g for 10 minutes, separate the supernatants and measure their optical density at 525 nm.

Calculations

A plot of the optical density (OD) as a function of incubation time gives the uptake at any time. The linear part of the curve allows the calculation of the rate of phagocytosis. A typical figure for the maximum uptake is 0.3 OD units per 10^8 cells and for the ingestion rate, 0.25 OD units/min/10^8 cells.

Interpretation

Compare the rates of ingestion of a range of normal (control) cells and the cells under investigation.

PHAGOCYTOSIS AND KILLING OF STAPHYLOCOCCUS AUREUS

Methods for phagocytosis and killing will be described separately. Both methodologies require the preparation of suitable suspensions of *S. aureus*; this will be dealt with first.

PREPARATION OF S. AUREUS FOR PHAGOCYTOSIS AND KILLING

Reagents

- *Staphylococcus aureus* (colonies on agar).
- Nutrient broth No. 2 (Oxoid).
- D-[6-^{3}H] glucose (Amersham International).
- Blood agar plates.
- Tricine-NaOH buffer, 100 mM (pH 8.5).
- Human immunoglobulin (150 mg protein/ml, Blood Products Laboratory).
- Saline.

Equipment

- ○ Magnetic stirrer and bar.
- ○ Syringes (5 ml).
- ○ Needles (21 G × 1.5).
- ○ Haemacytometer.

Methods

Culture and radiolabelling

1. *S. aureus* (Oxford strain NCTC 6571) are cultured overnight in nutrient broth (250 ml) containing radio-active glucose (1 μCi of [^{3}H] glucose/ml), at 37°C, with magnetic stirring.

2. Harvest by centrifugation at 1000 g for 15 minutes, at 10°C. Discard the supernatants.

3. Resuspend, combine and wash twice the bacterial pellets by resuspension in saline (50 ml) and centrifugation as in 2.

4. Resuspend the bacteria in saline, count and adjust concentration to about 10^{11}/ml. The concentration of bacteria is measured by placing dilutions of the suspension in a haemacytometer, allowing them to settle for 5 minutes before counting.

This suspension (live bacteria) will be either opsonised and used for phagocytosis and killing assays, or heat treated first (dead bacteria) and then opsonised for phagocytosis and digestion assays.

Heat treatment

1. Place an *S. aureus* suspension (step 4 above) in a boiling water-bath, for 20 minutes. Cool on ice.

2. Centrifuge at 1000 g for 15 minutes and resuspend the pellet in the original volume of saline. Count as in 4 above.

Opsonisation

1. Mix 1 ml of a suspension of *S. aureus* in saline (10^{11}/ml) with 1 ml of 100 mM tricine-NaOH buffer (pH 8.5) containing 30 mg human immunoglobulin, incubate at 37°C for 15 minutes and cool on ice.

2. Dilute with one volume of cold saline and centrifuge at 1000 g for 15 minutes.

3. Wash the pellet of bacteria by resuspension with saline (5 ml) and centrifugation as in 2.

4. Resuspend with 1 ml of saline and count as described above.

Live *S. aureus* may be stored for a week at 4°C or aliquoted out and stored at −20°C. Heat-killed *S. aureus* may be stored for 1–2 months at 4°C or aliquoted out and stored at −20°C.

PHAGOCYTOSIS OF S. AUREUS

Principle

The uptake (phagocytosis) of radiolabelled *S. aureus* is

determined by using an enzyme that differentially lyses extracellular bacteria, solubilising their radioactivity that can then be separated from the cells containing the ingested bacteria.

Reagents
- Radiolabelled bacteria, prepared and opsonised as described in the preceding section.
- RPMI 1640 medium containing N-ethylmaleimide (1 mM) and lysostaphin (0.1 mg/ml).
- RPMI 1640 medium.
- Sodium hydroxide (10 N).
- Scintillation fluid for radioactivity counting (Aquasol, NEN).

Equipment
- Incubation chamber (oxygen electrode), magnetically stirred.
- Microcentrifuge.
- Microcentrifuge tubes (1.5 ml).
- Vial inserts (5 ml).
- Glass scintillation vials.
- Beta radioactivity counter.

Method
1. Place 1 ml of a suspension of granulocytes ($0.5–1.0 \times 10^8$ per ml) in the incubation chamber. Leave 2–3 minutes, stirring.

2. Add an aliquot of the radiolabelled bacteria (10–20 μl, 10^{11}/ml). Take aliquots (50 μl) at various times (0, 0.5, 1, 2 and 4 minutes).

3. Pour each 50 μl aliquot into a microcentrifuge tube containing 0.5 ml of ice-cold RPMI with N-ethylmaleimide and lysostaphin and keep on ice until the lytic incubation (step 5).

4. Pipette 10 μl of the *S. aureus* suspension used into a microcentrifuge tube containing 0.55 ml of RPMI medium with N-ethylmaleimide and lysostaphin. This will be the control of efficiency of lysostaphin action. Keep on ice until step 5.

5. Incubate the microcentrifuge tubes from steps 3 and 4 at 37°C, for 30 minutes.

6. Centrifuge at 10 000 g for 3 minutes in a microcentrifuge.

7. Aspirate and transfer the supernatants to scintillation vial inserts. Add 50 μl of 10N NaOH.

8. Place 50 μl of the incubation mixture remaining from step 2 into a vial insert containing 0.5 ml of RPMI medium and 50 μl of 10N NaOH.

9. Place 10 μl of the suspension of radiolabelled bacteria used into a vial insert containing 0.5 ml of RPMI medium and 50 μl of 10N NaOH.

10. Add 4 ml of scintillation fluid to the vial inserts from steps 7, 8 and 9 and count in a β-radioactivity counter.

Calculation
The control incubation (step 4) containing only free *S. aureus* will give the efficiency (E) of lysostaphin action. The percentage of phagocytosis is calculated as follows:

$$E \text{ (usually 0.8–0.9)} = \frac{\text{CPM control supernatant (from step 4)}}{\text{CPM 10 } \mu\text{l bacterial suspension (step 9)}}$$

$$\% \text{ Phagocytosis} = 100 - \frac{100 \times \text{CPM supernatant (step 7)}}{E \times \text{CPM 50 } \mu\text{l incubation mixture (step 8)}}$$

The average number of ingested bacteria per neutrophil can also be calculated by knowing the number of radioactivity counts per bacterium and the number of cells.

Interpretation
Normal phagocytosis of adequately opsonised *S. aureus* reaches 80–90% in 4 minutes.

KILLING OF S. AUREUS

Principle
Killing is measured as the number of bacteria that survive intra- and extra-cellularly after incubation with the phagocytic cells as determined by growth of colonies on agar.

Reagents
- Bacterial suspension (non-radiolabelled microorganisms can be used, but these do not allow the simultaneous measurement of phagocytosis as described in the preceding section).
- Blood agar plates.

Equipment
- Incubation chamber (oxygen electrode), magnetically stirred.
- Colony counter.
- Vortex type mixer.
- Incubator (37°C).

Method
1. As for phagocytosis above.

2. As for phagocytosis above.

3. Pour each 50 μl aliquot into a tube containing 10 ml of ice-cold water and shake well. Leave for 1 hour on ice.

4. Vortex the tubes thoroughly and make dilutions (1:100, 1:500, 1:2500) from each.

5. Spread 100 μl from each dilution onto blood agar plates, in triplicate. Invert and incubate them at 37°C for 24–36 hours.

6. Count the number of colonies on the plates, either using a colony counter or by eye, dividing the plate in 4 sectors.

Calculation

The average number of colonies in the plates from the 0 time aliquot multiplied by the corresponding dilutions is used as the 0% killing reference value (RV). Hence, the percentage of killing can be calculated as follows:

% Killing =

$$= 100 \times \left(\frac{RV - \text{Av. number of colonies on plate} \times \text{dilution}}{RV} \right)$$

Interpretation

80–90% killing is achieved in 4 minutes by normal cells, provided the incubation mixture is rapidly stirred. This could be decreased to about 50% in some patients (e.g. chronic granulomatous disease).

Comments

— The proportion of bacteria killed depends on the incubation conditions and the ratio of organisms to phagocytes. It is therefore important to standardise the procedure and to run controls with phagocytes from a normal individual on every occasion.

— Killing can be measured with non-radiolabelled opsonised *S. aureus*. Decreased killing could be due either to impaired killing or diminished phagocytosis, in which event the latter must be measured independently.

— Bacterial clumps appear as a single colony on the agar plates. It is thus essential to ensure that the organisms are resuspended as homogeneously as possible before and after incubation with the cells.

DEGRANULATION

Principle

After an object has been engulfed by phagocytic cells the cytoplasmic granules release their contents into the phagocytic vacuole. Degranulation can be measured by incubating the cells with opsonised particles in the presence of cytochalasin B to inhibit microfilament function and hence phagocytosis. In these circumstances the granule contents are released onto the non-ingested particles to which the cells are attached, and, owing to the absence of phagocytosis, are found in the incubation medium. The latter is separated from the cells by centrifugation, and the granule components are subsequently measured in both supernatant (release products) and pellet (intracellular, i.e. non-degranulated material). The markers are cyanocobalamin-binding protein (specific granules); myeloperoxidase (azurophil granules); and lysozyme (both granules). A normal range of results must be established in each laboratory to allow the evaluation of presumed defective functions.

Reagents

- Saline containing N-ethylmaleimide (1 mM) and heparin (5 U/ml).
- Cytochalasin B (1 mg/ml, in dimethylsulphoxide).
- Opsonised latex (10^{10}/ml, in saline).
- Triton X-100 (10%, w/v).

Equipment

○ Plastic conical tubes, 10 ml.
○ Refrigerated centrifuge.

Method

All the procedures are carried out at 0–4°C.

1. Incubate neutrophils (2×10^8) with cytochalasin B (10 μl) for 5 minutes and then add opsonised latex particles (4×10^9), as described on p. 243, in a total volume of 2 ml.

2. Take 0.3 ml aliquots at different times (0, 1, 2, 4, 8, 16 min), pour into a conical tube containing 0.7 ml of ice-cold saline with N-ethylmaleimide and heparin, and centrifuge at 250 g for 10 minutes.

3. Separate the supernatants and add 10 μl of 10% Triton X-100. Store frozen if not to be used on the day.

4. Resuspend the pellets with 1 ml of saline containing N-ethylmaleimide and heparin and add 10 μl of Triton X-100. Shake vigorously and store frozen if not to be used on the day.

5. Measure the granule markers in both supernatants and resuspended pellets, as described below.

ASSAY OF GRANULE PROTEINS

The granule proteins are measured in the supernatants (released material) and pellets (intracellular material) from the aliquots taken at different times. Methods for cyanocobalamin-binding protein, myeloperoxidase and lysozyme will be described in full.

CYANOCOBALAMIN-BINDING PROTEIN

Principle

This protein binds radioactive cyanocobalamin which remains in the supernatant as a complex and can be measured. Unbound radiolabelled material is adsorbed and removed by activated charcoal.

Reagents

- Bovine serum albumin, fraction V.
- Activated charcoal.

- Triton X-100.
- Cyanocobalamin (vitamin B_{12}).
- [^{57}Co] cyanocobalamin (Amersham International).
- Sucrose, 20% (w/w).

Equipment
○ Magnetic stirrer.
○ End-over-end rotator.
○ Microcentrifuge tubes, 1.5 ml.
○ Microcentrifuge.
○ Gamma radioactivity counter.

Method
1. Prepare the stopping mixture, which contains bovine serum albumin (5 mg/ml) and activated charcoal (25 mg/ml), in water. This is magnetically stirred for 30 minutes and again during use.

2. Make up the radioactive substrate, which contains [^{57}Co] cyanocobalamin (50 ng, 0.2 mCi/ml) in 0.2% Triton X-100.

3. Place the test sample, or 20% sucrose to serve as blank (50 μl, in duplicate), and substrate (200 μl) in microcentrifuge tubes and mix well in an end-over-end rotator at room temperature, for at least 30 minutes.

4. End the incubations by the addition of 1 ml of the stopping mixture (step 1). Leave for a further 30 minutes at room temperature.

5. Centrifuge the tubes of 10 000 g for 2 minutes.

6. Carefully aspirate 1 ml of the supernatant and transfer to a plastic tube for γ-radioactivity counting.

Calculation
The results are calculated as follows:
  Average blank CPM values — B
  Average sample CPM values — S_s (value of supernatant) or S_p (value of pellet)
  V_s — volume of supernatant
  V_p — volume of resuspended pellet

% Degranulation =

$$= 100 \times \frac{(S_s - B) \times V_s}{(S_p - B) \times V_p + (S_s - B) \times V_s}$$

This is calculated for each incubation time of neutrophils with particles and plotted as percentage degranulation versus time. The time 0 value should be subtracted from the others.

Interpretation
Normal degranulation of cyanocobalamin-binding protein reaches 4–6% in 4 minutes. By 1 minute, half the maximal degranulation should have already occurred. The rate of degranulation is a better measure of the releasing activity of the neutrophil than the maximal degranulation achieved.

MYELOPEROXIDASE

Principle
The activity of this enzyme is measured by following spectrophotometrically the peroxidation of guaiacol by hydrogen peroxide.

Reagents
- Guaiacol.
- Hydrogen peroxide, 30% (w/v).
- Triton X-100.
- Sodium phosphate buffer pH 7.4, 50 mM.

Equipment
○ Double beam spectrophotometer, with a thermostat-controlled cell compartment and provided with a recorder.
○ Plastic cuvettes, 1 ml, disposable.

Method
1. Make up the substrate, which consists of 0.3 mM guaiacol, 0.2 mM H_2O_2 and 0.1% Triton X-100 in 50 mM sodium phosphate buffer (pH 7.4). It should be freshly prepared and warmed at 37°C for 15 minutes before use.

2. Set spectrophotometer at 436 nm and prewarm its cell compartment to 37°C.

3. Add 1 ml of substrate to each of 2 plastic cuvettes.

4. Start the reaction by adding sample (20 μl) to one of the cuvettes. Stir quickly and record absorbance continuously for about 2 minutes.

Calculation
The initial slopes (reaction rates) of the lines are measured in terms of absorbance per minute ($\triangle$A436 nm).
  $\triangle A_s$ — reaction rate with supernatant
  $\triangle A_p$ — reaction rate with pellet
  V_s — volume of supernatant
  V_p — volume of resuspended pellet

$$\% \text{ Degranulation} = 100 \times \frac{\triangle A_s \times V_s}{\triangle A_p \times V_p + \triangle A_s \times V_s}$$

This is calculated for each incubation time and plotted as percentage degranulation versus time. The time 0 value should be subtracted from the others.

Interpretation
As for cyanocobalamin-binding protein.

LYSOZYME

Principle
This enzyme is quantitated by the rate at which it lyses a suspension of *Micrococcus lysodeikticus*, followed spec-

trophotometrically as a decrease in absorbance at 450 nm.

Reagents
- M. lysodeikticus, dried cells (Sigma).
- Potassium phosphate buffer pH 6.2, 50 mM.
- Triton X-100, 0.2% (w/v).

Equipment
○ Sonicator.
○ Double beam spectrophotometer with a thermostat-controlled cell compartment and provided with a recorder.
○ Plastic cuvettes, 1 ml, disposable.

Method
1. Make up the substrate, which consists of a freshly prepared suspension of M. lysodeikticus (0.25 mg/ml) in 50 mM potassium phosphate buffer (pH 6.2), sonicated for 10 seconds at amplitude 4 μ. Warm at 37°C before use.

2. Set spectrophotometer at 450 nm and warm at 37°C.

3. Add 10 μl of sample and 10 μl of Triton X-100 (0.2%) to one of the cuvettes and 10 μl of Triton only to the other. Vortex both vigorously.

4. Add 1 ml of substrate to both of the cuvettes (start) and stir quickly. Record absorbance continuously for about 2 minutes.

Calculation
As described above for myeloperoxidase.

Interpretation
As for cyanocobalamin-binding protein, except that a greater extent of degranulation is to be expected since lysozyme is present in both primary and secondary granules.

DIGESTION

After phagocytosis, digestive enzymes are released from the cytoplasmic granules into the phagocytic vacuoles and the ingested organisms are then digested. Some of the products of digestion are released into the medium, while the rest remains within the phagocytic vacuoles.

Principle (Segal et al 1981)
S. aureus are grown in different radioactive substrates and then used to measure the digestion by neutrophils of the bacterial components into which these substrates have been incorporated.

Reagents
- [^{3}H] glucose-labelled S. aureus, grown, heat-killed and opsonised as described above.
- [^{14}C] aminoacid-labelled S. aureus, heat-killed and opsonised.
- Granulocyte suspension in RPMI medium containing heparin (5 U/ml), prepared as described on p. 280–281.
- RPMI medium containing heparin (5 U/ml).
- Saline containing N-ethylmaleimide (1 mM).
- Scintillation fluid for β-counting.

Equipment
○ Microcentrifuge tubes, 1.5 ml.
○ Rotating mixer.
○ Sodium hydroxide (1 N and 10 N).
○ [^{14}C] protein hydrolysate (Amersham International).
○ Vortex mixer.
○ Microcentrifuge.
○ Scintillation vial inserts.
○ Beta counter.

Method
1. Radiolabel S. aureus with [^{3}H] glucose, heat kill and opsonise as described on p. 372–373.

2. Radiolabel S. aureus with [^{14}C] protein hydrolysate as for [^{3}H] glucose, except add 0.5 μCi/μl [^{14}C] protein hydrolysate to the broth in which S. aureus are grown. Heat kill and opsonise as in 1.

3. Place 1 ml of a granulocyte suspension in RPMI medium (containing 5×10^7 cells) in a tube and pre-incubate at 37°C for 5 minutes.

4. Add 70 μl of a suspension of opsonised radiolabelled bacteria containing 5×10^8 organisms to the granulocyte suspension, to give a ratio of bacteria to phagocytes of 10:1. Vortex the tube and take immediately two aliquots of 100 μl for zero time values, which are poured into two microcentrifuge tubes containing 1 ml of cold saline with N-ethylmaleimide. Keep at 0–4°C until processed (step 10).

5. Place the tube containing granulocytes and bacteria on a rotary mixer, at 37°C.

6. Take two aliquots of 100 μl at 5, 20, 60 and 120 minutes, and pour them into microcentrifuge tubes containing 1 ml of cold saline with N-ethylmaleimide. Keep at 0–4°C until processed (step 10).

7. Add 70 μl of the bacterial suspension used in step 4 to 1 ml of RPMI medium containing heparin. Vortex and take two aliquots as in 4.

8. Place the tube containing only bacteria at 37°C, as in 5.

9. Take aliquots exactly as described in 6.

10. Stir thoroughly all the tubes where aliquots had been poured (steps 4, 6 and 9) and centrifuge in a microcentrifuge at 10 000 g for 1 minute. The super-

natants contain the egested products, while the intra-cellular digestion products are present in the pellets.

11. Transfer the supernatants after centrifugation to scintillation vial inserts, add 50 μl of 10 N NaOH and leave at room temperature overnight.

12. Subject the cell pellets from step 10 to hypotonic shock by addition of 0.5 ml ice-cold water. Vortex and centrifuge at 10 000 g for 5 minutes. Transfer the supernatants (intracellular digestion products) to vial inserts and add 50 μl of 10 N NaOH. Leave at room temperature overnight.

13. Solubilise the pellets from step 12 (undigested material) by addition of 0.5 ml 1 N NaOH. Leave over-night at room temperature and transfer to vial inserts.

14. Add 4 ml of scintillation fluid for radioactivity counting to the vial inserts from steps 11, 12 and 13. Count for β-radioactivity.

Calculations

Results are expressed as the percentage of radioactivity associated with the digestion products with respect to the total available.

$$100 \times \frac{\underset{\text{(step 11)} \quad \text{(step 12)} \qquad \text{(step 11)}}{\text{(Egested + intracellular) or egested only}}}{\underset{\text{(step 13)} \qquad \text{(step 12)} \quad \text{(step 11)}}{\text{undigested + digested + egested}}}$$

Interpretation

Normal values are:

Up to 15–20% egested + intracellular in 2 hours.

Up to 10% of egested products in 2 hours. Values for the digestion of ^{14}C-labelled bacteria are generally half the value of corresponding ^{3}H-labelled organisms.

Comments

— The spontaneous release of radioactivity from bacteria incubated in the absence of neutrophils is checked (steps 7–9).

— In chronic granulomatous disease, digestion is reduced by 50% or more.

— The analysis of digestion may require the measure-ment of phagocytosis, since an apparently decreased digestion may be the result of impaired phago-cytosis.

RESPIRATORY BURST

When phagocytic cells are stimulated by soluble agents such as phorbol myristate acetate (PMA) or by opson-ised particles, they undergo a large increase in oxygen consumption. This respiratory burst is produced by a specialised oxidase system and is important for the killing of microbes. The oxidase system is deficient in the cells of patients with chronic granulomatous disease (CGD), a rare inherited condition. The oxidase system is an electron transport chain that uses NADPH, initially coming from glucose and being generated through the hexose monophosphate shunt, to reduce oxygen with one electron to superoxide (O_2). Two superoxide molecules can then combine to form hydrogen peroxide.

$$2 H^+ + O_2^- + O_2^- = H_2O_2 + O_2$$

The only component of this electron transport chain that has been identified is a very unusual cytochrome b, b_{-245}.

Many different parameters can be measured as a means of assessing the integrity and rate of this oxidase system. These include the rate at which the hexose monophosphate shunt generates NADPH, the production of superoxide, and the consumption of oxygen. An impaired response either indicates the failure of acti-vation of the oxidase, for example by poor opsonisation or binding to receptors, or malfunction of one of its components. Complete failure in the face of adequate stimulation with PMA is diagnostic of CGD — the cells can then be tested to see if they are missing cytochrome b_{-245}, which is absent in most of these patients.

NITROBLUE TETRAZOLIUM TEST

Principle

Neutrophils are allowed to adhere to glass and stimu-lated with PMA. This activates the oxidase in normal cells, generating superoxide which reduces the yellow NBT to a dark blue formazan that is clearly visible under the microscope. It is useful for the diagnosis of patients with CGD (including antenatal diagnosis at 16 weeks of gestation) and heterozygote carriers of the X-linked variety of the disease.

Reagents

● Phosphate-buffered saline pH 7.4 containing glucose (5 mM) and albumin (0.5%).

● Nitroblue tetrazolium (Sigma).

● Phorbol myristate acetate (Sigma) — stock solution (1 mg/ml, in dimethylsulphoxide) kept at −20°C.

● Working solution: PMA, 1.25 mg/ml; albumin, 17 mg/ml; PMA, 1.0 mg/ml; glucose, 0.5 mM.

● Safranin (1%, in water).

Method

1. Blood is taken into heparin (5 U/ml or lithium heparin tube). An aliquot of this (50 μl) is taken into

cold PBS containing glucose and albumin and centrifuged at 200 g for 5 minutes. The pellet is resuspended in the PBS-glucose-albumin and centrifuged as before.

2. The pellet is resuspended in a small volume (25 μl) of the PBS-glucose-albumin and spread over a well on a multispot microscope slide and incubated at 37°C for 30 minutes in a moisture chamber (e.g. a petri dish containing wet tissues).

3. Unattached cells are gently flushed away with a stream of saline from a pipette and the attached cells in the well immediately covered with the NBT/PMA solution. Care must be taken to ensure that the cells are not allowed to dry.

4. After incubation for 30 minutes at 37°C, the slide is washed with physiological saline — which seems to give a cleaner end result than washing with any more complex solution — and air dried. Fix for 5 minutes in absolute methanol and stain in 1% Safranin for 1 minute.

5. View under the microscope at a magnification of × 200–400 to obtain an overall impression and then at × 1000 to observe detail.

Interpretation
In the absence of PMA, cells remain of normal size with a discrete nucleus and are light red in colour. After stimulation the cells become swollen, the nucleus loses its characteristic multilobed appearance and the cell becomes coloured a diffuse blue with spots of deeper intensity. This blue coloration is best seen in the absence of the red Safranin counter stain. In normal subjects, all the cells become swollen and blue coloured. In CGD, all the cells remain red and retain their normal architecture. The X-linked heterozygotes have a mixture of positive and negative cells.

Comments
— PMA is used as the stimulant because, being in solution, it reaches all the cells, and activates the oxidase without the need for opsonisation and receptor attachment.
— Multi-well glass slides are very convenient. However a much better picture is obtained if cells are adhered to dialysis membrane. The latter can be laid on filter paper moistened with medium and the cells applied in LP35 caps as described in the Raft technique for in-vitro locomotion. The membrane is treated in the same way as the slides except that it is finally mounted in water on a slide.

OXYGEN UPTAKE

Principle
The rate of oxygen consumption is determined with an oxygen electrode which is in contact with a closed, rapidly stirred and thermostatically controlled incubation chamber.

Reagents
- RPMI 1640 medium containing heparin (5 U/ml).
- Sodium dithionite.
- Latex particles opsonised with IgG, prepared as described on page 243.
- Phorbol myristate acetate (PMA) (10 μg/ml, in PBS containing 1% dimethylsulphoxide).

Equipment
○ Oxygen electrode (Clark type), with incubation chamber (Rank Bros.).
○ Chart recorder.
○ Water-bath, for the control of the temperature of the chamber.

Method

Calibration of the electrode
The electrode is calibrated to 100% air saturation of the medium and anaerobiosis before use. The 100% calibration is performed by equilibrating 1 ml of the medium with air at 37°C by stirring this solution with the lid off. The 0% calibration is then performed by the addition of a few grains of sodium dithionite to the medium and replacing the lid. The chamber is then emptied by suction and carefully washed to remove the reducing agent completely.

Oxygen uptake on ingestion of latex particles
1. Place 1 ml of a well-aerated suspension of granulocytes in RPMI 1640 medium (10^8/ml) in the thermostat-controlled electrode chamber, with the lid on, and leave to equilibrate at 37°C for 2–3 minutes with rapid stirring.

2. Switch on the chart recorder to obtain the basal rate of oxygen consumption (approximately 10 nmoles/ml/min per 10^8 cells).

3. After 1–2 minutes, add 0.1 ml of a prewarmed suspension of opsonised latex (5×10^{10} particles/ml) through the small hole in the chamber lid. The lid is lifted slightly to allow only the entry of the particle suspension but not of any additional air. After a lag period of approximately 30 seconds, a substantial oxygen uptake starts to take place and proceeds at a constant rate for at least 1 minute.

Oxygen uptake on stimulation by phorbol myristate acetate
1. Place 1 ml of a suspension of granulocytes (10^8/ml) in the electrode chamber and obtain the basal rate of oxygen consumption as described in 1 and 2 above.

2. Add 0.1 ml of 10 μg/ml phorbol myristate acetate to the chamber through the hole in the lid. A sustained

oxygen uptake is apparent after an initial lag of 20–30 seconds.

Calculations

The rate of oxygen uptake is calculated from the slope of the curve recorded ($\triangle$ reading in 1 min, within the linear portion of the tracing). The $\triangle$ reading is converted into amount of oxygen consumed by relating it to the difference between the 100 and 0% calibration levels recorded at the beginning of the procedure, which corresponds to the solubility of oxygen at 37°C, i.e. 184 nmoles/ml.

Therefore:

Rate of O_2 uptake =

$$= \frac{\triangle \text{ reading per min} \times 184 \text{ nmoles/ml}}{\triangle (100\% \text{ calib.level} - 0\% \text{ calib.level})}$$

Interpretation

The oxygen uptake rate of normal cells maximally stimulated is 300 ± 50 nmoles/min/10^8 cells. Submaximal stimulation, smaller cell concentrations and lower ratios of particles to cells will give lower uptake rates.

Comments

— The membrane above the oxygen electrode takes several hours to stabilise and is generally best fitted the day before use.
— Special care must be taken to ensure the absence of air from the chamber.
— Should the neutrophil suspension not consume oxygen, or consume it slowly, the pH of the suspension must be checked. If it has been prepared 2–3 hours before use, the medium might need to be changed.

SUPEROXIDE PRODUCTION

Principle

Superoxide (O_2^-) released by PMA-stimulated neutrophils is measured by the reduction of cytochrome c by O_2^-. This is accompanied by a colour change that is detected spectrophotometrically as an increase in absorbance at 550 nm. Cytochrome c can be reduced by other electron donors in the cell, and specificity is given to the reaction by the use of superoxide dismutase, an enzyme that removes O_2^- by converting it to O_2 and H_2O_2. A double beam spectrophotometer can be used to compare simultaneously the reduction in the absence and presence of superoxide dismutase and give a direct measure of superoxide generation.

Reagents

● Phosphate-buffered saline (PBS).
● Cytochrome c (type VI, from horse heart, 2 mM in PBS).
● Superoxide dismutase (from bovine blood, type I, 1 mg/ml in PBS).
● D-glucose (0.5 M, in water).
● Phorbol myristate acetate (PMA, 0.2 mg/ml, in dimethylsulphoxide).

Equipment

○ Double beam spectrophotometer, with temperature-controlled cuvette compartment and chart recorder.
○ Cuvettes (disposable, 1 ml).

Method

1. Add PBS (0.85 ml), cytochrome c (50 μl) and glucose (10 μl) to two cuvettes, which are warmed to 37°C (front and back positions).
2. Add superoxide dismutase (50 μl) to the back cuvette and an equal volume of PBS to the front one.
3. Add cells (usually 50 μl, containing 10^6 cells) to both cuvettes. Stir and record the absorbance at 550 nm as a function of time. This baseline recording from unstimulated cells should be relatively flat.
4. Add PMA solution (5 μl) to both back and front cuvettes to start the respiratory burst, stir immediately, and record the absorbance at 550 nm as a function of time.

Calculation

The rate of production of O_2^- is calculated from the rate of change in absorbance at 550 nm per minute within the linear portion of the curve as follows:

Rate of change at 550 nm (in OD units/min)/21.1, where 21.1 is the millimolar extinction coefficient of cytochrome c.

This gives the number of mmoles/ml/minute. It is multiplied by 1000 to give the result in nmoles/ml/minute and related to the exact number of cells used in the assay so as to express the rates of superoxide generation in nmoles/minute $\times 10^7$ cells.

Interpretation

Normal values are within 80 ± 20 nmoles/minute/10^7 cells.

Comment

It is possible to use a single beam spectrophotometer, in which case the reaction rates are determined in the absence and presence of superoxide dismutase and the difference calculated by subtraction.

REFERENCES

El-Maalem H, Fletcher J 1976 Defective neutrophil function in chronic granulocytic leukemia. British Journal of Haematology 34: 96–103

Segal A W, Jones O T G 1979 The subcellular distribution and some properties of the cytochrome b component of the microbiocidal oxidase system of human neutrophils. Biochemical Journal 182: 181–188

Segal A W, Geisow M, Garcia R, Harper A, Miller R 1981 The respiratory burst of phagocytic cells is associated with a rise in vacuolar pH. Nature 290: 406–409

Tan J S, Watanakunakorn C, Phair J P 1971 A modified assay of neutrophil function: use of lysostaphin to differentiate defective phagocytosis from impaired intracellular killing. Journal of Laboratory and Clinical Medicine 78: 316–322

16

Culture and analysis of human progenitor cells

The haemopoietic system, like other tissues which are called upon continually to produce a population of mature cells with limited lifespan, is organised in an hierarchical manner. The most primitive cells (stem cells) are also the least frequent cells. Stem cells have several important properties that include multipotentiality (i.e. the ability to give rise to cells of more than one lineage), the ability to self-renew (thus producing stem cells with identical or very similar properties), and the capacity for many cell divisions.

Stem cells give rise to committed progenitor cells which have a lower proliferative capacity, can only give rise to cells in a limited number of lineages and have limited capacity for self-replicative divisions. Committed progenitor cells give rise to cells with reduced or no proliferative potential and ultimately a fully-differentiated, functionally mature cell is generated. These latter stages of differentiation can occur in the absence of cell division.

Cells with proliferative potential can only be clearly identified on the basis of functional studies which demand expression of the ability to proliferate. In such studies of haemopoiesis in rodents, stem cells are identified by their ability to give rise to a nodule (colony) of cells in the spleen of an irradiated animal. Therefore, this stem cell has been called a CFU-S (colony-forming-unit-spleen). The committed progenitor cells are referred to as colony-forming-cells (CFCs) because of their ability to generate colonies of daughter cells in a semisolid culture medium such as agar or methylcellulose. The lineage to which a progenitor is committed is also only recognised in retrospect by examining the morphology of cells present in a particular colony. A prefix or suffix is used to denote a particular lineage, thus granulocyte-macrophage-CFC (GM-CFC), eosinophil-CFC (Eo-CFC) or, for the erythroid lineage, burst-forming-unit-erythroid (BFU-E), colony-forming-unit-erythroid (CFU-E).

It is possible to grow both murine and human colonies in vitro that consist of multiple haemopoietic lineages (multipotential colonies). Colonies of murine origin contain 'mature' CFU-S capable of a limited number of self-renewing divisions in vitro. Although human multipotential colonies consist of cells of more than one lineage and thus display one characteristic of stem cells (that of multipotentiality), human multi-CFC possess only limited self-renewal capacity and thus also represent relatively 'mature' cells in the hierarchy of stem cells.

Colonies of neutrophils, monocytes and eosinophils (clones of greater than 40 cells), can be grown from human blood or bone marrow cells when cells are stimulated by stimulatory factors called colony stimulating factors (CSFs). If cultures of marrow cells are examined after 7 days, most colonies are neutrophil in type, whereas after 14 days colonies of neutrophils, macrophages and eosinophils are present. The cells that give rise to colonies after 7 days of culture can be separated from, and are the progeny of, the cells giving rise to colonies after 14 days of culture. The purified human CSFs preferentially stimulate one or other subset of these cells. The growth of human erythroid colonies in vitro requires the addition of erythropoietin to CSF-stimulated cultures. There are two populations of erythroid progenitor cells — the more primitive giving rise to colonies after 14 days of culture (BFU-E), while the more mature cells generate colonies after 7 days of culture (CFU-E).

The proliferation and functional activation of haemopoietic cells in vitro is under the control of a family of glycoprotein hormones called colony-stimulating factors (CSFs), named because of their ability to stimulate progenitor cells to give rise to colonies in vitro. Some of the CSFs display specificity for particular lineages and this is indicated by a prefix, thus granulocyte-CSF (G-CSF), macrophage-CSF (M-CSF) and granulocyte-macrophage-CSF (GM-CSF). Two molecules that are active on specific haemopoietic lineages also display activity for lymphoid cells and stimulate B-cell growth and differentiation. One molecule is active on eosinophils ('Eosinophil-CSF' or Interleukin 5) and one molecule is active on mast cells (Interleukin 4). An additional molecule is named multipotential-CSF (multi-CSF) (or Interleukin 3) to indicate a broad spectrum of activity on all haemopoietic lineages, including activity on some stem cells.

Four actions have been established for the purified CSFs. These are:

1. the requirement for CSF for the survival of progenitor cells in vitro;

2. the requirement for CSF for cell division, with few cells even able to complete the cell-cycle in progress at the time of CSF withdrawal;

3. differentiation commitment, and

4. activation of mature cell function. This area has been extensively reviewed (Metcalf 1984).

The quantitation of progenitor cells in blood or bone marrow can be performed using CSF-stimulated semisolid cultures. These cultures may be useful in situations where knowledge of the frequency of progenitor cells is of value (e.g. bone marrow transplantation) and may provide additional information in some disease states. The frequency of progenitor cells (and multi-CFC) is decreased in aplastic anaemia and increased in diseases such as chronic myeloid leukaemia. In the acute myeloid leukemias the number of cluster-forming cells (generating clones of less than 40 cells) is markedly increased and colony-forming cells may be completely absent. Similar changes may be observed in the preleukaemic myelodysplastic syndromes (and chronic myeloid leukaemia undergoing acute transformation) many months before morphological evidence of frank leukaemia.

Although purified and recombinant human CSFs are available, these molecules stimulate only a subset of progenitor cells, therefore to maximally stimulate and thus quantitate all responsive progenitor cells requires the use of either mixtures of recombinant CSFs or crude conditioned-media which contain at least two and probably four or more different CSFs.

Liquid culture systems are more suited to studies which require cells for detailed morphological or surface antigen studies. Cells obtained from such cultures are also suitable for subsequent studies on the frequency of clonogenic cells and can be used as a technique for enriching for such cells. Studies that seek to analyse directly the action of CSFs, or the response of cells to stimulation, ideally require the use of both purified cell populations and purified CSFs.

SEMISOLID CULTURE METHODS FOR HUMAN PROGENITOR CELLS

Principle

Semisolid cloning methods are used for quantitation of granulocyte-monocyte progenitor cells present in blood and bone marrow. These cells proliferate and generate colonies of maturing progeny when stimulated by colony-stimulating factors (CSFs). Usually a known concentration of CSF is added to cultures, although significant CSF levels can sometimes be elaborated by macrophages and lymphocytes present in the cultured cell population. Detection of all the progenitor cells present in a cultured sample requires that culture conditions are optimal and that each colony is clearly separated from adjacent colonies. The principles involved and the various techniques used to grow human colonies have been extensively reviewed elsewhere (Metcalf 1984, Golde 1984).

Test samples

Blood and bone marrow samples are collected in a sterile tube containing preservative-free heparin. Bone marrow cells are dispersed by pipetting following the addition of tissue culture fluid. Buffy coat cells are prepared, or alternatively mononuclear cells are obtained following centrifugation for 20 minutes at 1000 g over Ficoll-Paque (Pharmacia). Interface cells are removed, washed, resuspended and counted.

Reagents

- Double-strength Dulbecco's modified Eagle's medium (DME) or Double-strength Iscove's modified Dulbecco's Medium (IMDM) (for erythroid progenitors and multi-CFC).
- Preselected fetal calf serum (FCS).
- Bacto-agar (Difco).
- Pretitrated, standard source of CSF (see below).

Equipment

- Cultures should be performed in a biohazard hood to protect the operator and maintain sterility.
- Glass ware and pipettes must be washed and sterilised.
- Culture medium and the source of CSF must be sterilised (e.g.0.22 μm filter, Millipore Corp).
- Tissue culture dishes (e.g.35 mm petri dishes) are required.

Incubator — temperature and CO_2 control.

Standards and controls

Three crude CSF preparations are commonly used and all contain at least two and probably four or more types of CSF:

1. Giant-cell-tumour (GCT) conditioned medium is commercially available (Gibco).

2. Human placental conditioned medium is obtained by incubating pieces of fresh placental tissue in single-strength DME and 10% FCS for 1 week. The supernatant is removed, concentrated and titrated to determine CSF activity.

3. Lectin-stimulated leucocyte conditioned medium can be prepared by stimulating peripheral blood mono-

nuclear cells with phytohaemagglutinin or concanavalin A in single-strength DME and 5% FCS. Conditioned medium is harvested after 7 days. All standard CSF preparations including recombinant material should be titrated and used at a concentration sufficient to deliver a maximal stimulus. This concentration is determined by preparing cultures of normal human cells stimulated by serial dilutions of the CSF-preparation. A sigmoid dose-response curve is obtained for the number of colonies stimulated by varying concentrations of CSF. That concentration of CSF which stimulates maximal (plateau) numbers of colonies is used subsequently.

Culture of control normal cells should be performed to confirm adequate culture conditions.

To identify erythroid and multipotential colonies, 1–2 units of erythropoietin are required per 1 ml culture.

Method

1. Prepare and count cell suspension. In general 5 $\times$ 10^4 normal bone marrow cells or 5 $\times$ 10^5 normal blood mononuclear cells are cultured per 1 ml culture.

2. Place empty sterile culture dishes on incubator tray and label lid with water insoluble ink.

3. Place required volumes of pretitrated stimulating material in culture dishes. This should not exceed 0.2 ml per 1 ml culture.

4. Boil 0.6% agar in double glass-distilled water for 2 minutes and allow to cool to 37°C.

5. Measure required volume of double-strength DME (or double-strength IMDM) and add FCS (in the ratio 3 volumes DME to 2 volumes FCS).

6. Add required volume of agar (ratio DME:FCS:agar = 3:2:5). Mix well.

7. Add required volume of cell suspension. Mix well.

8. Pipette 1 ml volumes of the mixture to each culture dish and mix with the stimulating material.

9. Allow cultures to gel and incubate at 37°C in a fully humidified atmosphere of 10% CO_2 in air. (5% CO_2 in air for erythroid colonies).

Scoring cultures

Colonies (of >40 cells) are quantitated after 7 and 14 days of incubation using a dissection (or an inverted) microscope. A normal bone marrow aspirate typically generates between 40–150 day 7 colonies per 10^5 cells and the ratio of clusters (of <40 cells) to colonies is 4–10:1. The number of day 14 colonies is usually half the number of day 7 colonies and approximately 20–30% are eosinophil colonies.

Colony numbers (with a normal cluster to colony ratio) are increased in chronic myeloid leukaemia and allied disorders. In acute myeloid leukaemia and the preleukaemic myelodysplastic syndromes the ratio of clusters to day 7 colonies is markedly increased and colonies may be absent. This latter pattern is also seen in some myeloproliferative disorders and prior to and during acute transformation of chronic myeloid leukaemia. In these disorders the number of cells cultured may need to be reduced to 10^3–10^4 cells per ml to allow accurate cluster counts.

Morphological analysis

Agar cultures can be fixed with 2.5% glutaraldehyde for 15 minutes–4 hours and the agar-gel floated onto a large microscope slide. The gel is allowed to dry and can then be stained (e.g. with Luxol Fast Blue for 60 minutes, non-specific or chloroacetate esterases). Slides are then washed in tap water and stained with Haematoxylin.

Comments

— Batches of FCS differ greatly in their ability to support haemopoietic colony growth and all candidate FCS batches must be pre-tested. This is particularly important in the selection of batches of FCS to support erythroid colony formation.

— Cell death will ensue either if agar temperature is >37°C or if cells are added to double-strength medium-FCS mixture prior to agar.

— Agar will not regel if premature gelling occurs during preparation of the culture, or gelling may fail to occur if large volumes of fluid containing the cell suspension or stimulus are used (i.e. >0.3 ml total per 1 ml agar-medium).

— The incubator must be checked regularly so that humidity, temperature (37°C) and pH (7.2–7.4) are maintained.

LIQUID CULTURE SYSTEMS

Such systems have the advantage of providing cells that are more suitable for morphological, cytochemical or monoclonal antibody studies. Liquid culture systems are also ideally suited to miniaturisation, so that small numbers of cells (e.g. 50–200) and small volumes of CSF (e.g. 5 μl) can be cultured in microtitre wells and monitored visually over several days.

A mixture of single-strength DME and 20% pre-selected FCS is prepared. A pretitrated source of CSF and similar concentrations are required as for semisolid clonal cultures. Cellular proliferation may be monitored by tritiated-thymidine uptake or by direct cell counts, although concomitant death of mature cells may mask cell proliferation if the latter method is used. The time of scoring or harvesting such cultures is determined by the population of cells under study, but often the culture period can be reduced compared with semisolid clonal cultures.

Composition of reagents

Dulbecco's modified Eagle's medium (double-strength)

Dulbecco's modified Eagle's medium HG16 Instant Tissue Culture Powder (Grand Island Biological co.) 10 g.

Double glass-distilled water 390 ml.

L-asparagine 3 ml of 6.7 mg/ml (final concentration 20 μg/ml).

DEAE dextran (Pharmacia, M. Wt. 500 000) 1.5 ml of 50 mg/ml (final concentration 75 μg/ml).

Penicillin 0.575 ml of 2×10^5 IU/ml).

Streptomycin 0.375 ml of 200 mg/ml.

NaHCO₃ 4.9 g.

Iscoves modified Dulbecco's medium (double-strength)

Iscove's modied Dulbecco's medium Tissue Culture Powder (Gibco) 35.32 g.

Double glass-distilled water 780 ml.

L-asparagine 0.4 g.

DEAE dextran (Pharmacia, M. Wt. 500 000) 3 ml of 50 mg/ml.

Penicillin 120 mg.

Streptomycin 200 mg.

NaHCO₃ 9.8 g.

2-mercaptoethanol (14.3 M; Calbiochem) 11.8 μl.

Luxol Fast Blue

Luxol Fast Blue MBS (0.1% w/v; G T Gurr) dissolved in 70% ethanol saturated with urea.

REFERENCES

Golde D 1984 Methods in haematology. Haematopoiesis. Churchill Livingstone, NY

Metcalf D 1984 The hemopoietic colony stimulating factors. Elsevier, Amsterdam

17

Marrow preservation

PREPARATION FOR BONE MARROW TRANSPLANTATION

An allogeneic bone marrow transplant involves collection of donor (usually sibling) marrow. Autologous bone marrow refers to the collection of the patient's own marrow which is stored for future return to the patient. Allogeneic BMT (allo-BMT) is employed for the treatment of certain immune deficiencies, for correction of incapacitating inborn errors of metabolism and for the treatment of chemoradiotherapy-responsive, usually haematological, malignancies.

Autologous BMT (ABMT), on the other hand, has been used exclusively for the treatment of malignant disease where, like allo-BMT, it provides a means of rescuing the patient from what might otherwise be supralethal chemoradiotherapy. ABMT, of course, avoids the need for an HLA-identical sibling and removes the dangers of allo-immune-based graft rejection and graft-versus-host disease (GVHD) (the latter danger increases rapidly with age). For these reasons, the technique is much more widely applicable than allo-BMT, but in the context of malignant disease has the serious disadvantage of being potentially contaminated by malignant cells. Currently, therefore, ABMT is usually only considered when no HLA-identical sibling is available or the patient is at particular risk of GVHD.

The techniques of allo-BMT and ABMT are very similar and will be considered together. Marrow, mixed with large quantities of blood, is harvested by multiple aspiration. Such material can be used without further manipulation, but some form of volume reduction with consequent concentration of progenitor cells is often incorporated. According to the clinical circumstances (see below), marrow is then subjected to freezing, perhaps preceded by selective removal (purging) of T cells or of contaminating malignant cells. Each of these procedures will be considered in turn.

BONE MARROW HARVEST

Principle
Aspirated marrow contains the relevant progenitor cells, along with other leucocyte types. Both allo-BMT and ABMT exploit the remarkable fact that progenitor cells infused intravenously are able to identify the marrow microenvironment, settle there, and rapidly re-establish haematopoiesis.

Method
1. Under a general anaesthetic, marrow is harvested aseptically — mainly from the posterior iliac crests, but additional material may also be obtained from the anterior iliac crests and the sternum.

2. Marrow is collected into a two-litre transfer bag (Travenol) containing 150 ml of ACD-A solution (also Travenol). The syringes and aspirate needles are used repeatedly, and between aspirates are rinsed with 0.9% physiological saline containing 5000 IU/l of preservative-free heparin; small amounts of saline are therefore transferred to the collection bag.

For both allo-BMT and ABMT, a total of 2×10^8 nucleated cells/kg recipient body weight is harvested. This is usually done by aspirating 800 ml of marrow in 5–10 ml aliquots and by then measuring the nucleated cell count on a cell counter (for a 70 kg man the minimum count in 800 ml should be of the order of 17×10^9/l).

VOLUME REDUCTION OF HARVESTED MARROW

Principle
Volume reduction serves to remove fat, clots and bone fragments as well as contaminating red cells and potential isohaemagglutinins, thus allowing BMT in the presence of ABH incompatibility. In addition, the procedure is necessary to reduce the total volume of aspirate to manageable proportions for cryopreservation (ABMT) and purging (allo-BMT and ABMT).

Various methods have been used for volume reduction and have employed centrifugation, density-gradient centrifugation, sedimentation with agents such as hydroxyethyl starch (HES), or combinations of these techniques.

We have found sedimentation with HES a simple and convenient method (Jones & Marcus 1985) and this is described here.

Method

1. The harvested marrow is divided into two 700 ml transfer bags (not more than 500 ml/bag).

2. Add hydroxyethyl starch (6%) in 0.9% physiological saline (Plasmasteril, Fresenius AG.) to a final concentration of 20% v/v. This is done via a three-way tap attached to the transfer line of the transfer bag.

3. The contents of the transfer bag are allowed to settle and the leucocyte-rich fraction separated from the sedimented red cells. This can be readily achieved with the sort of apparatus and procedure illustrated in Figure 17.1.

4. The product at this stage is suitable for re-infusion or cryopreservation. However, if purging is to be performed, washing and transfer to heparinised culture fluid is required. This is most easily performed by centrifugation in a standard laboratory centrifuge.

PURGING TECHNIQUES

Principle

Purging techniques are now widely used for both allo-BMT and ABMT, in the former being aimed at removing alloreactive T cells and in the latter being designed to remove residual tumour cells.

Purging has involved immunological, pharmacological

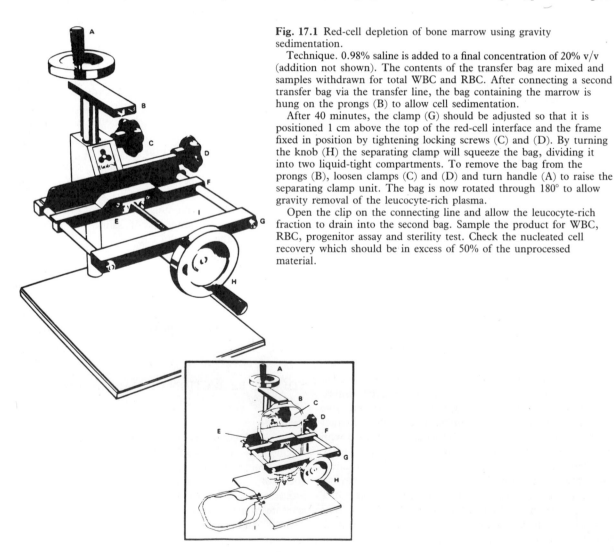

Fig. 17.1 Red-cell depletion of bone marrow using gravity sedimentation.

Technique. 0.98% saline is added to a final concentration of 20% v/v (addition not shown). The contents of the transfer bag are mixed and samples withdrawn for total WBC and RBC. After connecting a second transfer bag via the transfer line, the bag containing the marrow is hung on the prongs (B) to allow cell sedimentation.

After 40 minutes, the clamp (G) should be adjusted so that it is positioned 1 cm above the top of the red-cell interface and the frame fixed in position by tightening locking screws (C) and (D). By turning the knob (H) the separating clamp will squeeze the bag, dividing it into two liquid-tight compartments. To remove the bag from the prongs (B), loosen clamps (C) and (D) and turn handle (A) to raise the separating clamp unit. The bag is now rotated through 180° to allow gravity removal of the leucocyte-rich plasma.

Open the clip on the connecting line and allow the leucocyte-rich fraction to drain into the second bag. Sample the product for WBC, RBC, progenitor assay and sterility test. Check the nucleated cell recovery which should be in excess of 50% of the unprocessed material.

and physical methods. Immunological purging has mainly employed antibody-mediated mechanisms such as opsonisation and removal by the host reticuloendothelial system, complement-induced lysis, binding of cells to antibody-coated beads and antibody-mediated systems selectively delivering cell toxins.

Most immunological purging has involved monoclonal antibody (MAb) and complement lysis, and this methodology will be described here for CAMPATH 1 (Waldmann et al 1984), a rat anti-leucocyte MAb with which we have had experience.

Pharmacological purging has been investigated largely because of the lack of suitable MAb for removing AML cells. Most experience has been with derivatives of cyclophosphamide but the technique is limited by lack of selectivity, normal committed progenitors having a similar susceptibility to that of leukaemic cells.

Physical methods have involved various forms of density-gradient or counter current-centrifugation and seem to be cumbersome and relatively ineffective.

Method

1. Add 25 mg CAMPATH 1 to the volume-reduced marrow in 200–250 ml RPM1, all contained in a 700 ml transfer bag.

2. Leave at room temperature for 15 minutes, mixing occasionally.

3. Add previously collected autologous donor serum to give a final 25% v/v concentration.

4. Mix and incubate at 37°C for 45 minutes.

5. Wash once in physiological saline containing human plasma protein fraction (25% v/v) and heparin (2000 IU/l). Centrifuge at 400 g for 10 minutes at room temperature.

6. The product at this stage should be sampled for efficiency of T-cell removal and sterility and, if desired, for progenitor cell assay, before re-infusion (allo-BMT) or cryopreservation.

Comment

Many MAb are not good activators of complement and much effort has been directed towards developing relevant MAb with high titre lytic activity. IgM and IgG2 subclasses of mouse MAb are the most efficient activators of complement and are therefore preferred for this technique. However, mouse MAb, regardless of class, do not activate human complement adequately and rabbit serum is commonly employed as the complement source. Development of rat MAb (e.g. CAMPATH 1) which are suitable for use with human (donor) serum complement is thus of increasing interest. Relevant antibodies have been produced for purging of T and cALL cells but not for AML blasts because specific antibodies not toxic for normal progenitors have not been developed. The efficiency of removal

of particular cell types is enhanced by employing more than one appropriate MAb and highly effective panels of antibodies are now available for lysing T lymphocytes.

CRYOPRESERVATION FOR CLINICAL PURPOSES

Principle

Cryopreservation is mainly relevant to ABMT since it allows collection of autologous marrow or peripheral blood stem cells before ablative chemotherapy which may last for several days. Dimethyl sulphoxide (DMSO) is used as a cryoprotectant.

Method

1. A 20% v/v solution of DMSO in patient plasma or in tissue culture medium is prepared in a transfer bag. Volume-reduced marrow is placed on ice to cool (DMSO is cytotoxic at higher temperature) and mixed with an equal volume of cooled DMSO solution. The mixing is done slowly (e.g. 250 ml of each solution mixed over 15 min) via a syringe and an interconnecting system of taps and couplers.

2. The diluted marrow is transferred via the connecting system to freezing bags (Gambro Ltd.). Each is filled with not more than 120 ml, heat sealed, carefully labelled with a spirit-based marker pen, and then placed at 4°C. A small amount of the marrow is reserved in order to fill two 2 ml freezing vials which can be used to check the viability of the frozen marrow.

Comments

— DMSO is a solvent for many plastics, and care should be exercised in selecting compatible plastic ware (e.g. polypropylene transfer bags and Teflon storage bags).

— Various machines are available for programmed freezing. Some incorporate a facility for correction for latent heat of freezing (Fig. 17.2); but many workers feel this facility confers no advantage in terms of cell recovery; we have found a machine without this feature (Planer Biomedical Ltd.) entirely satisfactory.

STORAGE AND THAWING OF FROZEN MARROW

Principle

Marrow is stored temporarily while the patient is given chemotherapy. Marrow is sometimes stored for a prolonged period if it is to be used in the treatment of subsequent relapse.

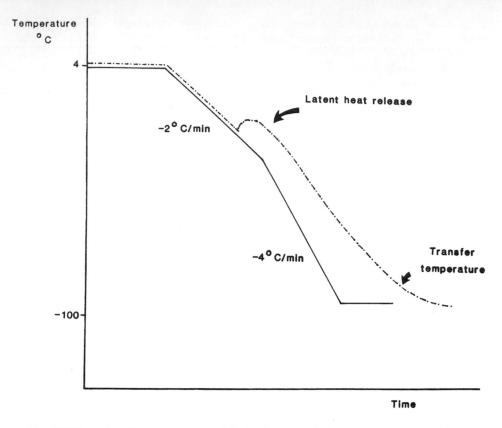

Fig. 17.2 Typical cooling curves recorded, (using thermocouples) when freezing bone marrow.

Method

1. Marrow is stored in specific containers employing liquid nitrogen.

2. As with any type of tissue banking, an accurate and fail-safe inventory control and donor record system is essential.

3. For thawing, frozen marrow is transferred to the ward in a dewar flask containing liquid nitrogen.

4. Marrow is removed from the dewar flask using long blunt forceps and thawed by total immersion in a water-bath (42°C) at the bedside. The bag should be agitated during thawing to ensure local refreezing does not occur and should thaw completely in 1–2 minutes.

5. Thawed marrow is then rapidly re-infused intra-venously.

Comment

Various styles and sizes of storage vessels are available and the type chosen by a given laboratory will depend on its particular needs. All have the disadvantage of requiring regular replenishment with liquid nitrogen.

Both the freezing machines mentioned above and the storage vessels must be operated in well-ventilated areas since the evaporated liquid nitrogen can potentially cause asphyxiation.

Quality control

Most laboratories incorporate controls to monitor the sterility of the preparations, the content of progenitor cells and the efficiency of any purging step(s). All these quality assurance procedures suffer the disadvantage of usually being retrospective in terms of clinical management.

REFERENCES

Jones H M, Marcus R E 1985 Red cell depletion of donor bone marrow using starch sedimentation and the Erytrenn plasma separator. Biotest Bulletin 2, (4), 197–200

Waldmann H, Hale G, Cividalli G et al, 1984 Elimination of graft versus host disease by a monoclonal rat anti human lymphocyte antibody (CAMPATH 1). Lancet 483: 483–486

Haemostasis

18

Physiology of normal haemostasis

The process of haemostasis involves protecting blood flow through a virtually closed circuit of blood vessels at various pressures and re-establishing vascular patency if any segments become occluded. Haemostatic reactions can be classified into several overlapping and sequential events; localised vasoconstriction at the site of injury, platelet adhesion to exposed subendothelial basement membrane and collagen fibres, formation of a platelet aggregate or plug, activation of the coagulation cascade leading to formation of fibrin which reinforces the platelet plug, and finally, activation of the fibrinolytic system which digests the haemostatic plug and allows growth of new vascular endothelial cells to complete the repair process (Sixma & Wester 1977). Also a complex system of physiological inhibitors and feed-back control mechanisms exists to control and limit any excessive or inappropriate activation of the haemostatic system (Bennett 1977).

Vessel wall

Following injury vasoconstriction is transient, lasting less than one minute, and seems to have little influence on the rate of bleeding. The lumen is not even reduced below two-thirds of its original diameter. The mechanism of vasoconstriction is unclear but is probably related to neurogenic contraction of the vessel wall and the release of various humoral substances, such as serotonin and thromboxane A_2 from activated platelets.

The various blood components are not activated to any significant extent by the healthy vascular endothelial surface. Following vessel wall damage the subsequent interactions with circulating platelets are summarised in Figure 18.1 (Vermylen et al 1983). When the vessel wall is damaged, subendothelial structures are exposed including basement membrane, collagen and microfibrils. Circulating platelets react with exposed collagen fibres and adhere to the damaged surface aided by fibronectin and high molecular weight multimers of factor VIII von Willebrand factor (VIIIvWF) binding to collagen fibres and the platelet surface (Zimmerman & Ruggeri 1983). This protein is synthesised mainly in

vascular endothelial cells but is also formed in megakaryocytes and is present in the platelet granules. The VIIIvWF protein consists of subunits with a M.Wt. of approximately 200 000–240 000 which readily form dimers and subsequently large multimers with molecular weights up to 20 million. It is the large multimeric forms of VIIIvWF with a M.Wt. in excess of 8 million which are essential for platelet adhesion to the damaged vessel wall.

In areas of non-linear blood flow, such as at the site of an injured vessel wall or atherosclerotic plaque, locally damaged red cells release adenosine-5-diphosphate (ADP) which further activates platelets and induces adhesion (Born et al 1976).

Platelets

Platelets circulate as non-nucleated discs and consist of a trilaminar phospholipoprotein membrane with submembrane circumferential contractile filaments, three types of granules and an irregular internal network of canaliculi whereby the granule contents can be released onto the platelet surface.

Following adhesion of a single layer of platelets to the damaged vascular endothelium, platelets stick to one another and form aggregates. Certain substances react with specific platelet membrane surface receptors and initiate platelet aggregation and further activation. These include exposed collagen fibres, ADP released from damaged red cells and other aggregated platelets, adrenaline, serotonin, thrombin and certain arachidonic acid metabolites including thromboxane A_2 (TXA_2). Upon the initiation of aggregation platelets immediately change shape losing their discoid shape, and form tiny spheres with numerous projecting pseudopods.

Human platelet aggregation may be activated by at least two and possibly three independent but related pathways. The first pathway of activation concerns arachidonic acid metabolism (Smith 1987). Activation of phospholipase enzymes releases free arachidonic acid from the membrane phospholipids. Approximately 50% of free arachidonic acid is converted initially by a lipoxy-

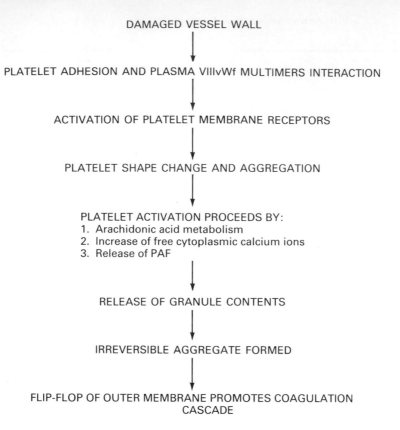

Fig. 18.1 Platelet involvement in the haemostatic process.

genase enzyme to a series of products including various leukotrienes which probably play very little role in the control of haemostasis. The remaining arachidonic acid is converted by the enzyme cyclo-oxygenase into the cyclic endoperoxides, PGG_2 and PGH_2 which are very labile products. Most of the endoperoxides are then rapidly converted by the thromboxane synthetase enzyme complex into thromboxane A_2 (TXA_2). TXA_2 has profound biological activity causing platelet granule release, local vasoconstriction and stimulation of other platelets to aggregate locally. Platelet granules are composed of three distinct groups. The granule types are: dense granules which release adenosine diphosphate (ADP), adenosine triphosphate (ATP), serotonin, and calcium ions; α granules whose release constituents include platelet derived growth factor, platelet factor 4 with heparin neutralising ability, β-thromboglobulin, factor VIII related antigen/von Willebrand factor; factor V, fibrinogen, fibronectin, and probably thrombospondin; and lysosomal granules.

The release of these various granule contents further supports platelet aggregate formation. TXA_2 is a very labile product with a half-life in vivo of approximately 45 seconds before being degraded to the inactive compounds thromboxane B_2 (TXB_2) and malondialdehyde. A small proportion of the cyclic endoperoxides are converted to the primary prostaglandins, PGE_2, PGD_2, and $PGF_{2\alpha}$. Platelet arachidonic acid metabolism is summarised in Figure 18.2.

The second pathway of platelet activation is completely independent of arachidonic acid metabolism and thromboxane A_2 generation. Various platelet activators including thrombin and collagen bring about a sudden increase in the amount of free cytoplasmic calcium (White 1980). Calcium is released from the dense tubular system and forms a complex with calmodulin, and the calcium-calmodulin complex acts as a coenzyme in a series of platelet reactions. It initiates granule release, liberates arachidonic acid from the membrane phospholipids so that it is available for conversion into thromboxane A_2 and activates the actomyosin contractile system of filaments beneath the platelet membrane.

The third pathway involves the release of a lysolecithin compound called PAF-acether (platelet activating factor) from the platelet membrane phospholipids which seems to activate platelets independently of thromboxane A_2 generation and calcium release (Chignard et

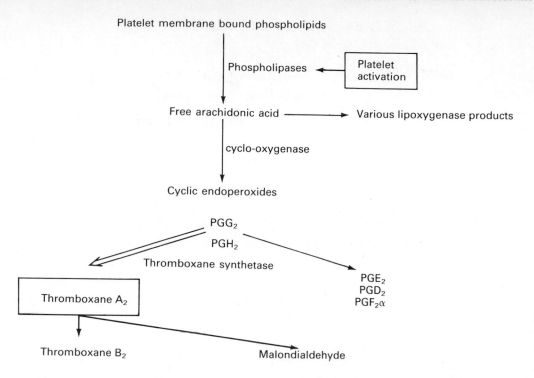

Fig. 18.2 Platelet arachidonic acid metabolism.

al 1980). The actual importance of PAF-acether activation of human platelets has not been fully determined.

The aggregating platelets align together into initially a rather loose reversible aggregate, but following the release reaction of the platelet granule constituents a larger interdigitating irreversible plug is formed. Changes in the configuration of the platelet membrane phospholipids now occur. This involves a flip-flop rearrangement whereby the negatively charged phospholipids, phosphatidyl serine and phosphatidyl inositol, become exposed in higher concentrations on the outer surface (Zwaal & Hemker 1982). Following activation of the coagulation cascade this enables certain reactions involving factors IXa, Xa and II to proceed much faster on the platelet surface by binding of the γ-carboxylated glutamic acid residues of these proteins with calcium ions and the exposed negatively-charged phospholipids. Platelets also possess specific membrane receptors for certain coagulation proteins such as factors X, XIII, Xa and V.

Coagulation

The coagulation mechanism, which consists of a multicomponent enzyme system of pro-enzymes, cofactors and inhibitors, is activated by contact with the negatively charged damaged endothelial surface (the intrinsic pathway) and local release of tissue thromboplastin (the extrinsic pathway). The coagulation reaction is shown schematically in Figure 18.3. The complex interaction of factor XII and high molecular weight kininogen, which are absorbed onto the negatively charged endothelial surface, and the binding of prekallikrein and factor XI to high molecular-weight kininogen lead to the activation of factor XI (Ratnoff 1985). Then follows a series of conversions of inert precursors into active serine proteases leading to fibrin formation. Diffusion of tissue juices into the circulation will activate the extrinsic pathway by converting factor VII into factor VIIa which subsequently activates factor X.

Two main clotting reactions are accelerated by the negatively charged phospholipid bilayer on the platelet surface — firstly, the interaction of activated factor IXa with factor VIII to activate factor X, and, secondly, that of activated factor Xa with factor V to form thrombin from prothrombin. Factors VIII and V are not serine proteases but play a role in orienting clotting factors on the platelet surface so as to accelerate proteolysis of factor X and prothrombin, respectively. Platelets may also actually trigger coagulation by directly activating factor XI and factor X.

Following thrombin formation, fibrinogen is cleaved to form fibrin monomers. These monomers polymerise

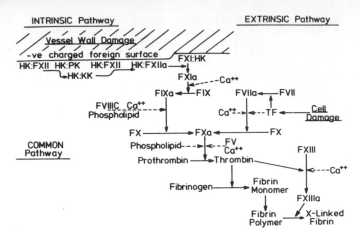

Fig. 18.3 Blood coagulation process.

to form a weak fibrin clot which is stabilised by factor XIII activity. Thrombin further reinforces the haemostatic mechanism by increasing factor VIII and V activity and causing platelet activation. Finally, the stabilised fibrin clot intertwines with the platelet clump, entrapping some red cells and forms a firm plug at the site of initial vessel wall damage.

Fibrinolysis

Once the haemostatic mechanism outlined above has been activated it is important that the reaction should be limited to the initial damaged area and that subsequent repair should be initiated with eventual regrowth of healthy endothelial cells. The digestion of the fibrin clot depends on activation of the fibrinolytic enzyme system which is shown schematically in Figure 18.4 (Gaffney 1987).

Plasminogen circulates as an inactive pro-enzyme and is converted by various different activators to the active serine protease, plasmin. Several different pathways of plasminogen activation exist.

The main source of plasminogen activator is from the vascular endothelial cell (tPA). The release of activator can be stimulated locally or systemically by a variety of physiological stimuli including venous occlusion, exercise, hyperpyrexia, stress and vaso-active agents. However, the vessel wall also releases a potent inhibitor to plasminogen activator activity and it is the overall balance which determines the degree of plasmin generation. The conversion of plasminogen to plasmin occurs most efficiently on the fibrin surface of a thrombus where activator and plasminogen are assembled (Collen 1985). Plasmin then hydrolyses fibrin into soluble split products and brings about gradual thrombus dissolution. Free plasmin in the bloodstream is very rapidly inactivated by α_2-antiplasmin, but plasmin generated at the fibrin surface is partially protected from inactivation. Certain organs, particularly the uterus and pros-

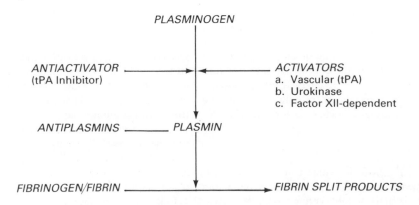

Fig. 18.4 The fibrinolytic system.

tate, release a tissue activator similar in structure and function to the main vascular activator locally after extensive trauma or extravascular fibrin deposition. The renal parenchymal cells synthesise and release a urinary activator, urokinase, which is excreted continuously in the urine and is probably important in maintaining patency of the urinary tract. Other less potent activating systems include a factor XII-mediated pathway which is inter-related with co-activation of kallikrein-kinin and complement systems (Stormorken 1977).

Inhibitors

To prevent uncontrolled activity in the intact circulation of the large number of inter-related reactions leading to fibrin formation, a powerful natural system of coagulation inhibitors exists. Antithrombin III (AT-III) is the major inhibitor of thrombin and factor Xa but also inhibits activated factor IXa, XIa, kallikrein and plasmin (Seegers 1978). Heparin binds to antithrombin III and alters its moleculer configuration so that inhibition of thrombin and factor Xa in particular are markedly accelerated (Rosenberg 1978). The other main plasma thrombin inhibitors are the recently discovered heparin cofactor II and alpha$_2$-macroglobulin. The latter is also an important inhibitor of the contact system, along with C$_1$-inhibitor, and inactivates plasmin when α_2-antiplasmin is overwhelmed by acute hyper fibrinolysis. Two vitamin K-dependent proteins, protein C and protein S, have recently been shown to have important inhibitory properties (Esmon 1983). Protein C is activated by the generation of small amounts of thrombin and inactivates the coenzyme activities of factor VIII:C and factor V. Protein S acts as a cofactor with protein C in inactivating factor V. As well as these inhibitory proteins, it seems likely that both coagulation pathways can control their own activity to some extent by a series of feedback proteolytic mechanisms.

Platelets do not adhere to undamaged endothelial cells, and in the last decade it has been shown that vascular endothelial cells play an important role in the control of the haemostatic process (Nawroth et al 1986). Endothelial cells synthesise prostacyclin from arachidonic acid which, when released into the circulation, causes local vasodilation and is the most potent known natural inhibitor of platelet adhesion and aggregation (Whittle & Moncada 1983). Prostacyclin probably does not circulate in biological quantities but is released locally when the vessel wall is stressed or injured so as to control any excessive platelet activation. Upon binding to specific platelet membrane receptors it activates membrane-bound adenylate cyclase which produces increased levels of cAMP. This inhibits platelet aggregation by inhibiting arachidonic acid metabolism and internal calcium flux. The vascular endothelial cell also synthesises, stores, and releases into the circulation prostaglandin E$_2$, plasminogen activator and inhibitor, factor VIIIvWF, fibronectin, a heparin-like material, and possesses a thrombin-induced binding site for protein C. All these processes control interactions between the blood and vessel wall and thus help to maintain vascular integrity and patency.

REFERENCES

Bennett B (1977) Coagulation pathways: inter-relationship and control mechanisms. Seminars in hematology XIV 3: 301–318.

Born G V, Bergguist D, Arfors K E (1976) Evidence inhibition of platelet activation in blood by a drug effect on erythrocytes. Nature 259: 233–235.

Chignard M, Le Couedic J P, Vergaftig B B, Benveniste J (1980) Platelet-activating factor (PAF-acether) secretion from platelets: effect of aggregating agents. British Journal of Haematology 46: 455–464.

Collen D (1985). Fibrinolysis: mechanism and clinical aspects. In: Bowie E J, Sharp A A (eds) Haemostasis and thrombosis, Butterworths, London, p 237–258.

Esmon C T (1983) Protein C: biochemistry, physiology and clinical implications. Blood 62: 1155–1158.

Gaffney P J (1987) Fibrinolysis. In: Bloom A L, Thomas D P T (eds) Haemostasis and thrombosis, 2nd edition. Churchill Livingstone, Edinburgh, p 223–244.

Nawroth P P, Mandley D A, Stern D M (1986) The multiple levels of endothelial cell-coagulation factor interactions. Clinics in Haematology 15: 2, 298–321.

Ratnoff O D (1985). The significance of contact activation. In: Bowie E J, Sharp A A (eds) Haemostasis and thrombosis. Butterworths, London, p 75–97.

Rosenberg R D (1978) Heparin, antithrombin and abnormal clotting. Annual Review of Medicine 29: 367–378.

Seegers W H (1978) Antithrombin III: theory and clinical implications. American Journal of Clinical Pathology 69: 299–359.

Sixma J J, Wester J (1977) The hemostatic plug. Seminars in Hematology XIV 3: 265–299.

Smith J B (1987) Prostaglandins in platelet aggregation and haemostasis. In: Bloom A L, Thomas D P (eds) Haemostasis and thrombosis, 2nd edition. Churchill Livingstone, Edinburgh, p 78–89.

Stormorken H (1977) Activation and interaction of some defence systems. Recent advances in blood coagulation, vol 2. Churchill Livingstone, Edinburgh, p 35–58.

Vermylen J, Badenhorst P N, Deckmyn H, Arnout J (1983) Normal mechanisms of platelet function. Clinics in Haematology 12: 107–152.

White G C (1980) Calcium-dependent proteins in platelets. Biochimica Biophysica Acta 631: 130–139.

Whittle B J R Moncada S (1983) Pharmacological interactions betweem prostacyclin and thromboxanes. British Medical Bulletin 39: 232–238.

Zimmerman T S, Ruggeri Z N (1983) Von Willebrand's disease. Clinics in Haematology 12: 175–200.

Zwall R F A, Hemker H C (1982) Blood cell membranes and haemostasis. Haemostasis II: 12–39.

19

Approach to a haemostatic problem

GENERAL APPROACH TO THE INVESTIGATION OF A BLEEDING TENDENCY

The haemostatic process is carefully balanced so that haemorrhage is promptly arrested and inappropriate thrombosis does not occur. The causes of haemostatic failure are numerous and it is useful to have a standardised initial approach to the clinical and laboratory diagnosis of any bleeding tendency.

The initial problem is to determine whether bleeding is due to a local factor, such as a peptic ulcer, or to an underlying haemostatic abnormality. Often a mild abnormality only becomes apparent after trauma or a local precipitating lesion. Any bleeding disorder may be inherited or acquired. This may result from one of the following mechanisms;

1. Thrombocytopenia
2. Functional platelet abnormality
3. Blood vessel defect
4. Coagulation factor (s) defect
5. Excess fibrinolysis
6. Combined defect

A careful clinical history, drug history and physical examination should be undertaken, and special care must be taken in patients with multi-system disease to recognise any bleeding tendency. In particular, continual oozing from venepuncture and drip sites, extensive petechiae and purpura at pressure areas, and steady blood loss from drainage tubes are often signs of impending haemostatic failure. Often the cause of the bleeding will then be strongly suspected but laboratory tests are always required to make a precise diagnosis and to define the severity of any abnormality.

Most patients with an inherited disorder present in childhood, often with a family history of a bleeding tendency and excessive bleeding in response to minor operations, dental extractions, or trauma. However, mild defects may sometimes not present until adult life, and occasionally in old age, often as a result of minor trauma or operative procedure. If an inherited disorder is suspected, no effort should be spared to investigate other family members who might also be affected.

Initially a series of simple screening tests which are easy to perform and give reliable results should be undertaken.

A suggested screening procedure is given below. The normal range for each test performed in the particular laboratory involved should be known before any results can be interpreted. If the screening tests suggest an abnormality, further specialised investigations should be followed as outlined below. If the screening tests are all within normal limits, it is unlikely that the bleeding tendency is related to a haemostatic disorder. In certain circumstances one should always be aware of the possibility of self-injury in the psychiatrically disturbed or mistreatment of the patient by relatives or other people in close attendance.

Screening tests for a bleeding tendency

1. For Coagulation disorders
   Prothrombin time (PT)
   Activated partial thromboplastin time (APTT)
   Thrombin time (TT)
   Fibrinogen assay

2. For platelet disorders
   Bleeding time
   Platelet count
   Fresh blood film inspection

3. For vascular disorders
   Bleeding time

GENERAL APPROACH TO THE INVESTIGATION OF A THROMBOTIC TENDENCY

Over the last decade important advances have been made in clinical diagnostic techniques, management and clinical trial methodology in arterial thrombotic disease and venous thrombo-embolism. In patients with severe, unexpected or repeated thrombotic episodes there are several important laboratory approaches to the investigation of the haemostatic system. Firstly, one must exclude a single specific inherited or acquired abnormality which might predispose to repeated thrombotic events. These defects include:

1. Abnormal fibrinogen
2. Antithrombin III
3. Protein C
4. Protein S
5. Heparin cofactor II
6. Lupus-type anticoagulant

Secondly, one must discover if a generalised hypercoagulable state exists and whether any particular part of the haemostatic system outlined previously is deranged. To answer these two important theoretical questions an initial screening test should be designed which is as complete as is locally feasible. A simplified screening test is outlined below. If a defect is suggested by the initial thrombotic screen more detailed studies should be performed as described in the following sections.

Lastly, it is often difficult clinically to confirm or exclude a diagnosis of on-going thrombosis. A sensitive and specific test to detect excessive intravascular thrombin generation and fibrin formation would be helpful. Unfortunately at the present time a reliable single blood test is not available. The details of laboratory control of antithrombotic therapy are dealt with separately.

Screening profile for a thrombotic or hypercoagulable state

1. Coagulation system
Prothrombin time
Thrombin time
Activated partial thromboplastin time with 50/50 mixture
Antithrombin III
Protein C
Protein S
Lupus anticoagulant test

2. Platelets
Platelet count
Platelet aggregation studies
Plasma β-thromboglobulin

3. Fibrinolytic system
Euglobin lysis time
Tissue plasminogen activator

GENERAL CONSIDERATIONS IN LABORATORY WORK

Certain items of equipment and materials are standard in coagulation laboratories and are used in many of the tests and assays described in this book. They are therefore described here, and only specialised reagents, samples and equipment will be noted under each individual method.

No written method can substitute for years of technical experience with a method at the bench. Many of the assay methods presented are merely intended as a guide; a certain level of knowledge is assumed and, where possible, the reader should visit a specialist laboratory for instruction. The competent investigator wishing to follow the more complex of these procedures is recommended to read the relevant literature, where certain experimental steps may be described in more detail.

Blood samples
Venous blood should be collected with minimal stasis, preferably from the antecubital fossa, using a large (19–21 gauge) needle. 'Butterflies' may often be helpful where multiple syringes must be filled. For many coagulation tests citrated blood is required. Blood is collected into 0.106 M Tri-sodium citrate in a ratio of 9:1. Plastic tubes should be used, where possible with accurate marks for filling. The tubes should not be stored for long periods of time as the anticoagulant may dry out. Blood should be mixed gently with the citrate by inverting the tube several times, shaking or violent mixing will cause lysis and activation. Where the haematocrit is grossly abnormal, the amount of citrate should be corrected to allow for the altered plasma volume (and consequent change in divalent cation concentration) as indicated in Table 19.1. Specimens

Table 19.1 Adjustment of citrate concentration for variations in PCV. Approximate volumes of citrate (ml) to add to 5 ml or 10 ml blood collection tubes.

PCV	5 ml tube	10 ml tube
0.20	0.70	1.40
0.25	0.65	1.30
0.30	0.61	1.22
0.35	0.57	1.14
0.40	0.52	1.05
0.45	0.48	0.96
0.50	0.44	0.88
0.55	0.39	0.78
0.60	0.36	0.72
0.65	0.31	0.62
0.70	0.27	0.54

should be examined for clots, fibrin strands, and haemolysis, as well as ensuring that the citrate/blood ratio is correct. Blood should generally be kept at room temperature prior to the separation of plasma, particularly in studies of platelets, factor VII and contact factors.

Preparation, handling and storage

Blood samples should be handled as quickly as possible after collection to avoid deterioration. They should be maintained at room temperature until centrifuged and separated. Centrifugation at 2000 g (approximately 4000 rpm in a standard bench centrifuge, see Fig. 19.1.)

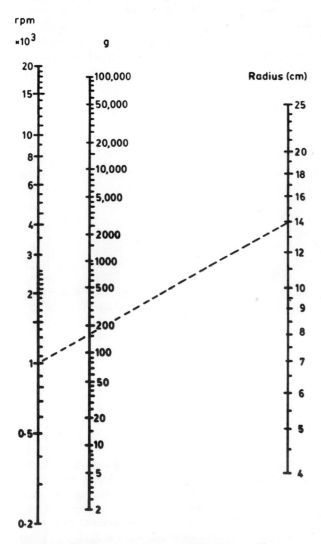

rpm

×10³

g

Radius (cm)

Fig. 19.1 Nomogram of relative centrifugal force. The centrifuge radius from the rotor centre to half-way along the specimen tube (with the bucket swung out) is measured. A line is drawn between this radius and the desired relative centrifugal force (g force) on the nomogram, and the centrifuge speed in rpm is read off.

gives a good separation of platelet-poor plasma, which can be pipetted off with a plastic Pasteur pipette into polystyrene tubes. These are capped and stored on ice or frozen below −20°C. Plasma should not come into contact with glass at this stage, or activation may occur. Generally, the colder the storage the slower the deterioration of the sample, and if long-term storage is required very low temperature freezers (below −70°C) or liquid nitrogen storage should be used. In the latter case, specialised plasma containers are needed. For the measurement of labile substances and storage of labile reagents during use, tubes should be kept in crushed ice (which is conveniently kept in polystyrene boxes) or 4°C water baths. Alternatively cryoracks may be used, these contain glycol, and after storing at −20°C overnight, they maintain a cold temperature on the bench during a working day.

Normal controls

Whenever possible, healthy laboratory staff should be bled as controls. A rota system makes this most convenient and fair for everyone. This means that one can work with a known and well-studied population, who are more aware of problems that may affect the tests for which they are controls and will, hopefully inform you of any acute medical problems. The risk from dangerous viruses is also limited. Subjects with a chronic illness should not be used, as their acute phase reactants (e.g. fibrinogen, factor VIIIC) may be increased, and similar problems occur if pregnant women are bled as controls. Age and sex will also affect clotting factor levels, and the stage of menstrual cycle or use of the contraceptive pill will modify results. For platelet function controls, diet, alcohol intake and use of patent medicines as well as prescription compounds must be checked. For many tests of coagulation it is best to use pooled normal plasma consisting of at least 10 donors, and as large as can be obtained.

Standards

National or internationally recognised standards should be used where available, otherwise commercial standards from reputable companies should be obtained. Failing the availability of these, local pooled normal plasmas should be used.

Water-baths

A 37°C water bath is required for thawing deep frozen plasmas, incubation steps, and for manual coagulation tests where the end point is a fibrin clot. The tolerance should be less than 0.5°C. Distilled water should be used to maintain the water level, to avoid furring of the heater and thermostat. Suitable mild antiseptics which are not contraindicated by the manufacturer's instructions should be used to keep the bath free from bacterial growth. Baths should be cleaned regularly, especially if there has been spillage of biological materials. A black tile in the water-bath and illumination from an Anglepoise lamp are desirable to help detect fibrin clot end points.

Reagents and buffers

Where the product of one manufacturer only is quoted it is because that particular product has been found suitable by the authors and is recommended. Where several products are cited the authors have tried them and any one of these would be suitable. Attention must be paid to the age and condition of solutions. Buffers should be inspected before use for bacterial growth, and whenever a solution is prepared it should be labelled with the date. Contamination with microorganisms can cause errors and assay failures due to the release of enzymes and other active biological substances into solution. Azide may be added as a preservative to some buffers, but should not be used in reagents for platelet studies or ELISA substrates. Chromogenic substrates should be reconstituted with sterile water, as bacterial enzymes may cause pNA release and a yellow discolouration of the reagent. Longterm storage should either be in the freeze-dried state, or frozen aliquots.

Plastic and glass tubes

For clotting tests, 75×10 mm glass rimless test tubes should be used and are referred to in the methods as 'glass clotting tubes'. Plastic tubes for sample dilutions, storage, and reagent preparation should usually be polystyrene, and a range of sizes with suitable caps should be kept.

Safety

Each laboratory should have its own safety recommendations, taking into account the use of specialised equipment, and procedures to follow in case of accident or contamination. Attention should be paid to fire, chemical, mechanical and microbiological safety aspects, and the handling of automated equipment.

Pipettes

A range of graduated glass and automatic pipettes must be obtained. The latter should be sufficiently accurate and durable, e.g. Gilson Pipetman, Eppendorf Finpipette, and SMI. Fluids should not be drawn into the pipette barrels and acids should not be pipetted with instruments containing metal piston assemblies, which may become pitted or corroded. Attention to technique is vital, as contamination of reagents with used pipette tips may occur, there may be errors of volume due to fluid on the exterior of the pipette tip, or the manner of addition of a reagent may alter the results obtained.

Stopwatches and clocks

Stopclocks are useful for timing incubation periods of several minutes or more, but stopwatches which may be easily held in the hand, and controlled should be used for measuring clotting times and for short incubations.

Glass ware

Where glass vessels are non-disposable, they should be washed in chromic acid or 2% Decon 90 (or similar detergent) and extensively rinsed afterwards. Residual detergent will have gross effects on clotting times, as will thrombin remaining stuck to used glass ware. It is recommended that glass tubes used for clotting times should be disposed of after use and not reused. Chromic acid is extremely caustic and must be used carefully; it will rapidly remove agarose gel blocking tubes and glass pipettes.

SCREENING TESTS

THROMBIN TIME (TT)

Principle

This test measures the formation of a fibrin clot in plasma by the action of thrombin on fibrinogen (Fig. 19.2).

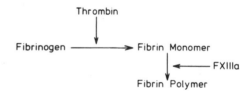

Fig. 19.2 The thrombin–fibrinogen interation.

Biochemical basis

Fibrinogen is composed of three pairs of non-identical polypeptide chains known as the alpha, beta, and gamma chains. These chains are interconnected by a series of disulphide bonds and the structure is denoted as (alpha$_2$, beta$_2$, gamma$_2$).

The molecule consists of a central domain with the amino-terminal segments of all 6 chains. Proceeding away from this central area there are two bundles, each consisting of three strands each (α, β, γ chains). These strands are gathered together at two nodes by disulphide rings and in between these two rings is an alpha-helical region. The terminal domain is composed of the carboxy two-thirds of the beta and gamma chains and the alpha chain protrudes as a highly polar appendage.

Thrombin catalyses the transformation of fibrinogen into fibrin by cleaving the alpha and beta chains at their amino terminals and releasing fibrinopeptides A and B. Release of fibrinopeptides A and B allows the central domain of one molecule (so-called fibrin monomer) to interact with the terminal domain of another molecule to form a dimer. Subsequently other fibrin monomers interact to form a polymerising oligomer which is the gelled and semisolid fibrin clot.

Reagents
- Bovine thrombin (e.g. Parke-Davis); dilute with isotonic saline (approximately 7 u/ml) to give a control thrombin time of 13–15 seconds; store in aliquots at −20°C.
- Isotonic saline

Controls
Pooled normal control plasma

Method
1. Add 0.1 ml of saline to duplicate glass tubes in a 37°C water-bath.
2. Add 0.1 ml of plasma to each tube.
3. Incubate for 30 seconds.
4. Add 0.1 ml of diluted bovine thrombin to each tube, mix immediately.
5. Record time for a visible fibrin clot to form.
6. Carry out the above procedure for both normal control plasma and test plasma.

Results
Express the thrombin time in seconds as the mean of the duplicates for the control and test plasmas.
The control thrombin time should be within 12–15 seconds.

Comments
- Detection of the end point may be difficult in samples with low levels of fibrinogen (hypofibrinogenaemia), an abnormal fibrinogen molecule (dysfibrinogenaemia) or excess of heparin. In these cases only a few fibrin strands rather than a solid clot will be seen.
- If no clot is seen after 120 seconds stop the test and express results as >120 seconds.
- Short control times should be avoided as mild abnormalities may be missed. If the control time is shorter than 12 seconds the bovine thrombin requires further dilution.

Interpretation
Normal range — within 2 seconds of control time. A prolonged thrombin time may be caused by:
  a. Deficiency of fibrinogen — this may be inherited (afibrinogenaemia or hypofibrinogenaemia) or acquired.

  b. Abnormal fibrinogen molecule (dysfibrinogenaemia) — inherited or acquired.
  c. Raised levels of FDPs.
  d. Presence of heparin in the sample. This may have been added inadvertently at the time of sample collection or the patient may be receiving heparin therapeutically.
  e. Grossly elevated fibrinogen levels. This effect disappears if the sample is diluted.
The approach to the further investigation of a prolonged thrombin time is discussed in the subsequent section.

PROTHROMBIN TIME (PT)

Principle
This test measures the extrinsic pathway of coagulation. Tissue factor (extracted from brain tissue) and calcium ions are added to plasma resulting in the activation of extrinsic clotting factors, thrombin generation and formation of a fibrin clot (Fig. 19.3). A number of modifications of the original PT (Quick 1935) have been described: P & P test, Normotest, and Thrombotest (see p. 333). The thromboplastins used in the modified systems contain added factor V and are therefore insensitive to a deficiency of factor V, but sensitive to the vitamin K-dependent factors, II, VII and X. They are used primarily in the monitoring of anticoagulant therapy. The method of Quick is the most suitable for investigation of an inherited or acquired coagulation defect of the extrinsic system.

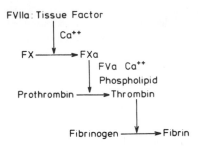

Fig. 19.3 Reactions involved in the prothrombin time test.

Biochemical basis
Tissue factor can be released from a wide range of cell types following rupture or damage, and activates the extrinsic pathway of coagulation. Tissue factor is usually retained on the surface of the damaged cell and forms a calcium-dependent complex with factor VII. In so doing, it alters the conformation of factor VII and exposes the active site; it then catalyses the activation of factor X by factor VII. The factor Xa thus generated cleaves prothrombin in a reaction catalysed by factor

Va, phospholipid and calcium ions, liberating thrombin (Fig. 19.3)

Reagents

- Brain thromboplastin — Manchester reagent or Diagen phenolised suspension. The International Sensitivity Index (ISI) of each batch must be noted.
- 0.025 M Calcium chloride — maintain at 37°C.

Controls

Pooled normal plasma or commercial quality control samples.

Method

1. Add 0.1 ml thromboplastin to duplicate glass tubes in a 37°C water-bath.
2. Add 0.1 ml normal control plasma to each tube.
3. Incubate for 1 minute.
4. Add 0.1 ml calcium chloride to each tube in turn and simultaneously start stopwatch.
5. Record time in seconds for a visible fibrin clot to form.
6. Repeat steps 1–5 with test plasmas.

Results

Express the prothrombin time in seconds as the mean of the duplicates for the control and test plasmas.
Control time should be 13–15 seconds.
When using the prothrombin time for oral anticoagulant control, the result should also be expressed as the International Normalised Ratio (INR) (see p. 329).

Comments

— Lightly shake tube prior to addition of calcium chloride to avoid sedimentation of thromboplastin particles.
— End-point detection may be difficult in samples with low fibrinogen levels or if there is an excess of heparin. In these circumstances a few fibrin strands may be seen instead of a solid clot.
— If no clot is seen after 180 seconds the test should be stopped and reported as >180 seconds.

Interpretation

Normal Range — within 2 seconds of control time. The phenolised rabbit brain suspensions described have excellent sensitivity to decreased levels of factors II, V, VII, and X activity and to the acarboxylated (PIVKA) forms of factors II, VII, and X found in patients on oral anticoagulants or suffering from vitamin K-deficient states.

A prolonged prothrombin time may be caused by:
a. Deficiency of factors II, V, X, or VII — inherited defects or acquired due to consumption (e.g. DIC), liver disease (vitamin K deficiency or lack of synthesis),

dilution (massive transfusion), anticoagulation (coumarin derivatives).
b. Presence of lupus anticoagulant.
c. Presence of specific inhibitors to coagulation factors.
d. High levels of heparin.
e. Very low levels of fibrinogen.
The approach to the further investigation of a prolonged prothrombin time is discussed in a following section.

ACTIVATED PARTIAL THROMBOPLASTIN TIME (APTT)

Principle

In this test an activator such as kaolin triggers the intrinsic coagulation pathway by activating the contact factors. In the presence of calcium ions and phospholipid (partial thromboplastin), the contact factors cause a cascade of enzyme reactions culminating in the generation of thrombin, and fibrin clot formation.

Biochemical basis

Kaolin binds to factor XII and alters its conformation, exposing the active site. Factor XIIa takes part in a positive feedback loop activating prekallikrein to kallikrein in the presence of high molecular weight kininogen (HK). This kallikrein feeds back onto factor XII generating more factor XIIa. In a second HK catalysed reaction, factor XIIa activates factor XI, which starts a series of reactions dependent on calcium ions and phospholipid, with factor VIIIa or factor Va as catalysts (Fig. 19.4).

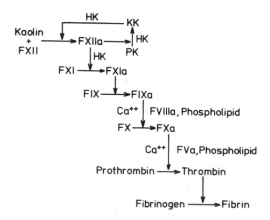

Fig. 19.4 Reactions taking place in the APTT system.

Reagents

- 0.05 g kaolin (light kaolin, BDH Chemical) in 10 ml Tris buffer.
- Tris buffer 0.2 M pH 7.4 — 24.23 g Tris base in 1 litre distilled water, pH adjusted with HCl.

- Platelet substitute (Diagen; Bell & Alton).
- 0.025 M Calcium chloride

Controls
Pooled normal plasma or commercial quality control samples.

Method
1. Add 0.1 ml plasma to duplicate glass tubes in 37°C water - bath.
2. Add 0.1 ml kaolin suspension, mix and start clock.
3. Remix kaolin at regular intervals.
4. After 9 minutes 45 seconds add 0.1 ml platelet substitute.
5. At 10 minutes add 0.1 ml calcium chloride and mix.
6. Record time for visible fibrin clot to form.
7. Carry out steps 1–5 for control and patient plasmas.

Results
Express the APTT in seconds as the mean of the duplicates for the control and test plasmas.

Comments
— It is convenient to perform a batch of tests together with a control.
— Decreased levels of clotting factors or presence of inhibitors may make the end point difficult to see. In these circumstances a few fibrin strands may be seen rather than a solid fibrin clot.
— Interpretation of prolonged APTTs is helped by testing mixtures of control and patient plasmas, particularly a 50:50 mix.
— A wide range of activators and reagents is available for APTTs, with varying sensitivity. The incubation time and order of addition of reagents also varies considerably between laboratories. Shorter incubation times appear to be more sensitive to contact factor deficiencies, but may miss mild coagulation factor deficiencies.

Interpretation
Normal range 30–40 seconds.
A prolonged APTT may be caused by:
  a. Deficiency of factors II, V, X, VIII, IX, XI, XII, PK, HK, or fibrinogen due to inherited defects (e.g. haemophilia), or acquired because of consumption (e.g. DIC), liver disease (vitamin K deficiency or decreased synthesis), dilution (massive transfusion), or anticoagulation (coumarin derivatives).
  b. Heparin therapy.
  c. Specific inhibitors.
  d. Lupus anticoagulant.
The performance of a mixing test with normal plasma helps to differentiate between a and c or d.

The further investigation of a prolonged APTT is outlined in a subsequent section.

REFERENCE

Quick A J 1935 The prothrombin in haemophilia and obstructive jaundice. Journal of Biological Chemistry 109: LXII–LXIV.

20

Investigation of a prolonged thrombin time

The thrombin time (TT) is prolonged in three basic situations: deficiency, molecular abnormality, and in the presence of an inhibitor. Deficiency may arise because of an inherited defect such as afibrinogenaemia or hypofibrinogenaemia, or acquired due to decreased synthesis in liver failure, or increased consumption as in DIC. Abnormal fibrinogen molecules, the 'dysfibrinogens', can arise because of congenital defects involving changes of primary sequence, or in liver disease, where there is an excess sialic acid portion of the molecule, which interferes with fibrin monomer polymerisation. Immunoglobulin inhibitors have been noted in paraproteinaemias and some auto-immune disorders, but inhibition is seen more often with heparin, or in the presence of FDPs which interfere in the thrombin/fibrinogen reaction, and can affect fibrin monomer polymerisation. The congenital defects, though rare, are important to diagnose, since fibrinogen deficiency can cause a marked bleeding diathesis which is easily correctable with fresh frozen plasma or cryoprecipitate. Congenital dysfibrinogens may cause thrombosis as well as a bleeding tendency and one should consider the use of antithrombotic prophylaxis if there is a thrombotic history, or a strong family history; however there is no proven treatment. Acquired abnormalities of fibrinogen, and other factors influencing the TT may often be seen together in severely ill patients, and must be delineated to allow suitable treatment.

Simple correction tests will often yield a great deal of information, the addition of normal plasma will demonstrate the presence of an inhibitor, protamine sulphate will correct in a dose-dependent manner for heparin contamination, as well as for FDPs. Toluidine Blue usually corrects thrombin times prolonged by liver dysfibrinogens, whereas protamine does not; it will also correct for heparin. A more specific test for heparin is to perform a reptilase time, since this test is not influenced by the anticoagulant; however care must be exercised in patients who have an underlying fibrinogen abnormality as well as heparin contamination. More specific tests of the fibrinogen molecule are of course available, and it is probably the easiest coagulation factor to measure. Apart from the specific assays, certain functional characteristics may be assessed such as fibrin monomer polymerisation and fibrinopeptide release.

CORRECTION TESTS

Principle
These tests utilise certain physicochemical properties of reagents to bind to inhibitors or abnormal molecules and normalise the thrombin time.

Biochemical basis
Protamine sulphate has a net electropositive charge and interacts with the sulphate groups on heparin, as well as binding to FDPs, neutralising the inhibitory effects of both. Toluidine Blue is also a charged reagent which will neutralise heparin, but not FDPs; it also normalises the thrombin time in dysfibrinogenaemia, probably by interaction with the excess sialic acid attached to these molecules.

Reagents
- 1 and 10 mg% protamine sulphate (Weddel Pharmaceuticals Ltd).
- 0.05 g Toluidine Blue in 100 ml saline.
- Bovine thrombin (Parke Davis).
- Isotonic saline.

Method
1. Place 0.1 ml plasma in a glass tube at 37°C.
2. Add 0.1 ml Toluidine Blue or protamine sulphate.
3. Warm for 1 minute.
4. Add 0.1 ml thrombin.
5. Record clotting time in seconds.
6. Carry out steps 1–5 for control and patient plasmas.
7. Also perform thrombin time on a 50/50 mix of control and normal plasmas plus saline.

Comments

— The end point may be particularly difficult to see in samples with low fibrinogen content in the toluidine correction owing to the dark colour of the reagent.

— If there is no correction with the 1 mg% protamine solution, the 10 mg% solution should be used.

— The use of calcium chloride instead of saline often improves the visualisation of end points, but one must adjust the system due to the shortening of the control time.

— Grossly elevated fibrinogen levels, or the presence of paraproteins can be a cause of prolonged TT; this can be eliminated by making doubling dilutions of test and normal plasma in saline, and performing the TT.

Interpretation

For interpretation see Table 20.1.

Table 20.1 Thrombin time correction tests. Influence of various reagents on the TT.

Reagent	Saline	NP	Protamine	Toluidine
Deficiency	INC	COR	NC	NC
High FG	COR	NC	NC	NC
Liver disease	NC	?	NC	COR
Heparin	NC	NC	COR*	COR*
FDPs	NC	?	COR	NC

Key: NP = normal plasma; FG = fibrinogen;
INC = increased; COR = corrected; NC = no correction;
* = dependent on dose of reagent/heparin concentration.

REPTILASE TIME

Principle

This test measures the formation of a fibrin clot in plasma by the action of reptilase on fibrinogen.

Biochemical basis

Reptilase is a brand name for a snake venom preparation from *Bothrops atrox*. This venom contains an enzyme very similar to thrombin, but which cleaves fibrinogen only on the alpha chain, without cleaving the beta chain so that only fibrinopeptide A is liberated — this is sufficient for the formation of a fibrin clot. The action of reptilase on other thrombin substrates differs, and it is not inhibited by heparin.

Reagents

Reptilase reagent (Paines & Byrne Ltd).

Controls

Pooled normal plasma.

Method

1. Place 0.2 ml of plasma in duplicate glass tubes at 37°C.
2. Warm for 1 minute.
3. Add 0.1 ml reptilase reagent.
4. Measure time in seconds for visible fibrin formation.
5. Carry out for control and patient plasmas.

Interpretation

Normal Range — within 2 seconds of control time.
The reptilase time may be prolonged by:

a. Decreased fibrinogen levels in inherited defects (afibrinogenaemia or hypofibrinogenaemia), or acquired defects (liver disease, DIC, etc.).

b. Inhibitors such as FDPs and specific immunoglobulin inhibitors of fibrinogen.

A completely normal reptilase time when the TT is significantly prolonged suggests the presence of heparin, which is not effective in this test.

FIBRINOGEN TITRE

Principle

A series of dilutions of plasma are made, so that the fibrinogen content is gradually diluted out to a point where a clot is no longer obtained. The dilution at which the fibrinogen is diluted out indicates the approximate concentration present. This is a rapid test for estimating the fibrinogen level, which may be incubated while a clotting screen is performed and read at the end. Though far less accurate than the assays described below, it can give extra information about inhibitors and fibrinolysis.

Reagents

- Saline 0.9% w/v.
- EACA 1 mg/ml in saline (6 amino-n-hexanoic acid).
- Protamine sulphate 40 mg in 100 ml saline (Weddel Pharmaceuticals Ltd.).
- Thrombin 10 u/ml (Parke Davis Ltd.).

Method

1. Place a row of 10 tubes in a 37°C water-bath.
2. Add 0.5 ml saline to tubes 2–10.
3. Add 0.5 ml plasma to tubes 1 and 2, then double dilute 0.5 ml from tube 2 through the row, discarding 0.5 ml from the last tube.
4. Add 1 drop of thrombin to each tube and mix.
5. After 10 minutes tilt the tubes and check for clot formation.
6. Find the highest dilution which has formed a clot.

Comments

— Heparin-contaminated plasma may show inhibition of clot formation in the first few tubes, and so all tubes should be read.
— The tubes should be read again after 1 hour, if increased fibrinolysis is present the result will drop by more than 1 tube.
— Hyperfibrinolysis may also be detected by comparing saline and EACA titres. Since the latter inhibits fibrinolysis, the titre will be at least 4-fold greater in the EACA row of tubes than in the saline row, if there is excessive fibrinolysis.
— When FDP levels are very high, e.g. in streptokinase therapy, their effect may be neutralised by making the 1/2 dilution in protamine sulphate and then diluting through the rest of the row in saline.

Interpretation

Normal fibrinogen titre — 1/64 or higher.
The fibrinogen titre may be influenced by:
  a. Decreased fibrinogen levels.
  b. Presence of inhibitors (specific immunoglobulin inhibitors, heparin, FDPs).
  c. Hyperfibrinolysis.

GRAVIMETRIC FIBRINOGEN ASSAY (CLOT WEIGHT ASSAY)

Principle

Excess thrombin is added to a fixed volume of plasma so that all clottable fibrinogen is removed from solution. If the remaining 'serum' is expressed, and the partially purified fibrin dried, its weight can be determined and related to the volume of plasma from which it was obtained. This test is accurate providing a sensitive chemical balance is available, and a good technique is used, but is slow to yield results. It is less affected by inhibitors and does not suffer from the difficult end-point detection of the Clauss assay.

Reagents

● 0.025 M calcium chloride.
● Bovine thrombin 10 u/ml (Parke Davis Ltd.).
● Saline.
● Acetone.

Equipment

○ Glass tubes 14 × 100 mm.
○ Applicator sticks.
○ Scalpel blade.
○ Petri dish.
○ Oven or incubator.
○ Microbalance (at least 4 decimal places).

Standard

Commercial standard or calibrated plasma.

Method

1. Place 1 ml plasma in a glass tube at 37°C.
2. Add 1 ml calcium chloride and 0.2 ml thrombin.
3. Mix well and incubate for 30 minutes.
4. Gently squeeze clot against test tube wall with 2 applicator sticks until all serum is expressed.
5. Carefully remove clot from sticks using a scalpel blade.
6. Wash clot twice in saline for 10 minutes.
7. Wash clot in distilled water for 10 minutes.
8. Dry clot in acetone for 10 minutes.
9. Place clot in a petri dish in an oven for at least 4 hours at 37°C or appropriate time at higher temperatures until dry.
10. Weigh clot on balance.

Calculation

If 1 ml of plasma was used, the weight is obtained in g/ml.
This is corrected to g/l and multiplied by 10/9 to correct for citrate to give the result as g/l plasma fibrinogen.

i.e. g/l Fibrinogen = weight in g $\times$ 1000 $\times$ 10/9

Comments

— For samples with excess heparin, protamine may be required for neutralisation.
— Samples with very low fibrinogen will yield small clots which are difficult to handle without loss and inaccurate to weigh. This may be resolved by using larger volumes of plasma and adjusting the calculation appropriately.
— Great care must be taken to ensure that no part of the clot is lost during handling.

Interpretation

Normal range — 1.5–4.0 g/l

FIBRINOGEN — CLAUSS ASSAY

Principle

Various dilutions of standard plasma with known fibrinogen concentration and of test plasma are clotted with an excess of thrombin. The relationship between fibrinogen level and clotting time is linear over a certain range of concentrations, and therefore the factor can be assayed. This assay is quick to perform, with good accuracy, but end-point detection may sometimes be difficult on low fibrinogen samples, and at high dilution; heparin and dysfibrinogens can yield erroneous results.

Reagents

- Imidazole (Glyoxaline) buffer 0.05 M pH 7.3–3.4 g imidazole, 5.85 g sodium chloride, 1 litre distilled water. Adjust pH with HCl.
- Bovine thrombin 100 u/ml (Parke Davis Ltd.).

Standard

Commercial standard or calibrated plasma.

Method

1. Prepare 1/5, 1/10, 1/20, and 1/40 dilutions of standard in polystyrene tubes at room temperature.
2. Pipette 0.2 ml of each dilution into duplicate glass tubes at 37°C.
3. Add 0.1 ml of thrombin and mix.
4. Record time in seconds for visible fibrin formation to occur.
5. Repeat for a 1/10 dilution of test plasma.

Calculation

A double logarithm plot of clotting time against dilution of standard is prepared. Taking the patients clotting time, the percentage activity is abstracted, and corrected to g/l.

Test potency (g/1)
= % activity × standard potency (g/l) / 100

Comments

— If the test sample has a high fibrinogen concentration, short clotting times will be obtained and the sample should therefore be further diluted and appropriate correction made at the end.
— If the test sample has a low fibrinogen concentration, a 1/5 dilution should be used and the result corrected.
— Heparinised samples may give false low results, but this may be counteracted by dissolving protamine sulphate in the diluting buffer to a concentration of 10 mg%.
— Dysfibrinogens may also give low results.

Interpretation

Normal range — 1.5–4.0 g/l.

FIBRINOGEN ANTIGEN (RADIAL IMMUNODIFFUSION)

Principle

An agarose gel containing precipitating antibody to fibrinogen is poured onto a glass plate or suitable support. After it has set, wells are made in the gel, and various dilutions of standard or test plasma are placed in the wells. As the plasma diffuses into the gel, fibrinogen binds antibody until equivalence is reached and the complex precipitates out giving a white ring. The diameter of this ring is proportional to the fibrinogen concentration. This assay is helpful when studying certain abnormal fibrinogen molecules, where false levels may be obtained in assays of clottable protein.

Reagents

- Agarose (LE) 1% (ICN Biomedicals Ltd.).
- Barbitone buffer pH 8.6 — 82.4 g sodium barbitone, 16 g diethyl barbituric acid, 2 g sodium azide. Dissolve in 20 litres distilled water, with gentle heating.
- Anti-human fibrinogen serum (Dako Ltd.).
- Normal saline.
- Coomassie stain — 5 g PAGE Blue 83 'Electran' (BDH Chemicals Ltd.) dissolved in: 450 ml methanol, 450 ml distilled water, 100 ml glacial acetic acid.
- Acid alcohol destain — as for stain, but without PAGE Blue.

Equipment

○ Glass plates 95 × 80 mm, or Gelbond film 75 × 100 mm.
○ Levelling table.
○ Moist chamber.
○ Well cutter — 2 mm diameter.
○ 56°C water-bath.
○ Glass tube 14 × 150 mm.
○ Parafilm.

Standards

Commercial standard or calibrated plasma.

Method

1. Dissolve 1% agarose in a boiling water-bath.
2. Place 13 ml of agarose in a glass tube at 56°C.
3. Add antisera (usually approx. 0.1–0.2 ml, depending on potency).
4. Mix and pour the solution onto a glass plate or Gelbond film on a levelling table.
5. When the gel sets (approximately 10 min), place it in a moist chamber at 4°C for at least 30 minutes.
6. Using the well cutter, make a series of wells in rows 2 cm apart down the plate.
7. Place the plate in a moist chamber and add 6.5 μl of plasma dilution to each well (standard 1/4–1/128; test 1/8–1/64).
8. Leave for 2 hours at room temperature and then at 4°C for 48 hours.
9. Measure diameter of precipitin rings.

Calculation

Plot a log/log graph of diameter squared against dilution

(concentration) for the standard. Read off the concentrations of each test dilution and multiply by the dilution factor. Correct potency to g/l.

Comments
— Dilutions of test must be adjusted according to the expected potency of the test sample, otherwise large numbers of dilutions must be tested.
— Visualisation of precipitin rings may be difficult and can be improved by pressing the gel and drying, followed by Coomassie Blue staining (see p. 311 Immunoelectrophoresis). Care should be taken if this is carried out, since the rings may become distorted.

Interpretation
Normal range — 1.5–4.0 g/l.

The presence of a higher fibrinogen antigen than clottable fibrinogen suggests the presence of a dysfunctional fibrinogen molecule if the presence of soluble fibrin monomer and FDP's has been ruled out.

FIBRINOGEN DEGRADATION PRODUCTS (FDPs) — THROMBOWELLCOTEST

Principle
Blood is collected into a mixture of an inhibitor to prevent fibrinolysis in vitro, and thrombin to ensure the removal of fibrinogen. Dilutions of serum are mixed with latex particles coated with antibody to fibrinogen and FDPs on a slide. If fibrinogen, fibrin, or their derivatives are present, they bind to the antibody, and cause agglutination of the latex, which can be read visually.

Biochemical basis
Plasminogen activator and plasmin bind to fibrin surfaces, where plasminogen can be cleaved to give the active enzyme plasmin. Attachment to the fibrin surface protects both proteins from their inhibitors and allows plasmin to sequentially degrade fibrin into successively smaller fragments known as FDPs. The larger of these, known as fragments X, Y, D, and E retain some common antigens with fibrinogen. These FDPs are free to diffuse from the clot, which gradually breaks down, and are removed by the reticuloendothelial system.

Test samples
2 ml of blood is collected into tubes containing thrombin and soybean trypsin inhibitor (Wellcome Diagnostics Ltd.). The blood is allowed to clot for 20 minutes at 37°C and then spun for serum.

Reagents
● Albumin glycine buffer pH 8.2 — 7.5 g glycine (0.1 M), 6.4 g NaCl, 0.1 g NaOH, 20.0 g bovine serum albumin (Sigma), 0.2 g sodium azide. Dissolve in 1 litre distilled water. Adjust pH with $NaCO_3$.
● Latex particles coated with antifibrinogen (Thrombowellcotest, Wellcome Diagnostics Ltd.).
● Positive and negative controls.

Equipment
○ Glass tile.
○ Applicator sticks.

Controls
Positive and negative control sera should be used on each run to check the activity of the antisera. These may be obtained commercially or stored from previous patients.

Method
1. 1/5 and 1/20 dilutions are prepared in plastic tubes using glycine buffer.
2. 1 drop of each dilution is placed on a section of the glass tile.
3. 1 drop of each control sera are placed on different sections of the tile.
4. 1 drop of latex particles are added to each section of the tile.
5. An applicator stick is used to mix and spread each sample out to a diameter of approximately 25 mm.
6. The tile is rocked gently for exactly 2 minutes and read for agglutination.

Calculation
Negative results at both dilutions indicate that less than 10 μg/ml FDP's are present. A positive result at 1/5 but not at 1/20 indicates 10–40 μg/ml; and positive results in both dilutions indicate >40 μg/ml. In the latter situation, the test should be repeated at higher dilutions to obtain a more accurate result.

Comments
— It is vital that all fibrinogen is clotted out of the serum sample before use, otherwise false positive results will occur.
— Results must be read at exactly 2 minutes, after longer periods false positivity may occur.

Interpretation
Normal range — <10 μg/ml.

The clinical relevance of raised FDP's measured by this technique is often difficult to determine. Mild elevations may be due to non-specific breakdown of fibrinogen or fibrin, and there are a wide range of causes of raised FDPs, which may not be related to the underlying pathology that the clinician is searching for. Patients with dysfibrinogenaemia can have falsely elevated FDP levels since not all of the fibrinogen is removed when the blood is clotted, leading to agglutination of the latex particles.

FIBRIN DEGRADATION PRODUCTS — D-DIMER LATEX ASSAY (DIMERTEST)

Principle
Patient samples are mixed on a glass slide with latex particles coated with monoclonal antibodies against the D-Dimer fragment of fibrin. If D-Dimer is present, it will bind to the antibodies and cause agglutination of the latex particles.

Biochemical basis
During fibrinolysis, plasmin degrades fibrin to progressively smaller fragments. If the fibrin chains have been crosslinked by factor XIII, the fragment D portion of two adjacent fibrin monomers remain crosslinked together as a D-Dimer. This fragment is not generated during the degradation of fibrinogen or non-crosslinked fibrin, and is therefore specific to the lysis of fibrin clots.

Test samples
1. Fresh citrated, heparinised, or EDTA plasma.
2. Serum prepared by clotting blood in a glass tube at 37°C for 30–60 minutes and centrifuging.
3. Serum prepared from blood collected into soybean trypsin inhibitor (2000 u/ml blood) and thrombin (10 NIH u/ml) may also be used.

Reagents
Dimertest latex kit (Porton Products Ltd.) — latex beads, phosphate buffer — dissolve in 100 ml distilled water.

Equipment
○ Clear glass slide.
○ Applicator sticks.

Standards and controls
Dimertest positive control — reconstitute with 0.2 ml phosphate buffer.

Method
1. Place 25 μl of latex beads on a glass slide.
2. Mix 10 μl undiluted sample with latex beads.
3. Rock slide gently for 3 minutes.
4. Look for agglutination by holding the slide over a black background.
5. If the test is positive, make doubling dilutions of sample in phosphate buffer and repeat steps 1–4 until a negative result is obtained.

Calculation
Results are calculated in ng/ml according to Table 20.2.

Table 20.2 Calculation of D-Dimer level.

D-Dimer (ng/ml)	Not diluted	1/2	1/4	1/8	1/16	1/32
<200	−	−	−	−	−	−
200–500	+	−	−	−	−	−
500–1000	+	+	−	−	−	−
1000–2000	+	+	+	−	−	−
2000–4000	+	+	+	+	−	−
4000–8000	+	+	+	+	+	−

+ = agglutination; − = no agglutination

Comments
— Latex should be pipetted onto the slide immediately before use to prevent drying out.
— The test should be read at exactly 3 minutes.
— Plasma samples are preferable to serum where possible, as entrapment of D-Dimer in the clot can occur in serum, giving slightly lower levels.
— Rheumatoid factor can cause non-specific agglutination of immunoglobulin-coated latex beads.
— The test is not affected by the presence of fibrinogen, therefore incompletely clotted samples or serum from patients with dysfibrinogenaemia will not give false positive results due to the presence of fibrinogen.

Interpretation
Normal value — < 200 ng/ml D-Dimer.

Elevated levels have been found in DVT, PE, DIC, and conditions associated with activation of coagulation and microvascular fibrin deposition.

Other FDP assays
Various radio-immunoassays for D-Dimer, Fragment E and other fibrin derivatives are available, but are more commonly used by research laboratories, and will not be described here.

FACTOR XIII ASSAY — CLOT SOLUBILITY TEST

Although factor XIII assays are not strictly performed in the investigation of a prolonged thrombin time, they are included here for convenience. Factor XIII deficiency is not detected by any of the global coagulation tests, and specific methods must be performed to ascertain its status.

Principle
A fibrin clot is formed, and either acetate or urea solutions are added and the sample incubated. Factor

XIII crosslinked fibrin is insoluble in these solutions, but non-crosslinked fibrin dissolves.

Biochemical basis

Factor XIII is a transglutaminase which, when activated by thrombin, and in the presence of calcium ions, forms crosslinks between parallel fibrin strands. It catalyses the formation of a linkage between glutamine and lysine residues in the gamma chains of different fibrin monomers. Crosslinked fibrin has greater tensile strength and is less likely to be swept away by flowing blood. Factor XIII circulates in blood as a dissociable complex of two pairs of different subunits, termed a and b (a2b2). Activation by thrombin results in dissociation of the complex and exposure of the active site on subunit a. Factor XIII may also have other physiological functions in anchoring macromolecules to fibrin clots and subendothelial surfaces (eg. alpha-2-antiplasmin to fibrin).

Reagents

- 2% acetic acid.
- 5 M urea.
- Calcium chloride 0.025 M.
- Thrombin 10 u/ml.
- Isotonic saline.

Equipment

○ Glass tubes 75 × 12 mm.
○ Metal spatula.

Controls

Normal citrated plasma is used as a positive control. Normal EDTA plasma provides a negative control.

Method

1. duplicate 0.2 ml amounts of normal or patient (citrated) plasma are placed in glass tubes at 37°C.

2. 0.2 ml of calcium chloride and 0.1 ml of thrombin are added, and mixed.

3. 0.2 ml of normal EDTA plasma is placed in a third pair of tubes at 37°C and 0.2 ml of saline and 0.1 ml of thrombin are added and mixed.

4. All six tubes are capped and incubated for 30 minutes.

5. 2.5 ml of urea is added to one tube from each pair, and 2.5 ml of acetate to the other tube.

6. Dislodge clots from the wall of the tube using a metal spatula.

7. Incubate at 37°C for 24 hours.

8. Inspect tubes for the presence of clots.

Comment

If there is a fibrinogen abnormality it may be difficult to form a clot. Small friable clots may be easily missed on inspection after 24 hours.

Calculation

At 24 hours there should be clots present in the normal citrated plasma tubes but absent in the normal EDTA plasma tubes. If factor XIII is absent in patient plasma, there will be no clots present at 24 hours either in acetate or urea. Low but detectable levels of factor XIII may give clots in urea but not in acetate. The test has poor sensitivity — urea only detects levels below approximately 1% and acetate below 2%. However, it is said that only severe deficiencies have clinical significance for haemostasis.

Interpretation

Abnormal clot solubility is caused by grossly decreased factor XIII levels, due to:

   a. Inherited deficiency or abormality.
   b. Consumption (DIC).
   c. Lack of synthesis (liver failure).

Factor XIII subunit concentrations may be determined by immunoelectrophoresis with commercial antisera (Behring Ltd.) using EDTA barbitone buffer pH 8.6. Similarly, their electrophoretic mobility may be determined by crossed immunoelectrophoresis using the above antisera and buffers in a method similar to that described on page 336.

21

Investigation of prolonged prothrombin time

The concept of an extrinsic and intrinsic system operating entirely independently of one another prior to activation of factor X is no longer accepted. In vivo there is a complex interaction and feedback mechanism between coagulation factors of the two pathways which ultimately results in the formation of thrombin (Fig. 21.1) (Triplett 1985).

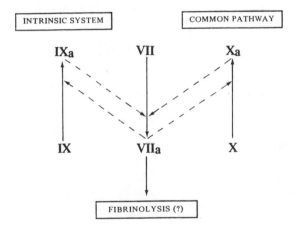

Fig. 21.1 Reactions involved in formation of thrombin.

The prothrombin time (PT) simply measures the time taken for a clot to form when thromboplastin (tissue factor) and calcium are added to plasma. For practical purposes the PT is sensitive to deficiencies of factors II, V, VII, and X, and is moderately sensitive to a low level of fibrinogen and to the presence of inhibitors of coagulation e.g. heparin and the lupus inhibitor. The PT gives limited information on its own: results are best interpreted in conjunction with results of an activated partial thromboplastin time (APTT) and thrombin time (TT) carried out at the same time.

Presence of heparin in plasma

Several situations may exist where the prothrombin time is prolonged by heparin:

1. The sample may have been taken from a heparinised line.

2. The patient may be on intravenous heparin.

3. A heparin-like inhibitor has been described in myeloma and in the newborn.

For further details, see Chapter 20.

CORRECTION TESTS

The correction to normal of a prolonged PT by the addition of normal control plasma is a useful method of establishing that the defect is due to a factor deficiency as opposed to the presence of an inhibitor. In the latter, the PT would be further prolonged due to the inhibitor in the test plasma, neutralising its specific coagulation factor present in the normal plasma (Table 21.1). Other correction reagents such as adsorbed human plasma and aged normal serum may give misleading results if not used with extreme care. It is probably better to proceed directly to specific assays now that the substrate plasmas are readily available.

Table 21.1 Prothrombin time correction test with normal plasma.

Sample	Prothrombin time	Interpretation
Control plasma	14 seconds	Normal
Test plasma	30 seconds	Abnormal
50/50 Mix test/control	15 seconds	Suggests factor deficiency
50/50 Mix test/control	40 seconds	Suggests presence of inhibitor

Storage of plasma for assays

The correct storage of plasma is important if valid assays are to be obtained. Table 21.2 gives an indication of the survival time of factor V and the vitamin K-dependent factors II, VII, and X (unpublished observations, Stirling & co-workers). The number of individual plasmas tested at ambient temperature, in ice and at −20°C was small; the conclusion for liquid nitrogen storage is the result of a study carried out on normal plasma in order to assess the long-term storage effect

Table 21.2 Survival time of factors detected by the prothrombin time test.

	Factor II	Factor V	Factor VII	Factor X
Ambient temperature	Up to 6 hours	Up to 6 hours	Up to 4 hours	Up to 6 hours
In ice	Up to 24 hours	Up to 24 hours	Subject to cold activation	Up to 24 hours
−20°C	4 weeks	4 weeks	4 weeks if rapidly frozen	4 weeks
Liquid nitrogen (−150°C)	No appreciable deterioration of II, V, VII, or X at 1 year			

on plasmas taken throughout pregnancy in one individual (Stirling et al 1984). Factor V and factor X, though surviving well in undiluted plasma for several hours, show fairly rapid deterioration on dilution in buffer. Factor V deteriorates much more quickly if taken into sodium oxalate as opposed to trisodium citrate.

FACTOR VII CLOTTING ACTIVITY ASSAY

Principle
Dilutions of a standard plasma (equivalent to 100% FVII) and dilutions of the test plasma are used in a one-stage assay based on the PT test to correct the clotting time of a plasma completely deficient in FVII.

Biochemical basis
The factor VII clotting activity (FVIIC) assay measures VII in its in vivo form consisting of both the single-chain protein and fully active double-chain form α VIIa. Tissue factor complexes with single-chain zymogen in vivo to activate both factor IX (FIX) and factor X. The active forms of these factors (FIXa and FXa) then feed back to FVII to generate the two-chain form α VIIa. This activated form of FVII which is many times more active than the single-chain form again acts on FX to form FXa. Thrombin and plasmin can also convert VII to VIIa. FXa with FV, phospholipid and calcium cleaves prothrombin to thrombin, which in turn acts on fibrinogen to form fibrin. FVII zymogen can also be indirectly converted to α VIIa during cold activation.

Reagents
- Factor VII-deficient plasma.
- Thromboplastin — diluted 1/4 in glyoxaline buffer pH 7.3.
- 25 mM calcium chloride.
- Thromboplastin/calcium mixture — mix equal parts of dilute thromboplastin and calcium chloride.
- Glyoxaline buffer pH 7.3.

Standard
Commercial standard (Immuno Ltd.) or pooled normal plasma.

Preparation of standard and test samples
Prepare 1/5, 1/25, 1/125 dilutions of standard and test samples in glyoxaline buffer in plastic tubes. Keep dilutions at room temperature to avoid cold activation.

Method (Brozovic et al 1974)
1. Add 0.1 ml glyoxaline buffer to two glass tubes to act as reagent blanks.
2. Transfer 0.1 ml amounts of each dilution of standard and test plasmas in duplicate to glass tubes.
3. Add 0.1 ml FVII-deficient plasma to each tube.
4. Place first two tubes in 37°C water-bath.
5. Add 0.2 ml thromboplastin/calcium mixture and record time for visible clot to form.
6. Repeat steps 4 and 5 for each pair of tubes.

Calculation
Plot results on double logarithmic paper (Fig. 21.2) or calculate using a programmable microcomputer.

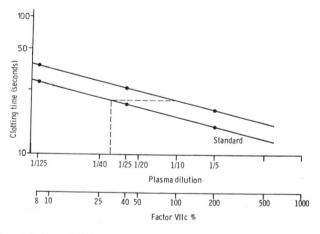

Fig. 21.2 Calculation of factor VII potency.

Comment
— Do not store plasmas or their dilutions at 4°C at any stage in order to avoid cold activation.

Interpretation
The lower limit of normal is 40% of standard.
　　Inherited factor VII deficiency is a rare disorder

transmitted by an autosomal incomplete recessive gene with variable expression and penetrance. Factor VII deficiency has been classified into five groups (Table 21.3) (Triplett 1984). A number of variant FVII molecules have also been described showing difference in FVII activity (FVIIC) depending on the thromboplastin species and type of assay used, e.g. chromogenic assay.

The methods for measuring factor VII Ag are complex procedures requiring reagents which are difficult to prepare or obtain and are generally carried out in specialised coagulation laboratories. An Elisa kit is now commercially available.

Table 21.3 Classification of factor VII deficiency.

Group	FVII C	FVII Ag	Clinical state
1	2%	2%	High incidence of intracerebral bleeding. Frequently die within first 2 years of life.
2	10%	100 ng by RIA	Recurrent haemarthroses and intramuscular haematoma.
3	Variable	100–250 ng by RIA	Easy bruising, epistaxis, genitourinary and gastrointestinal bleeds.
4	Variable	Variable	No clinical symptoms
5	1–20%	Variable	Thrombotic complications

Factor VII neutralising activity technique (Denson 1971)
This method, utilising an anti-FVII neutralising antibody, measures total FVII protein including the acarboxylated forms of the molecule. The Laurell rocket technique is not routinely possible due to the extreme difficulty in preparing a precipitating FVII antibody.

Release of activation peptide from tritiated Factor X by Factor VII
Total activatable FVII (FVIIT, Miller et al 1984) is determined by measuring the release of the activation peptide during the conversion of FX to Xa by FVII and tissue factor. Serum is prepared by clotting the standard and test plasmas with thromboplastin and calcium. As only the carboxylated forms of FVII take part in this reaction, the VIIT level is decreased in patients on oral anticoagulants.

Factor VII coupled two-stage amidolytic assay
(Unpublished modification of the method of Seligsohn 1978)
Total factor VII, independent of the activity state, is measured. Plasma, tissue factor, FX and calcium are incubated together at 37°C. The Xa generated releases

free pNA on addition of chromogenic substrate S2337 (Kabivitrum). The resultant yellow colour is colour-converted (Howarth et al 1985) and read in a spectrophotometer at 540 nm.

Factor VII variants
A number of FVII variants have been described on the basis of discrepant FVII clotting activity results depending on the choice of thromboplastin (i.e. different animal species) used. Refer to the paper by Triplett 1984 for list of published variants.

FACTOR II ASSAYS

Several methods for the measurement of FII are available. As prothrombin-deficient plasma is not readily available, techniques utilising prothrombin-converting snake venoms are generally employed. Taipan (*Oxyuranus scutellatus*) is in most common use. Others include *Echis carinatus*, *Notechis scutatus scutatus* and *Dispholidus typus*. (Bezeaud et al 1979).

TAIPAN VENOM CLOTTING ASSAY FOR FACTOR II

Principle
Taipan venom directly converts prothrombin to thrombin. The time taken for the thrombin to form a fibrin clot on the addition of adsorbed bovine plasma (as a source of fibrinogen) and platelet substitute is measured.

Biochemical basis
Taipan venom (*Oxyuranus scutellatus*) splits the same peptide as does FXa, the rate of reaction being dependent on calcium and phospholipid, but independent of FVa. The assay measures the functional activity of FII (carboxylated forms): decreased levels are found in patients on oral anticoagulants. Tiger snake venom (*Notechis scutatus scutatus*) also measures functional activity.

Reagents
- Taipan venom + calcium chloride (Diagen).
- Platelet substitute (Diagen).
- Adsorbed bovine plasma (Diagen).
- Glyoxaline buffer pH 7.3.

Dilute all reagents according to the instructions on the vial.

Standard
Commercial standard (Immuno Ltd) or pooled normal plasma.

Preparation of standard and test plasmas

Prepare 1/80, 1/160, and 1/320 dilutions of standard and test plasmas in glyoxaline buffer in plastic tubes. Keep all dilutions in ice.

Method (Modification of Denson et al 1971)

1. Transfer 0.1 ml amounts of each dilution of standard or test plasmas in duplicate to glass tubes.
2. Add 0.1 ml of platelet substitute and 0.1 ml of adsorbed bovine plasma to each tube.
3. Place the first 2 tubes in a 37°C water-bath.
4. To each tube in turn add 0.2 ml Taipan venom + calcium and record time for visible clot formation.
5. Repeat steps 3 and 4 for each pair to tubes.

Calculation

Plot results on log/log paper (see FVII assay) or calculate on a programmable calculator, microcomputer.

Comment

— Reagent blanks are not included as no clot is formed when buffer is substituted for standard or test plasma.

Interpretation

The lower limit of normal is 40% of standard.

Inherited factor II deficiency is extremely rare. Of the cases described the majority have reduced levels by both functional and immunological methods. A number of molecular variants have also been described. Total FII protein, i.e. carboxylated and acarboxy forms may be measured using *Echis carinatus* venom (see p. 335). The venom splits one peptide bond of prothrombin, but does not require accessory factors, calcium, phospholipid and FVa for its action.

Factor II antigen — Laurell technique

Total protein FII can be determined by using the electroimmunoassay of Laurell 1972.

In addition, suitable antisera can be used in two-dimensional electrophoresis to demonstrate abnormally migrating (including PIVKA) forms of FII (see p. 336). For a review of FII variants refer to Bloom 1981.

FACTOR V CLOTTING ACTIVITY ASSAY

Principle

The method is identical to the FVII assay, but using FV-deficient plasma. Dilutions of a standard plasma (equivalent to 100% FV) and dilutions of the test plasma are used in a one-stage assay based on the PT test to correct the time of a plasma completely deficient in FV.

Biochemical basis

The formation of thrombin from prothrombin by FXa requires cleavage of two peptide bonds in the prothrombin molecule. FXa alone can achieve this cleavage, but the effect is very greatly enhanced in the presence of Va (thrombin-activated V), phospholipid and calcium, this reaction taking place on the platelet surface membrane. The resultant thrombin acts on fibrinogen to form fibrin.

Reagents

- Factor V-deficient plasma.
- Thromboplastin — diluted 1/4 in glyoxaline buffer.
- 25 mM calcium chloride.
- Thromboplastin/calcium mixture — mix equal parts of dilute thromboplastin and calcium chloride.
- Glyoxaline buffer pH 7.3.

Preparation of standard and test plasmas

Prepare 1/5, 1/25, and 1/125 dilutions of standard and test plasmas in glyoxaline buffer in plastic tubes. Immediately place dilutions in ice.

Method (Brozovic et al 1974)

1. Add 0.1 ml glyoxaline buffer to 2 glass tubes to act as reagent blanks.
2. Transfer 0.1 ml amounts of each dilution in duplicate to glass tubes.
3. Add 0.1 ml FV-deficient plasma to each tube.
4. Place first 2 tubes in 37°C water-bath.
5. Add 0.2 ml thromboplastin/calcium mixture to each tube and record time for visible clot to form.
6. Repeat steps 4 and 5 for each pair of tubes.

Calculation

As for FVII.

Comment

— Factor V is very labile in dilution. Plasmas and dilutions must be kept in ice to avoid recording a falsely low level.

Interpretation

The lower limit of normal is 40% of standard.

Inherited factor V deficiency is a rare disorder with an autosomal recessive inheritance pattern. Patients presenting with bleeding and bruising are generally homozygotes, but some heterozygotes show mild symptoms and have a FV level below the lower limit of normal. Little work has been carried out on the classification of FV defects due to the lack of a precipitating antibody measuring FV Ag. A commercial reagent has, however, recently become available.

STYPVEN TIME TEST

Principle
The venom of the snake *Vipera russelli* (RVV) acts directly on FX to convert it to FXa in the absence of other clotting factors. This procedure is used to distinguish a FX from a FVII defect.

Reagents
- Russell's viper venom (Diagen).
- Platelet substitute (Diagen).
- 25 mM (M/40) calcium chloride.

Controls
Pooled normal plasma.

Preparation of working reagents
Dilute reagents according to instructions on vial. Further dilute RVV 1/5 in platelet substitute. Add an equal volume of 25 ml calcium chloride. This reagent should give a clotting time of around 15 seconds with normal plasma. Adjust RVV concentration if necessary.

Method
1. Add 0.1 ml pooled normal plasma to duplicate glass tubes in a 37°C water-bath.
2. Add 0.1 ml RVV/platelet substitute/calcium mixture and simultaneously start stopwatch.
3. Record time for formation of visible clot.
4. Repeat steps 1–3 using test plasma.

Results
Express the Stypven time as the mean of the duplicates of control and test plasmas.

Comment
— Keep RVV/platelet substitute mixture in ice as it tends to deteriorate if left at ambient temperature or at 37°C. Discard at end of day.

Interpretation
The result is abnormal if the test time is longer than the control time. A prolonged Stypven time in the presence of a prolonged prothrombin time is indicative of FX deficiency. A normal Stypven time does not rule out a FX variant, i.e. Friuli type.

Inherited FX deficiency is uncommon and passed as an autosomal recessive trait. Presumed homozygotes may present with severe bleeding, and there is evidence of consanguinity in some cases. Heterozygotes are often symptomless or have only mild symptoms. As factor X is involved in both extrinsic and intrinsic coagulation, both the prothrombin time and APTT are prolonged. Varying levels of factor X activity have been obtained depending on the type of assay used, resulting in the description of a number of molecular variants. Measurement of factor X antigen by different workers has given variable results, making classification of the factor X defect difficult. Girolami et al 1970, in a study of a group of patients in the Friuli valley in Italy, described a new variant of FX (FX Friuli) which is distinct from the Stuart and Prower defects (Table 21.4).

A number of specific assays for FX have been described. Human FX-deficient plasma being in short supply, a charcoal-adsorbed bovine plasma is generally used. This product which is depleted in FVII and FX, but contains FII, FV and fibrinogen is commercially available and relatively inexpensive.

Table 21.4 Factor X variants classified according to type of assay used.

Type	FX level (tissue extract)	FX level (RVV-cephalin)	FX Ag (immunological)
Prower	low	low	present
Stuart	v. low	v. low	absent
Friuli	low	normal	present

FACTOR X CLOTTING ASSAY USING TISSUE FACTOR

Principle
The principle of the test is identical to that for FVII clotting activity, but using substrate plasma deficient in FX.

Biochemical basis
Factor X can be activated to FXa by FIXa/FVIII, FVII/tissue factor or other proteases, including Russell's viper venom. Cleavage of a single, specific arginyl-isoleucine peptide bond in the heavy chain of FX is achieved regardless of the activation system involved. The amount of FX available to be activated to FXa and its subsequent interaction with FV, phospholipid and calcium determines the amount of thrombin formed and ultimately the time taken for a fibrin clot to form.

Reagents
- Factor X-deficient plasma (Diagen).
- Thromboplastin diluted 1/4 in glyoxaline buffer.
- Glyoxaline buffer pH 7.3.
- 25 mM (M/40) calcium chloride.

Standard
Commercial standard (e.g. Immuno Ltd.) or pooled normal plasma.

Preparation of standard and test plasmas
Prepare 1/20, 1/60, 1/180 dilutions of standard and test plasmas in glyoxaline buffer in plastic tubes.

Method
Proceed exactly as for FVII clotting activity assay.

Results
Plot results on log/log paper (Fig. 21.2) or calculate using a programmable calculator/microcomputer.

Comment
— Keep plasmas and dilutions in ice until ready for testing.

Interpretation
The lower limit of normal is 40% of standard.

FACTOR X CLOTTING ACTIVITY BY APTT METHOD

The method is identical to the one-stage factor VIII assay (p. 295), but using factor X-deficient plasma.

FACTOR X CLOTTING ACTIVITY USING RUSSELL's VIPER VENOM (Denson 1961)

Principle
The RVV assay is most generally used. Dilutions of a standard plasma (equivalent to 100% FX) and dilutions of the test plasma are used to correct the clotting time of a charcoal-adsorbed bovine plasma completely deficient in FX and FVII. As Russell's viper venom converts FX to FXa directly in the absence of any other clotting factor, only the FX level is measured.

Reagents
- Factor X-deficient plasma (Diagen).
- Russell's viper venom (Diagen).
- Platelet substitute (Diagen).
- 25 mM calcium chloride.
- Glyoxaline buffer pH 7.3

Standards
Commercial standard (e.g. Immuno Ltd.) or pooled normal plasma.

Preparation of reagents and plasmas
Dilute reagents according to instructions on vial. To 4.7 ml platelet substitute add 0.3 ml RVV. Add an equal volume (5 ml) 25 nM calcium chloride.

Prepare 1/50, 1/200, 1/800 dilutions of standard and test plasmas in glyoxaline buffer in plastic tubes, keep in ice.

Method
1. Add 0.1 ml glyoxaline buffer to two glass tubes to act as reagent blanks.
2. Transfer 0.1 ml amounts of each dilution in duplicate to glass tubes.
3. To each tube add 0.1 ml FX-deficient plasma.
4. Place first two tubes (i.e. 1/50 dilutions of standard) in 37°C water-bath.
5. Add 0.2 ml RVV/platelet substitute/calcium mixture to each tube and record time for visible clot to form. Clot off remainder of dilutions.

Results
Plot results on log/log paper (Fig. 21.2) or calculate using a programmeable calculator/microcomputer.

Comments
— Keep plasmas and their dilutions in ice.
— Keep RVV/platelet substitute/calcium mixture in ice. Discard at end of day.

Interpretation
The lower limit of normal is 40% of standard.

Other assays available for factor X estimation

Factor X assay with chromogenic substrate S2337
Factor X is activated by Russell's viper venom (in the presence of calcium) to FXa, which splits off the pNA from the chromogenic substrate to release a chromo-

Table 21.5 Causes of acquired prolonged prothrombin time.

Clinical state	PT	APTT	TT	Deficiency
Early liver disease	P	N	N	FVII
Advanced liver disease	P	P	N/P	FII, FV, FVII, FX
Vitamin K deficiency/oral anticoagulant therapy	P	P	N	Decreased FVII, normal FV
Paracetamol overdose	P	N	N	Decreased FVII
Amyloid	P	P	N	FX deficiency
Acute DIC	P	P	N/P	Decreased FV
Massive blood transfusion	P	P	N	Decreased FV
Lupus inhibitor	N/P	N/P	N	Inhibitor of prothrombinase
Gaucher's disease, Nieman-Pick disease	P	P	N	Decreased FV due to adsorption onto abnormal lipid

P = prolonged, N = normal

genic amine. The resultant yellow colour is colour-converted and measured in a spectrophotometer at 540 nm. An assay kit, Coatest FX, is available from Kabivitrum, using the substrate S2337 (Bz-Ile-Glu-Gly-Arg;pNA) which was reported by Aurell et al 1977 to be highly specific for the detection of FX in plasma. Only the intact FX is activated by RVV, and not the PIVKA variant. The assay has been assessed in the monitoring of oral anticoagulant therapy. Results are of value only in patients stabilised on warfarin and not in the early phase of treatment.

Factor X antigen
Factor X antigen can be determined in the same manner as FVII antigen (p. 287) using a suitable FX antibody.

Alternatively, FX antigen can be measured by Laurell rocket electrophoresis using a precipitating anti-FX antibody (see factor II antigen method). Results are reported as percentage of standard.

Acquired single or multiple coagulation factor deficiencies
Abnormal clotting test results with a deficiency of one or more factors are found in patients with a variety of disease states. It is extremely difficult to interpret the results in isolation and they should be examined in conjunction with the clinical details. The results of the APTT and thrombin time should be assessed at the same time as the prothrombin time. The more common causes of a prolonged prothrombin time are listed below (Table 21.5).

REFERENCES

Aurell L, Friberger P, Karlsson G, Claeson G 1977 A new sensitive and highly specific chromogenic peptide substrate for Xa. Thrombosis Research II: 595–609

Bezeaud A, Guillin M C, Olmeda F, Quintana M, Gomez, M 1979 Prothrombin Madrid: a new familiar abnormality of prothrombin. Thrombosis Research 16: 47–58

Bloom A L 1981 Inherited disorders of blood coagulation. Haemostasis and thrombosis. Churchill Livingstone, Edinburgh

Brozovic M, Stirling Y, Harricks C, North W R S, Meade T W 1974 Factor VII in an industrial population. British Journal of Haematology 28: 381–391

Denson K W E 1961 The specific assay of Prower-Stuart factor and factor VII. Acta Haematologica 25: 105–120

Denson K W E 1971 The levels of factors II, VII, IX and X by antibody neutralization techniques in the plasma of patients receiving phenindione treatment. British Journal of Haematology 20: 643–648

Denson K W E, Borrett R, Biggs R 1971 The specific assay of prothrombin using the Taipan snake venom. British Journal of Haematology 21: 219

Girolami et al 1970 A 'new' congenital haemorrhagic condition due to the presence of an abnormal factor X (factor X Friuli); Study of a large kindred. British Journal of Haematology 19: 179

Howarth D J, Samson D, Stirling Y, Seghatchian M J 1985 Antithrombin III 'Northwick Park': A variant antithrombin with normal affinity for heparin but reduced heparin cofactor activity. Thrombosis and Haemostasis 513: 314–319

Laurell C B 1972 Electroimmunoassay. Scandinavian Journal of Clinical and Laboratory Investigation 29 (suppl 124): 21–37

Miller G J, Walter S J, Stirling Y, Thompson S G, Esnouf M P, Meade T W 1985 Assay of factor VII activity by two techniques: Evidence for increased conversion of VII to VIIa in hyperlipidaemia with possible implications for ischaemic heart disease. British Journal of Haematology 59: 249–258

Seligsohn U, Osterud B, Rapaport S I 1978 Coupled amidolytic assay for factor VII: its use with a clotting assay to determine the activity state of factor VII. Blood 52: 978–988

Stirling Y, Woolf L, North W R S, Seghatchian M J, Meade T W 1984 Haemostasis in normal pregnancy. Thrombosis and Haemostasis 52: 176–182

Triplett D 1984 The extrinsic system. Clinics in Laboratory Medicine 4 (No 2): 221–244

22

Investigation of a prolonged activated partial thromboplastin time

There are many reasons for a prolonged APTT and often it may be due to some artefact or extraneous influence. The type of specimen container (see p. 271) may have an effect, as will the length of time since collection, the manner of storage, the quality of the venepuncture, contamination with heparin (from a venous line, the syringe, etc.) or other substance, or laboratory failure (technique or reagent quality). Before embarking on costly and time-consuming assays it is worthwhile checking the APTT on a fresh specimen collected under controlled conditions. If the APTT is genuinely prolonged, the clinical details and information may well give a guide as to the nature of the problem. The patient may be diagnosed as having a congenital bleeding tendency, or have SLE. Symptoms of bleeding or auto-immune disease should be checked and a family history of bleeding or lupus-like disease inquired about.

One must decide how far to proceed with the technology available to investigate this sort of problem, bearing in mind the clinical relevance. If the cause is acquired due to some underlying pathology, it may merely be enough to demonstrate a prolonged APTT which has obvious cause and does not need further investigation. This section will concentrate on the investigation of prolonged APTTs due to congenital coagulation deficiency, and acquired inhibitors will be discussed in a later section.

The approach to this type of problem differs between laboratories, some favouring mixing tests and others proceeding immediately with coagulation factor assays. In the case of factor VIIIC, several different assays are described (one- and two-stage clotting factor assays, chromogenic substrate assays, and immunological measurements), since each has its own advantages and disadvantages depending on the situation. The 1-stage assay is cheap if suitable haemophilic plasma is available; however, this is becoming increasingly difficult since not all severe haemophiliacs have plasma that gives good FVIIIC assays, many are on home treatment, and there is the risk of viral infection. The 2-stage assay is safer, using bovine reagents, but is technically more

difficult and more expensive than using local haemophilic plasma in a 1-stage assay. The 2-stage assay is also said to give a better estimate of in vivo recovery of FVIIIC after treatment, and is not usually affected by lupus anticoagulants. Perhaps the best assay of FVIIIC activity is the amidolytic assay, which is safe, inexpensive if performed by a microtitre technique, suitable for testing large numbers of samples, and correlates well with traditional assays on haemophiliacs and von Willebrand's disease patients. The FVIIIC:Ag assay is useful for carrier detection in haemophilia and for prenatal diagnosis of factor VIII coagulant protein defects.

CORRECTION TESTS

Principle
These test the ability of various reagents and known deficient plasmas (collected locally, or obtained commercially) to correct the clotting time of a patient plasma sample. Relatively small amounts of a clotting factor need to be added to a deficient plasma to obtain a correction. From the pattern of results with the various mixtures it is sometimes possible to determine the factor which is lacking.

Reagents
- Normal plasma
- Factor VIII-deficient plasma
- Factor IX-deficient plasma
- Factor XI-deficient plasma
- Factor XII-deficient plasma
- Fletcher trait plasma
- Fitzgerald trait plasma
- Aluminium hydroxide — 1 g moist gel (BDH Chemicals Ltd.) in 4 ml distilled water.
- Aged normal serum
- Other reagents as for APTT

Preparation of reagents

Aged normal serum
  1. Collect 10 ml of blood from each of 10 different

healthy volunteers into plain glass tubes.

2. Allow blood to clot and place at 37°C for 48 hours.

3. Centrifuge blood and pool the sera.

4. Store in aliquots below −20°C until needed.

Adsorbed normal plasma

1. Prepare fresh on the day of use.

2. Mix 1 ml of pooled normal plasma with 0.1 ml of well-mixed aluminium hydroxide suspension in a polystyrene test tube.

3. Incubate at 37°C for 3 minutes with frequent mixing.

4. Centrifuge at 2000 g (4000 rpm) for 10 minutes.

5. Pipette off the supernatant into a clean polystyrene tube, cap and store on ice.

Method

1. Place 80 μl of patient plasma in each of a series of glass clotting tubes.

2. Add 20 μl amounts of each correction reagent to duplicate tubes of patient plasma.

3. Perform an APTT on each mixture.

Interpretation

The amount of correction achieved should be compared to the result for patient plasma plus pooled normal plasma. If only one deficient plasma fails to give a correction, it suggests that the patient is lacking in that factor and one should proceed to a specific assay of that factor. Often the results are not clear and may lead to erroneous conclusions. Aged normal serum which lacks factor VIIIC, and adsorbed normal plasma, which lacks factor IX can sometimes be helpful as correction reagents, particularly in small centres where haemophiliac plasmas may not be available.

1-STAGE FACTOR IX ASSAY

Principle

This assay tests the ability of dilutions of patient plasma to correct the prolonged APTT of factor IX-deficient plasma. The degree of correction is compared to that obtained using dilutions of a standard plasma of known potency, so that a concentration can be calculated.

Biochemical basis

Factor IX activates factor X in the presence of factor VIII, phospholipid, and calcium ions, leading to subsequent thrombin generation and the formation of a fibrin clot. Factor IXa is a serine protease and a vitamin K-dependent protein, which binds to phospholipid surfaces in a calcium ion dependent mechanism. Its action on factor X is greatly accelerated by factor VIII.

Reagents

● Factor IX-deficient substrate plasma — severe factor IX-deficient patient plasma with <0.01 IU/ml local patient or commercial deficient plasma (Immuno, General Diagnostics, Dade). Alternatively, immune-depleted plasma (Diagnostic Reagents Ltd.).

● Tris buffer 0.2 M, pH 7.4.

● Kaolin 0.05 g in 10 ml Tris buffer.

● Diagen 'Bell & Alton' platelet substitute (Diagnostic Reagents Ltd.).

● Calcium chloride 0.025 M.

● Mix equal volumes of platelet substitute and calcium chloride and place at 37°C.

Standard

National standard or commercial standard, calibrated against the international standard.

Method

1. 0.1 ml of factor IXC-deficient plasma is placed in each of six pairs of glass clotting tubes on ice.

2. Standard plasma is diluted 1/10, 1/20 and 1/40 in Tris buffer in polystyrene tubes on ice.

	1/10	1/20	1/40
Buffer	0.9 ml	0.5 ml	0.5 ml
Plasma	0.1 ml	0.5 ml 1/10	0.5 ml 1/20

3. Warm the first 2 glass tubes at 37°C for 1 minute.

4. Add 0.1 ml of the 1/40 dilution to each tube, followed by 0.1 ml of kaolin, and start a clock.

5. Add duplicate 0.1 ml amounts of the other dilutions to the glass tubes on ice.

6. At one minute, the next pair of tubes are placed at 37°C, and at 2 minutes 0.1 ml of kaolin is added.

7. At 3 minutes the third pair of tubes are placed at 37°C, and at 4 minutes they receive kaolin.

8. During the above time intervals, the dilutions of test plasma are prepared in exactly the same way, and duplicate 0.1 ml amounts are added to the second 3 pairs of glass tubes on ice. These are placed at 37°C at 5, 7, and 9 minutes and receive kaolin at 6, 8, and 10 minutes respectively.

9. All tubes should be gently agitated at regular intervals to resuspend the kaolin.

10. At 10 minutes, after adding kaolin to tube pair six, 0.2 ml of platelet substitute/CaCl$_2$ mixture is added to the first pair of tubes and the clotting times determined.

11. Subsequent pairs of tubes are clotted off at 2-minute intervals.

Summary

0.1 ml deficient plasma

0.1 ml dilution.

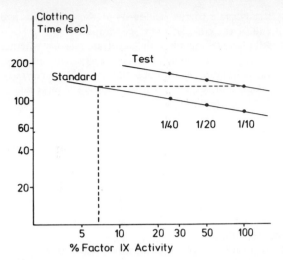

Fig. 22.1 1-stage factor IX assay, graph of clotting time against dilution.

0.1 ml kaolin.
Incubate for 10 minutes.
0.2 ml platelet substitute CaCl$_2$.
Read clotting time.

Calculation
A graph (Fig. 22.1) of log clotting time against log dilution (log concentration) is then plotted, and the activity of each test plasma is then determined as a percentage of the standard activity. A result in International Units can then be obtained after correcting for the potency of the batch of standard, e.g. standard = 0.69 IU/ml test plasma = 50% activity

$$\frac{50\% \times 0.69 \text{ IU/ml}}{100} = 0.35 \text{ IU/ml}$$

Different standards have different potencies and the calculation must be modified accordingly.

Interpretation
Normal range — 0.50–1.50 IU/ml (50–150 IU/dl).
Decreased factor IX levels are caused by:

a. Inherited defects (haemophilia B — Christmas Disease). Variant defects occur with normal antigen levels, or giving prolonged prothrombin times using ox brain thromboplastin e.g. thrombotest (factor IX Bm).

b. Haemodilution (massive transfusion).

c. Vitamin K deficiency or antagonism (intravenous feeding, gastrointestinal abnormalities, oral anticoagulation).

d. Acquired inhibitors (specific immunoglobulins to factor IX).

e. Inhibitors to other clotting factors involved in the assay system, or due to lupus anticoagulant. 2-Stage factor IX assays are said to overcome some of these problems.

1-STAGE FACTOR VIIIC ASSAY

Principle
This assay tests the ability of dilutions of patient plasma to correct the prolonged KPTT of factor VIII-deficient plasma. The degree of correction is compared to that obtained using dilutions of a standard plasma of known potency, so that a concentration can be calculated.

Biochemical basis
Factor VIIIC acts as a catalyst of the reaction of factor IX on factor X, increasing the reaction velocity. After activation by small amounts of thrombin, it binds to factor IXa and factor X on phospholipid surfaces, making the reaction more favourable. In the 1-stage assay test system thrombin generation is dependent on the factor VIII concentration, which thus influences the clotting time.

Reagents
- *FVIIIC-deficient substrate plasma*. Haemophilic plasma with less than 0.01 IU/ml factor VIIIC activity stored in aliquots below $-20°C$ and kept on ice when in use. Alternatively commercial freeze-dried haemophilic plasma may be used (e.g. Immuno, General Diagnostics Ltd., Dade), or immune-depleted plasmas are sometimes suitable (Diagnostic Reagents Ltd.).
- *Tris buffer 0.2 M pH 7.4*
    24.23 g Tris
    950 ml distilled water
    pH to 7.4 with conc.HCl and make to 1 litre.
- Kaolin — 0.5% BDH light kaolin suspended in Tris buffer.
- Phospholipid reagent — Diagen Bell & Alton platelet substitute (Diagnostic Reagents Ltd.) — reconstituted in 5 ml distilled water then diluted 1/3 with saline.
- Calcium chloride — 0.025 M

Standards
National standard for factor VIII, or commercial standard calibrated against the international standard.

Preparation of reagents
Equal volumes of phospholipid reagent and calcium chloride are mixed together and warmed to 37°C.

Method
1. 0.1 ml of factor VIIIC-deficient plasma is placed in each of six pairs of glass clotting tubes on ice.

2. Standard plasma is diluted 1/10, 1/20 and 1/40 in Tris buffer in polystyrene tubes on ice.

	1/10	1/20	1/40
Buffer	0.9 ml	0.5 ml	0.5 ml
Plasma	0.1 ml	0.5 ml 1/10	0.5 ml 1/20

3. Warm the first 2 glass tubes at 37°C for 1 minute.

4. Add 0.1 ml of the 1/40 dilution to each tube, followed by 0.1 ml of kaolin, and start a clock.

5. Add duplicate 0.1 ml amounts of the other dilutions to the glass tubes on ice.

6. At 1 minute, the next pair of tubes are placed at 37°C, and at 2 minutes 0.1 ml of kaolin is added.

7. At 3 minutes the third pair of tubes are placed at 37°C, and at 4 minutes they receive kaolin.

8. During the above time intervals, the dilutions of test plasma are prepared in exactly the same way and duplicate 0.1 ml amounts are added to the second 3 pairs of glass tubes on ice. These are placed at 37°C at 5, 7, and 9 minutes and receive kaolin at 6, 8, and 10 minutes respectively.

9. All tubes should be gently agitated at regular intervals to resuspend the kaolin.

10. At 10 minutes, after adding kaolin to tube pair six, 0.2 ml of platelet substitute/CaCl$_2$ mixture is added to the first pair of tubes and the clotting times determined.

11. Subsequent pairs of tubes are clotted off at 2-minute intervals.

Comments

— Plasma dilutions should be prepared on ice immediately before use as FVIIIC deteriorates in diluted form, and is heat labile.

— The range of dilutions should be adjusted according to the expected factor VIIIC activity of the sample. This may be roughly assessed by the APTT, e.g. for samples with very low factor VIIIC use 1/5, 1/10, 1/20; if raised factor VIIIC is likely, use 1/20, 1/40, 1/80, etc. Suitable dilutions are those which yield clotting times within the range of the standard times.

— It is useful to perform a buffer blank time to assess the sensitivity of the assay.

— The plasma of some haemophiliacs is more suitable as substrate than others, even though they may have similar factor VIIIC and factor VIIIC Ag levels.

— The contents of tubes should be mixed immediately after addition of a reagent, or bad precision will be obtained.

— Ideally 'reverse balance order' should be used. This helps to remove error due to factor VIIIC decay during the assay run. For large batches of assays it is advisable to run standards at the beginning and end of the run, or every six samples.

— All plasmas, including the substrate plasma (whether commercial or home produced) carry a risk of infection. Suitable safety precautions should therefore be taken, and reagents of human origin should not be used before virology testing.

Units

1 unit of factor VIIIC activity is the amount of activity in 1 ml of normal plasma.

Calculation

As for 1-stage factor IXC assay.

Interpretation

Normal range — 0.5–2.00 iu/ml (50–200 iu/dl).

Low factor VIIIC levels are due to:
   a. Haemophilia.
   b. von Willebrand's disease.
   c. Consumption (e.g. as in DIC).

High levels of factor VIIIC may be found in:
   a. Liver disease.
   b. Acute phase reactions.
   c. In the immediate post-operative period.

2-STAGE FACTOR VIIIC ASSAY

Principle

In the first stage, factor V, calcium chloride, phospholipid, and serum (a source of factors IX, X, XI and XII) are mixed together as the reagent (or may be obtained commercially as a combined reagent). Factor VIIIC is provided by adding a dilution of standard or patient plasma and factor Xa generation then proceeds. The rate of factor Xa generation therefore depends on the concentration of factor VIIIC provided in the plasma dilution. Factor II and fibrinogen are provided in the second stage by adding a substrate plasma. The rate of clot formation is therefore dependent on the amount of FXa generated in stage 1, and hence on the amount of FVIIIC available (Denson 1967).

Reagents

● Diagen combined factor VIII reagent (Diagnostic Reagents Ltd.)
● Substrate plasma — pooled normal plasma.
● *Citrate saline buffer*
   31.3 g Tri-sodium citrate dihydrate in 1 litre distilled water.
   8.5 g Sodium chloride in 1 litre distilled water.
   Mix 5 volumes of saline with 1 volume citrate.
● Aluminium hydroxide — 1 g aluminium hydroxide moist gel (BDH Chemicals Ltd.) suspended in 4 ml distilled water.

- Isotonic saline.
- Calcium chloride 0.025 M.

Standards
National standard for factor VIII or commercial standard calibrated against the international standard.

Preparation of reagents and test samples
Diagen combined reagent is reconstituted with 5 ml of saline and 5 ml of 0.025 M calcium chloride, and stored on ice.

Substrate plasma is diluted 1/2 with saline and stored on ice.

Standard and patient plasmas are adsorbed with aluminium hydroxide by adding 0.05 ml to 0.5 ml of plasma in a polystyrene tube and incubating at 37°C for 3 minutes with frequent mixing. The adsorbed plasmas are then centrifuged at 2000 g (4000 rpm) for 10 minutes and pipetted off into a clean polystyrene tube, capped and stored on ice.

Manual method
1. 0.2 ml of factor VIII reagent is placed in each of 12 glass clotting tubes on ice.
2. Adsorbed standard plasma is diluted 1/50, 1/100, and 1/200 in citrate saline buffer in plastic tubes on ice.
3. 2 glass tubes of reagent are placed at 37°C for 1 minute and duplicate 0.05 ml amounts of the highest standard dilution are added and a stopclock is started.
4. The next pair of glass tubes are placed at 37°C and 0.05 ml of the second dilution are added at 2 minutes.
5. The third pair of tubes are then warmed to 37°C and the lowest dilution is added at 4 minutes.
6. Adsorbed patient plasma is diluted as in step 2, and added to prewarmed glass tubes of reagent at further 2-minute intervals.
7. At 11 minutes, the first pair of standard tubes are clotted off with 0.1 ml of substrate plasma. Subsequent pairs of tubes are clotted off at 2-minute intervals.

Summary
1. 0.2 ml FVIII reagent.
2. 0.05 ml plasma dilution.
3. Incubate for 10 minutes.
4. 0.1 ml substrate plasma and clot off.

Calculation
Results are plotted on log/log graph paper, with clotting time (s) on the vertical axis and dilution (concentration) on the horizontal. Results are only valid if there is a suitable degree of parallelism between test and standard lines, and if the lines are straight. The result obtained as a percentage of standard is converted to IU/ml by multiplying by the standard potency in units and dividing by 100.

Comments
— The plateau of factor Xa generation of reagent should be determined for each batch. In practice it is usually found that the plateau runs from an incubation time of about 5–15 minutes, and therefore a 10 or 11 minute incubation period in the first stage is usually suitable. The plateau is determined by taking a dilution of standard plasma and varying the incubation time by 1-minute intervals, before adding the substrate plasma.
— It is said that thrombin-activated factor VIII, which may be present in hypercoagulable patients, is removed by the absorption step.
— Aluminium hydroxide adsorption can remove about 10% of factor VIII activity from normal plasma. Usually this is not a problem, since there is equal adsorption from standard and test plasmas. However, if factor VIII concentrates are assayed, there is high non-specific adsorption of factor VIII due to the loss of other plasma proteins normally present in excess. To avoid this problem, factor VIII concentrates should be prediluted 1/10 in haemophilic plasma, buffer-containing albumin, or specially prepared cryosupernatant, before the adsorption step.

Interpretation
Normal range — 0.50–2.00 IU/ml (50–200 IU/dl).
For deficiency states, see 1-stage factor VIIIC assay; lupus anticoagulants do not generally have any effect on 2-stage assays.

MICROTITRE AMIDOLYTIC FVIIIC ASSAY

Principle
This assay is similar to the first stage of the 2-stage clotting assay; a reagent is used which provides everything necessary except factor VIIIC in a factor Xa generation system. The amount of factor Xa generated is thus dependent on the factor VIIIC provided by a dilution of test plasma. The factor Xa is measured using a specific chromogenic substrate, and the influence of any thrombin generated is blocked with a synthetic thrombin inhibitor (Rosen 1984).

Biochemical basis
The generated factor Xa cleaves a specific tripeptide chromogenic substrate releasing an attached paranitroaniline (pNA) molecule, which gives the solution a yellow colour, and absorbs at 405 nm. A synthetic thrombin inhibitor is included to prevent any fibrin formation, and possible feedback reactions of thrombin.

Reagents

Coatest kit (Kabi Diagnostica) comprising:

- S-2222 + I-2581 20 mg chromogenic substrate and 335 μg synthetic thrombin inhibitor; reconstitute with 10 ml sterile water.
- Factor IXa + factor X reconstitute with 10 ml sterile water.
- 0.025 M calcium chloride.
- 0.05 M Tris pH 7.3 with 0.02% bovine albumin — provided as concentrate, dilute 1/10 to obtain working solution on day of assay.
- Phospholipid (porcine brain).
- 50% acetic acid.

Equipment

- Cooke microtitre plates (Type M29A, Sterilin).
- Microtitre plate reader (MR700, Dynatech Laboratories Ltd.).
- Multichannel pipettes (Labsystems Ltd.).

Standards

National standard for factor VIIIC or commercial standard calibrated against the international standard.

Preparation of test standards and reagents

For assays in the range 0.2–1.50 IU/ml, dilute standard according to Table 22.1, and for the range 0.01–0.20 IU/ml, according to Table 22.2. Store dilutions on ice until used.

Mix 5 volumes of factor IXa + X reagent with 1 volume phospholipid on ice. Just before use, add 3 volumes of calcium chloride to make a combined reagent and store on ice.

Method

1. Add 25 μl of buffer to wells A1 and B1 as blank.
2. Add 25 μl of each standard dilution to duplicate wells in rows A and B, columns 2 to 7.
3. Place 25 μl of each test sample in duplicate wells over the rest of the plate.
4. Add 75 μl of combined reagent to each well, mix gently, and cover plate.
5. Place plate in a 37°C incubator for 5 minutes (0.20–1.50 IU/ml range) or 10 minutes (0.01–0.20 IU/ml range).
6. Add 50 μl of chromogenic substrate, mix and cover.
7. Incubate at 37°C for 5 minutes (0.20–1.50 IU/ml range) or 10 minutes (0.01–0.20 IU/ml range).
8. Add 25 μl acetic acid to each well to stop the reaction.
9. Read the absorbance at 405 nm.

Calculation

Plot absorbances on linear graph paper and abstract test results from the standard curve. Correct the results to IU/ml by multiplying the percentage of standard by the standard potency and dividing by 100.

Comments

— Assays must be performed within 30 minutes of dilution of test samples and standards as factor VIII is particularly labile in dilute form.

Table 22.1 Standard and test dilutions for 0.20–1.50 IU/ml range. (Dilute test samples 25 μl in 3000 μl buffer).

Standard %	Predilution		Final dilution	
	Plasma (μl)	Buffer (μl)	Predilution (μl)	Buffer (μl)
150	—	undiluted	25	2000
120	100	25	25	2000
100	50	25	25	2000
75	50	50	25	2000
50	50	100	25	2000
21	50	300	25	2000

Table 22.2 Standard and test dilutions for 0.01–0.20 IU/ml range. (Dilute test samples 25 μl in 2000 μl buffer.)

Standard %	Predilution		Final dilution	
	Plasma (μl)	Buffer (μl)	Predilution (μl)	
20	50	200	25	2000
14.3	50	300	25	2000
9.1	50	500	25	2000
4.8	25	500	25	2000
1.2	25	2000	25	2000

— 1.0 M citrate buffer pH 3.0 (equal amounts of 1.5 M citric acid and 0.5 M trisodium citrate) can be used to stop the reaction instead of acetic acid.

— Factor VIII concentrates should be prediluted in buffer so that the factor VIII is within the range 0.20–1.50 IU/ml and the fibrinogen is less than 3 g/l. Alternatively a long series of dilutions must be tested and only the linear portion of the curve evaluated.

— Heparin levels above 0.2 IU/ml may interfere in the assay (e.g. patients on intravenous infusion), and samples should be diluted before assay to reduce the heparin concentration.

Interpretation

Several studies have shown a good agreement between the amidolytic assay and 1-stage clotting assays in haemophilic and von Willebrand's disease plasmas.

IRMA ASSAY FOR FACTOR VIII COAGULANT ANTIGEN (FVIII:Ag)

Principle

This assay measures the factor VIII:Ag activity in a sample through reaction with an excess of added radio-labelled anti-FVIII:Ag antibody (IgG) molecules to form high molecular weight immune complexes that can be selectively precipitated and separated from the excess untreated antibody. Radioactivity detected in the precipitated immune complexes is directly proportional to the amount of FVIII:Ag in the test sample.

Biochemical basis

Factor VIIIC is defined as the procoagulant activity of the factor VIII macromolecular complex. Classically haemophilia A manifests as a bleeding disorder caused by absence or low level of FVIIIC. A small proportion of severe haemophiliacs treated with FVIIIC concentrates experience an immunological response to the added 'foreign' protein whereby inhibitor IgG molecules, usually either subclass I or IV, directed against FVIIIC are observed. Inhibitors make subsequent treatment of bleeding episodes very difficult and often result in even higher inhibitor titres.

If the total IgG fraction is isolated from a subject exhibiting a very high titre inhibitor to FVIIIC, this can be utilised in a very sensitive immunoradiometric assay (IRMA) for measurement of the antigenicity of the FVIIIC molecule, FVIII:Ag (see references). Measurement of FVIII:Ag has proved useful for the antenatal diagnosis of haemophilia, and by determination of FVIII:Ag to FVIIIR:Ag (vWF:Ag) ratios for the evaluation of carrier status in haemophilia and von Willebrand's disease family studies.

Reagents

For assay

- ^{125}I-labelled Fab' prepared from the IgG of a haemophilia A subject with high titre inhibitor activity against normal FVIIIC (see below). Dilute to approximately 20 000 cpm/ml in borate-buffered saline.
- Borate-buffered saline pH 7.85–0.05 M boric acid, 0.15 M NaCl, 0.02% sodium azide.
- Normal human IgG solution 10 mg/ml in borate buffer (outdated clinical concentrates of human IgG may also be used).

Reagents for Fab' preparation and iodination

- 76% saturated $(NH_4)_2SO_4$ solution.
- 38% saturated $(NH_4)_2SO_4$ solution.
- Whatman DE52 cellulose anion exchanger.
- Sephadex G150, Sephadex G25, Sepharose 4B, CNBr-activated Sepharose 4B, Protein A Sepharose 4B (Pharmacia).
- Pepsin (Worthington).

Buffers

These are conveniently prepared as needed by mixing concentrated stock solutions of each compound, adjusting the pH and making up to volume with distilled water.

- 0.02 M Tris buffer pH 8.5.
- 0.02 M Tris 0.15 M NaCl pH 7.4.
- 0.05 M Tris 0.15 M NaCl pH 6.8.
- 0.05 M Tris 0.15 M NaCl pH 7.2.
- 0.1 M sodium acetate 1.0 M NaCl buffer pH 4.5.
- 0.1 M sodium acetate 1.0 M NaCl buffer pH 2.6.
- 0.1 M sodium acetate 0.01 M cysteine buffer pH 4.2.
- 0.1 M Na_2HPO_4 buffer pH 7.5.
- 0.1 M Na_2HPO_4 0.15 M NaCl buffer pH 7.5.
- 0.1 M Na_2HPO_4 1.0 M NaCl buffer pH 7.5.
- 0.1 M Na_2HPO_4 0.5 M NaCl buffer pH 7.5.
- 2 mCi $Na^{125}I$ (Amersham).
- 5 mg/ml chloramine T in 0.1 M Na_2HPO_4 pH 7.5 (unstable, make up just prior to use).
- 1.5 mg/ml sodium metabisulphite in Na_2HPO_4 pH 7.5.
- 200 μg/ml KI.
- Commercial factor VIII concentrate.
- 1.0 M ethanolamine 1.0 M NaCl buffer pH 8.0.
- 0.1 M borate 0.02% sodium azide buffer pH 7.85.
- 0.1 M borate buffer pH 7.5.
- 0.1 M NaOH.

Preparation of reagents

Preparation of Fab'
Stage 1
1. Citrated plasma from a haemophiliac with high

anti-FVIIIC inhibitor levels is converted to serum by the addition of 5 ml 1 M $CaCl_2$ per 95 ml plasma, and 1 u/ml thrombin, and allowing to clot overnight at room temperature. The fibrin clot is removed by filtering through glass wool.

2. Add equal volume of 76% saturated $(NH_4)_2SO_4$ to serum, and leave for 30 minutes at room temperature.

3. Centrifuge at 3000 g for 30 minutes at room temperature, then discard supernatant.

4. Dissolve pellet in approximately 5 ml H_2O.

5. Dialyse against several changes of 0.02 M Tris buffer pH 8.5.

6. Apply to 1.5 × 30 cm column of Whatman DE52 and elute with 0.02 M Tris buffer pH 8.5 at 30 ml/h at room temperature.

7. Collect void fractions which should contain all the IgG, including the inhibitor activity.

Stage 2. Most FVIIIC inhibitors are invariably of a single subclass, IgG I or IgG subclass IV. IgG III accounts for 50% of the total IgG and the specific activity of the anti-FVIII:Ag preparation can therefore be increased by removing subclass III.

1. Pour a 0.9 × 15 cm column with Protein A Sepharose 4B at 4°C.

2. Equilibrate with 0.02 M Tris 0.15 M NaCl pH 7.4 buffer at 4°C at 12 ml/h.

3. Apply IgG preparation from stage 1, collect fractions and continue eluting until the absorbance at 280 nm returns to baseline levels.

4. Elute column with 1 M NaCl, 0.1 M sodium acetate buffer pH 4.5 and collect fractions.

5. Assay the void fractions (subclass III) and the acid buffer eluent for FVIIIC inhibitor activity. Retain the inhibitor fraction for subsequent preparation.

6. If the inhibitor is located in both fractions, the column binding capacity may have been exceeded. The column should therefore be re-equilibrated as in step 2 and the void fraction re-applied, repeating steps 3–5.

Stage 3

1. Determine total protein concentration of the above prepared inhibitor using the Lowry method (Lowry et al 1951).

2. Dialyse against 0.1 M sodium acetate, 0.01 M cysteine buffer pH 4.2.

3. Digest with pepsin (2 mg/100 mg inhibitor preparation) at 37°C for 24–36 hours.

4. The resultant Fab' fragments are isolated by gel filtration on Sephadex G150 equilibrated and eluted with 0.05 M Tris, 0.15 M NaCl pH 6.8. Pool the inhibitor containing fractions (the major absorption peak at 280 nm).

5. Dialyse exhaustively against 0.1 M Na_2HPO_4 buffer pH 7.5.

6. Determine the total protein concentration by the Lowry method.

7. Dilute the Fab' preparation to 1.67 mg/ml with 0.1 M Na_2HPO_4 buffer pH 7.5 and store as 0.06 ml aliquots at −20°C for radiolabelling.

Radiolabelling of the Fab'

Fab' is radiolabelled with ^{125}I using a modification of the chloramine T method.

1. 0.06 ml Fab' (100 μg) in 0.1 M Na_2HPO_4 buffer pH 7.5 is mixed with 2 mCi $Na^{125}I$.

2. 0.01 ml chloramine T is added and mixed for 30 seconds.

3. Add 0.01 ml sodium metabisulphite followed by 1 ml KI.

4. Apply the whole reaction mixture to a 0.9 × 15 cm Sephadex G25 column pre-equilibrated with 0.1 M Na_2HPO_4 buffer pH 7.5 containing 1% (w/v) bovine serum albumin and elute with the same buffer.

5. Collect 0.5 ml fractions by hand.

6. Pool the fractions containing the highest radioactivity.

Immunopurification of [125I]-anti FVIII:Ag Fab'

The inhibitor [125I] Fab' is absorbed to FVIIIC immobilised on an inert support matrix, and then eluted from it.

Stage 1

1. 1800 IU of FVIIIC from commercial FVIII concentrate is redissolved in a total 30 ml distilled water.

2. The factor VIII is gel filtered on a 5 × 100 cm column of Sepharose 4B using 0.05 M Tris 0.15 M NaCl buffer pH 7.2 for the elution.

3. Pool the void fractions which contain the FVIII.

4. Precipitate the total protein in the combined fractions using 38% saturated $(NH_4)_2SO_4$.

5. Centrifuge at 3000 g at 4°C and discard the supernatant.

6. Dissolve the precipitate in the smallest possible volume of distilled water.

7. Dialyse against 0.1 M Na_2HPO_4 0.15 M NaCl buffer pH 7.5.

Stage 2

1. Wash 40 ml CNBr-activated Sepharose 4B with 0.1 M Na_2HPO_4 1.0 M NaCl buffer pH 7.5 and dry to a 'wet cake' using a sintered Buchner funnel.

2. Transfer the matrix to a 100 ml beaker and resuspend in 30 ml 0.1 M Na_2HPO_4 1.0 M NaCl buffer pH 7.5.

3. Add the factor VIIIC prepared above (approximately 10 ml).

4. Allow the protein-coupling reaction to proceed at room temperature with gentle mixing for 6 hours.

5. Allow the reaction mixture to stand at 4°C for 16–20 hours.

6. Wash the resin on a sintered Buchner funnel using 1 litre Na_2HPO_4 0.5 M NaCl buffer pH 7.5.

7. Transfer the resin back to a 100 ml beaker and continuously mix with 50 ml 1.0 M ethanolamine 1.0 M NaCl buffer pH 8.0 for 6 hours at room temperature.

8. Wash the resin free of ethanolamine using a sintered Buchner funnel with 0.1 M borate 0.02% sodium azide buffer pH 7.85.

9. Suspend the washed resin in an equal volume of 0.1 M borate 0.02% sodium azide buffer pH 7.85. Aliquot into universal tubes such that each contains approximately 2 ml settled resin, store indefinitely at 4°C.

Stage 3

1. Wash 2 ml factor VIII:Ag-Sepharose 4B resin prepared above by centrifugation at 1000 g in 0.1 M borate buffer pH 7.5.

2. Add [^{125}I]Fab′ prepared above and allow the immunoabsorption to the matrix-bound FVIIIC:Ag to proceed for 2 hours at 37°C with occasional shaking.

3. Separate the matrix-bound immunocomplex from the excess unbound [^{12}I]Fab′ by repeated centrifugation and resuspension of the resin in 20 ml changes of 0.1 M borate buffer pH 7.5. Continue the washing steps (about 5 washes) until the radioactivity in the supernatant is negligible.

4. Resuspend the 2 ml washed matrix in 10–20 ml 0.1 M sodium acetate 1.0 M NaCl buffer pH 2.6 and leave with occasional stirring at 37°C for 1 hour.

5. Centrifuge at 1000 g for 20 minutes at 4°C. Remove and retain the supernatant containing the re-eluted [^{125}I]Fab′.

6. Adjust the pH to between 7 and 8 with 0.1 M NaOH.

7. Add enough normal IgG to bring to approximately 10 mg/ml.

8. Add an equal volume of 76% saturated $(NH_4)_2SO_4$ solution.

9. Allow to stand for 30 minutes at room temperature.

10. Centrifuge at 3000 g for 30 minutes at 25°C.

11. Discard the precipitate and dialyse the supernatant solution at 4°C against several changes of 0.1 M borate buffer pH 7.85.

12. Store in suitable aliquots at 4°C for use in the immunoradiometric assay for FVIII:Ag.

Equipment

○ Rimless polystyrene test tubes 65 × 10 mm (RT25 tubes, Sterilin).

○ Vortex mixer.

○ Gamma radiation counter for quantitation of ^{125}I in precipitates.

Method

1. Label sufficient polystyrene test tubes to allow for duplicate tubes for each point on the standard curve (20 tubes), 2 tubes to measure the non-specific binding (NSB), 2 tubes to measure the total radioactivity, duplicates of each unknown sample to be tested.

2. Make serial doubling dilutions of pooled normal plasma standard down to 1/512 using borate-buffered saline.

3. Add 0.1 ml normal IgG solution (10 mg/ml) in borate-buffered saline to each tube.

4. Add 0.1 ml diluted standard or test plasma to their respective, labelled tubes.

5. To the NSB tubes add 0.1 ml borate-buffered saline.

6. Add 0.1 ml [^{125}I] to every tube including the two tubes designated for measurement of the total radioactivity used in the assay.

7. Stopper each tube and mix the contents.

8. Spin the tubes at 2500 g for 5 minutes.

9. Set aside the 2 tubes designated for measurement of total radioactivity. These will not be needed again until counting the rest of the tubes for radioactivity at the end of the assay.

10. Incubate tubes at 37°C for a minimum of 4 hours, preferably overnight at room temperature.

11. Add 0.3 ml 76% saturated $(NH_4)_2SO_4$ solution, mix and allow to stand for 30 minutes at room temperature.

12. Spin tubes at 2000 g for 20 minutes.

13. Remove supernatant and discard.

14. Break up the ammonium sulphate pellet with the aid of the vortex mixer.

15. Add 2 ml 38% saturated $(NH_4)_2SO_4$ solution and mix.

16. Spin tubes at 2000 g for 20 minutes and discard the supernatant.

17. Measure the radioactive content of each tube for 5 minutes.

Calculation

The NSB activity is subtracted from the radioactivity found in each tube. A double logarithmic curve of cpm against standard dilution is then plotted, and should give a straight line. The FVIII:Ag values of each test sample can then be read off.

Comments

— The assay is technically very easy to perform once the [^{125}I]Fab′ molecules have been prepared. Once the Fab′ molecules and FVIII-Sepharose 4B matrix have been prepared, they may be kept in aliquots over an extended period, and iodination can be performed (say once every 3 months). This would give sufficient [^{125}I]Fab′ to perform two large

FVIII:Ag IRMA runs per week with up to 200 test samples in each.

— Occasional errors and accidents may occur, especially in large assay runs, and for this reason it may be prudent to construct the standard curve from triplicate measurements instead of duplicates, so that ambiguities may be easier to sort out.

— For assays on test samples of unknown concentration range, it is preferable to perform assays at several dilutions, ensuring that some results fall on the linear part of the standard curve.

— The precipitates are washed with 38% saturated ammonium sulphate, a useful technique is to break up the wet precipitate using a vortex mixer before adding the 2 ml of wash liquid. Successful vortex mixing after adding the wash liquid is virtually impossible.

— The addition of normal IgG as carrier protein is essential to achieve quantitative recovery of the immune complex, and mandatory for the successful completion of the test.

FACTOR XI CLOTTING ASSAY

Principle
This assay tests the ability of dilutions of patient plasma to correct the prolonged KPTT of FXI-deficient plasma. The degree of correction is compared to that obtained using dilutions of a standard plasma of known potency, so that a concentration can be calculated.

Biochemical basis
Factor XI is activated on cell surfaces or charged artificial surfaces by factor XIIa, or at the platelet membrane by factor XII-dependent and independent mechanisms. Factor XIa then activates factor IX, initiating a chain of reactions leading to thrombin generation and fibrin formation. Factor Xa is a serine protease, but is not vitamin K-dependent.

Standard
Commercial standard (Immuno Ltd.).

Method
As for 1-stage factor VIIIC assay, but using factor XI-deficient substrate plasma.

Interpretation
Factor XI is decreased in:
  a. Inherited defects (haemophilia C). Deficiency has a particularly high incidence in Ashkenazi Jewish communities.
    b. Liver failure.
    c. DIC.

    d. Presence of specific inhibitors or interference by lupus anticoagulant.

FACTOR XI MICROTITRE AMIDOLYTIC ASSAY

Modification of the method of Scott et al 1985.

Principle
The inhibitors of factor XIa are neutralised, and SBTI is added to block kallikrein activity and stabilise the factor XI by forming a complex. After activation of factors XII and XI with kaolin, the factor XIIa is neutralised with corn inhibitor. A chromogenic substrate is then added, and colour generation is proportional to factor XIa concentration, since other relevant proteases have been blocked.

Reagents
- Soya bean trypsin inhibitor (SBTI) (Sigma Chemical Co.). 1 μM solution in sterile distilled water.
- Light kaolin (Aldrich Chemical Co.) — 1 mg/ml in buffer A.
- Corn trypsin inhibitor (Channel Diagnostics) — 0.1 mg/ml in sterile water.
- Chromogenic substrate S2366 (Kabi Diagnostica) — 25 mg dissolved in 25 ml of sterile water (1.9 mmol/l).
- Buffer A
  0.02 M Tris (2.4 g/l)
  0.15 M NaCl (8.8 g/l)
  1 mM EDTA disodium (0.37 g/l)
  Make up in distilled water and adjust to pH 7.4 with HCl.
- Buffer B — 0.1 M sodium phosphate, 0.15 M NaCl, 1 mM EDTA, pH 7.6.
- 0.167 M hydrochloric acid.
- 0.167 M sodium hydroxide.
- 50% acetic acid.

Equipment
○ Multichannel pipettes (Labsystems Ltd.).
○ Cooke microtitre plates (Type M29A, Sterilin).
○ Microtitre plate reader e.g. Dynatech MR700.

Standard
Commercial standard (Immuno Ltd.) or pooled normal plasma — at least 10 donors.

Preparation of standard and test plasmas
50 μl of standard or test plasma are incubated with 50 μl of 0.167 M HCl for 15 minutes at room temperature in polypropylene tubes. 50 μl of buffer B and 50 μl of 0.167 M NaOH are added to the acidified plasma.

Acidified standard plasma is diluted with buffer A in duplicate wells A2–A6 and B2–B6 of a microtitre plate, as shown below.

Standard %	Plasma μl	Buffer A μl
125	50	0
100	40	10
75	30	20
50	20	30
25	10	40

Acidified test plasmas were diluted in buffer A by adding 40 μl to 10 μl of buffer in wells A7B7 onwards of a microtitre plate.

Method

1. Plate 50 μl of buffer A in well A1B1.
2. In the other wells make dilutions of standard or test plasma in duplicate (see above).
3. Add 10 μl of SBTI to each well and mix by gently rocking plate.
4. Add 10 μl of 1 mg/ml kaolin and mix gently.
5. Cover plate and incubate at room temperature for 60 minutes.
6. Add 10 μl of corn trypsin inhibitor and incubate for 10 minutes.
7. Add 80 μl of substrate, cover with clingfilm and incubate for a final 30 minutes.
8. Stop the reaction with 100 μl of 50% acetic acid.
9. Read absorbance at 405–410 nm using a microtitre plate reader.

Units

1 unit of factor XI is the activity contained in 1 ml of normal plasma.

Calculation

Plot absorbance against standard concentration and abstract the test values from the standard curve.

Comments

— During the 30 minutes incubation with substrate it is advisable to cover the plate, making it airtight.
— The plate reader should be blanked on well A1.
— The assay may be affected by deficiency of factor XII.
— Small quantities of heparin have no effect on the assay system.
— If samples are lipaemic or icteric, a plasma blank should be performed with buffer substituted for chromogenic substrate. Blank absorbance should be subtracted from that of test before calculation.

Interpretation

Normal range (males) — 0.65–1.45 u/ml (mean ± 2SD).

Normal range (females) — 0.75–1.55 u/ml (mean ± 2SD).
The discrepancy between males and females is probably due to the oral contraceptive pill.

FACTOR XII CLOTTING ASSAY

Principle

This assay tests the ability of dilutions of patient plasma to correct the prolonged KPTT of FXII-deficient plasma. The degree of correction is compared to that obtained using dilutions of a standard plasma of known potency, so that a concentration can be calculated.

Biochemical basis

Factor XII may be activated by exposure to charged surfaces such as subendothelial components, or, in vitro, glass, kaolin, or ellagic acid etc. This protein acts as a pivot between a number of enzyme cascades, i.e. the intrinsic and extrinsic coagulation pathways, complement, fibrinolysis, and kinin systems. The 1-stage clotting assay depends on its activation of factor XI, and subsequent reactions leading to clot formation. This activation of factor XI takes place in the solid phase, with high molecular weight kininogen acting as a cofactor and catalyst.

Standard

Commercial standard (Immuno Ltd.).

Method

As for 1-stage factor VIIIC assay, but using factor XII-deficient substrate plasma.

Interpretation

Normal range 0.56–1.48 u/ml.
Factor XII deficiency is not usually associated with any bleeding diathesis. Decreased levels are found in:
a. Inherited defects.
b. Liver failure.
c. DIC.
d. Apparent deficiencies may be found in the presence of lupus anticoagulant.

Increased levels may be found in women taking oral contraceptive pills (personal observation).

FACTOR XII MICROTITRE AMIDOLYTIC ASSAY

Principle

Factor XII is readily activated by exposure to extravascular surface or activated platelets, and occupies a key position, initiating several different enzyme cascades. It is the pivot between the intrinsic and extrinsic coagulation systems, the fibrinolytic, complement and kinin systems. Which of these systems is triggered depends on the molecular form of factor XII following its cleavage by other proteases. Factor XII deficiency is not usually associated with any marked haemorrhagic tendency, but its role and importance in the other cascade systems remains to be fully elucidated. The measurement of contact factors and their inhibitors may be relevant to both the management and prognosis of critically ill patients.

Factor XII assays are most frequently performed by one-stage coagulation assays, which are time-consuming and dependent on congenitally deficient plasma as substrate. The latter is both expensive and may have viral contamination. A chromogenic substrate assay for factor XII has recently been described (Gallimore et al 1987) which overcomes some of these problems. This assay system depends on the conversion of factor XII to an active form and the specific cleavage of a chromogenic peptide substrate in the presence of suitable inhibitors of other contact proteins. We describe here a modification of this system to a microtitre technique which makes the assay rapid, safe and inexpensive.

Reagents
- Factor XII activator (Channel Diagnostics).
- Chromogenic substrate S2222 (Kabi Diagnostica).
- Kallikrein inhibitor (Channel diagnostics).
- Buffer A Tris-HCl 0.05 mol/l pH 7.9 containing 0.12 M methylamine and 3.36 g/l EDTA.
- Buffer B — Tris-HCl 0.05 mol/l pH 7.9.
- 50% acetic acid.
- Acetone.

Equipment
- Cooke microtitre plates (Type M29A, Sterilin Ltd.).
- Microtitre plate reader — Dynatech MR700.
- Multichannel pipettes (Labsystems).
- Polypropylene Microcentrifuge Tubes (Sarstedt Ltd.).

Standards
Commercial standard (Immuno Ltd.) or pooled normal plasma (at least 10 donors).

Preparation of reagents, standard and test plasmas

Preparation of plasma 1 volume of acetone was added to 3 volumes of plasma in polypropylene microfuge tubes. After mixing, the tubes were left for at least 30 minutes at 4°C. A standard curve was prepared by diluting acetone-treated pooled normal plasma in buffer A as follows;

Standard %	Plasma (μl)	Buffer (μl)
200	200	200
150	150	250
100	100	300
75	75	325
50	50	350
25	25	375

Test plasmas were diluted 1/4 in buffer A.

Reagent preparation Factor XII activator was reconstituted with 2.5 ml sterile water and left to stand for 5 minutes before mixing and storing on ice.

25 mg chromogenic substrate S2222 was dissolved in 22 ml of sterile water (1.5 mmol/l).

Kallikrein inhibitor was reconstituted in 10 ml sterile water and stored at 4°C. Immediately before use, 2 ml of kallikrein inhibitor was diluted in 98 ml of buffer B.

Prewarm factor XII activator, substrate and buffer B to 37°C in a water-bath.

Method
1. 25 μl of buffer A (buffer blank) or plasma dilution are pipetted into each well of a microtitre plate and 25 μl of factor XII activator added.
2. After gently mixing, the plate is covered and incubated for 10 minutes at room temperature.
3. 75 μl of dilute kallikrein inhibitor is added to each well and the plate incubated for a further 1 minute at room temperature.
4. Add 50 μl of substrate, cover and incubate for exactly 10 minutes.
5. Stop the reaction with 50 μl of 50% acetic acid.
6. Read absorbance at 405–410 nm against buffer blank on a microtitre plate reader.

Calculation
A graph of absorbance against standard concentration is plotted and the concentrations of test samples abstracted from this standard curve.

Comments
— For plasmas with a high bilirubin level, a plasma blank is prepared, using 75 μl of buffer A instead of substrate and factor XII activator.
— The assay is not affected by deficiency of factor XI, prekallikrein or high molecular weight kininogen.

Interpretation
Normal range — 0.73–1.45 u/ml.

Factor XII deficiency is rarely associated with a bleeding tendency, the significance of its contribution to other enzyme systems in the clinical setting is currently poorly understood. Factor XII levels may be raised in women taking the oral contraceptive pill (personal observation).

PREKALLIKREIN ASSAY

Principle

Prekallikrein (PKK) is converted to kallikrein (KK) by an activator mixture, containing ellagic acid, which activates factor XII, and a plasma fraction providing factor XII and high molecular weight kininogen (HK). The amount of KK liberated is determined by measuring its amidolytic activity on a specific chromogenic peptide substrate (Gallimore and Friberger, 1982). The release of p-nitroaniline (pNA) from the substrate is determined at 405 nm.

Biochemical basis

Plasma kallikrein circulates in the blood as an inactive precursor PKK. Approximately 75% circulates bound to high molecular weight kininogen (HK), only 25% exists as free PKK. Activation of human plasma KK involves limited proteolysis. Plasma KK cleaves the single chain proenzyme factor XII (FXII) into an active enzyme (αFXIIa), which itself is further cleaved to liberate a 28 000 molecular weight active enzyme (βFXIIa). It has been suggested that both activated FXII and Hageman factor fragments (βFXIIa) are potent PKK activators. Plasma KK also liberates biologically active polypeptide fragments from HK, known as kinins, and these include bradykinin.

The activation of PKK in plasma is difficult to effect when the plasma is undiluted. This is because the rapid generation of FXIIa is needed to convert the PKK to KK and stimulate the feedback activation of FXII before inhibitors can interfere. One approach to overcome this problem is acid treatment of the plasma before dilution. Reasonable concentrations of FXII, PKK, and HK are required for activation of FXII and subsequent activation of PKK. To overcome this problem the activator used contains FXII and HK.

Reagents

- Prekallikrein activator (Channel Diagnostics).
- Chromogenic substrate S2302 (Kabi Diagnostica) 25 mg in 20 ml sterile water.
- Buffer A — Tris-HCl 0.05 mol/l, pH 7.9 + 0.1% PEG 6000.
- Buffer B
    0.1 M sodium phosphate pH 7.6
    0.15 M sodium chloride
    1 mM disodium EDTA.
- 0.167 M HCl.
- 0.167 M NaOH.

Equipment

- Cooke microtitre plates (Types M29A, Sterilin).
- Microtitre plate reader e.g. Dynatech MR700 (Dynatech Laboratories Ltd.).
- Multichannel pipettes (Labsystems Ltd.).

Standard

Pooled normal plasma (at least 10 donors).

Preparation of standard and test plasmas

Acidification of plasma:
1. Add 50 μl of 0.167 M HCl to 50 μl of plasma in a polypropylene tube.
2. Incubate for 15 minutes at room temperature.
3. Add 50 μl of buffer B and 50 μl of 0.167 M NaOH to the acidified plasma.

Dilute the acidified standard plasma with buffer A as follows:

Standard %	Acid-treated diluted plasma	Buffer μl
125	50 μl	270
100	100 μl	700
75	300 μl of 100%	100
50	200 μl of 100%	200
25	100 μl of 100%	300

Dilute acidified test plasmas 1/8 (100 μl plasma + 700 μl buffer).

Method

1. Place 50 μl of plasma dilution or buffer in each well of the microtitre plate and add 50 μl of prekallikrein activator.
2. Cover plate and incubate at room temperature for 5 minutes.
3. Add 50 μl of substrate and incubate for a further 10 minutes at room temperature.
4. Stop the reaction with 50 μl of 50% acetic acid.
5. Read the absorbance at 405–410 nM using a microtitre plate reader.

Calculation

Plot a graph of absorbance against standard concentration and abstract the test values from the curve.

Comment

— May be performed by a tube technique if four times the reagent volumes are used, and results are read in a spectrophotometer cuvette.

Interpretation

Normal range — 0.78–1.26 u/ml.

PKK deficiency is not usually associated with a bleeding diathesis, the clinical significance of its absence on fibrinolytic, kinin and other systems is uncertain.

High molecular weight kininogen assay

High molecular weight kininogen (HK) may be assayed by a coagulation method using congenital deficient plasma (Immuno Ltd.), or by immunological assay for heavy or light chains (Behring).

REFERENCES

Denson K W E 1967 The simplified two stage assay for factor VIII using a combined reagent. Transactions of the International Committee on Haemostasis and Thrombosis, Chapel Hill, North Carolina, p 197

Gallimore M J, Friberger P 1982 Simple chromogenic peptide substrate assays for determining prekallikrein, kallikrein inhibition and kallikrein 'like' activity in human plasma. Thrombosis Research 25: 293–298

Gallimore M J, Rees W A, Fuhrer G, Heller W 1987 A direct chromogenic substrate assay for Hageman factor (FXII). Fibrinolysis 1: 123–128

Hunter W H, Greenwood F C 1962 Preparation of iodine-131 labelled human growth hormone of high specific activity. Nature 194: 495–496

Lazarchick J, Hoyer L W 1978 Immunoradiometric measurement of the factor VIII procoagulant antigen. Journal of Clinical Investigation 62: 1048–1052

Lowry O H, Rosebrough N J, Parr A L, Randall R J 1951 Protein measurement with the Folin-Phenol reagent. Journal of Biological Chemistry 193: 265–275

Peake I R, Bloom A L 1978 Immunoradiometric assay of procoagulant factor VIII antigen in plasma and serum and its reduction in haemophillia. Lancet 1: 473–475

Reisner H M, Barrow E S, Graham J B 1979 Radioimmunoassay for coagulant factor VIII-related antigen (VIII:Cag). Thrombosis Research 14: 235–239

Rosen S 1984 The assay of factor VIII with a chromogenic substrate. Scandinavian Journal of Haematology 33: Supplement 40: 139–145

Scott C F, Sinha D, Seaman F S, Walsh F N, Colman R W 1985 Amidolytic assay of human factor XII in plasma: comparison coagulant assay and a new rapid radioimmunoassay. Blood 63: 42–50

23

Von Willebrand factor assay

RISTOCETIN COFACTOR ASSAY — FIXED WASHED PLATELET AGGREGOMETRY METHOD

Principle
The ristocetin cofactor activity of a plasma may be determined in an assay using formalin-fixed, washed platelets agglutinated in the presence of von Willebrand factor, using the antibiotic ristocetin.

Biochemical basis
Von Willebrand factor (vWF) is an adhesive protein mediating the adhesion and spreading of platelets to the subendothelium, particularly in the small vessels where there is a high shear rate. The importance of this action to haemostasis is reflected by the marked bleeding tendency seen in von Willebrand's disease, where it is congenitally absent or abnormal. It is a very large protein of varying molecular size existing in plasma as a series of multimers of molecular weight $1-20 \times 10^6$. The multimers are built from protomers of 10^6 daltons, which are in turn composed of subunits each of molecular weight 2.3×10^5. Using monoclonal antibodies and competitive inhibition studies, two types of platelet-binding site have been defined, as well as a discrete collagen binding site. vWF also acts as a carrier for factor VIII coagulant activity, the two proteins circulating in plasma as a complex. vWF is synthesised by megakaryocytes (and thus circulates in platelets) and vascular endothelial cells. Each of these cell types is able to release vWF under suitable stimulus.

vWF may be measured by several types of immunological method, but functional assays of its adhesive properties are beyond the scope of most laboratories; instead vWF 'function' is assessed by its property of causing platelet agglutination in the presence of the antibiotic ristocetin. The mechanism of this interaction is poorly understood, and a physiological counterpart of ristocetin has not been found, although thrombin has been suggested as a mediator of vWF binding.

Test samples
The test lends itself to a batched assay approach, and plasma samples are aliquoted and stored at $-80°C$ until processed. For reasons of standardisation even 'urgent' samples are treated to a 'freezing' step before assay. Frozen samples may only be thawed once before processing.

Reagents
- Sterile 109 mM tri-sodium citrate dihydrate — 32.35 g in 1 litre distilled water. Sterilise in glass 50 ml ampoules.
- Normal Saline 0.9%.
- 50 mM Tris buffer pH 7.4 — 6.06 g Tris in 990 ml distilled water, adjust pH to 7.4 with concentrated HCl and make to 1 litre.
- Buffered saline pH 7.4 — 2.2 g of sodium chloride in 1 litre of 50 mM Tris pH 7.4 containing 0.05% w/v sodium azide.
- Buffered saline containing bovine albumin — 30% bovine albumin (ICN Biomedicals Ltd.) is added to buffered saline to give 50 mg/buffer.
- 20 g/l ristocetin (Lundbeck & Co. Ltd.) — 100 mg dissolved in 5 ml 0.9% sodium chloride, store in aliquots at $-80°C$.
- Formalin-fixed washed platelets (FWP).
- Formalin.

Equipment
- Venesection bags, transfer bags and plasma aspirator (Fenwal Products, Travenol Laboratories).
- Large capacity centrifuge (e.g. Mistral 4l).
- A selection of plastic tubes and containers (25–500 ml capacity).
- Rotating mixing apparatus (e.g. Matburn Ltd.).
- Aggregometer (e.g. 300BD, Centronic Sales Ltd.).
- Chart recorder (e.g. Series 28000, Bryans Southern Instruments Ltd.).
- $-80°C$ deep freeze (e.g. Denley Instruments Ltd.).

Standard

Pooled normal plasma from at least 20 normal individuals, preferably with a 50:50 sex distribution, aliquoted in 500 μl volumes at $-80°C$.

Preparation of fixed washed platelets (FWP)

(Process may be scaled down for preparation of smaller quantities as required).

1. Collect four pints of blood from normal or polycythaemic individuals into 109 mM tri-sodium citrate (1 volume anticoagulant: 9 volumes blood), mixing constantly.

2. Without delay, centrifuge at 60 g for 15 minutes at room temperature to produce platelet-rich plasma (PRP).

3. Separate PRP into transfer bags and place in a 37°C water-bath for 1 hour.

4. Dilute PRP with an equal volume of 2% formalin in normal saline using plastic containers.

5. This mixture is placed at 4°C and left undisturbed for 18 hours.

6. Slowly decant the supernatant into plastic centrifuge containers, leaving most of the sedimented red blood cells.

7. The platelets are centrifuged at 2000 g for 20 minutes at 4°C.

8. Pour off and replace the supernatant with cold normal saline to resuspend the platelets. Some mechanical mixing is necessary.

9. Sedimentation and resuspension in fresh normal saline is repeated three times.

10. Transfer the suspension to universal containers and remove remaining red cells with a slow centrifugation at 60 g for 10 minutes at room temperature.

11. After red cell contamination has been removed the FWP are centrifuged at 2000 g for 10 minutes at room temperature and the supernatant discarded.

12. The sedimented platelets are reconstituted with approximately 10 ml of buffered saline containing bovine albumin. The reconstitution is achieved slowly by using a rotating mixer.

13. Pool the platelets and aliquot into universal containers so that when they are spun and resuspended (in step 14) with 6 ml of diluent a platelet count between 300 and 500 $\times$ 10^9/l is achieved.

14. The FWP aliquots are centrifuged at 2000 g for 10 minutes, the supernatant discarded, and the platelet 'button' maintained at $-80°C$.

Preparation of working reagents, test and standard samples

All plasma samples are thawed at 37°C before assay and maintained on ice until processed.

Stock ristocetin is thawed, diluted to 10 g/l in 0.9% sodium chloride and left on ice.

FWP are left at 37°C for 5 minutes on removal from $-80°C$ storage, and then reconstituted with 6 ml of isotonic buffered saline, after which they are left to equilibrate at room temperature for 30 minutes before processing, and maintained at that temperature during the assay.

Doubling dilutions of standard and test plasma (1/2–1/32) are made in buffered saline containing bovine albumin. The dilutions are prepared just prior to individual testing.

A 'blank' dilution is prepared consisting of 300 μl of buffered saline with albumin and 100 μl of FWP. This is used in conjunction with the dilution of 1/2 standard plasma to set the sensitivity limits of the aggregometer system.

Method

1. One recorder channel is used, removing channel/channel variability.

2. Place 200 μl of the standard 1/2 dilution and 250 μl of FWP in a cuvette, and stir in the aggregometer. Set the 0% light transmission.

3. Set 100% light transmission using 400 μl of the 'blank' dilution.

4. Add 50 μl dilute ristocetin to the cuvette from step 2 and record agglutination.

5. Repeat steps 1–4 with subsequent dilutions of test and standard.

Units

The standard is arbitrarily designated with a 100% potency, 1 unit/ml for vWF.

Calculation

The steepest angle of deflection is plotted against the plasma concentration on log/linear graph paper (Fig. 23.1). The dilutions of test samples which give the best fit graphically are used in the dose response curve.

Comments

— Platelets for FWP must be processed as freshly as possible after donation and maintained at room temperature. Outdated platelet concentrates have not been found useful for this procedure.

— Examine the platelets after reconstitution for agglutinates before and after the assay procedure.

— Quality control checks should be performed on FWP, to screen for spontaneous agglutination, to ensure a sensitive dose response curve, and a severe vWF plasma control sample should be tested with each new batch prepared.

— Make plasma dilutions separately and then transfer to cuvettes without the production of air bubbles.

— Lyophilised plasma samples produce inhibitory activity using this method. This may be corrected

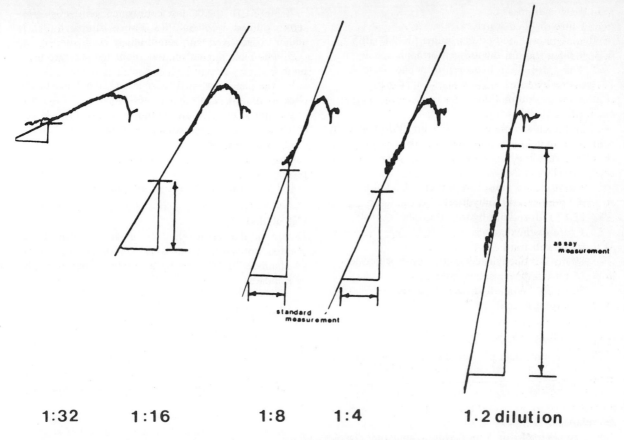

1:32   1:16   1:8   1:4   1.2 dilution

Fig. 23.1 Ristocetin cofactor assay. Aggregometer responses obtained with varying dilutions of test or standard samples.

by dilution and the results extrapolated from the standard graph.
— It is essential that a dilution series is constructed on test plasma, as lipaemic samples may produce inhibition.

Interpretation

Normal range — 38–261%.

ENZYME-LINKED IMMUNOSORBENT ASSAY (ELISA)

Principle

A heterologous multivalent factor VIII antibody is adsorbed to the solid phase (Fig. 23.2). After an incubation period sample dilutions are applied to the plate, and specific antigen attaches to the antibody. Following a further incubation, enzyme-labelled specific antibody attaches to the bound antigen. Finally, an enzyme substrate is added and the level of hydrolysis is found to be proportional to the amount of antigen present (Short et al 1982).

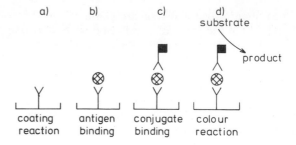

Fig. 23.2 ELISA technique: a) microtitre plate is coated with the primary antibody by adsorption, b) antigen from test sample is bound to antibody, c) second antibody conjugated to enzyme is bound to antigen, d) substrate is converted to a coloured product by the enzyme.

Reagents

- Rabbit anti-human factor VIII serum and rabbit anti-human factor VIII serum horseradish peroxidase conjugate (Code No's A082 and P226, Dako Ltd.).
- 50 mM carbonate buffer pH 9.6
    1.59 g sodium carbonate anhydrous
    2.93 g sodium hydrogen carbonate

0.2 g sodium azide
1 litre distilled water.
- 10 mM phosphate-buffered saline pH 7.2 (PBS)
   0.345 g sodium dihydrogen orthophosphate
   2.68 g di-sodium hydrogen orthophosphate dodecahydrate
   8.474 g sodium chloride
   1 litre distilled water.
- PBS Tween sample buffer — 1 litre PBS containing 1 ml Tween 20.
- PBS Tween washing buffer — 1 litre PBS containing 0.5 ml Tween 20.
- 100 mM citrate phosphate buffer pH 5.0
   7.3 g citric acid anhydrous
   23.87 g di-sodium hydrogen orthophosphate
   1 litre distilled water.
- Enzyme substrate
   80 mg 1,2-phenylenediamine dihydrochloride
   15 ml citrate phosphate buffer
   30 μl 20 volume hydrogen peroxide.
- 1 M sulphuric acid.

Equipment
○ Titertek multiskan plate reader (Flow Laboratories).
○ Microtitre plates (M129B, Dynatech Laboratories).
○ Multichannel pipette (Titertek, Flow Laboratories).

Standard
Standard (British or other) for coagulation factors (NIBSC), or commercial standard.

Preparation of test and standard plasmas
Standard and test plasmas are diluted from 1/10 to 1/80 in doubling dilutions, in PBS Tween sample buffer.

Method
1. 100 μl of unconjugated antifactor VIII, diluted 1/500 in carbonate buffer is added to each well of the microtitre plate using a multichannel pipette.
2. The plate is incubated for 1 hour at room temperature in a moist chamber.
3. The plate is washed 3 times by immersion in PBS Tween washing buffer for 1–2 minutes.
4. 100 μl of sample buffer is added to each well of column 1 to act as a reagent blank. Column 2 contains the standard dilutions; 100 μl of 1/10 standard is added to wells A and E, followed by 1/20 dilution in wells B and F, 1/40 in wells C and G, and 1/80 in wells D and H. Columns 3–12 incorporate quality control and test plasma dilutions.
5. All dilutions are incubated for 1 hour at room temperature in a moist chamber.
6. The plate is washed as in stage 3.

7. 100 μl of peroxidase-conjugated antifactor VIII serum diluted 1/500 in PBS Tween sample buffer is added to each well with a multichannel pipette.
8. The plate is incubated at room temperature for 1 hour.
9. The plate is washed twice as in stage 3 and finally once in 10 mM citrate buffer pH 5.0.
10. 100 μl of substrate solution is added to each well and incubated for approximately 20 minutes.
11. Stop the reaction by adding 150 μl of 1 M sulphuric acid to each well with the multichannel pipette.
12. Read the absorbance at 492 nm.

Calculation
Determine the relative potency of samples using incorporated software, a bioassay computer programme (Williams et al 1978) or by a graphical log/linear plot of standard.

Comments
— The optimal dilutions of both antibodies must be ascertained using a 'chequer board' technique before test samples are incorporated. This needs to be repeated occasionally when using the same batch of antibody, and always when new batches are introduced.
— The incubation time with substrate will vary, since an optimal OD should be achieved before stopping the reaction.
— The volume of hydrogen peroxide added to the substrate may alter if the container is exposed to the air. To overcome this problem, seal the container with a rubber bung, and penetrate this with a needle attached to a syringe on the day of assay.
— The Titertek plate reader has a linear OD reading between 0 and 1.5, and it has been found to be convenient if the colour development of the standard 1/10 dilution is stopped when the OD is approximately 0.2, thereby causing the final OD reading to be of the order of 1.2–1.3.
— 3,3′ 5,5′ — Tetramethylbenzidine (TMB) is an alternative substrate for use with horseradish peroxidase conjugates in ELISA techniques. This compound, unlike OPD, is non-mutagenic and non-carcinogenic. It can be obtained from ICN Biomedicals Ltd.

Interpretation
Normal range — 45.0–160.0 iu/dl.
   Plasma levels below the normal range are suggestive of von Willebrand's disease; with borderline values it is advisable to repeat the estimations on plasma samples taken at repeated intervals.

LAURELL TECHNIQUE

Principle

The method employs xenogeneic antibody to human factor VIII incorporated into agarose gel. Measured volumes of antigen are placed in wells cut into the agarose and electrophoresis is performed to induce migration of antigen towards the anode.

Antigen antibody interaction occurs and precipitation arcs are formed with the appearance of ascending rockets. The area enclosed by the rocket varies with the concentration of antigen applied to the well, and consequently the height of the rocket is empirically assessed to be proportional to the antigen concentration (Laurell 1966).

Reagents

- Barbital buffer 50 mM pH 8.6
  51.5 g sodium barbitone
  10 g barbitone (diethylbarbituric acid).
  Dissolve in distilled water on a hotplate. When cool add 0.25 g sodium azide.
  Make up to 5 litres with distilled water.
- Barbital buffer 20 mM pH 8.6 — take 2 volumes of barbital buffer 50 mM and make up to 5 volumes with distilled water.
- 1% Agarose LE (ICN Biomedicals Ltd.) — suspend in 20 mM barbital buffer in a conical flask and heat until a clear solution is achieved. Decant into 25 ml glass universals and store at 4°C until needed.
- Rabbit anti-human factor VIII (Dako Ltd. or Hoechst).
- Coomassie Brilliant Blue stain R250 (Gurr: Hopkins and Williams Ltd.) — 5 g stain dissolved in 450 ml methanol, 100 ml glacial acetic acid, and 450 ml distilled water, overnight. Filter and keep at room temperature.
- Decolourising solution — as above, but without stain.

Equipment

- Electrophoresis power pack and tank. The tank should be connected to a water source to enable cooling.
- Clean glass plates 200 × 110 × 1 mm.
- U-Frames (the same external dimensions as the glass plates, the base of the frame corresponding to the long axis of the plate, 10 mm wide and 1 mm thick, made of non-conducting material).
- Cutting templates for making wells in the agarose.
- Well cutter 3 mm diameter, connected to a Venturi pump.
- Filter paper sheets 200 × 100 mm for wicks (Whatman, chromatography paper 3 MM).
- Bull-dog clips.
- Glass universal bottles.
- 56°C incubator and water-bath.
- Hotplate or Bunsen burner.
- X-ray viewing box.

Standards

Standard for coagulation factors (NIBSC), or commercial standard.

Preparation of test samples, standard and working reagents

Antibody concentration

The optimum concentration of antibody in the gel must be determined for each batch by trial and error, with voltage variations, to obtain rockets with clearly defined peaks and minimal diffusion around the wicks and application sites of samples. A peak height of 25 mm using a 1/2 dilution of factor VIII standard would appear to give the best sensitivity in the assay system.

Agarose plates

Boil the appropriate number of 25 ml agarose bottles, allow to cool in a 56°C water-bath, and add the predetermined volume of antiserum to the agarose. Mix the suspension and pour between two prewarmed glass plates with a 1 mm U-frame between them. The plates are securely held in position by means of bull-dog clips. When the plates have set (20 minutes) transfer to the refrigerator at 4°C for a further 20 minutes. Remove the bull-dog clips and the upper glass plate from the gel in an easy horizontal sliding movement, keeping the U-frame in position. 18 × 3 mm wells are cut into each plate at a uniform distance apart (5 mm) along a horizontal plane. The wells are cut far enough in from the long edge of the plate to allow for wick overlap in the electrophoretic tanks. With the aid of the cutter, the guide and Venturi pump, the wells should come out cleanly.

Electrophoresis tank

Freshly prepared 50 mM barbital buffer is placed in the tanks. Filter-paper wicks are cut carefully so that the leading edge is straight.

Test samples and standard

Thaw test samples at 37°C just prior to the assay and reconstitute freeze-dried standard. Replicate dilutions of each plasma are made in 50 mM barbital buffer from 1/2 to 1/8.

Method

1. The agarose plate is laid on the central rack of the electrophoresis tank, so that the edge of the plate near the wells is on the cathodic side.

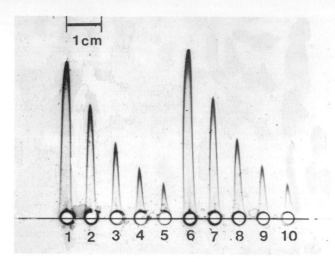

Fig 23.3 Immunoelectrophoretic assay of factor VIII related antigen showing rockets. Wells 1–10: various samples containing vWF:Ag. Anode at top figure

2. A wick is applied to each of the long sides of the plate, overlapping the agarose by 10–15 mm, and allowing the free edges of the wicks to dip into the buffer tanks.

3. Apply a 50 v charge through the tank to prevent diffusion problems when applying the standard and tests.

4. Starting at one edge of the plate fill the first three wells with 8 μl of each standard dilution, then the next three wells with dilutions of the first patient's plasma, and the next three with dilutions of the second patient's plasma. Using replicate dilutions, the subsequent three wells are filled with dilutions of standard, the next three with the first patient's dilutions, and the final three with the second patient's dilutions.

5. The water cooling circuit is switched on and the lid of the electrophoresis tank applied. The current is raised to 90 v and electrophoresis continued overnight.

6. The electricity and water are turned off, the plate is removed and placed on the bench, gel uppermost.

7. The gel is covered with a moistened filter paper (soaked in 3% sodium chloride) taking care to avoid trapping air bubbles. This is covered with several layers of paper towels and a glass plate placed on top. A weight of about 3 kg is then applied to the glass plate.

8. After 1 hour the towels and filter paper are removed and the plate placed in a 56°C oven for about 20 minutes or until dry.

9. The U-frame is removed and the dried gel is immersed in Coomassie Blue in a flat dish for 20 minutes.

10. The plate is transferred to a translucent dish containing the decolourising solution, and rocked gently over a horizontal light source until the optimal differentiation of the precipitin arcs (rockets) have been obtained.

11. Air dry the plate (this can be hastened with a hairdryer) and measure the height of each rocket from the centre of its well (Fig. 23.3).

Calculation

The heights of the rockets are handled as in a parallel line bioassay obtaining the potency of the patient's antigen as a proportion of that of the standard on log/log graph paper or by computer programme (Williams et al 1975).

Comments

— The order of sample application helps eliminate bias caused by irregularities in the setting of the gel or in current flow.

— The polarity of the power pack can be reversed a few times between runs to conserve the buffer, providing that the method is not being used for a different protein.

— The potential difference across the gel is measured in v/cm between the edges of the wicks lying on it. This can vary according to whether one applies current during sample loading or not, and is finally set at 10 v/cm.

— The first and last wells should be cut approximately 2 cm from the shortest side of the glass plate to enable a uniform flow of current, producing vertical rocket formation.

— Many variables can influence Laurell electrophoresis: gel thickness, sample volume, well size, high or low voltages, pH and ionic strength, temperature, non-uniform current, electrophoretic mobility of test sample, antibody specificity.

Interpretation
Normal range 53.6–169.4 IU/dl.

IMMUNORADIOMETRIC ASSAY (IRMA)

Principle
The immunoradiometric (IRMA) assay for von Willebrand factor antigen (vWF:Ag) in a given sample depends upon reaction with an excess of radiolabelled heterologous antibody molecules with specificity directed against human vWF:Ag, separation of the high molecular weight immune complexes from the low molecular weight excess, unreacted, labelled antibody (by an ammonium sulphate precipitation step) and measurement of the radioactivity. The amount of radioactivity found in the precipitate is directly proportional to the amount of vWF:Ag in the test sample which can be quantitated by reference to a standard curve (Hoyer 1972; Girma et al 1979).

Reagents
- Normal rabbit plasma.
- Normal rabbit serum.
- Normal human plasma.
- Radio-iodinated immune-purified rabbit IgG with high titre antibody against human vWF:Ag (e.g. Dako Ltd.). Dilute in borate-buffered saline pH 7.85 to give 1000 cpm per 0.2 ml.
- 50% saturated ammonium sulphate.
- 25% saturated ammonium sulphate.
- Borate buffer pH 8.4
   6.4 g boric acid
   9.5 g sodium borate
   4.4 g sodium chloride
   1 litre distilled water.
- Borate-buffered saline pH 7.85
   2.2 g boric acid
   0.2 g sodium hydroxide
   9.29 g sodium chloride
   1 litre distilled water.
- 0.05 M glycine 0.1 M saline buffer pH 2.4.
- 4 M NaOH.
- 0.04 M Na_2HPO_4 buffer pH 8.0.
- 0.1 M Na_2HPO_4 buffer pH 7.5.
- DE-52 cellulose anion exchanger (Whatman).
- Sepharose 6B & Sephadex G2000 (Pharmacia Ltd.).
- [^{125}I]Na 1 mCi (Amersham).
- Chloramine T — 1 mg/ml in 0.1 M Na_2HPO_4 buffer pH 7.5 — prepare fresh, immediately before use.

- Sodium metabisulphite — 1 mg/ml in 0.1 M Na_2HPO_4 buffer pH 7.5.
- 5% KI in distilled water.

Preparation of reagents

Isolation of IgG
1. An equal volume of 50% saturated ammonium sulphate is added to the anti-human vWF:Ag serum.
2. The pH is adjusted to 8.0 with 1 M NaOH, and the precipitate is stirred for 30 minutes.
3. Centrifuge at 3000 g for 30 minutes; discard the supernatant.
4. Dissolve the precipitate in distilled water to bring to one-half the volume of the original antiserum.
5. Dialyse against 0.04 M Na_2HPO_4 buffer pH 8.0.
6. Equilibrate a column of DE-52 cellulose resin (30 ml/100 mg globulin to be chromatographed) with 0.04 M Na_2HPO_4 buffer pH 8.0.
7. Apply the dialysed proteins to the chromatography column and elute with 0.04 M Na_2HPO_4 buffer pH 8.0. Collect and pool the void volume fractions containing the IgG and other proteins not absorbed to the column.
8. Precipitate the IgG fraction with an equal volume of 50% saturated ammonium sulphate solution.
9. Dissolve the precipitate in distilled water to bring the protein concentration to approximately 10 mg/ml.
10. Dialyse against borate-buffered saline pH 7.95 and store as 1 ml aliquots frozen at $-20°C$.

Radiolabelling the IgG (Hunter & Greenwood 1962)
1. Dilute purified IgG to 2 mg/ml with 0.1 M Na_2HPO_4 buffer pH 7.5. Mix 10 μl protein with 10 μl [^{125}I] Na 1 mCi in a polystyrene test tube.
2. Add 50 μl chloramine T at room temperature, rapidly mix and allow the reaction to proceed for 30 seconds exactly.
3. Stop the reaction by adding 100 μl sodium metabisulphite followed by 0.2 ml KI.
4. Separate the radiolabelled protein from the excess free ^{125}I on a 0.9 × 10 cm column of Sephadex G25. Equilibrate and elute with 0.9% sodium chloride containing 0.1% bovine serum albumin at a flow rate of 9 ml/h, collecting 0.5 ml fractions.
5. Screen the fractions for radioactivity using a gamma radiation counter and pool the void volume fractions which should contain the ^{125}I IgG.
Comments
— The extent of iodination of the IgG should be 70–80% of the total ^{125}I used. Compare the total radioactivity in the pooled fractions with the total radioactivity used.
— Determine the TCA precipitability by mixing 10 μl of a 1/100 dilution of the iodinated protein, 50 μl normal serum (human or rabbit), 240 μl borate-

buffered saline and 300 μl of 20% TCA. Stand at 4°C for at least 2 hours, centrifuge to remove precipitate and measure the radioactivity remaining in the supernatant (should be <5%).

Purification of the radiolabelled anti-vWF:Ag

1. Mix the ^{125}I IgG prepared above with 5 ml normal citrated plasma for at least 30 minutes at 37°C.

2. Apply the mixture to a 1.5 × 60 cm column containing Sepharose 6B which has been equilibrated with borate-buffered saline pH 7.85. Elute at 20 ml/h, collect 5 ml fractions.

3. Take 0.02 ml aliquots of each fraction to screen for radioactivity. 3–7% of the total applied radioactivity should be recovered in the void volume fractions, corresponding to the [^{125}I] IgG/vWF:Ag high molecular weight complexes. Pool these fractions.

4. Add 0.25 ml normal rabbit serum to the pool to act as a source of carrier protein.

5. Dialyse against 1 litre of 0.05 M glycine 0.1 M NaCl buffer pH 2.4 for 1 hour at room temperature.

6. Remove the material from the dialysis sack, estimate the volume and remove 0.01 ml for radioactivity determination.

7. Chromatograph the material on a 2.6 × 100 cm column of Sephadex G200 which has been equilibrated with a glycine-saline buffer pH 2.4. Apply the sample to the bottom of the column and upwards elute at a flow rate of 10–15 ml/h, collecting 5 ml fractions into tubes containing 3 ml borate buffer pH 8.4.

8. Pool the fractions corresponding to the second peak of radioactivity. There is often overlap with the first peak which contains undissociated immune complexes and dissociated vWF:AG. It is important not to include a significant amount of the first peak material in the pooled fractions.

9. Add 2 ml normal rabbit serum plus enough ammonium sulphate to bring to 50% saturated.

10. Bring to pH 8.0 with 4 M NaOH and mix for one hour at room temperature.

11. Centrifuge at 3000 g for 45 minutes, so that the supernatant contains very little radioactivity and can be discarded.

12. Dissolve precipitate in 5 ml distilled water and add 2.5 ml normal rabbit plasma and 2.2 ml saturated ammonium sulphate solution.

13. Mix for 1 hour at room temperature.

14. Centrifuge at 3000 g for 1 hour or 9000 g for 20 minutes at room temperature. Discard the precipitate.

15. Dialyse the supernatant against three changes of 1 litre each of borate saline buffer pH 7.85. After dialysis, store the material in 1 ml aliquots at −20°C.

Sample dilutions

Serial doubling dilutions of standard are made, down to 1/512 in borate-buffered saline pH 7.85. Test plasma are diluted if necessary in the same buffer.

Equipment

○ Rimless stoppered polystyrene test tubes 12 × 75 mm (RT30 tubes, Sterilin Ltd.).
○ Gamma counter.

Method

1. Label tubes for each dilution of standard in duplicate, each test sample in duplicate, and 3 tubes in which buffer will be substituted for test or standard plasmas to measure non-specific binding (NSB), and a further 3 tubes to measure the total amount of radioactivity used in the assay.

2. Add 0.1 ml aliquots of test and standard samples to their respective labelled tubes.

3. Add 0.1 ml borate-buffered saline alone to each of the NSB tubes.

4. Add 0.1 ml normal rabbit plasma to each tube.

5. Add 0.2 ml [^{125}I] rabbit anti-vWF:Ag IgG preparation to each tube, including the tubes for total radioactivity measurement.

6. Mix the contents of each tube and incubate at 37°C for 30 minutes.

7. Add 0.4 ml of 50% saturated ammonium sulphate solution to each tube at room temperature and mix with a vortex mixer.

8. Separate the precipitates by centrifugation at 2500 g at room temperature for 30 minutes.

9. Discard the supernatants and wash the precipitates by adding 1 ml 25% saturated ammonium sulphate solution to each tube. Mix with the vortex mixer and repeat the centrifugation step at room temperature.

10. Discard the supernatants and measure the radioactivity in each tube by counting on the gamma counter for 10 minutes.

Calculation

Plot a graph of radioactivity against dilution for standard and abstract test plasma results from the standard curve.

Comments

— The purification of anti-vWF:Ag IgG yields sufficient aliquots to last most operators for several years.

— The iodination will have to be performed at a regular frequency, but enough is usually made in one iodination to last for 3–4 months. After this period, the natural rate of radioactive decay of the isotope will probably necessitate iodination of a new aliquot of the IgG.

— Test samples containing very high concentrations of vWF:Ag will probably require dilution in buffer before assay.

MULTIMERIC SIZING

Principle

This test measures the degree of multimerisation of vWF:Ag in plasma by discontinuous SDS electrophoresis. vWF:Ag is visualised by either established autoradiographic methods (Ruggeri & Zimmerman 1981, Enayat & Hill 1983) or via a more novel approach utilising enzyme-linked antibodies (Chow & Savidge 1985, Brosstad et al 1986, Lombardi et al 1986, Aihara et al 1986, Miller et al 1985, Dalton et al, 1988).

Reagents

- Sample buffer — 10 mM Tris HCl, 1 mM EDTA, 8 M urea, 2% SDS, 0.1% Bromophenol Blue pH 8.0.
- Stacking gel buffer — 0.125 M Tris HCl, 0.1% SDS pH 6.8.
- Stacking gel — 0.8% Seakem HGT (P) agarose (ICN Biomedicals Ltd.) in stacking gel buffer. Store in glass tubes in aliquots at 4°C, heat in a boiling water-bath to dissolve, when required.
- Running gel buffer — 0.5 M Tris HCl, 0.1% SDS pH 8.8.
- Running gel agarose — 1.07% Seakem HGT(P) agarose in running gel buffer. Store in glass universal containers in aliquots at 4°C. Heat in a boiling water-bath to dissolve, when required.
- 6.4% TEMED.
- Polyacrylamide solution (20% solution with 5% cross-linking) — 19 g acrylamide + 1 g bis-acrylamide in 100 ml distilled water) — make fresh.
- 2% ammonium persulphate (must be made fresh).
- Electrophoresis buffer — 0.05 M Tris, 0.38 M glycine, 0.1% SDS pH 8.35.
- Acid isopropanol — 25% isopropanol + 10% acetic acid.

For peroxidase-antiperoxidase (PAP) staining

PBST washing buffer — 0.01 M phosphate-buffered saline (0.1% Tween 20) pH 7.2.

- Rabbit anti-human vWF:Ag, swine anti-rabbit IgG, and rabbit PAP (Dako Ltd.).
- Substrate — 50 mg diaminobenzidine in 100 ml 0.05 M Tris buffer pH 7.6. Filter and add H_2O_2 to a final concentration of 0.02% immediately before use. Avoid skin contact with substrate.

For autoradiography

- Bovine IgG.
- Normal rabbit serum.
- ^{125}I-labelled anti-human vWF:Ag IgG.
- 0.5 M NaCl.
- 0.025 M barbitone buffer pH 8.6.

Equipment

- LKB Multiphor (2117) system.
- Gel cassette.
- Gelbond PAGFilm (ICN Biomedicals).
- Whatman No. 3MM chromatography paper.
- 56°C oven.

For autoradiography

- Dupont Cronex 4 film.
- Dupont Quanta II intensifying screen.
- −70°C freezer or liquid nitrogen.

Standards and controls

Pooled normal control plasma. Purified IgM (dimethyl suberimidate crosslinked) (Davies & Stark 1970).

Preparation of gels and samples

The gel cassette consists of a siliconised template with wells (0.6–0.8 mm thick) placed onto gel-bond film adhered to a glass plate. The sandwich is held together by bull-dog clips and warmed to 56°C. Running gel is prepared by mixing 7.5 ml running gel agarose (heated and dissolved), 0.15 ml distilled water, 0.60 ml TEMED, and 1.25 ml polyacrylamide solution at above 56°C, and adding 0.5 ml of ammonium persulphate immediately before pouring the gel. Running gel is injected into the cassette using a syringe, until the level is 1 cm below the wells. Leave the plate to set for 15 minutes and then warm to 56°C before addition of stacking gel by a similar method. The template is then left at 4°C for 20 minutes and prised apart carefully with the gel remaining on the gel-bond.

Samples are diluted 1/10 with diluting buffer and heated at 56°C for 30 minutes.

Method

1. The gel is placed on the cooling platten of the Multiphor tank so that the wells are nearest the cathode. Three layers of chromatography paper, cut to the size of the plate, act as wicks. They are soaked in electrophoresis buffer, and placed on each side of the plate so that 1 cm of gel is covered and the wick edges are parallel.

2. 15 µl of pooled normal plasma, test plasma, or crosslinked IgM is placed in each well, and electrophoresis started at 0.8 mA/sample. Once the samples have migrated into the stacking gel, the wells are filled with agarose and the current reapplied.

3. Electrophoresis is stopped when the tracking dye reaches the far wick (approximately 18 h).

4. The gel is fixed in acid isopropanol for 1 hour, then washed in water (3 times) over 1 hour. The gel is then dried onto the gel-bond sheet using a hairdryer.

Peroxidase-antiperoxidase (PAP) staining

1. 100 µl of rabbit anti-human vWF:Ag is added to 10 ml of phosphate-buffered Tween (PBST) and layered

onto the dried gel, placed horizontally in a moisture chamber, and incubated overnight at room temperature.

2. The antibody solution is tipped off and the gel washed three times in 200 ml of PBST over 1 hour.

3. 75 μl swine anti-rabbit IgG in 10 ml PBST is layered onto the washed gel and again incubated overnight at room temperature in the same way.

4. The gel is washed as in step 6, and 75 μl of rabbit PAP in 10 ml PBST are layered onto the gel and incubated overnight at room temperature.

5. The gel is washed as in step 6, and substrate is then poured onto the gel. The peroxidase reaction is allowed to take place until the protein bands can be visualised (within 1 h), and then washed and dried.

Autoradiography

1. Cover dried, fixed gel after electrophoresis with 10 mg/ml bovine IgG in barbitone buffer for 20 minutes.

2. Wash gel in barbitone buffer and incubate with normal rabbit serum diluted 1/10 in barbitone buffer for 20 minutes.

3. Wash gel in barbitone buffer and incubate overnight with rabbit anti-human vWF:Ag IgG labelled with ^{125}I via the chlorine gas method (Butt et al 1972). The labelled antibody should be diluted in barbitone buffer to give 1×10^6 cpm/ml.

4. Wash gel in 0.5 M NaCl (6 changes over 24–48 h), and then dry.

5. Carry out autoradiography at −70°C for 2–3 days to allow clear resolution of bands.

Comments

— Optimum antibody incubation times for the PAP system are 12 hours or more.

— The PAP system has similar specificity and sensitivity to the autoradiography system. However, the higher molecular weight multimers seem to be stained to a lesser degree in the PAP system and this may be important in classification of type IIB disease.

— A low molecular weight band appears in all samples and even in severe von Willebrand's disease, von Willebrand inhibitor patients and in acquired von Willebrand's disease, which is of unknown origin. It is likely to be non-specific binding of antibodies to IgG or IgM. This does not affect the overall interpretation, since the majority of multimers are of high molecular weight.

— The agarose acrylamide mix (0.8%:2.5%) employed is only one of many discontinuous systems that can be employed (for review of methods see Mannucci et al 1985).

— Recently the method has been made more rapid by the introduction of electroblotting techniques, where the proteins are transferred onto nitrocellulose before adding antibodies (Lombardi et al 1986).

— Due to its large size vWf tends to transfer slowly, but rapid blotting can be achieved (16 minutes) using high currents in a semidry method (Dalton et al, 1988).

— Nitrocellulose can be cheaply and conveniently blocked with a 5% solution of powdered milk (Marvel, Cadbury's).

— Staining of vWf on nitrocellulose gels with peroxidase linked antibodies (1/750 dilution) can be

Table 23.1 Multimeric distributions of von Willebrand factor in various subtypes.

vWD subtype	Multimeric distribution
I (mild)	All present in reduced amount
I (severe)	No protein at all
IIA	Largest and medium sized absent
IIB	Largest absent
IIC	Largest absent plus abnormal triplet structure
IID	Largest absent plus aberrant bands

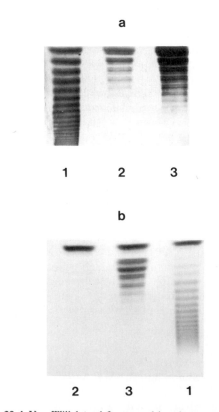

Fig. 23.4 Von Willebrand factor multimeric patterns: a. immunoblot, b. autoradiogram of 1.6% agarose gel. lane 1 = normal plasma, 2 = Type IIA vWD, 3 = Type IIA vWD post-DDAVP infusion. Origin at bottom of Fig.

achieved with relatively short incubation periods (1–2 Hours).

— Use of direct staining with peroxidase conjugated 1st antibodies, conjugated 2nd antibodies, PAP and avidin-biotin systems are all effective with varying degrees of sensitivity.

Interpretation

Von Willebrand factor multimer patterns need careful analysis as abnormalities can occur in the number of bands present, their density, mobility and presence of subsidiary bands (Table 23.1). The change in pattern seen after certain treatments such as DDAVP infusion may also be relevant (Fig. 23.4). Multimeric sizing alone should not be used for diagnosis of von Willebrand's disease. It is useful to clarify the exact classification when a whole range of vWF assays have been performed.

REFERENCES

Aihara M, Sawada Y, Veno K et al 1986 Visualization of vWF multimers by immunoenzymatic stain using Avidin-Biotin peroxidase complex. Thrombosis and Haemostasis 55: 263–267

Brinkhous K M, Read M S 1978 Preservation of platelet receptors for platelet aggregating factor/von Willebrand factor by air drying, freezing, or lyophilization: new stable platelet preparations for von Willebrand factor assays. Thrombosis Research 13: 591–597

Brosstad F, Kjonniksen I, Ronning B, Stormorken H 1986 Visualization of von Willebrand multimers by enzyme conjugated antibodies. Thrombosis and Haemostasis 55: 276–278

Butt W R 1972 The iodination of follicle stimulating and other hormones for RIA. Journal of Endocrinology 55: 453–454

Chow R, Savidge G F 1985 Enzyme linked antibody systems for the visualization of factor VIII multimers. Thrombosis and Haemostasis 54: 75

Dalton R G, Lasham A, Savidge G F 1988 A new rapid semi-dry blotting technique for multimeric sizing of von Willebrand factor. Thrombosis Research 50: 345–349

Davies G E, Stark G R 1970 Use of dimethyl suberimidate, a cross-linking reagent, in studying the subunit structure of oligomeric proteins. Proceedings of the National Academy of Sciences 66: 651–656

Enayat M S, Hill F G H 1983 Analysis of the complexity of the multimeric structure of factor VIII related antigen/von Willebrand protein using a modified electrophoretic technique. Journal of Clinical Pathology 36: 915–919

Girma J-P, Ardaillou N, Meyer D, Lavergne J-M, Larrieu M-J 1979 Fluid-phase immunoradiometric assay for the detection of qualitative abnormalities of factor VIII/von Willebrand factor in variants of von Willebrands disease. Journal of Laboratory and Clinical Medicine 93: 926–939

Hoyer L W 1972 Immunologic studies of antihemophilic factor (AHF, factor VIII); IV — Radioimmunoassay of AHF antigen. Journal of Laboratory and Clinical Medicine 80: 822–833

Hunter W H, Greenwood F C 1962 Preparation of iodine-131 labelled human growth hormone of high specific activity. Nature 194: 495–496

Laurell C B 1966 Quantitative estimation of proteins by electrophoresis in agarose gel containing antibodies. Analytical Biochemistry 15: 45–52

Lombardi R, Gelfi C, Righetti P S, Cattuada A, Mannucci P M 1986 Electroblot and immunoperoxidase staining for rapid screening of abnormalities of multimeric structure of vWF in vWD. Thrombosis and Haemostasis 55: 246–249

Macfarlane D E, Stibbe J, Kirby E P et al 1975 A method for assaying von Willebrand factor (ristocetin cofactor). Thrombosis et Diathesis Haemorrhagica (Stuttgart) 34: 306–308

Mannucci P M, Abildgaard C F, Gralnick H R et al 1985 Multicenter comparison of von Willebrand factor multimer sizing techniques. Thrombosis and Haemostasis 54: 873–877

Miller M A, Palascak J E, Thompson M R, Martelo O J 1985 A modified SDS agarose gel method for determining factor VIII/von Willebrand factor multimers using commercially available reagents. Thrombosis Research 39: 777–780

Ruggeri Z M, Zimmerman T S 1981 The complex multimeric composition of factor VIII/von Willebrand factor. Blood 57: 1140–1143

Short P E et al 1982 Medical Laboratory Sciences 39: 351–355

Williams K N, Davidson J M F, Ingram G I C 1975 A computer programme for the analysis of parallel line bioassays of clotting factors. British Journal of Haematology 31: 13–23

24

Quality control of blood coagulation

Quality control, according to Harper (1971), is concerned with ensuring that the quality of goods and services remains within predetermined quality standards. *External quality control* involves periodic testing of samples of known value provided by an outside reference centre. *Internal quality control* monitors day-to-day variation within a particular laboratory. The former has been dealt with extensively by Poller (1980). Each laboratory should set up its own internal quality control procedures which, once established, must be rigidly adhered to.

Coagulation factors are, in the main, determined by biological assay which can be defined as the method for the estimation of the nature, constitution or potency of a material (Finney 1971). Although similar to a quantitative chemical analysis in that one is providing a numerical assessment of the test material, it differs in the lack of pure substances being available for use as primary standards. The standards used in coagulation are made up of a large pool of normal plasmas which has been assayed against the national and/or international standards and has an assigned potency.

INTERNAL QUALITY CONTROL

This is applied to:

The monitoring of screening tests and assays undertaken for clinical purposes.

The monitoring of large numbers of assays carried out over a long period of time as part of a research study.

Production of clinical concentrates e.g. factor VIII and IX concentrates for the treatment of haemophilia.

Screening tests and assays performed for clinical diagnosis

Most laboratories perform tests on normal plasmas for the prothrombin time (PT), activated partial thromboplastin time (APTT) and thrombin time (TT) daily before commencing the testing of patient samples. There are a number of preparations that are suitable as normal controls.

a. Pool of plasmas freshly collected from normal individuals. Four or five plasmas should be tested individually before pooling to avoid inclusion of samples which are either activated and have very short clotting times or those with prolonged times. It is inadvisable, to use a single plasma.

b. Freeze-dried normal plasma. Freeze-dried plasmas are excellent, but need meticulous care in preparation to avoid activation or loss of potency during the freeze-drying process. Commercial plasmas are available, but tend to be expensive.

c. Liquid nitrogen stored plasma. A suitable pool of plasma stored in small aliquots in liquid nitrogen is satisfactory. Some deterioration takes place eventually, but plasmas can be stored usefully for up to about one year (Stirling et al 1984).

The combination of testing both a freeze-dried plasma and a fresh pool daily would appear to be the most satisfactory system. The freeze-dried plasma is used to control the reagents; the fresh pool is available for use during the day for correction tests and other procedures requiring normal plasma such as inhibitor testing. The clotting time of liquid-nitrogen stored pool tends to shorten slightly on storage and is not entirely suitable for correction tests.

Factors affecting coagulation assays

Availability of plasmas for use as standards
Commercially available standards which have been calibrated against the national and international standard (where potency for a particular factor has been assigned) are the most suitable. However, these tend to be expensive. An alternative is for the laboratory to prepare and calibrate its own 'house standard' using either freeze-dried or liquid-nitrogen stored pooled plasma (Table 24.1). A single plasma or small pool is invalid, and most animal plasmas are unsuitable. In preparing a 'house standard' the following points are pertinent and careful selection of the donors is required.
— There is a rise in factor VIII after exercise or stress (Iatridis & Ferguson 1963).

Table 24.1 Statistical design for calibrating 'house standard' in terms of national or current standard for factor VII activity (two operators using two automated instruments). Each assay run consists of:

Assay run no.	Ampoule of house standard			Instrument	Operator	Instrument	Operator
1	A_1	A_2	A_3	1	1	2	2
2	A_4	A_5	A_6	1	1	2	2
3	A_7	A_8	A_9	1	1	2	2
4	A_{10}	A_{11}	A_{12}	1	2	2	1
5	A_{13}	A_{14}	A_{15}	1	2	2	1
6	A_{16}	A_{17}	A_{18}	1	2	2	1

1. Duplicates of current standard diluted $\frac{1}{10}, \frac{1}{20}, \frac{1}{40}, \frac{1}{80}, \frac{1}{160}$, in glyoxaline buffer.
2. Duplicate blanks (buffer only in place of plasma dilution).
3. Duplicates of Ampoule A_1 diluted $\frac{1}{10}, \frac{1}{20}, \frac{1}{40}, \frac{1}{80}, \frac{1}{160}$ in glyoxaline buffer.
4. Duplicates of Ampoule A_2 diluted $\frac{1}{10} - \frac{1}{160}$.
5. Duplicates of Ampoule A_3 diluted $\frac{1}{10} - \frac{1}{160}$.
6. Duplicates of current standard $\frac{1}{10} - \frac{1}{160}$.

Design of programme allows for calculation of
1. polency of House Standard
2. variability between operators
3. variability between instruments.

Operator No. 1 makes the dilutions for run 1; operator No. 2 makes the dilutions for run 2 and so on. All dilutions are assayed by one-stage factor VII assay. The design of this programme allows for calculation of the potency of the 'house standard; variability between operators and between instruments.

— A number of coagulation factors are considerably altered in pregnancy (Stirling et al 1984).
— There are ethnic differences in coagulation factor levels; blacks have higher factor VIII level than whites (Meade et al 1978).
— There is an increase of factor V, VII and VIII with increasing age (Meade et al 1976).
— Some animal plasmas have extremely high levels of factors V and VIII (Garner and Conning 1970; Stirling, unpublished observations).

Provision of internal reference plasma
Freeze-dried normal plasma or a large amount i.e. the pooled plasma from one to two units of blood snap-frozen in small aliquots in liquid nitrogen is suitable. A new vial should be opened and assayed with each batch of tests assayed.

Standardised reagents
The availability of human congenital factor-deficient plasma is limited and consequently expensive to purchase. Plasmas prepared by the use of monoclonal antibodies may eventually prove to be cheaper. The preparation of a number of artificial factor-deficient substrate plasmas is possible but is a time-consuming process and requires very careful testing to ensure that each batch compares exactly with the previous batch. i.e. factor V-deficient (Wolf 1953), factor VII-deficient (Lechner & Deutsch 1967) and factor VIII-deficient (Essien and Ingram 1967, Nyman 1970). The reagent must be stable and behave as human congenital-deficient plasma.

All newly prepared reagents, buffers, calcium chloride etc. should be tested against the existing batch before being put into routine use.

Meticulous care in performing the tests
From the taking of the blood sample through to the calculation of the results, all procedures must be carried out with meticulous attention to detail.

a. It is essential to work on a blood sample which has been obtained by 'clean' venepuncture without stasis (wherever possible) and added to the correct amount of anticoagulant.

b. The sample must be centrifuged at the correct temperature and speed and the plasma transferred to a plastic tube using a plastic pipette to avoid activation.

c. If assays are not to be performed immediately, plasma should be stored — preferably in liquid nitrogen. Slow cooling of plasma to minus 20°C can result in increased levels of factor VII activity due to cold activation. Keeping the plasma in an ice bucket all day will also cold-activate factor VII. Factor VIII cryo-precipitates after several hours in ice, resulting in falsely low levels.

d. Dilutions of plasma (the greatest source of error) are most accurately made with Eppendorf or Oxford type pipettes or a computed diluter. Repetitive amounts of reagent can be delivered from a calibrated syringe attached to a reservoir.

e. Blanks (buffer substituted for plasma dilution) should be included at the beginning and end of each run to check on the deterioration or activation of the reagents.

Relevant and adequate calculation
It is now customary for assay results to be calculated by computer, using methods based on plotting parallel lines of standard and test dilution clotting time on log paper. Should a large number of tests have been carried out within one batch, the programme should allow for

the gradual deterioration of the standard plasma over time, the first batch of tests being computed between the first and second standard, the next batch between the second and third standard, and so on.

Recognition of trends
Examination of the clotting times for the standard and blanks and the value obtained for the internal reference plasma will allow an immediate assessment of the validity of the assay run. The whole procedure should be repeated if there is considerable difference in clotting times of the standard and blanks from previous runs. Excess lengthening or shortening of clotting times of the final standard and blanks in comparison with those at the start is also an indication that the assays should be repeated. The values for successive internal reference plasmas can be plotted on a means and standard deviation chart or on a cusum chart.

Means and standard deviation chart
The chart is constructed by calculating the mean factor VII activity for the internal reference plasma from the first five assay runs performed. (Recalculate the mean as more batches are carried out.) Calculate one and two standard deviations (SD) from the mean and plot as shown, Table 24.2, Figure 24.1. Values of up to one SD from the mean are acceptable; between one and two

Table 24.2 Construction of mean and standard deviation chart. Values of internal plasma for factor VII activity (as per cent of standard).

100	98	78
90	96	95
102	104	
110	92	

Mean of first 5 values = 100% factor VII.
One standard deviation from the mean — 7.211.

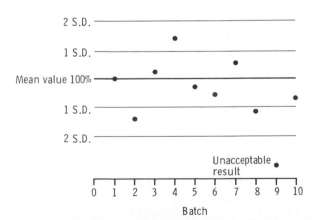

Fig. 24.1 Means and standard deviation chart. Factor VII activity of internal reference plasma.

SD suggest that the assay system could be improved. Those values outside two SD are unacceptable.

Cusum chart
The essential features of the cusum chart (Cumulative sum chart) Table 24.3, Figure 24.2, are that the current mean value of the series is represented by the slope (a zero slope representing the target value) and that a change in slope is immediately apparent to the eye, in spite of the random fluctuations of individual terms. Small variations around the target value are to be expected. A gross change in direction indicates a cumulative change in the mean value, which requires investigation. The slope change seen in Figure 24.2 was due to the introduction of a new standard which had a lower potency than the previous one.

Table 24.3 Construction of cusum chart. Values of internal reference plasma for factor VII activity (as per cent of standard): 100   90   102   110   98
Mean value (i.e. target value) = 100% factor VII.
Subtract target value from each internal reference factor VII value:

100 − 100 = zero
 90 − 100 = −10 Add to zero = −10
102 − 100 = +2 Add to − 10 above = −8
110 − 100 = +10 Add to −8 above = +2
 98 − 100 = −2 Add to +2 above = zero
112 − 100 = +12 Add to zero above = +12
113 − 100 = +13 Add to + 12 above = +25
112 − 100 = +12 Add to + 25 above = +37

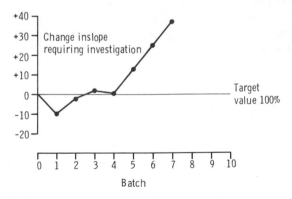

Fig. 24.2 Cusum chart. Factor VII activity of internal reference plasma.

Quality control of a long-term study
Quality control of a long-term study differs from day-to-day monitoring of screening tests and assays carried out for clinical purposes. As a generalisation, in the latter the main interest is determining abnormal values which may lead to diagnosis and treatment. Coagulation

factor levels are expressed as percentage of the standard which has been accorded a value of 100%. In a study spanning, quite often, many years, all results must ultimately be comparable with one another. A number of standards, each with a life of around 18 months, will be used during this time. Due to their biological nature, standards do not all have a value of 100% but tend to vary in their potency. Consequently, conversion factors to allow for this differing potency have to be calculated.

Three methods for this purpose have been described by North et al (1982):

a. Assay of the new standard against the current standard.

b. Comparison of internal reference plasma values, one plasma spanning the use of two successive standards.

c. An epidemiological method based on the assumption that the mean value for any given coagulation factor would be the same in comparable groups of study participants. This method appears to be the most reliable in providing conversion factors, though it is limited to those studies having a large enough group of subjects for this purpose.

Quality control of a long-term study is best served by plotting a cusum chart (Fig. 24.2) or quangle (North 1980). Inter-batch variation can be viewed retrospectively and gross changes due to e.g. change of standard, extremes of ambient temperature or alteration of the sensitivity detection of an instrument due to servicing can be pinpointed. Allowances for this variation can be made in the final analysis. It is not practicable, however, to allow for intra-batch variation (North et al 1982).

Quality control in the production of clinical concentrates

The potency of each batch of factor VIII concentrate is assessed by assay against the current (3rd) International standard for FVIII. The concentration of antithrombin III in ATIII concentrate is determined by Laurell rocket technique against an 'in-house' plasma standard.

REFERENCES

Conard J, Bousser M G, Samama M 1976 Contraceptifs oraux et thromboses. Epidemiologie. Anomalies biologiques. Revue de Medicine 34: 1849–1862

Essien E M, Ingram G I C 1967 Diagnosis of haemophilia: use of an artificial factor-VIII-deficient human plasma system. Journal of Clinical Pathology 20: 620

Finney D J 1971 In: Statistical Method in Biological Assay. Griffin, London

Garner R, Conning D M 1970 The assay of human factor VII by means of a modified factor VII deficient dog plasma. British Journal of Haematology 18: 57

Harper W M 1971 In: Statistics, 2nd edn. MacDonald and Evans, London

Iatridis S G, Ferguson J H 1963 Effect of physical exercise on blood clotting and fibrinolysis. Journal of Applied Physiology 18: 337–344

Lechner K, Deutsch E 1967 Ein einfache Methode zur Herstellung von menschlichem Factor-VII-Mangel plasma. Thrombosis et Diathesis Haemorrhagica 18: 252

Meade et al 1976 An epidemiological study of the haemostatic and other effects of oral contraceptives. British Journal of Haematology 34: 353–364

Meade T W, North W R S, Chakrabarti R, Haines A P, Stirling Y 1977 Population based distribution of haemostatic variables. British Medical Bulletin 33: 283–288

Meade T W, Brozovic M, Chakrabarti R, Haines A P, North W R S, Stirling Y 1978 Ethnic group comparisons of variables associated with ischaemic heart disease. British Heart Journal 40: 789–795

North W R S 1980 The quangle — a modification of the cusum chart. Applied Statistics 31: 155–158

North W R S, Stirling Y, Meade T W 1982a Common units for clotting factors assayed against different standards. Thrombosis and Haemostasis 48: 270–273

North W R S, Stirling Y, Meade T W 1982b Variation between batches in clotting factors assays. Thrombosis and Haemostasis 48: 274–276

Nyman D 1970 The preparation of an artificial reagent for the one-stage factor VIII assay. Thrombosis et Diathesis Haemorrhagica 23: 206

Poller L, Thomson J M 1966 Clotting factors during oral contraception. British Medical Journal 2: 23–25

Poller L 1980 Quality control in blood coagulation. In: Blood Coagulation and Haemostasis. Churchill Livingstone, Edinburgh

Stirling Y, Woolf L, North W R S, Seghatchian M J, Meade T W 1984 Haemostasis in normal pregnancy. Thrombosis and Haemostasis 52: 176–182

Wolf P 1953 A modification for routine laboratory use of Stefanini's method of estimating factor V activity in human oxalated plasma. Journal of Clinical Pathology 6: 34

25

Automation in coagulation

Automation of coagulation testing was introduced primarily to:

1. Increase the throughput of samples.

2. Increase precision of results by reducing operator error.

3. Relieve the strain and tedium of manual clotting.

Many forms of instrumentation with varying principles of end-point detection have been devised in recent years. A number of independent reviews have been published (Wujastyk & Triplett 1983, Messmore 1983, Walenge et al 1983, Italian CISMEL study group 1983, Drewinko et al, 1977, Koepke 1977). Although difficult to establish precisely, probably the three types most widely used are (not necessarily in order of usage):

1. Optical density change detection.

2. Electromechanical detection of a fibrin thread across an electrode.

3. Impedance. Displacement of a revolving steel ball by a fibrin thread, thereby triggering an impulse in the magnetic sensor.

Detailed discussion will be confined to these three types. The instruments available vary considerably in sensitivity, precision, complexity of use, speed, operator time needed and cost. The majority, including the types listed above, are semi-automated, requiring constant operator monitoring and expertise. The more generally used smaller instruments can accommodate from two to ten samples at a time. The tests are accomplished speedily, and the problem of deterioration of test plasmas and reagents does not arise. Loss of potency can occur, particularly of the labile factors V, VIII and X, by 50 to 60 samples being loaded onto the turntable of the larger (generally optical density detection) instruments, the last dilutions being incubated for around an hour prior to testing. Plasma dilutions should be made up and fed on at intervals. Recently developed instruments overcome this problem by reading a number of samples simultaneously. As factor VII is relatively stable, larger numbers of assays can be left to proceed without significant loss of potency.

Manual methods may require modification for some forms of instrumentation. Dilution of reagents or the mixing of two or more reagents to accommodate the design of the machine may be necessary i.e. delivery of three reagents when only two pumps are available. In addition, the dilutions for the standard curve may not be the same as for the manual technique and should be established for each instrument by construction of a

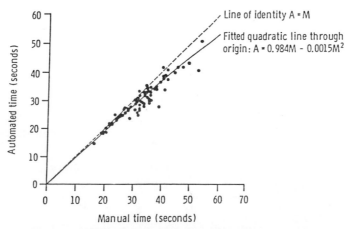

Fig. 25.1 Relationship between automated (Schnitger & Gross coagulometer) and manual clotting times.

complete sigmoid. Modification of the sensitivity detection of the instrument should be avoided. Manual reference (normal) ranges should not be used. A reference range for each test or assay should be established for each instrument used.

The testing of anticoagulated plasma presents the greatest problem. The suggested therapeutic range used in the United Kingdom is based on the provision of thromboplastin by a reference centre and manual prothrombin times. The clotting times on the majority of instruments do not compare exactly with manual times. Figure 25.1 and Table 25.1 demonstrate for one instrument, the Schnitger and Gross coagulometer, that the automated times become shorter as the prothrombin ratio (INR) increases. Either an extrapolation curve or an alteration of the therapeutic range is needed to avoid the overdosing of a patient as indicated by a falsely low prothrombin ratio. Care should also be taken if more than one type of instrumentation is used within a laboratory, as different machines may give differing clotting times for the same plasma sample.

It is clear that considerable thought should go into the type of instrumentation best suited to the needs of the laboratory concerned. Not every laboratory needs

Table 25.1 Increase in % difference between automated (Schnitger and Gross coagulometer) and manual clotting times.

Manual time (s)	Predicted automated time (s)	% difference
15	14.4	3.9%
25	23.7	5.4%
35	32.6	6.9%
45	41.2	8.4%
55	49.6	9.9%

large-scale automation. Those performing minimal numbers of prothrombin times probably do not need automation at all. However, carefully chosen instrumentation can reduce operator time and increase precision of results.

TYPES OF AUTOMATION

OPTICAL DENSITY DETECTION

Large-scale automation can be defined as those instruments having a turntable onto which 50–60 plasmas or plasma dilutions are placed in cuvettes or tubes.

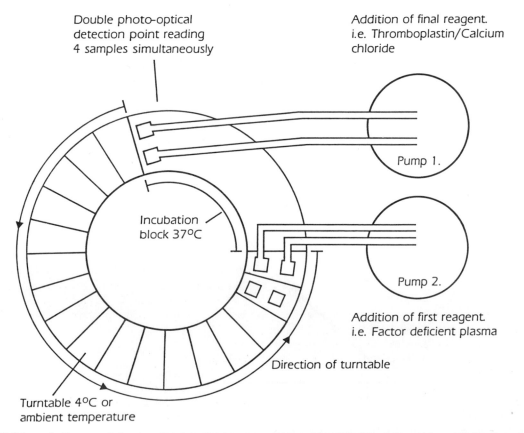

Fig. 25.2 Schematic diagram of photo-optical detection instrument Coag-a-Mate X2. (Reproduce with permission from General Diagnostics)

Reagent, i.e. factor-deficient plasma is delivered at pre-set intervals from a secondary pump. Samples move on to the incubation block maintained at 37°C and the final reagent is delivered from the primary pump, initiating clot formation and also triggering the timing mechanism (Fig. 25.2).

Principle

The change in optical density which occurs on clot formation is detected, the clotting time being recorded on a print-out.

Comments

— Semi-automated, requiring samples to be fed on to the turntable at intervals (factor VII assays excepted).
— An over-riding timer is required to ensure that all samples have an equal incubation time. The turn-table, in some instruments, moves on as soon as the clot is formed, giving random incubation time at 37°C.
— Turntable should be operable at 4°C or ambient temperature.
— Reagent reservoirs should be operable at 37°C or ambient temperature.
— Safety mechanism should be incorporated so that the pumps deliver only when the cuvette is correctly placed to receive reagent.

Example
Coag-a-Mate X 2 (General Diagnostics)

ELECTROMECHANICAL DETECTION OF A FIBRIN THREAD ACROSS A HOOK-TYPE ELECTRODE

This is an example of a small-scale instrument. Plasmas and reagents are fed by the operator into tubes placed on the instrument. A hook-type electrode is placed in the incubating mixture as soon as the final reagent has been added (Fig. 25.3).

Principle

The hook-type electrode moves in and out of the incubating mixture. The first fibrin thread formed across the electrode completes the electrical circuit and stops the timer. The clotting time in seconds is shown on a display panel.

Comments

— Semi-automated.
— Clinical concentrates with very high levels of fibrinogen (1000 mg/dl) stop the timer prematurely,

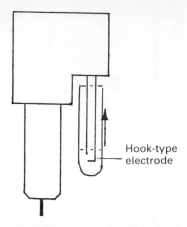

Fig. 25.3 Schematic diagram of hook-type electrode. Schnitger & Gross coagulometer. (Reproduced with permission from Heinrich Amelung)

giving falsely high levels in the factor VIII assay (Stirling et al 1978).
— Results of prothrombin times on anticoagulated plasmas do not compare exactly with those obtained by manual method, the difference becoming greater above the therapeutic range INR 2.0–4.0.
— Good duplication. Suitable for most assay procedures.

Example
Schnitger and Gross coagulometer (Heinrich Amelung).

IMPEDANCE: REVOLVING STEEL BALL DISPLACEMENT BY FIBRIN THREAD FORMATION

Plasmas and reagents are fed by the operator into cuvettes containing a steel ball. The timer is triggered by delivery of final reagent from attached pipette (Fig. 25.4).

Principle

The incubating mixture is situated in an inclined cuvette that rotates around its longitudinal axis. A steel ball runs on a given point in the mixture. As coagulation occurs, the fibrin filament displaces the ball and trips a magnetic sensor which automatically records the time of clot formation on a display panel.

Comments

— Semi-automated.
— Excellent precision.
— Results of prothrombin time on anticoagulated plasmas compare exactly with those obtained by manual method.
— Suitable for all clotting assays.

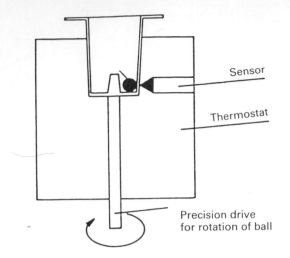

Fig. 25.4 Schematic diagram of clot detection by impedance. KC10 coagulometer. (Reproduced with permission from Heinrich Amelung)

Example
Coagulometer KC10 (Heinrich Amelung).

Testing of new instrumentation
Each new instrument acquired should be systematically tested to determine whether the following are required:

a. Modification of the method to fit the requirements of the instrument.

b. Modification of reagents.

c. Modification of standard and test dilutions.

Results from the new instrument must be comparable with results obtained using the manual technique, and comparable with results from existing instrumentation within the laboratory, if reference ranges and anticoagulant therapeutic range are to remain unaltered.

Provision of new ranges may be required, as previously discussed.

Recent developments in automation
Of particular interest are the types of instrumentation now becoming available.

FP910 Coagulation Analyzer (Lab Systems UK Ltd.)
Although semi-automated, this is a versatile instrument having a vertical light path and detection system. Particulate reagents such as suspensions of thromboplastin which may, in other instruments, prematurely trigger the end-point detection mechanism, can be used. In addition to conventional clotting methods, by incorporating a variety of wave length filters, both end-point and kinetic studies using chromogenic substrates can be performed. Initial work on the instrument suggests that ELISA methods can also be successfully carried out (George, J 1986 personal communication).

Ortho Koagulab 40-A (Ortho Diagnostic Systems)
Prothrombin times (PT) and activated partial thromboplastin times (APTT) are performed by direct sampling from the centrifuged blood which is placed on the instrument, thereby considerably reducing operator time.

MCA100WP (BioData International Corporation, USA)
Whole blood placed on the machine is filtered through a membrane to provide plasma. Vertically oriented micro-optics allow a full 360° view of the clot during its formation. Samples can be tested on a random basis thus avoiding having to batch PTs and APTTs etc. Only micro amounts (around 25% of the amount normally required) of both plasma and reagents are used. This instrument can save in cost of reagents and is particularly useful for paediatric work.

REFERENCES

Drewinko B, Roe E, Hasler D, Wallace B, Johnston D 1980 Evaluation of automatic and semi-automatic coagulation assay instruments. Clinical Laboratory Haematology 2: 215–226

Italian CISMEL study group 1983 Multicentre comparison of nine coagulometers and manual tilt-tube methods for prothrombin time performance. Clinical Laboratory Haematology 5: 177–184

Koepke J A 1977 Evaluation of materials and methods for coagulation testing. In: Henry J B, Giegel J L (eds). Quality control in laboratory medicine, Masson, New York

Messmore H L Jr 1983 Automation in coagulation testing.

Clinical applications. Seminars in Thrombosis and Hemostasis 9(4): 341–345

Stirling Y, Howarth D J, Vickers M V, North W R S, Meade T W 1978 Automation of two-stage factor VIII assay. Thrombosis and Haemostasis 39(2): 455–465

Walenge J M, Hoppensteadt D, Fareed J, Silberman S, Shelvin P 1983 Automated clot-based methods in coagulation testing: current and future considerations. Seminars in Thrombosis and Hemostasis 9(4): 245–249

Wujastyk J, Triplett D A 1983 Selecting instrumentation and reagents for the coagulation laboratory. Pathologist XXXVII: 398–403

26

Laboratory control of anticoagulant therapy

Venous thrombo-embolism is a major cause of mortality and morbidity. Heparin and oral anticoagulants are the main antithrombotic agents in use and they require careful and regular laboratory control so as to achieve maximal clinical benefit with minimal risks of side effects.

HEPARIN

Mechanism of action

Heparin is an anionic mucopolysaccharide of varying molecular weight from 4000–40 000, averaging approximately 15 000. Activity is determined by biological assay against a reference international standard and expressed as BP units (British Pharmacopea) which are equivalent to the European Pharmacopeal Assay. The USP (United States Pharmacopea) method gives values differing from the international standard by about 7–10%. It has to be administered intravenously, when it has an effective half-life of $1\frac{1}{2}$ hours. When given by subcutaneous injection, its half-life is 4–6 hours. Metabolism occurs in the liver and a degraded form is excreted in the urine. Heparin does not cross the placental barrier or enter maternal milk.

Heparin exerts most of its anticoagulant effect by its interaction with the plasma inhibitor antithrombin III (ATIII). Heparin binds to lysine residues on the ATIII molecule thus causing a conformational change of the ATIII molecule. This binding markedly accelerates the inhibitory action of ATIII by approximately 1000-fold. ATIII combines with and inactivates certain activated coagulation factors; namely factors XIIa, XIa, IXa, Xa and thrombin. ATIII forms an irreversible 1:1 stoichiometric complex by arginine residues interacting with serine on the activated clotting factor. Following this reaction both coagulation factor and inhibitor are inactivated, but heparin will dissociate from this complex and is then able to bind with other ATIII molecules.

Recently a variety of low molecular weight heparin fractions and fragments with a mean molecular weight of 4–6000 have been introduced. Compared to unfractionated heparin which has an anti-Xa/APTT ratio of approximately 1, these fractions have ratios of between 2 and 4. These substances were thought to maintain their antithrombotic effect through anti-Xa activity but to cause less clinical bleeding by reduced action on the APTT and overall clotting. However, this hypothesis has not been substantiated by clinical trials (Thomas 1986). Their main advantage is a prolonged half-life after subcutaneous injection of approximately 12 hours, so enabling once-daily prophylactic administration.

Clinical usage of heparin

The clinical indications for the use of heparin are:

Treatment of an acute thrombotic event

The immediate treatment of newly diagnosed deep vein thrombosis and/or pulmonary embolism must be by continuous intravenous infusion and should ideally continue for 4–7 days as this duration of treatment has been shown to maximally prevent extension of thrombus formation. Heparin is given as an initial bolus of 5000 units followed by a maintenance infusion of 20 000–30 000 units every 24 hours. The exact dosage is controlled by daily tests, usually aiming to maintain a plasma heparin level of 0.2–0.5 u/ml, which is approximately equivalent to an APTT 1.5–2.5 greater than the control value. During the last four days of heparin therapy oral anticoagulation with warfarin should be started and the heparin infusion should not be stopped until the oral anticoagulant effect is within the expected therapeutic range.

Prophylaxis of venous thrombo-embolism

Heparin is given subcutaneously in a dosage regime usually of 5000 units 8- or 12-hourly as prophylaxis for post-operative thrombosis and in other high risk clinical situations (see Table 26.1). Heparin should be maintained at a plasma level of 0.02–0.05 u/ml. Most users of low dose heparin do not perform any laboratory test to monitor the response, but at these plasma levels the APTT should remain within the normal range. Similarly the PT and TT should remain within the normal

Table 26.1 Clinical risk factors associated with a high incidence of venous thrombosis.

High risk factors	Uncommon diseases with a high incidence
Surgical & non-surgical trauma	Homocystinuria
Age	Myeloproliferative disorders
Malignancy	Polycythaemia
Immobilisation	Systemic lupus erythematosus
Heart failure	Behçet's disease
Previous venous thrombosis	Paraproteinaemias
Myocardial infarction	Nephrotic syndrome
Paralysis of lower limbs	
Varicose veins	
Obesity	
Oestrogen therapy	
Pregnancy and the puerperium	
Diabetes mellitus	

range. However, an increase in post-operative wound haematoma has been reported with this form of prophylaxis and is more likely to occur if the heparin levels exceed 0.2 u/ml.

Pregnancy
There is considerable controversy over the ideal way to manage prophylaxis of thrombosis during pregnancy (Drugs and Therapeutics Bulletin 1987). Patients with diseased or prosthetic heart valves and other high risk situations should receive heparin prophylaxis subcutaneously 10 000 units 12-hourly up to 16 weeks and from 36 weeks to delivery, but oral anticoagulants are probably safer from 16–36 weeks. Heparin does not cross the placenta and can be rapidly reversed if necessary.

Extra-corporeal circulation
Heparin is the anticoagulant of choice to prevent thrombosis when blood is passed around an external artificial circuit such as in cardiac bypass surgery and renal dialysis. Sufficient heparin is given intravenously to approximately double the activated whole blood clotting time, and at the end of the procedure the heparin effect is reversed by a protamine sulphate injection. Heparin is rapidly cleared with a plasma half-life of 60–90 minutes. These procedures nowadays only very rarely develop post-neutralisation bleeding events, and if they do any bleeding is only short-lived and readily controlled.

Side effects
The major side effect of a continuous intravenous infusion of heparin is bleeding. This is usually due to excessive dosage and withdrawal is usually sufficient. If bleeding continues, protamine sulphate by slow intravenous infusion will neutralise the heparin effect (1 mg protamine neutralises approximately 150 units of

heparin). Bleeding is not troublesome with subcutaneous prophylaxis although some surgeons do report an increase in wound haematomas. Other rarely reported side effects include thrombocytopenia, alopecia, local skin necrosis from hypersensitivity and anaphylactic shock. Occasionally patients receiving long-term therapy of over one month's duration may develop osteoporosis, and this is a particular risk when prophylaxis is given during pregnancy.

ORAL ANTICOAGULANTS

These compounds are competitive vitamin K antagonists and are well absorbed from the gastrointestinal tract. There are two main types available; the coumarin and indanedione derivatives. The coumarin warfarin is the most widely used in clinical practice. Following absorption, approximately 95–99% of warfarin is loosely bound to albumin in the circulation and only the unbound fraction is pharmacologically active. Upon uptake by the liver warfarin inhibits vitamin K 2–3 epoxide reductase activity, causing decreased synthesis of the biologically active γ-carboxylated forms of the vitamin K-dependent clotting factors, factor II, VII, IX, X, protein C and S. Warfarin is degraded to inactive metabolites by liver enzymes and subsequently excreted in the urine.

The main clinical indications for oral anticoagulant therapy are:

1. The treatment of established deep vein thrombosis and/or pulmonary embolism. This should follow a 5–7 day course of continuous intravenous heparin therapy. For a first episode this should continue for approximately 12 weeks but if recurrent venous thrombotic episodes occur treatment should probably be lifelong.

2. Long-term therapy to prevent systemic embolisation in patients with artificial heart valve implants, mitral valve disease or atrial fibrillation.

3. As prophylaxis of venous thrombosis following surgery in certain patients with a high risk of developing thrombosis (i.e. hip replacement operations) until the patient is fully mobile again.

4. There are a variety of other conditions including transient ischaemic attacks, post-arterial graft surgery and post-myocardial infarction where the value of long-term warfarin therapy has not been clearly established but is still advocated by some physicians.

The initial dosage of warfarin therapy should be 10 mg orally for 2 days, 5 mg on the third day and on the fourth day the dosage adjusted according to the results of the laboratory screening test. The prothrombin time or thrombotest are the most reliable and widely used screening tests, but whichever test is used all the results should be reported as an International Normalised Ratio (INR) and the results recorded on a special card or booklet which is carried by the patient. The INR scheme of reporting results was introduced in 1985 to avoid the confusion which had previously arisen due to the many different methods of laboratory test systems and the different sensitivity of the varying human and animal thromboplastins used worldwide (Lewis 1987). The INR is derived from the equation:

$$INR = ratio^c$$

where ratio is the prothrombin time ratio derived by the patient PT/control normal PT.

and ^{c} is the International Sensitivity Index (ISI) of the thromboplastin used.

When choosing a thromboplastin for oral anticoagulant control, check the ISI of each batch of material, which must be stated by the manufacturer.

As animal preparations of thromboplastin have differing sensitivity, calibration of each batch of reagent in terms of an ISI allows the same therapeutic ranges to be applied by using the INR reporting system. The patient should regularly attend an anticoagulant clinic, where the warfarin dosage will be adjusted. The ideal therapeutic range at which the INR should be maintained for the various clinical conditions as recommended by the British Society of Haematology (BSH) is shown in Table 26.2. The average regular daily dosage of warfarin is 6 mg, but this may vary considerably from 1–20 mg.

Table 26.2 Therapeutic ranges for oral anticoagulation.

INR	Clinical state
2.0–2.5	Prophylaxis of deep vein thrombosis including high risk surgery. 2.0–3.0 for hip surgery and operations for fractured femur
2.0–3.0	Treatment of deep vein thrombosis, pulmonary embolism, transient ischaemic attacks.
3.0–4.5	Recurrent deep vein thrombosis and pulmonary embolism; arterial disease including myocardial infarction; arterial grafts; cardiac prosthetic valves and grafts.

The major side effect of anticoagulant therapy is bleeding. This is unlikely to occur providing the INR remains within the overall range of 1.0–4.5. If the INR becomes grossly prolonged over 5.0 spontaneous bleeding episodes may occur. Haematuria and bruising after minor trauma occur most frequently but there is always the risk of a severe intracerebral haemorrhage and the prothrombin time must be checked immediately the patient reports any haemorrhagic event. The most important factor leading to a grossly prolonged INR and fluctuating anticoagulant control is the interaction of oral anticoagulants with a large variety of drugs. The mechanisms of interactions include the following:

1. Reducing absorption of vitamin K (i.e. cholestyramine).

2. Reducing or increasing warfarin absorption.

3. Reducing warfarin binding to albumin so resulting in an increased level of free, unbound warfarin (i.e. phenylbutazone, sulphonamides).

4. Altering the rate of hepatic inactivation of warfarin (i.e. barbiturates).

5. Increasing the rate of hepatic synthesis of the vitamin K-dependent proteins, so producing a relative resistance to warfarin therapy (i.e. oestrogens, oral contraceptives).

6. Increasing the breakdown of the vitamin K-dependent proteins (i.e. thyroxine).

7. Any other drug which affects the haemostatic mechanism will potentiate the action of oral anticoagulants (i.e. aspirin).

8. Changes in the dietary sources of vitamin K (i.e. patients receiving long-term intravenous nutrition).

Patients receiving oral anticoagulants should avoid other drugs, especially those compounds known to increase or decrease the anticoagulant effect. Commonly used drugs reported to interfere with oral anticoagulation are listed in Table 26.3. Obviously, when a change in a patient's medication is made, the INR should be regularly monitored and the daily dose of warfarin therapy appropriately adjusted. Other medical causes which may potentiate oral anticoagulation are:

Alcohol excess
Liver damage
Cardiac failure
Cholestasis
Diarrhoea
Fever and infection
Gastro-colic fistulae
Malnutrition
Renal impairment
Thyrotoxicosis

Table 26.3 Commonly used drugs which interfere with oral anticoagulant control.

Drugs which increase the effect of oral anticoagulants	Drugs which decrease the effect of oral anticoagulants
Acetylsalicylic acid	Barbiturates
Allopurinol	Cholestyramine
Ampicillin	Diuretics
Anabolic steroids	Oestrogens
Chloramphenicol	Oral contraceptives
Clofibrate	Phenytoin
Neomycin	Rifampicin
Phenylbutazone	
Sulphonamides	
Thyroxine	
Tricyclic antidepressants	

Poor compliance with irregular tablet taking is particularly dangerous and such patients are unsuitable for long-term oral anticoagulation. If the prothrombin time becomes grossly prolonged and spontaneous bleeding develops, the warfarin effect must be temporarily reversed. An intravenous dose of vitamin K_1 takes 6 hours before any synthesis of biologically active factors occurs and then subsequently the prothrombin time will shorten. Complete correction is not obtained until 24 hours later. 1 mg of vitamin K_1 intravenously allows temporary correction, whereas a higher dose of 5–10 mg precludes effective oral anticoagulation for the next 2–3 weeks. To control serious acute bleeding an infusion of fresh frozen plasma or factor II, IX and X concentrate is required. Obviously patients who require surgical procedures or dental extractions should have the anticoagulant effect temporarily reversed by a small dose of vitamin K_1 and/or an infusion of fresh frozen plasma prior to the procedure, or omission of one or two doses of warfarin.

Non-haemorrhagic side effects to warfarin are extremely rare but include skin necrosis (especially during the first few days of therapy), dermatitis and hypersensitivity reactions. The indanedione compounds (i.e. phenindione) have a much higher incidence of serious hypersensitivity reactions and are only rarely used today. Because all oral anticoagulants cross the placenta, and especially during the first trimester may cause fetal malformations (chondrodysplasia punctata and mental retardation), their use should be discontinued at the first signs of pregnancy and replaced by subcutaneous heparin prophylaxis until 16 weeks gestation.

HEPARIN CONTROL

Activated partial thromboplastin time

The APTT method is detailed on page 274.

The dosage of intravenous heparin should be based on the therapeutic range of 1.5–2.5 times the control APTT time (Thomson & Poller 1986). This represents a heparin concentration of approximately 0.2–0.5 IU/ml. The normal value from which the APTT ratio should be calculated is a matter of controversy, some laboratories taking the mean normal time, others the upper limit of the normal range, or the patient's own pre-treatment value. The former is probably the safest, since the APTT may be shortened due to activation or acute phase reaction in the patient, and such a sample may not always be available; the mean control time offers a standard reference point. Daily monitoring of continuous intravenous heparin therapy is advised, preferably at the same time of day.

CALCIUM THROMBIN TIME AND PROTAMINE CORRECTION

Principle

Difficulty of clot detection in the standard thrombin time can be a problem with intravenous heparin therapy. Poor clot formation or undetectable end points can make interpretation of tests and control of therapy difficult. The dilution of thrombin in calcium chloride (O'Shea et al 1971) makes it easier to detect an end point in heparinised samples which would be unclottable in the ordinary thrombin time.

A more accurate estimation of the heparin level may be obtained by adding various concentrations of protamine sulphate to plasma and performing the calcium thrombin time. The heparin level may be calculated assuming that 1 mg protamine sulphate neutralised 1 mg heparin, and that 1 mg heparin has 100 units of activity. This also allows for the in vivo correction of over-anticoagulation with heparin, when required in emergency situations.

Reagents

- 0.025 M calcium chloride.
- Bovine thrombin 50 NIH u/ml.
- 0.05 M imidazole buffer pH 7.3
     3.4 g imidazole
     5.85 g NaCl
     1 litre distilled water.
     Adjust pH with HCl.
- Protamine sulphate (Weddel Pharmaceuticals Ltd.) diluted in imidazole buffer to give: 0.125, 0.5, 0.75, 1.0, 1.5, and 2.0 mg/100 ml solutions.

Preparation of working reagent
Thrombin is diluted in calcium chloride to give a clotting time of 12–15 seconds control plasma in the method below.

Method

1. 0.1 ml control or test plasma is placed in a glass clotting tube at 37°C.

2. 0.1 ml of imidazole buffer is added, followed by 0.1 ml calcium thrombin, and the clotting time is recorded.

3. Steps 1 and 2 are repeated on test plasma if the clotting time is longer than the control, substituting the dilutions of protamine for imidazole buffer. Increasing protamine concentrations are used until a correction of the clotting time is obtained.

Calculation

If the 1.5 mg/100 ml protamine solution gives a correction, and assuming that 1 mg protamine neutralises 1 mg heparin, and that 1 mg heparin contains 100 units activity (these figures will vary slightly according to specific activity):

1.5/1000 mg protamine were required

1.5/1000 mg heparin/0.1 ml plasma i.e. 15/1000 mg/ml

Plasma heparin concentration was 15 × 100/1000 u/ml = 1.5 u/ml

Therefore 15/1000 mg protamine per ml plasma must be given to correct the heparin.

The exact amount of protamine to inject may be determined by the equation:

$$\frac{P \times 75 \times \text{Body weight (kg)} \times (1\text{-PCV})}{1000}$$
= mg protamine to be given

where P = neutralising dose of protamine in mg/ml plasma (from calcium TT).

Comments
— Great care must be taken in detecting the clot on prolonged thrombin times. The tube should be tilted very gently and less frequently as the time prolongs.
— Where very high levels of heparin occur and are not expected, there may be contamination of the sample by collection through a heparinised line, from the same vein as the heparin i.v., into a heparinised syringe.

ANTI Xa ASSAYS FOR HEPARIN

Prophylactic heparin is administered in low dosage e.g. 5000 IU/ml subcutaneously, 2–3 times daily. The resulting blood heparin level is very low (usually less than 0.05 IU/ml) and is therefore difficult and often impossible to monitor by the APTT. A more sensitive method is to use an anti-Xa assay for heparin, either by a coagulation assay or, more conveniently, by amidolytic assay.

Either International Standard Heparin, or the heparin being received by the patient should be used as the standard for the assay, since heparin preparations vary tremendously according to batch, brand, tissue, and species, and newer preparations of fractionated heparin are also available.

ANTI Xa CLOTTING ASSAY FOR HEPARIN

Principle
Test plasma is mixed with excess factor Xa and then residual factor X is assayed. The ability of the test plasma to neutralise factor Xa is compared to that of a standard heparin preparation (Denson & Bonnar 1973) dilute in normal plasma.

Reagents
- Citrate imidazole albumin buffer
    75 ml imidazole buffer pH 7.3
    15 ml sodium citrate 3.13% (0.106 M)
    0.5 ml bovine albumin (20%).
- Activated bovine factor X (Diagnostic Reagents Ltd.).
- Factor X-deficient substrate plasma (Diagnostic Reagents Ltd.).
- Platelet substitute (Diagnostic Reagents Ltd.).
- Calcium chloride 0.05 M.
- Pooled normal plasma (PNP) — at least 10 donors.

Preparation of working reagents
1. Dilute factor Xa 1/50 or 1/100 before use in citrate imidazole albumin buffer, so that heat-treated PNP gives a clotting time of 18–28 seconds in the test system and approximately 60 seconds in the presence of 0.2 u/ml heparin.
2. Reconstitute International Standard Heparin in distilled water to give 10 u/ml, store at 4°C.
3. Prepare dilutions of heparin in pooled normal plasma to give: 0.02, 0.04, 0.06, 0.08, 0.1, 0.15, 0.2 heparin u/ml plasma.
4. Heat the heparin dilutions, an aliquot of plasma without heparin, and test plasmas in a 56°C water-bath for 15 minutes. Centrifuge at 2000 g for 5 minutes.
5. Make an equal volume mixture of factor X-deficient substrate plasma and platelet substitute.

Standard
International Heparin Standard or heparin that patient is receiving.

Method
1. Place 0.3 ml of diluted factor Xa in a series of polystyrene tubes.
2. Incubate 1 tube at 37°C and add 0.1 ml heat-treated plasma, start stopwatch.
3. Mix contents, and at 4 minutes 45 seconds, transfer duplicate 0.1 ml amounts to clotting tubes containing 0.1 ml calcium chloride.
4. At 5 minutes add 0.2 ml of factor X-deficient plasma/platelet substitute mixture.
5. Record clotting time.
6. Repeat steps 2–5 for all dilutions of heparin standard and test samples.

Calculation
A standard curve of heparin concentration against log clotting time is plotted and the patient's heparin

concentration interpolated according to the clotting time.

Comment

The patient's own pre-treatment plasma sample may be used as the diluent in heparin standard curve preparation.

ANTI Xa AMIDOLYTIC ASSAY FOR HEPARIN

Principle

Test plasma is mixed with purified antithrombin III (ATIII), to form a heparin: ATIII complex. The sample is then diluted in EDTA buffer to avoid coagulation and then incubated with an excess of factor Xa. Factor Xa is neutralised in proportion to the amount of heparin: ATIII complex present. The residual factor Xa is then assayed by adding a specific chromogenic peptide substrate and measuring the rate of pNA release by colour formation. The reaction rate decreases linearly with increasing heparin concentration. (Teien et al 1976, Teien & Lie 1977).

Reagents

Reagents may be bought in kit form or separately from Kabi Diagnostica, or from other suppliers of similar quality reagents.

- Tris EDTA saline buffer pH 8.4
    6.1 g Tris   (50 mmol/l)
    2.8 g $Na_2EDTA.2H_2O$ (7.5 mmol/l)
    10.2 g NaCl   (175 mmol/l)
    800 ml distilled water, adjust pH with 1 M HCl, bring to 1 litre with distilled water.
- Chromogenic substrate S-2222 — reconstitute a 25 mg vial with 34 ml sterile water (1mmol/l). Place at 37°C for assay.
- 71 nkat bovine factor Xa (Kabi Diagnostica) reconstituted with 10 ml sterile water, or 1 ampoule 'Diagen' bovine factor Xa (Diagnostic Reagents Ltd.) is dissolved in 0.8 ml sterile water. Leave at room temperature for assay.
- Antithrombin III — 10 *u* human ATIII reconstituted with 10 ml sterile water.
- Pooled normal plasma (at least 10 donors).
- Isotonic saline.
- Acetic acid 50%.

Equipment

○ Spectrophotometer.
○ Microcuvettes.

Standard

The heparin used in the patient or International Standard Heparin should be used to construct the standard curve.

Preparation of standard and test samples

A complete standard curve should be made for each set of equipment and new types or batches of heparin. Heparin standard is diluted to 10 IU/ml with saline. 100 μl of the heparin dilution is further diluted with 4.9 ml buffer to obtain 0.2 IU/ml heparin. The standard curve is then constructed according to Table 26.4.

For daily control use the 0.2 and 0.6 IU/ml standards.

Immediately before use, dilute 100 μl of test plasma in 800 μl of buffer and 100 μl of ATIII in a polystyrene tube.

Method

1. Place 200 μl of standard or test dilution in a polystyrene tube, in a 37°C water-bath, incubate for 3 minutes.
2. Add 100 μl factor Xa, mix and incubate for 30 seconds at 37°C.
3. Add 200 μl substrate S-2222, mix and incubate for 180 seconds.
4. Stop the reaction with 300 μl acetic acid.
5. Read the absorbance at 405 nm against a sample blank (200 μl test or standard dilution, 300 μl acetic acid, and 300 μl distilled water added in place of factor Xa and substrate) in a spectrophotometer.

Calculation

Plot a graph of absorbance against heparin concentration, and read off test values. Alternatively use the formula:

IU heparin / ml plasma
= [0.4/(A1-A2)] [(3A1-A2)/2]-Ax

where A1 is the absorbance for 0.2 IU/ml heparin standard

Table 26.4 Standard curve for amidolytic assay of heparin.

Standards IU/ml plasma	Buffer μl	ATIII μl	Pooled normal plasma μl	Heparin 0.2 IU/ml μl
0	800	100	100	0
0.2	700	100	100	100
0.4	600	100	100	200
0.6	500	100	100	300
0.8	400	100	100	400

A2 is the absorbance for 0.6 IU/ml heparin standard

Ax is the absorbance for the unknown sample.

Comments
— For samples that are not lipaemic and have a bilirubin level less than 100 μmol/l, the sample blank will be constant and may be omitted.
— If the test plasma contains more than 0.8 iu heparin per ml, dilute it 1/2 with pooled normal plasma and multiply the obtained heparin value by two.

ORAL ANTICOAGULANT CONTROL

Prothrombin time

The prothrombin time is the most widely used method of oral anticoagulant control, for method see page 273.

MANCHESTER CAPILLARY TEST

Principle
Capillary blood from a finger-prick sample is added to a reagent comprising seitz-filtered adsorbed plasma, thromboplastin, and calcium chloride. The method is calibrated against the PT on venous samples, and an INR may be obtained after using a calibration curve.

Test samples
Collect 50 μl capillary blood from the first drop of blood obtained after pricking the skin with a sterile lancet, into a disposable micropipette.

Reagent
- Rabbit brain thromboplastin (National UK Reference Laboratory For Anticoagulant Reagents and Control).
- Lyophilised plasma.
- Calcium chloride 12.5 mM.

Preparation of working reagent
Reconstitute the lyophilised plasma with 2 ml of the calcium chloride. Invert gently to suspend.

Add 1 ml thromboplastin and invert gently. Leave at room temperature for 5 minutes prior to use. After reconstitution, the reagent is stable at 4°C for at least 48 hours.

Method
1. Pipette 0.25 ml capillary reagent into duplicate glass clotting tubes at 37°C. (Incubate for at least 1 min but do not keep at 37°C for >30 min).
2. Blow 0.05 ml capillary blood into reagent, mix and tilt to determine clotting time.

Calculation
The INR (and British Ratio) of the resulting clotting time are determined by reference to the table provided with each batch of reagent.

Interpretation
The oral anticoagulant ratio should be adjusted according to the INR result as outlined above.

THROMBOTEST

Principle
The Thrombotest reagent consists of bovine brain thromboplastin and adsorbed bovine plasma with excess factor V. It is reconstituted with calcium chloride, and the test sample therefore provides the vitamin K-dependent factors necessary for coagulation to occur. This reagent is claimed to have a high sensitivity to factors VII and X, and to the inhibitory effect of PIVKA proteins. It is also sensitive to the variant form of factor IX deficiency, factor IX Bm. The method may be performed on whole blood or plasma, or by a capillary technique, and lends itself to the assessment of large numbers of patients in anticoagulant clinics, where space and resources are limited.

Test samples
For the venous blood and plasma methods, citrated blood is collected and prepared in the normal way (p. 270). For the capillary method, a skin puncture is made in the finger using a sterile lancet to produce a free flow of blood. The first few drops of blood are used, and 50 μl are collected using a capillary pipette held horizontally with its tip in the drop of blood. Final adjustment of the volume is made by placing the point of the pipette against filter paper.

Equipment
○ Siliconized capillary pipettes for blood collection.
○ Filter paper.

Reagents
- Thrombotest reagent (Nycomed Ltd.).
  For venous blood and plasma methods:
- Sterile calcium chloride 3.2 mmol/l.
  For capillary method:
- Sterile distilled water.

Preparation of reagent
For venous blood and plasma methods:

Add 11 ml of 3.2 mmol/l calcium chloride to a large vial of Thrombotest reagent (240 tests) or 2.2 ml to a small vial (96 tests). Leave for a few minutes and then mix well by shaking. Aliquot 0.25 ml amounts into glass clotting tubes, cap and freeze below $-20°C$, thaw when required. Stable at $-20°C$ for 2 months.

For capillary method: add 11 ml of sterile distilled water to a large vial of Thrombotest reagent or 2.2 ml to a small vial. Mix and aliquot as above.

Method for plasma
1. Add 30 μl of plasma to 0.25 ml of reagent in a glass clotting tube at $37°C$.
2. Mix and determine clotting time.

Method for venous whole blood
1. 50 μl of citrated blood is added to 0.25 ml of Thrombotest reagent in a glass clotting tube at $37°C$.
2. Mix and determine clotting time.

Method for capillary blood
1. Expel 50 μl of blood from the capillary into 0.25 ml Thrombotest reagent in a glass clotting tube at $37°C$.
2. Mix and determine clotting time.
Calculation. Calculate the Thrombotest percentage coagulation activity using the clotting time and the calibration curve provided. Use the upper curve for citrated venous blood and plasma, and the lower curve for capillary blood. These values may be converted to an INR by reference to the ISI and a table provided with each batch of Thrombotest reagent.

Comments
— It is essential that the batch number on the correlation curve matches the number on the vial.
— Thrombotest reagent should not be left at $37°C$ for longer than 60 minutes.
— The Thrombotest percentage must be multiplied by a correction factor using a chart provided by the manufacturers if there is severe anaemia or polycythaemia.

Interpretation
Normal subjects generally have Thrombotest values above 70%. The therapeutic range for anticoagulant control may either be used as an INR value (see above), or as the Thrombotest activity:
$<5\%$ — the patient is over-anticoagulated and a prothrombin time value should be determined and warfarin therapy reduced or stopped.
5–10% for antithrombotic prophylaxis in atherosclerotic diseases and for treatment of established venous thrombosis.
10–15% for prophylaxis during surgery and in the postoperative period.
$>15\%$ — under-anticoagulated.

NORMOTEST

Principle
Normotest reagent contains rabbit brain thromboplastin and a bovine plasma modified to contain all coagulation factors except II, VII, IX, and X. Normotest, unlike Thrombotest, is almost insensitive to endogenous coagulation inhibitors (i.e. PIVKA's) and accelerators, but is sensitive to changes in the levels of II, VII, and X.

Test samples
For the venous blood and plasma method, citrated blood is collected and prepared in the normal way (p. 270). For the capillary method, a skin puncture is made in the finger using a sterile lancet to produce a free flow of blood. The first few drops of blood are used, and 50 μl are collected using a capillary pipette held horizontally with its tip in the drop of blood. Final adjustment of the volume is made by placing the point of the pipette against filter paper.

Equipment
○ Siliconised glass capillaries.
○ Filter paper.

Reagents
● Normotest reagent (Nycomed Ltd,).
● Sterile water.

Preparation of working reagent
Add 11 ml of sterile water to a large vial of Normotest reagent (240 tests) or 2.2 ml to a small vial (96 tests). Leave for a few minutes and then mix well by shaking. Aliquot 0.25 ml amounts into glass clotting tubes, cap and freeze below $-20°C$, thaw when required. Stable at $-20°C$ for 2 months.

Method
For venous blood:
1. Add 25 μl of citrated blood to 0.25 ml Normotest reagent in a glass tube prewarmed to $37°C$ in a waterbath.
2. Mix and time clot formation.
For capillary blood:
1. Blow 25 μl capillary blood into 0.25 ml Normotest reagent in a glass tube prewarmed in a $37°C$ water-bath.
2. Flush capillary by drawing up blood/reagent mixture and expelling again.
3. Time clot formation.
For diluted plasma:
1. Dilute 6 volumes of citrated plasma with 4 volumes of saline in a plastic tube.
2. Add 25 μl diluted plasma to 0.25 ml Normotest reagent in a glass tube prewarmed in a $37°C$ water-bath.
3. Time clot formation.

Calculation

Calculate the Normotest percentage coagulation activity using the clotting time and the calibration curve provided on the green paper. Use the upper curve for citrated venous blood and plasma, and the lower curve for capillary blood. These values may be converted to an INR by reference to the ISI and a table provided with each batch of Normotest reagent.

Comments

— For paediatric samples, 10 μl of blood or diluted plasma may be used, and the result must then be read from the graph on the yellow paper.
— It is essential that the batch number on the correlation curve matches the number on the vial.
— Normotest reagent should not be left at 37°C for longer than 60 minutes.
— The Normotest percentage must be multiplied by a correction factor using a chart provided by the manufacturers if there is severe anaemia or polycythaemia.

Interpretation

The normal range in healthy adults is usually 70–130%, although slightly lower values are sometimes encountered.

Normotest may be used for the investigation of congenital and acquired deficiencies of factors II, VII, and X; and for the control of oral anticoagulant therapy.

Therapeutic range for oral anticoagulation:
12–20% for antithrombotic prophylaxis in atherosclerotic diseases and for treatment of established venous thrombosis.
20–28% for prophylaxis during surgery and in the post-operative period.

ECARIN ASSAY FOR PROTHROMBIN

Principle

Ecarin is an enzyme purified from the venom of *Echis carinatus*, which converts prothrombin to an active thrombin-like form, meizothrombin. This product can be measured using a chromogenic peptide substrate (Bergstrom & Egberg 1978).

Biochemical basis

Ecarin converts prothrombin to ecarin-thrombin, or meizothrombin, which retains some of the proteolytic activities of thrombin, but is not inhibited by heparin. This activation occurs in the absence of factor V, calcium ions and phospholipid, and therefore PIVKA (proteins induced by vitamin K antagonism) forms of prothrombin, which lack the calcium binding Gla residues, can be activated as well as normal prothrombin.

This allows the estimation of total prothrombin in patients on oral anticoagulants, or who are vitamin K-deficient, and the difference between this assay and other prothrombin assays has been said to be a measure of PIVKA-II.

Reagents

- 0.15 M Tris-imidazole buffer pH 7.9 is prepared from 3 stock solutions:
  - A. 0.85 g imidazole in 250 ml 0.1 M HCl and 250 ml distilled water.
  - B. 2.02 g Tris
    1.135 g imidazole
    0.975 g NaCl
    in 500 ml distilled water.
  - C. 5.825 g NaCl in 500 ml distilled water.
    Mix solutions A and B to pH 7.9 and add an equal volume of solution C.
- Ecarin (Pentapharm Ltd.) — 50 μ vial (approximately 10 μg) reconstituted in 1 ml sterile water, and diluted 1/10 with buffer.
- Chromogenic substrate S-2238 (Kabi Diagnostica) — 1 mmol/l.
- Glacial acetic acid.

Equipment

○ Spectrophotometer.
○ Microcuvettes.

Standard

Commercial standard (Immuno Ltd.) or pooled normal plasma (at least 10 donors).

Preparation of standard and test samples

The standard is diluted 1/10, 1/20, 1/40, and 1/80 in buffer immediately before the assay. Test samples are similarly diluted to 1/20.

Method

1. Mix 50 μl of each standard dilution in 750 μl buffer, in polystyrene test tubes at 37°C.
2. Add 100 μl Ecarin, and mix.
3. Incubate for 60 seconds and add 100 μl S-2238, mix.
4. Incubate until a gradation of colour is seen in the standard dilutions and stop reaction with 100 μl acetic acid.
5. Repeat steps 1–4 for test dilutions, using the same substrate incubation time as for the standard dilutions.
6. Read absorbance at 405 nm against a distilled water blank in a spectrophotometer.

Units

1 unit of activity in this assay is defined as the amount of activity in 1 ml of normal plasma.

Calculation

A graph of absorbance against concentration for the standard is plotted, and the test values abstracted from the curve.

Comments

— Care must be taken to ensure good mixing of reagents at each stage of the assay.
— Very high or low concentrations of prothrombin/PIVKA-II in samples may require adjustment of the test sample dilutions.
— A test sample blank should be used for samples with a high bilirubin level. This may be made by substituting 200 μl distilled water for the Ecarin and substrate.

Interpretation

The results should be compared to those obtained by functional assays for prothrombin. A discrepancy occurs when PIVKA-II is present, since the latter is measured in the Ecarin assay. The ratio of Ecarin assay: prothrombin assay may be increased in:

a. Patients on oral anticoagulants.

b. Vitamin K-deficient patients (parenteral feeding, obstructive jaundice).

c. Congenital abnormality of the vitamin K-dependent carboxylase system in the liver.

Low values in the Ecarin assay may be obtained in:

a. Congenital deficiency of prothrombin.

b. Hepatocellular failure.

c. Patients stabilised on oral anticoagulants.

CROSSED IMMUNOELECTROPHORESIS — DETECTION OF PIVKA

Principle

Plasma proteins are separated in agarose gel by their electrophoretic mobility, which is a function of their size and electrostatic charge. They are then electrophoresed into a gel containing specific antisera which precipitate the protein of interest, and allow its visualisation as a protein peak (Laurell 1965). If calcium ions are present in the first stage of electrophoresis, normal vitamin K-dependent factors may be separated from PIVKA on the basis of calcium binding and the resultant decrease in electrophoretic mobility.

Reagents

● Calcium lactate buffer
    2.0 g calcium lactate
    20.6 g sodium barbitone
    4.0 g diethyl barbituric acid
    0.5 g sodium azide
    5 litres distilled water.
● Agarose LE (ICN Biomedicals Ltd.).
● Antisera to Factor II, IX, or X (Dako Ltd.).
● Tracking dye — 10% bovine serum albumin containing 1% Bromophenol Blue.
● Coomassie Blue stain — 5 g PAGE Blue 83 'Electran' (BDH) dissolved in 450 ml methanol, 450 ml distilled water, 100 ml glacial acetic acid.
● Destain — 450 ml methanol, 450 ml distilled water, 100 ml glacial acetic acid.

Equipment

○ 10 cm square 'U' formers (Mercia Diagnostics Ltd.).
○ 0.2 mm Gelbond film (ICN Biomedicals Ltd.).
○ Bull-dog clips.
○ Glass plates 10 × 10 cm.
○ 20 ml hypodermic syringe and needle.
○ Magnetic stirrer/hotplate.
○ 56°C water-bath.
○ Electrophoresis wicks — J cloths (Johnson & Johnson) 4 layers cut to size of gel (10 cm), and evenly layed together.
○ Electrophoresis tank with cooling plate.
○ Gel cutting template (Fig. 26.1) — prepare using graph paper.
○ Well cutter 4 mm.
○ Filter paper.
○ Paper towelling.
○ 37°C incubator or hairdryer.

Method

1. Add 150 ml calcium lactate buffer to 1.5 g agarose LE in a 25 ml conical flask.

2. Heat flask gently and stir continuously on a magnetic stirrer/hotplate.

3. When completely dissolved, remove flask to a 56°C water-bath.

4. Place hydrophilic side of Gelbond film next to plastic 'U' former and sandwich between 2 glass plates, fasten with bull-dog clips and stand in a vertical position on a level bench (Fig. 26.1).

5. Pour agarose solution into gap between 'U' former and Gelbond film using a hypodermic syringe. and needle.

6. Allow to set at room temperature, and then place at 4°C for at least 20 minutes to harden.

7. Carefully remove bull-dog clips and glass plates, place agarose gel supported by Gelbond film on template.

8. Cut sample well 1.5 cm in and 1.5 cm up from bottom left hand corner of plate. Cut tracking dye well 1.5 cm in and 5 cm up from bottom left hand side corner.

9. Lay gel face up on the cooling plate of the electrophoresis tank with the sample well nearest the cathode.

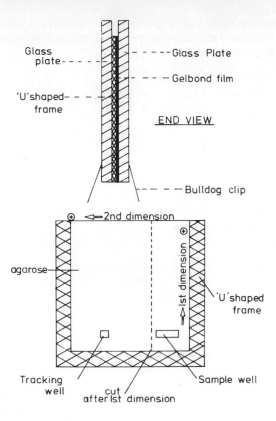

Fig. 26.1 Crossed immunoelectrophoresis: preparation of gel and sample wells.

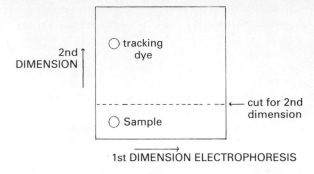

Fig. 26.2 Crossed immunoelectrophoresis: preparation of gel for second dimension.

19. Next morning, the gel is removed and washed gently by immersion in isotonic saline for 30 minutes.

20. The gel is removed to a flat surface and covered with a square of filter paper, followed by several layers of paper towelling. A flat board is placed on top and a 1 kg weight. The towelling is changed at regular intervals until the gel is pressed flat.

21. The gel is then dried at 37°C in an incubator, or using a hairdryer.

22. The dry plate (with the filter paper peeled off) is stained in Coomassie Blue for 10 minutes, and then destained until the protein peaks are clearly seen (Fig. 26.3).

Comments
— Bubbles in the agarose gel should be avoided as they will interfere with electrophoresis.
— The buffer pH should be preserved by reversing the polarity of the tank after the first dimension of electrophoresis.
— A normal plasma should be run with every set of test plates.
— Electrophoresis should be continued for each plate until the tracking dye has reached 1 cm from the anode edge of the gel, so that the mobility of proteins on each plate is being compared to the mobility of albumin.
— Crossed immunoelectrophoresis is difficult to perform for factor VII, owing to the difficulty in obtaining suitable precipitating antisera.

Interpretation
Normal plasma from subjects not receiving oral anticoagulants should give a single peak of protein. Patients receiving the coumarin derivatives usually show this peak plus an additional, faster moving peak of protein (Fig. 26.3). The relative levels of the peaks depend on vitamin K reserves and the degree and length of time anticoagulated. Similar fast moving peaks of protein

10. Pour calcium lactate buffer into electrophoresis tank (at least 500 ml each side).

11. Soak wicks in buffer and use them to cover a 1 cm strip of gel each side of the plate. Ensure that the layers and edge of wick are even.

12. Apply 15 μl of plasma to the sample well and 15 μl of tracking dye to its well.

13. Apply electric current at 10 v/cm gel, constant current; and circulate water through cooling plate.

14. Continue electrophoresis until slower moving patch of tracking dye reaches a point 1 cm from the end of the gel.

15. Remove gel to template, and cut off and remove agarose so that only a 2.5 cm strip of gel is left, containing the separated plasma sample (Fig. 26.2).

16. Add approximately 50–100 μl antisera (this will depend on antibody potency) to 10 ml agarose gel at 56°C, mix and pour onto bare area of gel plate.

17. When the gel has set, place on the cooling plate of the electrophoresis tank so that the separated sample strip is nearest the cathode, and attach wicks as before.

18. Electrophorese overnight at 2.5 v/cm gel, constant current.

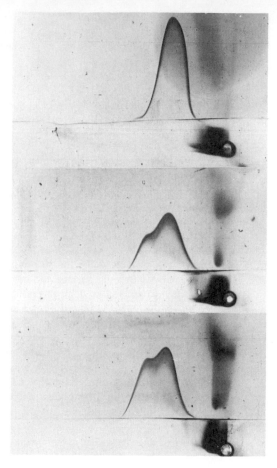

Fig. 26.3 Crossed immunoelectrophoretic pattern for prothrombin. Upper = normal plasma; middle & lower = patients on oral anticoagulant treatment.

may be seen in liver disease, vitamin K deficiency due to poor diet or obstructive liver disease, and in certain congenital defects of the vitamin K-dependent proteins.

MEASUREMENT OF PLASMA WARFARIN OR OTHER ORAL ANTICOAGULANTS

Plasma measurements of warfarin (or other oral anti-coagulants) have no place in routine anticoagulant control but are sometimes useful for specific investigations of suspected drug (or rodenticide) abuse, suspected resistance (hereditary or acquired) or simply to check therapeutic compliance.

Principle

Plasma or serum is extracted with methyl *tert*-butyl ether after acidification with HCl. After brief centrifugation, the upper ether phase is analysed directly by normal-phase high performance liquid chromatography (HPLC). Quantification is by the method of internal standardisation.

Reagents
- Warfarin [3-(α-acetonylbenzyl)-4-hydroxycoumarin] (Sigma) : 100 μg/ml in 1,2-dichloroethane stored at 4°C.
- Acenocoumarin [3-(α-acetonyl-*p*-nitrobenzyl)-4-hydroxycoumarin] (Geigy) : 20 μg/ml in 1,2-dichloro-ethane stored at 4°C.
- HPLC grade solvents : methyl *tert*-butyl ether, hexane, propan-2-ol and dichloromethane.
- Acids : 5 M HCl and glacial acetic acid (analytical grades).

Equipment
- Standard HPLC equipment to include a pump, a UV photometer able to operate near 305 nm, a chart recorder and a syringe loading injection valve (Rheo-dyne model 7125) fitted with a 100 μl loop.
- Microcentrifuge (Eppendorf model 5415).

Preparation of calibration standards

Prepare stock calibration standards in 1,2-dichloroethane with 2, 10, 20, 30, 40, 60 and 80 μg/ml of warfarin together with 20 μg/ml of acenocoumarin and therefore containing known weight ratios of warfarin to acenocoumarin ranging from 0.1 to 4.0. Prepare working calibration standards of 10-fold dilution by evaporation of aliquots of stock solutions under N_2 and reconstitute in methyl *tert*-butyl ether. Similarly, prepare a working internal standard solution of aceno-coumarin with a concentration of 2 μg/ml in methyl *tert*-butyl ether.

Method

1. *Plasma Extraction*. Pipette 100 μl of plasma into a micro, capped, centrifuge tube (polypropylene, 1.5 ml capacity) and add 100 μl (0.2 μg) of the working internal standard solution of acenocoumarin. Add 100 μl of methyl *tert*-butyl ether and 50 μl of 5 M HCl. Mix contents briefly but vigorously on a vortex mixer. Centrifuge for 5 minutes to separate an upper ether phase from a lower aqueous phase with a precipitated protein interphase.

2. *HPLC Conditions*.

Column :	Spherisorb nitrile, particle size 5 μm (Phase Separations) dimensions 250 × 5 mm (i.d.).
Mobile phase :	82–84% hexane, 10–12% propan-2-ol, 5% dichloromethane and 1% acetic acid.
Flow rate :	2 ml/min.
Detection :	UV, 305 nm.

3. *Sample Injection*. Allow column to equilibrate with mobile phase and detector to stabilise. Inject (30–70 μl) of the upper methyl *tert*-butyl ether phase and record chromatogram (chart speed 0.5 cm/min).

4. *Calibration*. Inject (30–70 μl) of the working calibration standards and record chromatograms.

Calculation of results and normal range

A typical chromatogram of a plasma extract from a patient taking warfarin is shown in Figure 26.4. Quantification of the plasma warfarin concentration is made by reference to the peak given by the known amount of acenocoumarin which was originally added to the plasma as an internal standard. This is done by first calculating the peak height ratio (PHR) of warfarin to acenocoumarin from the chromatograms. The linear calibration graph is obtained by plotting the PHRs given by the standards against their known weight ratios. For the unknowns the PHR of warfarin to acenocoumarin may then be converted to an equivalent weight ratio by reference to the calibration graph. Multiplication of this weight ratio by the amount of internal standard (0.2 μg) originally added gives the amount of warfarin in 100 μl of plasma extracted.

The normal range of plasma warfarin in patients whose anticoagulant control was both stable and within the therapeutic range was 0.7–3.2 μg/ml (mean 1.6 μg/ml).

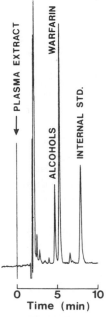

Fig. 26.4 Chromatogram illustrating the assay of warfarin in plasma including the detection of warfarin alcohol metabolites (two possible pairs of diastereoisomers eluting as a single peak). The column was Spherisorb 5 nitrile, the mobile phase 84% hexane, 10% propan-2-ol, 5% dichloromethane and 1% acetic acid and the flow rate 2 ml/min. The internal standard was acenocoumarin (sintrom).

Comments

— Further technical details and an alternative procedure using reversed-phase HPLC may be found elsewhere (Shearer 1986a).

— Advantages of this normal-phase method are the high column stability, its ability to simultaneously resolve the hydroxylated and alcohol metabolites of warfarin which, if present in sufficient concentrations, may be detected (Figure 26.4) and the ease with which the methodology may be used for the assay of other coumarin anticoagulants such as acenocoumarin (sintrom), tromexan (ethyl biscoumacetate) and phenprocoumon (marcoumar).

— Methyl *tert*-butyl ether is the preferred extracting solvent because it can be injected directly onto the HPLC column, has a high boiling point and low risk of peroxide formation.

Interpretation

The few clinical situations in which a plasma measurement of warfarin may be of value have been reviewed (Breckenridge & Orme 1973). One of these is to detect warfarin abuse, especially to confirm the often difficult diagnosis of surreptitious self-administration. The method described here is highly specific and may be used to screen for several coumarin anticoagulants including rodenticides.

A second use of this methodology is to investigate warfarin resistance. An exceedingly rare condition is hereditary resistance in which plasma levels as high as 55 μg/ml are necessary to achieve anticoagulant control and hence may be diagnosed on this basis. An acquired resistance may be due to the simultaneous ingestion of drugs that increase the rate of warfarin metabolism leading to a fall in the steady state plasma concentration and lack of anticoagulant effect (Breckenridge & Orme 1973). Although a low plasma warfarin is characteristic, in practice it is impossible from a single plasma measurement to differentiate an acquired resistance from poor compliance. Some situations may therefore require more detailed plasma warfarin measurements.

MEASUREMENT OF PLASMA PHYLLOQUINONE (VITAMIN K_1)

Vitamin K exists in nature as a number of molecular forms. Phylloquinone (vitamin K_1), synthesised by plants, has a phytyl side chain whereas the multiple series of menaquinones (vitamins K_2), synthesised by bacteria, have multi-prenyl side chains; they are designated menaquinone-n (MK-n) according to the number of prenyl units. The major forms thought to be important to human nutrition are vitamin K_1 and MKs 7–10.

Principle

Plasma or serum is extracted with hexane after flocculation of proteins with ethanol. This hexane extract is subjected to an intensive purification procedure to remove interfering lipids before the final separation of vitamin K_1 by reversed-phase high performance liquid chromatography (HPLC) and redox mode electrochemical (EC) detection using a cell with two porous graphite electrodes arranged in series. The principle of the detection method is to reduce the quinone moiety of vitamin K_1 at the upstream (generator) electrode and to re-oxidise the hydroquinone product at the downstream (detector) electrode. The electrolysis current generated by the re-oxidation step is detected and recorded as a chromatographic peak. Quantification is by the method of internal standardisation. For plasma measurements another K vitamin (menaquinone-6) is a suitable internal standard.

Biochemical basis

Traditional methods of assessing vitamin K status are indirect and rely either on the assessment of the procoagulant activity of the vitamin K-dependent factors (II, VII, IX and X) or the detection of abnormal, des-γ-carboxy forms of prothrombin (PIVKAs). The limitation of coagulation-based tests is their poor sensitivity. Immunoassays of PIVKA are sensitive, even to subclinical vitamin K deficiency, but may reflect a past rather than an existing deficiency. No method currently in use is specific to a nutritional deficiency of vitamin K. PIVKAs may be present as a consequence of liver disease or vitamin K antagonists. The measurement of plasma levels of vitamin K offers a more direct and specific way of assessing vitamin K status. To date, plasma measurements are limited to vitamin K_1 and have been used mainly in a research context. Expected future developments should offer the opportunity for more routine measurements.

Reagents

- Vitamin K_1 [2-methyl-3-phytyl-1,4-naphthoquinone] (Sigma): stock solution of about 25 μg/ml stored in ethanol at $-20°$C.
- Menaquinone-6 [2-methyl-3-farnesyl-farnesyl-1,4-naphthoquinone] (gift from Hoffmann-La Roche): stock solution of about 30 μg/ml stored in ethanol at $-20°$C.
- Solvents : hexane, dichloromethane, methanol and water (all HPLC grade); diethyl ether (Analar grade); ethanol (GPR, absolute).
- Sodium acetate (anhydrous) and acetic acid (both Aristar grade).

Equipment

○ Equipment for HPLC. Two dedicated systems are recommended. The semi-preparative purification stage requires a standard pump and a UV photometer. The analytical stage requires a high quality pump (to minimise sensitivity of EC detection to pump noise) and a model 5100 A Coulochem detector equipped with a model 5011 dual electrode analytical cell (Environmental Sciences Associates). Each system requires a syringe loading injection valve (Rheodyne model 7125) and a chart recorder.
○ Water-bath and gas-manifold arrangement to hold tubes for evaporation of solvents under N_2 at 50°C.

Preparation of calibration standards

Prepare stock calibration solutions in ethanol of K_1 and MK-6 with accurately known concentrations in the range 100–300 ng/ml. These are stable indefinitely at $-20°$C. From these, prepare a series of working calibration standards in ethanol such that the weight ratio of K_1 to the MK-6 internal standard ranges from 0.1 to 4.0 and the final concentration of the internal standard is about 50 ng/ml. Similarly, prepare a working internal standard solution of MK-6 in ethanol (typical concentration 3 ng/ml) by accurate dilution of the stock calibration solution.

Method

1. Plasma extraction

Pipette 1–2 ml of plasma into a glass, stoppered centrifuge tube, add 2 volumes of ethanol including an appropriate volume (typically 0.5 ml) of the MK-6 internal standard solution and vortex mix briefly. Add 4 volumes of hexane and mix the contents vigorously by alternate hand shaking and vortex mixing for 5 minutes. Centrifuge at 1500 g for 10 minutes to separate an upper hexane layer from a lower aqueous-ethanolic layer and precipitated proteins. Transfer the upper hexane layer with a Pasteur pipette to a glass, stoppered tube. Evaporate the hexane extract to dryness under a stream of nitrogen at 50°C.

2. Sorbent extraction using silica cartridges.

Dissolve the lipid extract in 2 ml of hexane and introduce into a glass syringe with a Luer end fitting. Attach the Luer end fitting to a Sep-Pak silica cartridge (Waters Associates) and push the hexane solution through the cartridge to load the extract at the head of the cartridge. Rinse the lipid extract tube with a further 2 ml of hexane and load in the same way. Elute the cartridge with successive volumes of 10 ml of hexane (discard eluate) and 10 ml of 3% (v/v) diethyl ether in hexane. Collect this eluate into a glass, stoppered, tapered tube and evaporate to dryness.

3. Semi-preparative HPLC.

a. HPLC conditions.

Column: Spherisorb-5 nitrile, particle size 5 μm (Phase Separations), dimensions 250 × 5 mm (i.d.).

Mobile phase: 3–6% (v/v) of 50% water-saturated dichloromethane in hexane.

Flow rate: 1 ml/min.

Detection: UV, 254 or 270 nm.

b. *Procedure.* Adjust the mobile phase composition so that the retention of a standard solution containing K_1 and MK-6 is constant with the retention of K_1 in the range of 8–10 minutes. Note that MK-6 elutes after K_1. Thoroughly wash the valve injector with mobile phase. Dissolve the vitamin K fraction isolated by sorbent extraction in 70 μl of mobile phase, vortex mix briefly and inject the total volume onto the column. Collect the eluate fraction which encloses K_1 and the MK-6 internal standard into a glass, stoppered, tapered tube and evaporate to dryness.

4. Analytical HPLC

a. HPLC conditions.

Column: Spherisorb octyl, particle size 5 μm (Phase Separations), dimensions 250 × 5 mm (i.d.)

Mobile phase: 3–5% (v/v) of 0.05 M acetate buffer (pH 3.0) in methanol and containing 0.1 mM EDTA.

Flow rate: 1 ml/min.

Detection: Series dual-electrode EC detection with the upstream electrode set at − 1.3 v and the downstream electrode set at 0 v or + 0.05 v.

b. *Sample injection.* Dissolve the fraction from semi-preparative HPLC in methanol (50–70 μl), warm and vortex mix briefly. Inject a suitable volume (typically 20 μl) onto the column and record chromatogram.

c. *Calibration.* Inject 10–20 μl of the working calibration standards containing K_1 and MK-6 and record chromatograms.

Calculation of results and normal range

A typical chromatogram of a plasma extract is shown in Figure 26.5. To quantify the plasma concentration of K_1 the peak height ratios (PHR) of K_1 to MK-6 given by the samples and calibration standards are first calculated. A calibration graph is obtained by plotting the PHRs of the standards against their known weight ratios. The sample PHR may then be converted to an equivalent weight ratio by reference to the calibration graph. Multiplication of this weight ratio by the amount

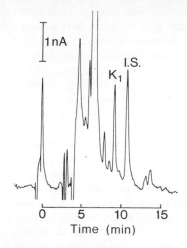

Fig. 26.5 Chromatogram illustrating the assay of phylloquinone (vitamin K_1) in plasma. The column was Spherisorb 5 octyl, the mobile phase 3% 0.05 M acetate buffer (pH 3.0) in methanol and the flow rate 1 ml/min. The upstream electrode was set at −1.3 v and the downstream electrode at 0 v. The internal standard (IS) was menaquinone-6.

of internal standard originally added gives the amount of K_1 in the volume of plasma extracted.

The normal adult range by this method is 0.17–0.68 ng/ml (median 0.37, mean 0.41, n = 45) in fasting subjects and 0.15–1.55 ng/ml (median 0.53, mean 0.66, n = 22) in non-fasting subjects.

Comments

— Further technical details of this method may be found elsewhere, (Hart et al 1985, Shearer 1986b).

— Accurate concentrations of K_1 and MK-6 in stock solutions may be determined by UV absorption spectroscopy (EmM at 248 nm = 18.9).

— Vitamin K_1 in pure solutions and plasma is stable for months when stored at −20°C. All vitamin K compounds are unstable to light and alkaline conditions: all manipulations should be carried out in subdued light and glass ware should be free from all traces of detergents. Care should be taken to avoid contamination of samples with extraneous sources of lipids such as rubber stoppers and lubricants.

— At the sorbent extraction stage, care should be taken to avoid deactivation of the silica cartridges by traces of water or ethanol (e.g. from storage condensation or incomplete evaporation after extraction) otherwise K_1 and MK-6 will be lost in the hexane wash.

— At the semi-preparative HPLC stage, rigorous precautions need to be taken to avoid cross-contamination of samples (from syringes or injection valve) with the K_1 and MK-6 standard used to determine the retention time. Since the collection of the eluate from sample injections is carried out 'blind', generous allowance should be made to ensure complete collection of K_1 from the later eluting MK-6.

— At the analytical HPLC stage, the applied potentials are designed to give maximum selectivity rather than maximum sensitivity. If changes in the electrode response cause a shift in the hydrodynamic voltammogram, some adjustments to the potentials may be necessary (Hart et al 1985, Shearer 1986b). The addition of 0.1 mM EDTA to the mobile phase improves the stability and delays electrode passivation. With a new pump, column and/or mobile phase, the time taken for the baseline to stabilise may be several hours or days. In the long term, high stability and low background currents are best achieved by recycling the mobile phase. Extreme loss of sensitivity, due to electrode passivation, may be restored by a cell washing procedure (Hart et al 1985, Shearer 1986b).

Interpretation

Although the relationship of plasma concentrations of vitamin K_1 to total tissue stores (i.e. including menaquinones) has not yet been established, evidence to date does suggest that low plasma levels reflect a reduced vitamin K status. Substantially reduced plasma levels have been detected in patients with a reduced vitamin K_1 intake (malnourishment or parenteral feeding), an impaired absorption (chronic gastrointestinal disease) or impaired plasma transport (abetalipoproteinaemia). An association has been shown between low plasma levels and susceptibility to antibiotic-induced hypoprothrombinaemia. Low values have also been found in osteoporotic patients. An extremely low normal range (4–45 pg/ml) is a physiological feature in newborn babies and may account for their increased susceptibility to vitamin K deficiency.

Apart from the diagnosis of hypovitaminosis K from low plasma levels, the finding of normal values may usefully differentiate a nutritional deficiency from a mild congenital deficiency of the vitamin K-dependent factors or an acquired deficiency produced by antagonists to vitamin K. Elevated plasma levels of vitamin K_1 may be seen in hyperlipoproteinaemia, particularly in hypertriglyceridaemia.

REFERENCES

Bergstrom K, Egberg N 1978 Determination of vitamin K sensitive coagulation factors in plasma. Studies on three methods using synthetic chromogenic substrates. Thrombosis Research 12: 531–547

Breckenridge A, Orme M L 'E 1973 Measurement of plasma warfarin concentrations in clinical practice. In: Davies D S, Prichard B N C (eds) Biological Effects of Drugs in Relation to their Plasma Concentrations. Macmillan, New York, p 145–154

British Society for Haematology 1987 Guidelines on the use and monitoring of heparin therapy

Denson K W E, Bonnar J 1973 The measurement of heparin method based on the potentiation of anti-factor Xa. Thrombosis et Diathesis Haemorrhagica 30: 471–479

Drugs and Therapeutics Bulletin 1987 Use of anticoagulants in pregnancy 25: 1–4

Hart J P, Shearer M J, McCarthy P T 1985 Enhanced sensitivity for the determination of endogenous phylloquinone (vitamin K_1) in plasma using high-performance liquid chromatography with dual-electrode electrochemical detection. Analyst 110: 1181–1184

Laurell C B 1965 Antigen-antibody crossed electrophoresis. Analytical Biochemistry 10: 358–361

Lewis M 1987 Thromboplastin and oral anticoagulant control. British Journal of Haematology 66: 1–4

O'Shea M J, Flute P T, Pannell G M 1971 Laboratory control of heparin therapy. Journal of Clinical Pathology 24: 542–546

Shearer M J 1986a Assay of coumarin antagonists of vitamin K in blood by high performance liquid chromatography. In: Chytil F, McCormick D M (eds) Methods in Enzymology Vol 123. Academic Press, Orlando p 223–234

Shearer M J 1986b In: Lim C K (ed) HPLC of Small Molecules — A Practical Approach. IRL Press, Oxford, p 157–219

Teien A N, Lie M 1977 Evaluation of an amidolytic heparin assay method: increased sensitivity by adding purified antithrombin III. Thrombosis Research: 10, 399

Teien A N, Lei M, Abildgaard U 1976 Assay of heparin in plasma using a chromogenic substrate. Thrombosis Research: 8, 413

Thomas D P 1986 Current status of low molecular weight heparin. Thrombosis and Haemostasis 56: 241–242

Thomson J M, Poller L 1985 The activated partial thromboplastin time. In: Thomson J M (ed) Blood Coagulation and Haemostasis, A Practical Guide. Churchill Livingstone, Edinburgh

27

Naturally occurring inhibitors

Haemostasis is a well-maintained biological system, containing self-regulating enzyme pathways, inhibitors of various steps, as well as counter systems balancing or neutralising the effects of others. Thus there are procoagulant pathways as well as anticoagulant and fibrinolytic pathways; specific inhibitors of procoagulant enzymes and inhibitors of fibrinolytic enzymes, 'wheels within wheels'. The inhibitors themselves may be divided into enzyme inhibitors which block the active site by forming a complex with it — e.g. antithrombin III, those which compete and interfere with reactions — e.g. FDPs in fibrin monomer polymerisation, and inhibitors which act by degrading a substance, such as protein C. There are also various cofactors of these inhibitors, e.g. heparin for ATIII, protein S for protein C. The clinical importance of these substances is seen in their deficiency states: antithrombin III and protein C deficiencies causing venous thrombosis; C1 inhibitor deficiency causing angioneurotic oedema. The physiology and biochemistry of many of these inhibitory systems are poorly understood, and some only recently discovered, such as tissue thromboplastin inhibitor.

The advent of specific peptide chromogenic substrates and new purification techniques coupled with modern immunological methods is helping to expand our knowledge of plasma inhibitors. The scope of this section, however, is limited to the methods available in a routine laboratory.

ANTITHROMBIN III AMIDOLYTIC ASSAY

Principle

Antithrombin III (ATIII) from standard or test plasmas is activated with heparin and incubated with excess thrombin. A proportion of this thrombin will be inhibited and any residual free enzyme can then be measured using a specific peptide chromogenic substrate. The assay may also be performed as an anti-factor Xa assay rather than as an antithrombin assay, using purified factor Xa and a specific peptide chromogenic substrate for this enzyme.

Biochemical basis

ATIII forms 1:1 stoichiometric complexes with serine proteases, binding to and blocking their active sites. This action is accelerated by heparin which binds to a specific lysine binding site on ATIII. In the circulation, it is probably accelerated by glycosaminoglycans such as heparin sulphate attached to cell surfaces. ATIII is the major plasma inhibitor of thrombin and factor Xa, but is also able to inhibit factors VII and IX, XI and kallikrein. Enzyme inhibitor complexes are removed from the circulation by the reticulo-endothelial system.

Reagents

Test kits are available commercially from several companies, or individual reagents may be purchased.
- Tris EDTA saline buffer
    175 mM Sodium chloride (10.2 g/l)
    50 mM Tris (6.1 g/l)
    7.5 mM disodium EDTA (2.8 g/l)
    Dissolve in distilled water, adjust to pH 8.4 with HCl.
- Sodium heparin (Weddel Pharmaceuticals Ltd.)
- Buffer with heparin — dilute heparin in Tris EDTA saline buffer to 3 IU/ml.
- Bovine thrombin (Diagnostic Reagents Ltd) — dilute in saline to approximately 10 NIH u/ml leave at room temperature during assay.
- Chromogenic substrate S-2238 (Kabi Diagnostica) — dissolve 25 mg in 53 ml sterile water, store in aliquots at −20°C until required.
- Polybrene (Sigma) — 1 mg/ml in sterile water, store at 4°C.
- Substrate/polybrene mixture — mix 2 volumes S-2238 with 1 volume polybrene, bring to 37°C immediately before assay.
- 50% Acetic acid.

Equipment

○ Microtitre plate reader (e.g. Dynatech MR700) or spectrophotometer (for tube assay — see comments).
○ Cooke microtitre plates — (Type M29A, Sterilin).
○ 37°C incubator.

○ 12 channel microtitre pipette (50–200 μl) (Labsystems Ltd.)
○ 37°C water-bath.

Standards
National standard or commercial standard (Immuno Ltd.) calibrated against the international reference preparation.

Preparation of standard and test plasmas
Dilute 12.5 μl test plasma in 875 μl buffer with heparin.

Dilute 150 μl standard plasma in 1625 μl buffer with heparin, further dilute as indicated in Table 27.1.

Table 27.1 Standard curve preparation for ATIII assay.

% ATIII	Buffer with heparin (μl)	Diluted standard (μl)
25	575	25
50	550	50
75	525	75
100	500	100
125	475	125

Method
1. Place duplicate 100 μl amounts of standard or test plasma dilutions in the wells of rows A and B of a microtitre plate.
2. Add 25 μl thrombin using a 12 channel pipette and incubate at room temperature for 30 seconds.
3. Add 75 μl substrate/polybrene mixture to each well using a multichannel pipette, and incubate for 120 seconds at room temperature.
4. Add 75 μl 50% acetic acid to each well with a multichannel pipette.
5. Repeat with further samples in other rows of plate.
6. Read absorbance at 405–410 nm.

Calculation
Results may be calculated using software available on the microtitre plate reader or spectrophotometer, or plotted on a linear graph of absorbance against ATIII concentration, and abstracting the results from the standard curve. Alternatively, they may be calculated from the following formulae:

$$\% \text{ ATIII} = a \times b$$

where   a $= 75/(A1{-}A2)$
        b $= (4A1{-}A2)/3{-}Ax$
        A1 $=$ absorbance of the 25% standard
        A2 $=$ absorbance of the 100% standard
        Ax $=$ absorbance of the test sample

$$\text{ATIII (IU/ml)} = \% \text{ ATIII} \times \text{standard potency}/100$$

Comments
— The assay may be performed as a tube technique using polystyrene tubes and 4 times the volume of reagents; the incubation time with chromogenic substrate/polybrene mixture is shortened to 30 seconds; all incubations are at 37°C.
— Care must be taken to ensure mixing of reagents by adding them rapidly from the pipette.
— Plasma with high bilirubin should have a blank subtraction. This may be carried out by measuring the absorbance of 100 μl test dilution plus 75 μl 50% acetic acid plus 100 μl distilled water.

Interpretation
Normal range — 0.80–1.20 IU/ml; patients with levels below 0.70 IU/ml are at a significant risk of developing spontaneous venous thrombosis.
ATIII may be reduced in:
  a. Congenital deficiency.
  b. Consumption coagulopathies.
  c. Nephrotic syndrome.
  d. Patients receiving 1-Asparaginase therapy.
  e. Individuals taking the oral contraceptive pill.
  f. After long periods (several days) on i.v. heparin therapy.

ANTITHROMBIN III IMMUNOLOGICAL ASSAY

Principle
This assay is based on the method of Laurell 1966, and is described in detail on page 311.

Reagents
● Barbitone/EDTA buffer pH 8.6
    82.4 g sodium barbitone
    16 g diethyl barbituric acid
    10 g disodium EDTA
    2 g sodium azide.
    Dissolve in 20 litres distilled water by gently heating.
● Agarose LE — 1% in buffer (ICN Biomedicals Ltd.).
● Rabbit antihuman ATIII — Dako Ltd.
● Coomassie stain — 5 g PAGE Blue 83 'Electran' (BDH Chemicals Ltd.) dissolved in 450 ml methanol, 450 ml distilled water, 100 ml glacial acetic acid.
● Destain — as for stain, but without PAGE Blue.

Equipment
○ Gelbond film.
○ Magnetic stirrer/Hotplate.
○ 56°C water-bath.

○ Glass test tubes 16 × 148 mm.
○ Gel 'U' formers.
○ Electrophoresis tank with cooling platten.
○ Electrophoresis wicks
○ Well cutter 2.5 mm.
○ Moist chamber.
○ Staining bath.
○ Flat board.
○ 37°C incubator.

Standard

National standard or commercial standard (Immuno Ltd.) calibrated against the international reference preparation.

Preparation of standards and test samples

Doubling dilutions of test and standard are made in buffer to give 1/4, 1/8, and 1/16 of standard, and 1/8 and 1/16 of each test.

Method

1. 1.5 g of agarose is placed in a 250 ml conical flask, and 150 ml buffer is added.

2. The flask is placed on a hotplate, and stirred magnetically while heating.

3. As soon as the agarose has dissolved, leaving a clear solution, the flask is removed to a 56°C water-bath.

4. 13 ml of 1% agarose is pipetted into a prewarmed glass test tube at 56°C.

5. Antiserum is added, the tube is covered with parafilm and the contents mixed by inverting 5 or 6 times.

6. A piece of Gelbond film is cut to 10 × 10 cm and sandwiched between the 'U' shaped gel former and glass plates using bull-dog clips (see Fig. 26.1, p. 337).

7. Agarose with antibody is injected into this template using a syringe and tubing, and the assembly is left to set at room temperature and then stored at 4°C for 30 minutes.

8. The 'U' former and glass plates are then removed and the gel, on its Gelbond backing, is laid flat on the bench, and a row of wells are cut 15 mm from one end of the plate using the well cutter.

9. After ensuring that residual pieces of agarose have been removed from the wells, the plate is placed on the cooling platten of the electrophoresis tank, so that the wells are on the cathodal side of the tank.

10. Wicks soaked in buffer are attached to each side of the gel so that 1 cm strips of gel are covered.

11. 6.5 μl of sample is placed in each well.

12. A voltage of 3 v/cm gel width is applied at constant current overnight, cooling the platten at 10°C.

13. Next morning, the power is turned off, and the gel is removed from the tank.

14. The gel is covered with filter paper and holes are made through the paper and over the wells using a hypodermic needle.

15. Several layers of paper towelling are placed on top, followed by a flat board and a 1 kg weight.

16. The paper towel is changed 2 or 3 times, until the gel is pressed flat and dried; it is then placed in a 37°C incubator until completely dry, when the filter paper peels off.

17. The gel is then stained for 10 minutes in Coomassie stain, and destained until the precipitin lines are clearly visible.

Calculation

The height of each rocket is measured from the top of the well to the tip of the rocket. A log/log graph of rocket height against ATIII concentration is plotted and the test values abstracted from the standard curve.

This percentage of standard value is corrected to IU/ml by multiplying the percentage by the standard potency and dividing by 100.

Comments

— Agarose should not be heated for too long, or at too high a temperature, or it may char and take on a brown discolouration.

— Higher or lower test dilutions must be made if levels are very high or very low.

— The correct volume of antiserum to use must be determined for each batch, but is usually in the region of 100 μl per 10 ml of agarose.

Interpretation

Normal range — 0.80–120 IU/ml.

ATIII Ag may be decreased in:

a. Type I congenital deficiency (decreased levels of ATIII protein).

b. Consumptive coagulopathies.

c. Nephrotic syndrome.

ATIII Ag may be higher than ATIII functional levels in:

a. Type II congenital deficiency (ATIII is present in plasma but does not function normally).

b. Situations where coagulation has been activated, before frank acute DIC occurs.

PROTEIN C AMIDOLYTIC ASSAY (THROMBIN ACTIVATED)

Principle

Protein C is absorbed on to aluminium hydroxide to separate it from its inhibitor and from certain other proteins; the absorbent is washed, and the protein C eluted. Thrombin is added to cause activation, and the protein C concentration is determined from the rate of cleavage of a specific synthetic tripeptide chromogenic substrate, while residual thrombin is neutralised with a synthetic inhibitor (Bertina et al 1984).

Biochemical basis

Protein C (PC) is a vitamin K-dependent protein synthesised in the liver, which circulates in a precursor, zymogen form, which can be activated to give a serine protease. PC is activated by thrombin, in the presence of a source of phospholipid and thrombomodulin (a catalyst). Once activated, PC cleaves factors V and VIII, inactivating them, these reactions are catalysed by protein S. A specific, but poorly studied inhibitor of active PC circulates in plasma.

Reagents

Kabi Coaset Kit (Kabi Diagnostica), comprising:
- S-2366 + I-2581 chromogenic substrate — 6 mg S-2366 and 1 mg I-2581 reconstituted with 2 ml sterile water.
- Elution buffer — 0.25 mol/l sodium/potassium phosphate buffer pH 8.0.
- Hydrolysis buffer — 0.25 mol/l Tris, 0.5 mol/l caesium chloride and 1% PEG 6000 pH 8.0.
- Aluminium hydroxide suspension — 6% w/v aluminium hydroxide moist gel.
- Bovine thrombin — 9 NIH-u/ml (23 nkat/ml) reconstituted with 8.0 ml sterile water.
- Human antithrombin III — reconstituted with 4 ml sterile water to 2.5 IU/ml.
- Heparin 60 iu/ml.
- ATIII/heparin solution — mix 2 volumes ATIII with 1 volume heparin, store on ice.
- S-2366 + I-2581 working solution — 1 volume S-2366 + I-2581 plus 2 volumes hydrolysis buffer, store on ice.
- Protein C-deficient plasma (Kabi Diagnostica).

Equipment

- Microtitre plate reader — e.g. Dynatech MR700 (Dynatech Laboratories Ltd.).
- Microtitre plates — (Type M29A, Sterilin).
- Microcentrifuge.
- 37°C incubator.
- Conical polypropylene microcentrifuge tubes.
- 'End-over-end' mixer.

Standards

Commercial standard or pooled normal plasma (minimum of 10 donors), diluted in protein C-deficient plasma (Table 27.2).

Table 27.2 Protein C assay standard curve preparation.

PC %	PC def. plasma (μl)	Pooled normal plasma (μl)
0	500	—
25	375	125
50	250	250
75	125	375
100	—	500
125	—	625

Preparation of standard and test samples

1. Place 500 μl test or standard plasma in a microcentrifuge tube.
2. Add 100 μl aluminium hydroxide suspension and mix for 30 minutes on an end-over-end mixer.
3. Centrifuge for 5 minutes at 3000 g.
4. Discard supernatant and dry by inverting onto adsorbent paper.
5. Resuspend precipitate in 500 μl sterile water at 4°C using a vortex mixer.
6. Mix for 5 minutes.
7. Centrifuge for 5 minutes at 3000 g.
8. Repeat steps 4–7.
9. Discard the supernatant and dry against absorbing paper.
10. Resuspend precipitate in 100 μl elution buffer.
11. Mix for 15 minutes at room temperature.
12. Centrifuge for 5 minutes at 3000 g, transfer supernatant to a fresh microcentrifuge tube.
13. Assay directly or store at −20°C. Keep fresh or thawed eluate at room temperature to avoid buffer precipitation.

Method

1. Place 12.5 μl of eluate into duplicate wells on a microtitre plate, e.g. wells A1 and A2, B1 and B2, etc., so that the top 2 rows of the plate are full.
2. Add 100 μl thrombin to each well using a 12 channel pipette, cover plate and incubate at 37°C for 10 minutes.
3. Add 100 μl ATII-heparin solution with a 12 channel pipette, cover and incubate at 37°C for 5 minutes.
4. Add 100 μl chromogenic substrate working solution, cover and incubate at 37°C for 5 minutes.
5. Add 100 μl 20% acetic acid.
6. Repeat on further batches of 12 eluates in rows C and D, E and F, G and H.
7. Read absorbance at 405–410 nm on a microtitre plate reader.

Calculation

Results may either be calculated using software packages on the microtitre plate reader or spectrophotometer, or by plotting absorbance against protein C concentration on linear graph paper, and abstracting test results from the standard curve.

Comments
— Care must be taken when discarding supernatants and blotting excess buffer that no aluminium hydroxide precipitate is lost.
— Resuspension and mixing must be performed thoroughly and carefully to prevent contamination with unwanted proteins.
— It is important to add the reagents to the microtitre plate with some force so as to ensure immediate mixing.
— The assay may be carried out in polystyrene tubes by doubling the volumes of reagents and reading colour in a spectrophotometer.
— Colour is stable for 4 hours providing evaporation is prevented.

Interpretation
Normal range — 0.70–1.40 u/ml.
    Decreased levels of protein C are found in:
    a. Congenital deficiency.
    b. Liver disease.
    c. Vitamin K deficiency.
    d. Oral anticoagulant treatment.
    e. Consumptive coagulopathies.
    Many patients are already on oral anticoagulants before protein C can be assayed, which complicates diagnosis. Congenital deficient patients may be differentiated from patients with low protein C levels due to oral anticoagulant therapy by comparing the levels of protein C and factor VII, which have a similar in vivo half-life. If there is a congenital protein C deficiency, the levels of this factor will be significantly lower than those of factor VII. Assays should be compared like with like, i.e. antigen with antigen or functional with functional. The antigen assays are often more helpful due to the very low factor VII levels that are often obtained by clotting assays during anticoagulation, but factor VII antigen techniques are not currently widely used, although there are some commercial kits available. The other vitamin K-dependent factors may also be used as a comparison, if the degree of anticoagulation is taken into account.

PROTEIN C AMIDOLYTIC (SNAKE VENOM ACTIVATED) ASSAY

Principle
An enzyme from the venom of the Copperhead snake (*Agkistrodon contortrix*) is able to activate protein C which can subsequently be measured by the cleavage of a tripeptide chromogenic substrate.

Test samples
Citrated plasma.

Standard
Commercial standard or pooled normal plasma (20 donors).

Preparation of standards
A standard curve is prepared by diluting pooled normal plasma in buffer as follows:

Activity (%)	0	20	40	60	80	100
Plasma (μl)	0	20	40	60	80	100
Buffer (μl)	100	80	60	40	20	0

Reagents
• Snake venom — Protac C reagent (Pentapharm), reconstitute in 6 ml sterile distilled water and store in aliquots at $-20°C$ until required.
• Chromogenic substrate — 2 AcOH-H-D-Lys (Cbo)-Pro-Arg-pNA (Pentapharm) — reconstitute in 5 ml sterile distilled water (2 mM solution) and aliquot at $-20°C$ until required.
• Tris imidazole buffer pH 8.4
    7.07 g Tris
    3.97 g imidazole
    25.35 g NaCl
    100 ml distilled water
    50 ml 1 M HC1.
    Adjust pH and make to 200 ml with distilled water.
    Dilute 1/10 before use.
• 50% acetic acid.

Equipment
○ Microtitre plates.
○ Multichannel or multi-delivery pipettes.
○ Microtitre plate reader.
○ Incubator 37°C.

Method
1. Starting with the 0% standard, pipette triplicate 12 μl amounts into wells ABC1 to ABC6. Place triplicate 12 μl amounts of each test plasma into the remaining wells of the 3 rows, and into rows DEF of the plate.
2. Add 25 μl of buffer to all wells in rows A and D.
3. Add 25 μl Protac C reagent to all wells in rows B, C, E, F, mix gently, cover plate, and incubate at 37°C for 5 minutes.
4. Add 200 μl buffer to each well.
5. Add 50 μl of substrate to all 6 rows, mix, cover and incubate plate at 37°C for 15 minutes.
6. Add 50 μl of 50% acetic acid to all wells and mix.
7. Measure the absorbance at 405–410 mm on a microtitre plate reader using well A1 as a blank.

Units

1 unit of protein C is the amount of activity in 1 ml of pooled normal plasma.

Calculation

Plot a graph of absorbance against concentration of standard and abstract test sample values from the curve. In certain samples — the blanks where Protac C reagent was omitted, there will be high background colour; in this situation the standard curve should be replotted after subtracting the appropriate blank value, and the test sample read from the curve, after deducting its own blank measurement. If this correction is not performed, false high values may be obtained.

Interpretation

Normal range — 0.7–1.3 u/ml.
  Decreased levels of protein C are found in:
  a. Congenital deficiency.
  b. Liver disease.
  c. Vitamin K deficiency
  d. Oral anticoagulant treatment.
  e. Consumptive coagulopathies.

PROTEIN C IMMUNOLOGICAL (ELISA) ASSAY

Principle

Microtitre plates are coated with antisera against protein C, and dilutions of standard and test plasmas are added. After incubation, during which time protein C binds to the antibody, the plates are washed in buffer, and a second antibody directed against protein C, but coupled to an enzyme (peroxidase), is added. After a final wash, a substrate for peroxidase is added which generates a yellow colour on reaction. The greater the colour, the more protein C bound to the plate and therefore the higher the plasma level.

Reagents

- Buffer A — PBS coating buffer pH 7.2
    0.345 g $NaH_2PO_4.H_2O$ (0.0025 M)
    2.680 g $Na_2HPO_4.12H_2O$ (0.0075 M)
    8.474 g NaCl   (0.145 M)
    in distilled water.
- Buffer B — washing and dilution buffer. PBS/0.5 M NaCl/0.1% Tween 20 pH7.2
    1 litre PBS (buffer A)
    0.372 g $Na_2EDTA.2H_2O$ (1 mM)
    20.75 g NaCl
    1 ml Tween 20.
- Rabbit anti-human protein C serum and rabbit anti-human protein C conjugated to horse radish peroxidase (HRP: anti-protein C) (Dako Ltd.).
- 1,2-phenylenediamine dihydrochloride (orthopheny-

lenediamine, OPD) (Sigma) or 2 mg tablets from Dako Ltd.
- 0.1 M citrate phosphate buffer pH 5.0
    7.3 g citric acid.H_2O (0.0347 M)
    23.87 g $Na_2HPO_4.12H_2O$ (0.0667 M)
    1 litre distilled water.
- Hydrogen peroxide 3%.
- Sulphuric acid 2 M.

Equipment

○ Microtitre plate reader e.g. Dynatech MR700.
○ Microtitre plates (Dynatech Laboratories Ltd., Gibco Ltd.).
○ Multichannel pipettes (Labsystems Ltd.).
○ Dark chamber.

Standard

Commercial standard or pooled normal plasma (at least 10 donors).

Preparation of standard and controls

Doubling dilutions of standard are made from 1/10 to 1/160 in buffer A. Doubling dilutions of test samples are made from 1/20–1/80 in buffer A. The substrate is prepared by mixing the following reagents just before use:

  8 mg OPD
  12 ml citrate phosphate buffer
  5 μl 3% H_2O_2.

Method

1. 100 μl of 1/1000 anti-human protein C (diluted in buffer A) is placed in each well of a microtitre plate.
2. The plate is covered and placed at 4°C overnight.
3. The wells are emptied by inversion and blotting on paper towels, and washed 3 times for 3 minutes each with 150 μl buffer B.
4. After the final blotting, 100 μl samples are placed in duplicate wells, in rows A and B.
5. The plate is covered and left at room temperature for 1 hour.
6. The plate is emptied and washed 4 times with 150 μl buffer B.
7. 100 μl of HRP: anti-protein C (diluted 1/250 in buffer B) is placed in each well, the plate is covered and incubated for 1 hour at room temperature.
8. The plate is washed 3 times for 3 minutes with 150 μl buffer B.
9. 100 μl fresh substrate is added to each well and the plate placed in the dark until optimum colour development has occurred.
10. 150 μl sulphuric acid is added to each well.
11. Absorbance at 490 nm is measured on a microtitre plate reader.

Units

1 unit of protein C antigen is the amount of protein C measured in 1 ml of normal plasma.

Calculation

A graph of log concentration against absorbance is plotted, and the test values read from the standard curve.

Comments

— If protein C levels are very low, 1/5 or 1/10 dilutions should be used.
— The substrate is very toxic, and mutagenic; bodily contact, inhalation, and general contamination should be avoided.
— The substrate should be prepared fresh, immediately before use, and kept in the dark until used, otherwise it may become discoloured due to oxidation.
— The time taken for optimal colour development will vary, but is usually between 15 and 30 minutes. The reaction is stopped when a gradation of yellow colour can be seen through the dilutions of standard.
— The incubation periods with antibody or samples may be extended by a few hours without loss of activity, providing the plate is sealed to prevent evaporation.
— For further general comments about the ELISA technique, see page 310.

Interpretation

Normal range — 0.7–1.3 u/ml.

Decreased levels of protein C antigen may be found in:

   a. Congenital deficiency.
   b. Treatment with oral anticoagulants.
   c. Hepatocellular failure.
   d. DIC.

DETERMINATION OF KALLIKREIN INHIBITORS IN PLASMA

Principle

Dilutions of standard and test plasmas are incubated with purified kallikrein, and then residual kallikrein is measured by cleavage of a specific chromogenic peptide substrate (Gallimore 1985).

Biochemical basis

C_1 inhibitor (previously termed C_1 esterase inhibitor) and alpha-2-macroglobulin account for over 90% of the kallikrein inhibitory activity in plasma, the former being the predominant inhibitor. Antithrombin III also inhibits, but very slowly, and there is an unidentified low molecular weight inhibitor (Gallimore et al 1979, Schmaier & Colman 1985). Formation of a complex between kallikrein and high molecular weight kininogen reduces the rate of inhibition of kallikrein. Alpha-2-macroglobulin inhibits kallikrein's kinin-forming activity but not esterolytic or amidolytic activity. C_1 inhibitor forms a 1:1 stoichiometric complex with kallikrein, resulting in loss of both proteolytic and amidolytic activity. When C_1 inhibitor levels are low, alpha-2-macroglobulin and the low molecular weight inhibitor act as a 'backup' pool of inhibitor.

Reagents

● Plasma kallikrein (Channel Diagnostics) — reconstituted in 10 ml of sterile water containing 0.2% albumin and stored at 4°C.
● Chromogenic substrate S2302 (Kabi Diagnostica). 25 mg in 20 ml of sterile water.
● Buffer — Tris-HCl 0.05 mol/l, pH 7.8 containing 0.15 mol/l NaCl. The stock buffer was diluted 100 ml plus 900 ml distilled water.
● 50% acetic acid.

Equipment

○ Microtitre plates (Type M29A, Sterilin).
○ Multichannel pipettes (Labsystems Ltd.).
○ Microtitre plate reader e.g. Dynatech MR700 (Dynatech Laboratories Ltd).
○ 37°C incubator.

Preparation of standard and test plasmas

The standard plasma was diluted with buffer as follows:

Standard %	Plasma (μl)	Buffer (μl)
200	100	900
150	300 μl of 200%	100%
100	100	1900
75	300 of 100%	100
50	200 of 100%	200
25	100 of 100%	300

100 μl of test plasma was diluted with 1900 μl of buffer.

Method

1. Add 50 μl of buffer or plasma dilution prewarmed to 37°C to each well of a microtitre plate.
2. Add 50 μl of plasma kallikrein, mix, cover and incubate at 37°C for 10 minutes.
3. Add 50 μl substrate, cover and incubate for 5 minutes at 37°C.
4. Stop the reaction with 50% acetic acid.
5. Read the absorbance at 405–410 nm using a microplate reader.

Calculation

Plot absorbance against standard concentration and read off the test values.

Interpretation

Normal range — 0.85–1.29 u/ml.

Decreased levels may be found in hereditary angioneurotic oedema, septic shock, polytrauma, pancreatitis, and adult respiratory distress syndrome. Increased levels may be found in cirrhosis and carcinoma.

Good correlations have been obtained between kallikrein inhibitor assays and C_1 inhibitor antigen in normals and clinical materials, except where samples with low C_1 inhibitor levels were tested. This is because of the influence of other inhibitors; the effects of alpha-2-macroglobulin can be overcome in this instance by diluting in methylamine-containing buffer, to block the kallikrein binding site of alpha-2-macroglobulin. C_1 inhibitor and alpha-2-macroglobulin may also be assayed immunologically using commercially available antisera.

DETERMINATION OF βXIIa INHIBITORS IN PLASMA

Principle

Kallikrein causes further proteolysis of the factor XIIa molecule (αXIIa), generating a 28 000 M.Wt. fragment, βXIIa. This has litttle activity on factor XI, but is able to activate factor VII, prekallikrein, and fibrinolysis.

Standard and test plasma dilutions are mixed with a specific inhibitor of kallikrein, and then purified βXIIa is added. After incubation, residual βXIIa not complexed to its plasma inhibitor is measured using a chromogenic peptide substrate (Gallimore 1985).

Biochemical basis

C_1 inhibitor accounts for over 90% of the αXIIa and βXIIa inhibitory activity in plasma (Friberger et al 1984, Schmaier & Colman 1985). Antithrombin III will also bind and inactivate βXIIa, but at a much slower rate.

Reagents

- βXIIa (Channel Diagnostics) — reconstitute with 15 ml of sterile water containing 0.2% albumin.
- Chromogenic substrate S2222 (Kabi Diagnostica) — 25 mg dissolved in 22 ml of sterile water.
- Kallikrein inhibitor (Channel Diagnostics) — reconstituted with 10 ml sterile water, store at 4°C.
- Tris HCl buffer 0.05 mol/l pH 7.9.
- 50% acetic acid.

Equipment

○ Multichannel pipettes (Labsystems Ltd.).
○ Microtitre plates (Type M29A, Sterilin).
○ Microtitre plate reader e.g. Dynatech MR700 (Dynatech Laboratories Ltd.).

Standard

Pooled normal plasma (at least 10 donors).

Preparation of reagents, standard and test plasmas

Immediately before use, dilute 2 ml of kallikrein inhibitor in 98 ml buffer.

Dilute the standard plasma with buffer containing kallikrein inhibitor as follows:

Standard %	Plasma (μl)	Buffer (μl)
200	100	1900
150	75	1925
100	50	1950
75	300 μl of 100%	100
50	200 μl of 100%	200
25	100 μl of 100%	300

50 μl of test plasmas were diluted in 1950 μl of buffer plus kallikrein inhibitor.

Method

1. Add 50 μl of plasma dilution or buffer to each well of the microtitre plate and incubate at 37°C for 2 minutes.
2. Add 50 μl of βXIIa, mix gently, cover and incubate at 37°C for exactly 5 minutes.
3. Add 50 μl of substrate, cover and incubate for a final 5 minutes at 37°C.
4. Stop the reaction with 50 μl of 50% acetic acid.
5. Measure absorbance at 405–410 nm on a microtitre plate reader.

Calculation

Plot a graph of absorbance against standard concentration and read off the test values.

Interpretation

Normal range — 0.64–1.52 u/ml.

ALPHA-2-MACROGLOBULIN — AMIDOLYTIC ASSAY

Principle

Excess trypsin is added to diluted plasma, where part of it forms a complex with alpha-2-macroglobulin; this complex retains its amidolytic activity. The remaining uncomplexed trypsin is blocked with soy bean trypsin inhibitor. The complex can then be measured in terms of cleavage of a specific chromogenic peptide substrate (Gallimore et al 1983).

Reagents

Available in kit form from Kabi Diagnostica comprising:
- 0.05 mol/l Tris buffer pH 8.0.
- Porcine trypsin 0.2 mg reconstituted with 10 ml 1 mM HCl.
- Soy bean trypsin inhibitor (SBTI) 20 mg reconstituted with 10 ml sterile water.
- Chromogenic substrate S-2677 7 mg reconstituted with 10 ml sterile water.
- 50% acetic acid.

Equipment

- Cooke microtitre plates (Type M29A, Sterilin).
- Microtitre plate reader (e.g. MR700, Dynatech Laboratories Ltd.).
- Microtitre pipettes (Labsystems Ltd.).

Standard

Pooled normal plasma (at least 10 donors), or suitable commercial standard.

Preparation of working reagents, standard and test plasmas

A standard curve should be prepared for each batch of reagents, but for day-to-day use only the 25 and 100% standards are required.

Alpha-2-m (%)	Normal plasma (μl)	Buffer (μl)
25	50	150
50	100	100
75	150	50
100	Undiluted	
200	Undiluted	

The 25–100% standards should be further diluted in buffer by adding 25 μl of the mixtures in the table above to 3975 μl buffer. The 200% standard is obtained by diluting 50 μl normal plasma in 3950 μl buffer. Test plasmas are diluted 25 μl in 3975 μl buffer. Warm substrate to 37°C immediately before use.

Method

1. Pipette 50 μl of buffer (blank), standard or test plasma dilution into duplicate wells of a microtitre plate, cover and warm for 2 minutes at 37°C.

2. Add 50 μl trypsin to each well, cover and incubate for 2 minutes at 37°C.

3. Add 50 μl of SBTI to each well, cover and incubate for 2 minutes at 37°C.

4. Add 50 μl substrate to each well, cover and incubate for a final 2 minutes.

5. Add 50 μl of acetic acid to each well to stop the reaction.

6. Read the absorbance at 405–410 nm using a microtitre plate reader.

Comments

— The assay is sensitive to about 10% (0.10 u/ml).
— The assay may be performed using a tube technique if 4 times the reagent volumes are used, and results are read in a spectrophotometer.

Calculation

Plot the absorbance against concentration of standard on linear graph paper. Read off test plasma results and obtain percentage activity.

Units

1 unit of alpha-2-macroglobulin is the amount of activity in 1 ml of normal plasma.

Interpretation

Normal range — 0.67–1.51 u/ml.

Alpha-2-macroglobulin may be reduced in septic shock and adult respiratory distress syndrome.

ALPHA-1-ANTITRYPSIN (A-1-AT)

Principle

Plasma is diluted in buffer containing methylamine, which inactivates alpha-2-macroglobulin. After further dilution, trypsin is added in excess, and a proportion of this is inhibited by alpha-1-antitrypsin. The remaining free trypsin is measured with a specific chromogenic peptide substrate (Gallimore et al 1983).

Reagents

Available in kit form from Kabi Diagnostica comprising:
- Tris buffer — 0.05 mol/l Tris buffer pH 8.0.
- Buffer with methylamine — 0.05 mol/l Tris, 0.15 mol/l methylamine pH 8.9.
- Porcine trypsin 0.2 mg reconstituted with 10 ml 1 mM HCl, store in 1 ml aliquots at −20°C. For assay dilute 1/40 in 1 mM HCl for working solution.
- Chromogenic substrate S-2677 7 mg reconstituted with 10 ml sterile water.
- 50% acetic acid.

Equipment

- Cooke microtitre plates (Type M29A, Sterilin).
- Microtitre plate reader (e.g. MR700, Dynatech Laboratories Ltd.).
- Microtitre pipettes (Labsystems Ltd.).

Standard

Pooled normal plasma (at least 10 donors), or suitable commercial standard.

Preparation of working reagents, standard and test plasmas

A standard curve should be prepared for each batch of

reagents, but for day-to-day use only the 25 and 100% standards are required.

A-1-AT (%)	Normal plasma (μl)	Buffer with methylamine (μl)
25	50	150
50	100	100
75	150	50
100	Undiluted	
195	Undiluted	

The 25–100% standards should be further diluted in buffer by adding 25 μl of the mixtures in the table above to 975 μl buffer with methylamine. The 195% standard is obtained by diluting 50 μl normal plasma in 950 μl buffer with methylamine. Test plasmas are diluted 25 μl in 975 μl buffer with methylamine. All test and standard dilutions are then further diluted 50 μl in 1950 μl buffer without methylamine. Warm substrate to 37°C immediately before use.

Method

1. Place 50 μl of buffer (blank), test or standard dilutions in duplicate wells of a microtitre plate cover and incubate at 37°C for 3 minutes.

2. Add 50 μl trypsin to each well, cover and incubate for 5 minutes at 37°C.

3. Add 50 μl substrate, cover and incubate for 1 minute at 37°C.

4. Add 50 μl acetic acid to stop the reaction.

5. Read absorbance at 405–410 nm on a microtitre plate reader.

Comments

— The assay is sensitive to about 10% (0.10 u/ml).
— The assay may be performed using a tube technique if 4 times the reagent volumes are used, and results are read in a spectrophotometer.

Units

1 unit of alpha-1-antitrypsin is the amount of activity in 1 ml of normal plasma.

Calculation

Plot a graph of log absorbance against concentration for the standard and abstract the test plasma values from this curve.

Interpretation

Normal range — 0.69–1.53 u/ml.

IMMUNOLOGICAL ASSAYS

Immunological assays for alpha-2-macroglobulin, C_1 inhibitor, and alpha-1-antitrypsin are possible by immunoelectrophoresis or ELISA using commercially available antisera.

REFERENCES

Bertina R M, Broekmans A W, Krommenhoek-Van E S C, Van Wijngaarden A 1984 The use of a functional and immunological assay for plasma protein C in the study of the heterogeneity of congenital protein C deficiency. Thrombosis and Haemostasis 51: 1–5

Friberger P, Aurell L, Rees W, Gallimore M J 1984 Studies on synthetic peptide substrates for FXII enzymes. In: Abstracts Kinin 84 Savannah, USA

Gallimore M J 1985 Chromogenic peptide substrate assays for determining components of the plasma kallikrein system. Scandinavian Journal of Clinical and Laboratory Investigation 45: 127–132

Gallimore M J, Amundsen E, Larsbraaten M, Lyngass K, Fareid E 1979 Studies on plasma inhibitors of plasma kallikrein using chromogenic peptide substrate assays. Thrombosis Research 16: 695

Gallimore M J, Aurell L, Friberger P, Gustavsson S, Rees W A 1983 Chromogenic peptide substrate assays for determining functional activities of a alpha-2-macroglobulin and alpha-1-antitrypsin using a new trypsin substrate. Thrombosis and Haemostasis 50: 230

Laurell C B 1966 Quantitative estimation of proteins by electrophoresis in agarose gel containing antibodies. Analytical Biochemistry 15: 42–52

Odegaard O R, Lie M, Abildgaard U 1975 Heparin cofactor activity measured with an amidolytic method. Thrombosis Research 6: 287–

Schmaier A H, Colman R W 1985 The contact phase of coagulation: a review and specific techniques to study its components. In: Thomson J M (ed) Blood Coagulation and Haemostasis A Practical Guide. Churchill Livingstone, Edinburgh

28

Acquired inhibitors of coagulation

Acquired inhibitors of coagulation have been reported in a variety of conditions. They may occur in association with certain auto-immune diseases such as systemic lupus erythematosus (SLE), and rheumatoid arthritis; in monoclonal gammopathies (e.g. myeloma, macroglobulinaemia) and lymphoproliferative disorders; in association with the congenital deficiency of a coagulation factor, such as in haemophilia and von Willebrand's disease; or spontaneously and transiently during or immediately after pregnancy, and in old age. The effects of these inhibitors vary tremendously; the lupus anti-coagulant in SLE is rarely associated with any bleeding tendency, but many patients suffer a thrombotic history; the inhibitors that can arise in haemophilia cause severe bleeding problems, but those in pregnancy are rarely known to cause problems. It is therefore important to screen for inhibitors in conditions where they are known to occur and to define the specificity and potency of the inhibitor.

Global coagulation tests such as the PT and APTT, along with mixing studies using normal plasma, are often useful screening tests. These and the clotting factor assays stemming from them have been developed into inhibitor assays to determine potency. The most common inhibitors, and often the most clinically significant ones, affect the APTT, but inhibitors to other haemostatic components have been noted, such as fibrinogen and von Willebrand factor, as well as platelet antibodies (which will be covered in a later section), and antibodies against components of the fibrinolytic system.

Most clinically significant inhibitors are antibodies of varying class and subclass, and bind to the active or functional sites of a coagulation protein or cofactor. The reaction kinetics (where known) are usually second order (e.g. haemophilia), but can be complex (factor VIIIC inhibitors in macroglobulinaemia).

APTT MIXING STUDIES

Principle

The APTT is performed on a variety of mixtures of normal and patient plasma. If one or more coagulation factors are deficient, one would expect that small amounts of normal plasma would correct a prolonged time, since clotting factors are generally present in relative excess. If an inhibitor is present, far more normal plasma must be added to correct the clotting time, and sometimes if the inhibitor is potent enough, no correction can be obtained.

Test samples
Citrated plasma.

Reagents and equipment
As for APTT method.

Method
Plasmas are mixed in the following way:

Normal plasma (μl)	0	10	20	30	40	50	60	70	80	90	100
Patient plasma (μl)	100	90	80	70	60	50	40	30	20	10	0

An APTT is then performed on the mixtures.

Interpretation
The results may be assessed either visually or after plotting on graph paper. Complete or partial (to a time less than half-way between patient and normal time) correction with a 50/50 mixture suggests a clotting factor deficiency, whereas failure of any correction or only a few seconds shortening suggests the presence of an inhibitor. This type of test can give false results, and where possible, if an inhibitor is suspected for some other reason, or if there is any doubt, a more specific test should be performed.

Concentrates of certain clotting factors can also be useful in correction tests, but it must be remembered that mild inhibitors could be swamped out by very high levels of clotting factors.

'SEPARATELY AND TOGETHER' TESTS OF PROGRESSIVE INHIBITION

Principle

Normal plasma and patient plasma are incubated

separately and together as a mixture. At various incubation times aliquots of the two plasmas are mixed and tested alongside an aliquot of the incubated mixture, and a clotting time performed. Thus, if there is a progressive inhibition, the clotting time of the incubated mixture will become progressively longer than that of the fresh mixture.

Method

1. 75 × 15 mm polystyrene tubes are filled and stoppered as follows:

Tube 1 — 0.6 ml normal plasma
Tube 2 — 0.6 ml patient plasma
Tube 3 — 0.6 ml normal plasma + 0.6 ml patient plasma.

2. Place tubes at 37°C.

3. Remove 0.05 ml amounts of plasma from each of tubes 1 and 2 and mix them in duplicate glass clotting tubes. Remove 0.1 ml from tube 3 and place in each of a further two tubes.

4. Perform an APTT on the four tubes immediately (0 min incubation).

5. Repeat this procedure at 30, 60, 120, and 240 minutes.

Comment

Sensitivity may be improved by incubating or mixing plasmas in the ratio of 4 parts patient plasma to 1 part control.

Interpretation

Immediate acting inhibitors such as lupus anticoagulants will give prolonged APTT's in the incubated and non-incubated mixtures (as compared to normal plasma alone) even at 0 minutes incubation.

Other inhibitors, such as those found in haemophiliacs, are usually progressive and the clotting time of the incubated mixture as compared to the separately incubated plasmas becomes progressively longer as the incubation goes on.

Some inhibitors display little activity in the first 1 to 2 hours, and so it is vital to continue the tests for the full 4 hours to avoid missing them.

KAOLIN CLOTTING TIME

Principle

In this test an APTT is performed in the absence of a phospholipid reagent. This makes the test very sensitive for lupus anticoagulants, presumably because the small residual amounts of platelets and other phospholipid remaining in plasma even after centrifugation for PPP become rate-limiting for the clotting time, and are readily blocked by a lupus anticoagulant.

Reagents

● Kaolin — 0.5% in 0.2 M Tris buffer pH 7.4.
● Calcium chloride 0.025 M.

Method

1. Duplicate 0.1 ml amounts of normal or patient plasma are placed in glass clotting tubes; 0.05 ml of each plasma is mixed in a further pair of tubes.

2. 0.1 ml of kaolin is added, and the mixture incubated for 10 minutes at 37°C.

3. 0.1 ml of calcium chloride is added and the clotting time determined.

Interpretation

The patient's clotting time may be prolonged due to the presence of an inhibitor or due to a clotting factor deficiency. If the time of the mixture is close to the patient's time, it suggests the presence of an inhibitor. If it is nearer the control time, a deficiency or weak progressive inhibitor may be present. The test is not specific for lupus anticoagulant but is very sensitive.

HEAT STABILITY TEST

Principle

This test basically detects immunoglobulin inhibitors by virtue of the fact that they are not absorbed to aluminium hydroxide and are stable at 56°C, whereas most clotting factors are removed or inactivated by this treatment. The treated plasmas may then be mixed with fresh normal plasmas and an APTT performed.

Reagents

● Aluminium hydroxide suspension.
● Kaolin 0.5% in 0.2 M Tris buffer pH 7.4.
● Phospholipid — 'Bell & Alton', platelet substitute (Diagnostic Reagents Ltd).
● Calcium chloride 0.025 M.

Equipment

○ 56°C water-bath.

Method

1. 0.5 ml of normal or patient plasma is placed in a polystyrene 75 × 15 mm round bottomed tube.

2. 0.05 ml aluminium hydroxide suspension is added and the tubes incubated at 37°C for 3 minutes.

3. The tubes are centrifuged at 2000 g for 15 minutes.

4. The supernatant is carefully pipetted off into a fresh plastic tube, capped, and placed at 56°C for 30 minutes.

5. The plasmas are centrifuged for 10 minutes at 2000 g.

6. 0.1 ml of treated patient or control plasmas are mixed with 0.1 ml of fresh normal plasma in a glass clotting tube at 37°C, and an APTT is performed.

Interpretation

If an immunoglobulin inhibitor is present, the clotting time of the mixture of treated patient plasma and fresh normal plasma will be at least 2 seconds longer than that of treated and fresh normal plasma. This test is not specific for lupus anticoagulants and will detect haemophilic and other inhibitors but is useful in patients receiving oral anticoagulants.

DILUTE THROMBOPLASTIN TESTS

Principle

Brain thromboplastin contains massive amounts of phospholipid; if this is diluted out, the concentration becomes critical, and so lupus anticoagulants may inhibit the phospholipid component, thereby prolonging the clotting time in a PT system.

Reagents

- Brain thromboplastin.
- Imidazole buffer pH 7.3, 0.05 M
    3.4 g imidazole
    5.85 g sodium chloride
    1 litre distilled water.
    Adjust pH with HCl.
- Calcium chloride 0.025 M.

Method

1. Brain thromboplastin is diluted 1/4, 1/32, and 1/256 in imidazole buffer.
2. This diluted brain is then used as the thromboplastin source in a prothrombin time on control and patient plasmas.

Calculation

The ratio of patient time to control time is calculated at each dilution of thromboplastin.

Comment

Not all lupus anticoagulants, whatever their potency, will prolong the dilute thromboplastin time. Of the ones that do, there is some dependence on the antibody strength.

Interpretation

Deficiencies of prothrombin, factors V, X, or VII will prolong the clotting times, and give a high ratio, but the ratio will remain approximately the same at each dilution of thromboplastin. Lupus anticoagulants cause a progressive increase in the ratio as the dilution of thromboplastin becomes higher.

DILUTE RUSSELL's VIPER VENOM TIME (DRVT)

Principle

Russell's viper venom, phospholipid and calcium ions are added to plasma and the clotting time recorded. Lupus anticoagulant will prolong the clotting time, but it is corrected if the phospholipid reagent is replaced by washed and activated platelets. These latter are resistant to the action of lupus anticoagulant for unknown reasons. Dilution of the venom and phospholipid make it a particularly sensitive test (Thiagarajan & Shapiro 1983).

Biochemical basis

The venom from the Russell's viper contains a series of enzymes, some of which act on factors V, IX, and X. The latter enzyme is particularly useful as a laboratory reagent, since its direct action on factor X limits the part of the coagulation cascade being studied. It requires phospholipid and calcium ions to function. If the phospholipid reagent is dilute, anti-phospholipid activities block the cofactor activity of the phospholipid surface, slowing the activation of factor X. The system is thus limited to factors II, V, X, and fibrinogen, so that interference by specific anticoagulation factor antibodies or deficiencies of factors are less likely to influence the test. The phospholipid suspension may be replaced by washed platelets which have been thermally ruptured to expose the coagulant active phospholipid on the inner half of their plasma membranes. This material is insensitive to the action of lupus anticoagulant, probably because of steric hindrance, since the clotting factor complex sits tightly together on the surface, binding to specific receptor sites with a higher affinity than the anti-phospholipid.

Reagents

- Imidazole buffer — 0.05 M pH 7.3.
- Russell's viper venom (Diagnostic Reagents Ltd.) — 1 mg/ml in saline, dilute approximately 1/200 in imidazole buffer.
- Phospholipid — 'Bell & Alton', platelet substitute (Diagnostic Reagents Ltd.). Reconstitute according to manufacturer.
- Calcium chloride — 0.025 M.
- Washed platelets — normal platelets washed 3 times in Tyrode's buffer by centrifugation and resuspended to a count of $200–400 \times 10^9/l$. Platelets are stored in aliquots at −20°C.

Reagent preparation

1. Washed platelets are freeze/thaw lysed (5 cycles) to expose coagulant active phospholipid.
2. The RVV concentration is adjusted to give a clot-

ting time of 30–35 seconds when 0.1 ml of RVV is added to 0.1 ml of normal plasma and 0.1 ml of undiluted phospholipid.

3. The test is then repeated using normal plasma, diluted RVV and a range of doubling dilutions of phospholipid reagent. The last dilution of phospholipid before there is a significant prolongation of the clotting time is chosen for the test (usually 1/4–1/8; with a clotting time of 35–40 s).

4. Step 3 is repeated using dilutions of washed activated platelets instead of phospholipid reagent.

Method

1. In a glass tube at 37°C place 0.1 ml normal plasma and 0.1 ml dilute phospholipid reagent.

2. Add 0.1 ml dilute RVV and incubate for 30 seconds.

3. Add 0.1 ml calcium chloride and time clot formation.

4. Repeat steps 1–3 using dilute washed platelets instead of phospholipid reagent.

5. Repeat steps 1–4 using patient plasma.

Calculation

Calculate the ratio of patient/control clotting times, for both platelet substitute and washed platelets.

Comment

Very potent lupus anticoagulants may sometimes be difficult to correct with washed platelets, and a more concentrated suspension must be used to shorten the clotting times.

Interpretation

Normal ratio — 0.9–1.05.

Ratios greater than 1.10 with phospholipid reagent, which decrease with washed platelets, are suggestive of lupus anticoagulants. The presence of heparin may give false positive results. Marked deficiency of factors II, V, X, or fibrinogen, or treatment with oral anticoagulants will prolong clotting times with both phospholipid reagent and washed platelets and make identification of lupus anticoagulants difficult. Testing an equal volume mixture of patient and control plasmas may help identification, since normal plasma will not correct abnormal ratios caused by lupus anticoagulants.

CARDIOLIPIN ANTIBODY ASSAY

Principle

Microtitre plates or polystyrene tubes are coated with purified cardiolipin. Serum samples are then applied, and if any antibody to cardiolipin is present it will bind to the cardiolipin. A detector antibody, anti-human IgG, IgM, or IgA conjugated to alkaline phosphatase enzyme is then applied, and binds to any antibody present, so that when an enzyme substrate is used, antibody is detected by colour formation (Loizou et al 1985; Harris et al 1987).

Biochemical basis

Cardiolipin is effectively a double phosphatidic acid molecule; it is found in cells, predominantly in the inner mitochondrial membrane. To find an auto-antibody against it is therefore unusual in the absence of extensive tissue damage. However, in lupus, antibodies are formed which interact with the phosphodiester linkage found in certain negatively charged phospholipids and nucleic acids, hence the apparent antibodies against these macromolecules. Since cardiolipin has the correct molecular spacing of phosphorus and oxygen atoms, and is a doublet of a common membrane phospholipid, it makes it a sensitive substrate for a test of anti-phospholipid activities in systemic lupus and similar disorders.

Test samples

Serum (plasma may be used if necessary).

Reagents

- Cardiolipin — (product no. C-1649, Sigma Chemical Co.).
- Ethanol (absolute alcohol).
- Phosphate-buffered saline pH 7.3 (PBS).
- Adult bovine serum (Sigma) — 10% in PBS (ABS buffer).
- Alkaline phosphatase conjugated goat anti-human IgG, IgM, and IgA (Sigma). IgG and IgM diluted 1/1000, and IgA diluted 1/500 in 10% ABS buffer.
- Diethanolamine buffer
    97 g Diethanolamine
    0.1 g magnesium chloride hexahydrate
    0.2 g sodium azide
    1 litre distilled water, pH 9.8 with 1 M HCl.
- Substrate — p-nitrophenyl phosphate disodium hexahydrate (phosphatase tablets, Sigma), 1 mg/ml in Diethanolamine buffer.

Equipment

○ Microtitre plates — M129 Dynatech Ltd.
○ Plate reader.

Standards and controls

Purified IgG from an SLE patient with a high titre antibody, or high titre sera for IgM and IgA. Suitable reference sera are available from some specialist laboratories and commercial sources calibrated in IgG and IgM anti-phospholipid units (GPLu and MPLu respectively).

Method

1. Microtitre plates are coated with $30\mu l$/well of $50\mu g$/ml cardiolipin in ethanol.

2. The plates are incubated overnight at 4°C, allowing the ethanol to evaporate.

3. The plates are washed 3 times with PBS $100\mu l$/well.

4. $75\mu l$ of 10% ABS buffer is added to each well to block excess active sites.

5. The plate is incubated for 1 hour at room temperature, and then the well contents are discarded and the plate washed once with $100\mu l$ PBS.

6. $50\mu l$ aliquots of doubling dilutions of reference sera, or 1/50 diluted test samples in 10% ABS buffer are added to each of duplicate wells. The plate is incubated for 3 hours at room temperature.

7. Sample aliquots are then discarded and the plates washed 3 times with $100\mu l$ PBS.

8. $50\mu l$ aliquots of alkaline phosphatase conjugated goat anti-human IgG, IgM, or IgA in 10% ABS buffer are added to each well and the plates incubated for 90 minutes at room temperature.

9. The conjugate is discarded and the plates washed 3 times with $100\mu l$ PBS.

10. $50\mu l$ of 1 mg/ml substrate in diethanolamine buffer is added to each well, and the the plate placed in a dark chamber at 37°C for 45 minutes, or until suitable colour has developed.

11. $50\mu l$ of 3 M NaOH is then added to each well to stop the reaction.

12. The absorbance is then read at 405 nm using a plate reader.

Calculation

The results are plotted on log/log graph paper, and the test results calculated as a percentage of the reference serum, which is assumed to be 100%. If calibrated standards are used, results are obtained in GPL or MPL units.

Interpretation

Care must be taken in the selection of reference sera, and in the setting of the cut-off limits for normal values (usually at least 2SD from the mean). Where calibrated standards have been used, results are usually considered positive when >3 GPLu or >5 MPLu. Positive results for cardiolipin antibodies are frequently found in several auto-immune conditions, including systemic lupus erythematosus (SLE), related collagen disorders and idiopathic thrombocytopenia purpura (ITP). Very often, positive antibody levels correlate with the presence of a lupus-type anticoagulant and are associated with recurrent thrombotic episodes and repeated spontaneous abortions in early pregnancy. The use of this test should be considered as a screening procedure for

patients with thrombotic events. Serial determination of antibody levels may be useful in monitoring the response to specific therapy. Anti-cardiolipin antibodies have also been seen after vaccination or during infectious mononucleosis, and post myocardial infarction, and may not always be indicative of SLE.

BETHESDA ASSAY

This is used for the assay of inhibitors against specific coagulation factors.

Principle

Patient plasma is mixed with normal plasma, which acts as a source of clotting factors. After a 2-hour incubation, a factor assay is performed on the mixture and this is compared to an assay on normal plasma mixed and incubated with buffer. If an inhibitor is present against the clotting factor assayed for, it will have neutralised some of that clotting factor during the incubation, and the residual activity will be low when compared to control. By incubating suitable dilutions of patient plasma with normal, inhibitor units can be calculated (Kasper et al 1975).

Biochemical basis

Specific antibodies against coagulation factors vary in heavy and light chain class and differ in specificity and reaction kinetics. The inhibitors arising in classical haemophilia are usually IgG, but occasionally IgM, with only a single light chain type present. These inhibitors arise in less than 10% of haemophiliacs. Inhibitors arising in non-haemophiliacs are more diverse with both light chain types present and mixtures of gamma chain subtypes. Most haemophiliac inhibitors display simple reaction kinetics (Kasper & Ewing 1982), whereas most other patients with inhibitors to FVIII have inhibitors with complex reaction kinetics.

Antibodies can be directed against various parts of the clotting factor molecule, some binding to the active site, others interacting with phospholipid or cofactor binding regions. The ones acting against active sites are most often discovered since they lead to more severe clinical problems, particularly a lack of response to appropriate factor VIII replacement therapy.

Reagents

Reagents as for 1-stage factor assay (e.g. VIII, IX, XI, etc.).

Method

1. A series of doubling dilutions of test plasma in buffer are prepared.

2. Place 0.2 ml of each dilution in a polystyrene tube.

3. Add 0.2 ml pooled normal plasma, mix and cap.

4. Incubate tubes for 2 hours at 37°C, along with a control (0.2 ml buffer + 0.2 ml pooled normal plasma).

5. Perform a 1-stage factor assay on control and dilute test plasma/normal plasma mixtures.

Units

One Bethesda unit is the amount of inhibitor in 1 ml of plasma that will neutralise 50% of the clotting factor activity.

Calculation

The clotting times for control are plotted on log/log graph paper; each test mixture is plotted against the control, and the residual clotting factor activity determined as a percentage of control. The number of Bethesda units is then determined by reference to a graph (Fig. 28.1), and correction for test plasma dilution.

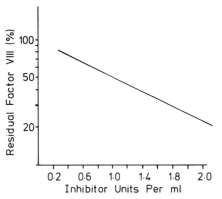

Fig. 28.1 Graph of residual factor VIII: C activity against Bethesda Inhibitor Units.

Comments

— The range of dilutions to set up will depend on the expected potency of the inhibitor, which may be known from past experience with the patient, or estimated from the degree of prolongation of the screening test.

— The amounts of test dilution and normal plasma mixed together should be increased if more than one factor is to be assayed after the incubation, i.e. if the inhibitor is unknown.

— The residual activity must be between 25 and 75% for accurate results.

NEW OXFORD ASSAY

Principle

The New Oxford assay (Rizza & Biggs 1973) differs from the Bethesda method in the source of clotting factor used (a concentrate instead of plasma) and incubation time (4 h instead of 2). It is generally only applied to factor VIII and IX inhibitors, and has been improved from the original Oxford assay (Biggs & Bidwell 1959).

Reagents
- Diluent — buffer containing 5% albumin, factor-deficient plasma, or (for factor VIII inhibitors only) cryosupernatant that has been further cryoprecipitated two times to remove FVIII.
- Clinical concentrate of factor VIII or IX.
- Reagents for factor VIII or IX assay.

Standards and controls

National standard for factor VIII or IX.

Method

1. A range of dilutions of test plasma are made, and 0.2 ml of each are placed in polystyrene tubes.

2. 0.05 ml of clinical concentrate (diluted to about 5 u/ml) is added to each tube.

3. The tubes are capped and incubated at 37°C for 4 hours.

4. A control tube containing 0.2 ml diluent and 0.05 ml concentrate is also incubated for 4 hours.

5. After incubation, all tubes are assayed against standard.

Units

One New Oxford Unit is the amount of inhibitory activity which will neutralise 0.5 units of factor VIII or IX.

Calculation

The potency of control is calculated from the British Standard using a log/log graph. The residual activity of each test dilution is calculated on a similar graph against the control.

The dilution of test plasma giving 50% residual activity (D) was determined graphically and New Oxford Units calculated from the following formula:

$$N.O.units = 1/D \times 5/4 \times control\ u/ml$$

Comments

— The range of dilutions of test incubated depends on the expected inhibitor potency. For low and moderate potency inhibitors, dilutions of 1/5, 1/10, 1/25, 1/50, 1/100, 1/150, 1/200, 1/500, 1/750, and 1/1000 will usually produce a result.

— Staggering the timing of incubation helps prevent excessive variation in incubation time of each tube when a number of tubes must be assayed.

Interpretation

The New Oxford assay has the advantage that it looks at the potency of the inhibitor against a clinical therapeutic material, since a concentrate is used as the source of clotting factor. By varying the type of clinical concentrate used in the test, one can determine for example the most effective human variety of factor VIII concentrate to give, or whether a porcine or bovine concentrate would be haemostatically effective, or merely swamped by the inhibitor. Bethesda and New Oxford units are not equivalent, they differ by approximately a factor of two, but there is considerable variation between patients, and this factor cannot be relied upon.

REFERENCES

Biggs R, Bidwell E 1959 A method for the study of antihaemophilic globulin inhibitors with references to six cases. British Journal of Haemotology 5: 379–395

Harris E N, Gharavi A E, Patel S P, Hughes G R V 1987 Evaluation of the anti-cardiolipin antibody test: report of an international workshop held 4th April 1986. Clinical Experimental Immunology (in press)

Kasper C K et al 1975 A more uniform measurement of factor VIII inhibitors. Thrombosis et Diathesis Haemorrhagica 34: 869–872

Kasper C K, Ewing N P 1982 Measurement of inhibitor to Factor VIIIc (and IXC). In: Bloom A L (ed) The Haemophilias, Methods in Haematology, Vol 5. Churchill Livingstone, Edinburgh

Loizou S, McCrea J D, Rudge A C, Reynolds R, Boyle C C, Harris E N 1985 Measurement of anti-cardiolipin antibodies by an enzyme-linked immunosorbent assay (ELISA): standardization and quantitation of results. Clinical Experimental Immunology 62: 738–745

Rizza C R, Biggs R 1973 The treatment of patients who have factor VIII antibodies. British Journal of Haematology 24: 65–82

Thiagarajan P, Shapiro S S 1983 Lupus Anticoagulants. In: Colman R W (ed): Methods in Hematology: Disorders of thrombin formation other than haemophilia. Churchill Livingstone, Edinburgh

29

Fibrinolysis

In recent years our knowledge of the fibrinolytic system has expanded dramatically, but many problems remain currently unresolved. Fibrinolysis is the system by which plasminogen activators convert a zymogen, plasminogen, into an active serine protease, plasmin, which degrades fibrin clots, culminating in their dissolution. Various mechanisms of plasminogen activation have been described, and there are also a variety of inhibitors and modulators of the system (Collen 1985, Walker & Davidson 1985, Hessel & Kluft 1986). Patients with decreased fibrinolytic activities, either for congenital or acquired reasons, often have an increased incidence of venous thrombosis, and it is important to identify the level of the problem, since a variety of pharmacological agents are becoming available to correct the abnormalities. Tissue plasminogen activator has been produced by recombinant DNA technology, while urokinase and streptokinase (of bacterial origin) are fairly readily purified, and in some cases have been derivatised. These have been used as thrombolytic agents for the treatment of massive pulmonary embolus and for the restoration of coronary blood flow after myocardial infarct and occlusion of coronary arteries. There are also a variety of profibrinolytic drugs which promote plasminogen activator synthesis and release in vivo; these include bezafibrate, phenformin, ethyloestrenol, and stanozolol. Increased fibrinolysis can also cause clinical problems and may be treated with inhibitory substances such as tranexamic acid.

Three systems of plasminogen activation have been described, an extrinsic system and two intrinsic systems (factor XII-dependent and -independent). The extrinsic system involves tissue plasminogen activator (tPA) secreted by vascular endothelial cells, and the action of this protease on plasminogen (Fig. 18.4). tPA is the major component of plasminogen activator activity measured by euglobin clot lysis and fibrin plates, but may also be measured more specifically by immunological assays or functional assays using chromogenic substrates. The action of tPA appears to be modified by a specific inhibitor (PAI-1), released mainly by the vascular endothelium and liver, which rapidly complexes

with tPA in blood, inactivating it. PAI-1 is usually present in excess, but has a very short half-life; many of the changes in fibrinolytic activity measured in tests such as the euglobin clot lysis time reflect alterations in PAI-1 level rather than changes in tPA concentration. Thus the dramatic fall off in fibrinolytic activity seen after surgery, the diurnal variation in activity, and the poor responsiveness to stress such as exercise or venous occlusion, as well as to agents such as DDAVP, in certain patients with thrombotic histories is due to alteration in PAI-1 rather than tPA levels. Specific immunological assays for tPA may yield more useful information than clot lysis times or fibrin plates in studying patients before and after stress tests. Better still would be the inclusion of a specific assay for PAI-1, but these are not widely available and there is much controversy over normal plasma levels for this activity owing to wide interlaboratory discrepancies, depending on the method used and the amount of tPA employed (in functional assays).

With such an excess inhibitory capacity, special mechanisms must occur in the locality of the fibrin clot to ensure its lysis. tPA has a strong affinity for fibrin, and may be protected from its inhibitor when bound. Plasminogen is also bound to fibrin, and when plasmin is formed, it is less readily inhibited by alpha-2-antiplasmin. Fibrin thus causes marked acceleration of fibrinolysis. Local release of tPA from endothelial cells may be stimulated by substances such as thrombin, bradykinin, and PAF-acether. Platelets release additional PAI-1, probably to help localise the fibrinolytic response, but its decay is accelerated by activated protein C and thrombin.

The intrinsic pathways of plasminogen activation account for about 50% of the total activity. The factor XII-dependent pathway involves the action of factor XII on prekallikrein, with the liberation of kallikrein. This reaction is catalysed by high molecular weight kininogen and occurs most readily at surfaces. There is a positive feedback cycle with kallikrein generating more factor XIIa and thus more kallikrein, and the latter can directly convert plasminogen to plasmin. However there may well be a further protease involved, and it has been suggested that kallikrein converts a proactivator to activator, and that the latter is a more important plasminogen activator. Activated factor XI may also have some direct action on plasminogen. These reactions are modulated by C_1 inhibitor and alpha-2-macroglobulin which block kallikrein and factor XIIa activity. The contribution of factor XII-dependent plasminogen activation may be assessed by comparing clot lysis before and after activation of plasma with kaolin. The factor XII-independent pathway is due to urokinase (uPA) activity, the origin of which is unknown, although leucocytes are able to release the protein. uPA has a direct action on plasminogen.

Plasmin formed by activation of plasminogen is the key enzyme of fibrinolysis, and its broad protease spectrum is limited to action on fibrin clots by the presence of excess circulating inhibitors, the most important of which is alpha-2-antiplasmin. Deficiency of the latter results in a severe bleeding diathesis. Alpha-2-macroglobulin is a slower inhibitor of plasmin, and its role is probably to inhibit plasmin generated in excess of the inhibitory capacity of alpha-2-antiplasmin. About 60% of plasminogen is available for activation, the rest is reversibly bound to histidine-rich glycoprotein (HRG), which prevents plasminogen binding to fibrin. A further plasminogen binding protein is known as tetranectin, and this stimulates plasminogen activation by tPA in the presence of polylysine. At sites of fibrin deposition, platelets are able to release further HRG as well as thrombospondin, which binds both HRG and plasminogen, and is a non-competitive inhibitor of plasminogen activation by tPA. Fibrin accelerates the action of tPA on plasminogen, and congenital dysfibrinogens which lack this activity and have a thrombotic history have been described. Plasmin cleaves fibrin, yielding a number of degradation products (FDP's) of varying sizes, and these are progressively proteolysed giving smaller fragments.

EUGLOBIN CLOT LYSIS TIME

Principle
The euglobin clot lysis time (ELT) is a global test of the fibrinolytic system, but in the presence of normal levels of plasminogen and fibrinogen, is mainly a measure of plasminogen activator. A euglobin fraction is precipitated from plasma by acidification, and this fraction contains fibrinogen, plasminogen, and plasminogen activator. However, inhibitors such as alpha-2-antiplasmin remain in the supernatant and are thus removed from the test system. The euglobin fraction is suspended in buffer and clotted with thrombin; during incubation plasminogen is converted to plasmin, which cleaves the fibrin to FDPs. The time taken for lysis of

the fibrin clot may be determined by observation, and is a rough measure of plasminogen activator activity.

Test samples
Blood should be collected with minimal venous stasis and taken into plastic tubes containing tri-sodium citrate which have been chilled in ice. The anticoagulated blood should be kept in ice until processing, which should be as rapid as possible. The blood is centrifuged at 2000 g for 10 minutes at 4°C to obtain platelet-poor plasma, which is separated and kept in ice.

Reagents
- 0.27 M acetic acid (3.2 ml of 1% acetic acid diluted to 200 ml).
- Phosphate buffer pH 7.4
     1.515 g Na_2HPO_4
     0.483 g KH_2PO_4
     6.8 g NaCl
     1 litre distilled water.
- Bovine thrombin 4 NIH u/ml (Parke-Davis, Warner Lambert Co.).

Equipment
○ 12 ml polystyrene conical centrifuge tubes (Sterilin Ltd.)
○ Plastic transfer pipettes.
○ Glass test tubes 75 × 12 mm.

Method
1. 9.5 ml of chilled acetic acid is placed in each of two plastic centrifuge tubes in ice, and 0.5 ml of plasma is added to each.
2. After 15 minutes (but less than 120 min) the tubes are centrifuged at 4°C for 10 minutes at 1000 g.
3. The supernatant is poured off and the tubes inverted onto tissues, and then carefully dried inside using further paper tissues, before replacing in ice.
4. 0.5 ml of cold phosphate buffer is added to each tube, and the precipitate redissolved by drawing it up and down in a plastic pipette.
5. The redissolved precipitates are transferred to glass test tubes in ice, and 0.5 ml thrombin is added.
6. After a few minutes, the solution clots and should then be transferred to a 37°C bath.
7. The tubes are observed at intervals of about 15 minutes for the first 2 hours and then every 30–60 minutes until the clots have completely lysed. The time from placing at 37°C until lysis is calculated.

Comments
— The end point may alternatively be monitored using automated clot lysis monitors, or by recording photographically with an automatic camera which takes pictures at regular intervals.

— Various methods for preparing euglobin precipitates have been described, but for optimum fibrinolytic recovery pH values in the final solution of about 6.0 are desirable, and dilution during acidification helps prevent coprecipitation of C_1 inhibitor. Alteration of pH may either be achieved by adding fixed volumes of acetic acid, or by monitoring the pH and gradually adding acetic acid, or blowing carbon dioxide over the surface of the solution.

— It is essential to maintain solutions and fractions at 4°C throughout the handling as some components of the fibrinolytic system are labile.

— Detection of the end point needs care as the solution surrounding a dissolving fibrin clot will not always be clear, and may be confused with solid clot.

— In patients with very low fibrinogen levels, it may be difficult to obtain a fibrin clot unless exogenous purified fibrinogen is added.

Interpretation

Normal values should be determined in each laboratory, but will usually lie within the range 60–270 minutes. The lysis time varies with age, sex, exercise, alcohol and smoking habits. The ELT may be expressed as reciprocal clot lysis time units.

FIBRIN PLATE TECHNIQUE

Principle

A plasminogen-rich fibrinogen solution is clotted in a petri dish using thrombin, so that an even layer of fibrin is formed. Euglobin fractions of plasma are layered onto the gel and incubated for 18 hours at 37°C. Since excess plasminogen and fibrinogen are provided, and most of the inhibitors removed by euglobin precipitation, the amount of lysis of the gel depends mainly on plasminogen activator concentration. The latter may be estimated by measuring the area of the zone of lysis after incubation.

Test samples

Citrated blood is collected and processed as described above in the ELT method.

Reagents

- Lyophilised fibrinogen (Kabi Diagnostica).
- Combined salt solution
  0.33 M calcium chloride dihydrate
  0.014 M magnesium chloride hexahydrate
  1.87 M sodium chloride
  distilled water.
- Plate buffer
  20.62 g sodium diethyl barbiturate in 1350 ml distilled water

500 ml 0.1 M HCl
100 ml combined salt solution.
Adjust pH to 7.8 with 0.1 M HCl.
Make to 2 litres with distilled water.

- Bovine thrombin (Parke Davis Ltd., Warner Lambert Co.) — 20 NIH u/ml in saline.

Preparation of fibrinogen solution

Solid fibrinogen is dissolved in fibrin plate buffer to give a final fibrinogen concentration of 0.1% w/v and ionic strength of 0.15. The ions present in the fibrinogen starting material must be taken into account, and the plate buffer diluted with distilled water accordingly, so that the ionic strength of 0.15 is achieved.

Equipment

- Petri dishes (Sterilin Ltd.) — 90 × 15 mm.
- 37°C incubator.
- Spirit level.

Standards

Euglobin fraction prepared from pooled normal plasma handled as described above for test samples is used, and for quantification of plasminogen activator a range of dilutions of the euglobin fraction may be made and applied to plates.

Method

1. Euglobin fractions are prepared as described above.

2. 6 ml of fibrinogen solution is pipetted into clean plastic petri dishes on a levelling table (check and adjust with spirit level).

3. Add 0.2 ml thrombin solution to each dish and carefully but thoroughly mix by swirling.

4. Leave on the levelling table for at least 30 minutes to allow an even layer of fibrin to form.

5. Apply 30 μl drops in triplicate, of each test and standard solution carefully to the surface of the fibrin, allowing sufficient space between each application site to allow for the zone of lysis.

6. Leave undisturbed for 30 minutes at room temperature.

7. Incubate for 18 hours at 37°C on exactly horizontal shelves in an incubator that will not be disturbed by vibrations.

Calculation

Measure the diameter of each zone of lysis by two perpendicular measurements. This may be facilitated by placing the plate over graph paper with millimetre squares, or better still, a photographic negative of such graph paper placed on a light box. Find the mean diameter of the triplicate applications.

Comments

— Avoid bubble formation when preparing the fibrin plates.
— All plates used in a run must be poured at the same time from the same fibrinogen solution and using the same thrombin. Therefore the necessary number of plates and volumes of reagents needed must be calculated before beginning the assay.

Interpretation

The result may be expressed in mm and each laboratory should determine its own normal range of lysis zone diameter. Alternatively, percentage activity of standard may be calculated if a range of dilutions of standard euglobin fraction are applied to the plate.

Factor XII-mediated activity

The contribution of the factor XII-dependent pathway of fibrinolysis may be investigated by incubating diluted, acidified plasma (as in the prekallikrein method), with kaolin at 37°C prior to measuring fibrinolytic activity (Ogston 1976).

TISSUE PLASMINOGEN ACTIVATOR — ELISA ASSAY

Principle

Two monoclonal antibodies recognising different epitopes on the tPA molecule are used on a solid phase matrix to capture the antigen. EDTA is included in the sample buffer to chelate calcium ions and thus dissociate tPA complexes with its inhibitor, so that total plasma tPA is measured. A monoclonal antibody recognising a third epitope of the tPA molecule is conjugated with peroxidase enzyme and used as the detector antibody. A substrate is then applied, and the amount of colour generated is proportional to the amount of antigen bound (Holvoet et al 1985).

Reagents

- Coating antibody (a mixture of antibodies MA-62E8 and MA-3B6) — dilute to 4 μg/ml in coating buffer.
- Conjugated antibody (MA-29B9 conjugated to horse radish peroxidase) — Diluted 1/1000 in conjugate buffer.
- PBS
    0.04 M phosphate/0.14 M saline pH 7.4
    18 ml $NaH_2PO_4.2H_2O$ (6.24 g/l)
    82 ml Na_2HPO_4 (5.68 g/l)
    8.18 g NaCl (0.14 M).
- Coating buffer — 1 litre PBS containing 10 g PEG 6000 and 60 g sucrose.
- Blocking buffer — coating buffer plus 0.3% (w/v) gelatine — prepare fresh at 37°C.
- Washing buffer (PBS Tween) — 1 litre PBS containing 0.002% Tween 80.
- Sample buffer — PBS Tween containing 0.3% (w/v) gelatine and 5 mM EDTA — prepare fresh at 37°C.
- Conjugate buffer — PBS Tween containing 0.3% (w/v) gelatine — prepare fresh at 37°C.
- Substrate buffer
    0.1 M citrate/0.2 M $NaPO_4$ pH 5.0
    21.01 g/l citric acid
    35.6 g/l $Na_2HPO_4. 2H_2O$.
    Mix appropriately equal volumes of each to give pH 5.0.
- Substrate — dissolve 6 mg o-phenylene-diamine (OPD) in 30 ml substrate buffer and add H_2O_2 to give a final concentration of 0.003%. Prepare fresh each day.
- 4 M sulphuric acid.

Equipment

○ Cooke microtitre plates (NUNC, Gibco Ltd.).
○ Multichannel pipettes (Labsystems Ltd.).
○ Microtitre plate reader (e.g. MR700, Dynatech Laboratories Ltd.).

Standard

A large pool of normal plasma provides a working standard and can be calibrated by assaying against the International Reference Preparation (IRP 83/517, NIBSC), and storing in aliquots at −70°C.

Preparation of standard and test dilutions

Standard and test plasmas are normally diluted in the range 1/4–1/128, and purified materials such as the IRP to 0.2–5.0 ng/ml in sample buffer. Three dilutions of each test sample and six dilutions of standard are normally applied to the plate in duplicate.

Method

1. Add 200 μl of coating antibody to each well of a microtitre plate.
2. Cover plate and incubate for 48 hours at 4°C.
3. Empty wells and blot, then add 200 μl of blocking buffer to each well.
4. Incubate for 2 hours at room temperature.
5. Wash twice with 200 μl coating buffer.
6. Add 180 μl of standard or test plasma dilution to each well, except A1, which gets 180 μl sample buffer as blank.
7. Incubate for 18 hours at 4°C in a moist chamber.
8. Empty plate and blot, then wash 4 times for 3 minutes each with PBS Tween Washing buffer.
9. Add 160 μl HRP conjugate to each well and incubate for 2 hours at room temperature.
10. Wash 6 times for 3 minutes each with PBS Tween Washing buffer.

11. Add 160 μl of substrate to each well and develop for 10–30 minutes (or until there is suitable colour development in the standard curve) at room temperature in the dark.

12. Stop the reaction by adding 50 μl 4 M sulphuric acid to each well.

13. Read the absorbance against the sample blank at 492 nm using the plate reader.

Comments

— The antibodies to tPA used in our laboratory were kind gifts from Dr Holvoet, Leuven, Belgium, but other suitable monoclonal antibodies may be obtained commercially (e.g. Bioscot Ltd. American Diagnostica Inc.) and used in a similar fashion.

— Gelatine comes out of solution at 4°C and solutions containing it should therefore be made fresh on the day of use.

— The substrate must be prepared immediately before use or it will oxidise and undergo a colour change.

— The EDTA concentration of test samples is critical, decreased EDTA levels affect tPA binding to the plate, and this may cause non-parallelism if samples are not diluted at least 1/4.

Interpretation

The normal range should be established in each laboratory, and may vary depending on the type of monoclonal antibodies used. The tPA antigen level may be of use in the investigation of patients with recurrent thrombosis and abnormal fibrinolysis, particularly if studied before and after venous occlusion or DDAVP infusion. Some patients have a discrepancy between the increase in tPA antigen and fibrinolytic activity suggesting that they have higher tPA inhibitor levels.

TISSUE PLASMINOGEN ACTIVATOR (tPA) AMIDOLYTIC ASSAY

Two main types of amidolytic assay for tPA have been described. The first relies on the activation of purified plasminogen to plasmin in the presence of fibrinogen fragments which stimulate tPA activity; the plasmin is then measured with the chromogenic substrate S-2251 (CoaSet kit, Kabi Diagnostica). In the second method tPA is captured on specific antibodies bound to a solid phase matrix such as a microtitre plate, plasminogen is added along with a stimulator of tPA activity, and the plasmin produced is measured with chromogenic substrates (Mahmoud & Gaffney 1985). Alternatively, chromogenic peptide substrates which measure the proteolytic activity of tPA directly may be used, but there can be problems of specificity with these, particularly in plasma assays.

Tissue plasminogen activator inhibitor (PAI-1)
Several PAI-1 assays have been described using chromogenic peptide substrates or monoclonal antibodies. However, there are many problems with reproducibility and interlaboratory error, and the monoclonal antibodies are not widely available. No doubt these problems will soon be overcome, and suitable commercial kits will be available.

PLASMINOGEN AMIDOLYTIC ASSAY

Principle

An excess of streptokinase is added to diluted plasma and a 1:1 stoichiometric complex is formed between plasminogen and streptokinase. This complex has enzymatic activity which can be measured by the cleavage of pNA from a chromogenic peptide substrate, which results in formation of a yellow colour. As the streptokinase is added in excess, there is no free plasminogen to be converted to plasmin, and therefore the activity is not inhibited by plasma protease inhibitors.

Reagents

These may be obtained in kit form (Kabi Diagnostica), or as individual reagents as listed below.

- Substrate S-2251 — contents of 25 mg vial dissolved in 15 ml sterile distilled water.
- Streptokinase — Kabikinase reagent reconstituted in distilled water to a concentration of 10 000 IU/ml.
- Tris buffer pH 7.4
    6.1 g Tris (50 mM)
    0.7 g NaCl (12 mM)
    800 ml distilled water.
    Adjust pH to 7.4 with HCl.
    Bring to 1 litre with distilled water.
- Substrate buffer mixture — 2 volumes of S-2251 mixed with 5 volumes buffer.
- 50% acetic acid.

Equipment

○ Cooke microtitre plates (Type M29A, Sterilin Ltd.).
○ Microtitre plate reader (e.g. MR700, Dynatech Laboratories Ltd.).
○ Multichannel pipettes (Labsystems Ltd.).
○ 37°C incubator.
For tube type assay:
○ Polystyrene test tubes.
○ Spectrophotometer.
○ 37°C water-bath.

Standards

Pooled normal plasma or commercial standard (e.g. Immuno Ltd.).

Table 29.1 Standard curve preparation for plasminogen assay.

% Plasminogen	Standard plasma (μl)	Buffer (μl)
25	25	175
50	50	150
75	75	125
100	100	100
125	125	75
150	150	50

Preparation of standard and test plasmas
50 μl of each standard concentration (Table 29.1) is diluted with 1250 μl buffer; 50 μl of each test sample is diluted with 2500 μl of buffer.

Method

1. Pipette duplicate 50 μl amounts of each standard and test dilution into wells on a microtitre plate, placing 50 μl of buffer in well A1 as blank.

2. Cover plate and warm to 37°C in an incubator for 5 minutes.

3. Using a multichannel pipette, add 25 μl streptokinase to each well, mix gently, cover and incubate at 37°C for 10 minutes.

4. Add 175 μl substrate buffer solution to each well and incubate at 37°C for 180 seconds or until sufficient colour has developed.

5. Stop the reaction by adding 25 μl of acetic acid to each well.

6. Read the absorbance at 405–410 nm.

Calculation

Plot the absorbance of the standard dilutions against concentration on linear graph paper, and abstract the test results. Alternatively use software in microplate reader where available.

Comments

— The assay may be performed as a tube technique using polystyrene tubes for the reaction, in a 37°C water-bath and 4 times the reagent/plasma dilution volumes. Results are read in a spectrophotometer using semi-microcuvettes.

— If test samples are lipaemic or have high bilirubin levels, the absorbance of the test plasma blank should be subtracted. The latter can be performed by adding the equivalent volume of distilled water instead of streptokinase and substrate.

Interpretation

Plasminogen levels are low in full-term infants and may be undetectable in premature neonates. Congenital deficiency has not been described, and may be incompatible with life, but there are inherited variant plas-minogen molecules, which have abnormal activation to plasmin, and are associated with an increased incidence of thrombosis. Decreased levels are also found in liver disease, since this organ is the site of synthesis.

Plasminogen levels increase during pregnancy, in women on the oral contraceptive pill, and with age, and are higher in Africans than Caucasians.

Various other assays of plasminogen activity are available, using casein as substrate, or plasminogen-free fibrin plates.

PLASMINOGEN IMMUNOLOGICAL ASSAY

Plasminogen antigen may be assayed by radial immuno-diffusion, Laurell rocket immunoelectrophoresis, and ELISA assay; commercial antisera are widely available. The immunological methods tend to overestimate plasminogen levels when compared to functional methods, probably because they measure molecules which are not readily available for activation, such as the histidine-rich glycoprotein-bound pool. Immunological assays are useful in the investigation of suspected plasminogen variants, where a low value has been obtained in the amidolytic assay, and it may be helpful to perform crossed immunoelectrophoresis to look for changes in electrophoretic mobility.

ALPHA-2-ANTIPLASMIN AMIDOLYTIC ASSAY

Principle

Plasma dilutions are incubated with excess plasmin, and a proportion of the plasmin will be inhibited by anti-plasmins. Residual plasmin is then measured using a specific chromogenic peptide substrate from which plasmin cleaves pNA, giving the solution a yellow colour which may be measured in a spectrophotometer. Alpha-2-antiplasmin is the major circulating inhibitor of plasmin; it forms an irreversible inhibitory complex, acting at a much faster rate than other inhibitors. If the reaction times are kept short, this assay is therefore effectively a measure of alpha-2-antiplasmin.

Reagents

A commercial kit is available from Kabi Diagnostica, but components may be obtained individually and are listed below.

● Substrate S-2251 — the contents of a 25 mg vial are dissolved in 13 ml sterile distilled water.

● Glycerol/HCL solution — 50% glycerol in 2 mM HCl with 5 g/l Carbowax 6000.

● Human plasmin — dissolve in glycerol/HCl solution to give 0.25 CU/ml. Store below −20°C, and warm an aliquot to room temperature for at least 1 hour before use.

- Tris buffer
    6.1 g Tris (50 mM)
    6.5 g NaCl (110 mM)
    800 ml distilled water.
    Adjust pH to 7.4 with HCl.
    Make to 1 litre with distilled water.
- 50% acetic acid.

Equipment
○ Cooke microtitre plates (Type M29A, Sterilin Ltd.).
○ Microtitre plate reader (e.g. MR700, Dynatech Laboratories Ltd.).
○ Multichannel pipettes (Labsystems Ltd.).
○ 37°C incubator.
For tube type assay:
○ Polystyrene test tubes.
○ Spectrophotometer.
○ 37°C water-bath.

Standard
Pooled normal plasma.

Preparation of standard and test plasma dilutions
50 μl of the 25–100% standards (Table 29.2) and all test plasmas are diluted in 1500 μl of buffer.

Table 29.2 Standard curve preparation for alpha-2-antiplasmin assay.

Antiplasmin activity (%)	Normal plasma (μl)	Buffer (μl)
25	25	75
50	50	50
75	75	25
100	100	—

Method
1. Add 150 μl of buffer to the first well on a microtitre plate, and duplicate 150 μl amounts of each standard and test plasma dilution to the other wells of a double row.
2. Cover the plate and place in a 37°C incubator for 5 minutes.
3. Using a multichannel pipette, add 50 μl plasmin to each row of wells, leaving a 10 second gap between each row, and mix gently.
4. Incubate at 37°C for 30 seconds and add 50 μl of substrate to the wells of each row, again leaving a 10-second gap between each row, mix gently.
5. Cover plate and incubate at 37°C for 120 seconds, add 25 μl acetic acid to each row, staggered by 10 seconds, mix gently.
6. Read absorbance at 405–410 nm.

Calculation
Plot the absorbance of the standard dilutions against concentration on linear graph paper, and abstract the test results. Alternatively use software in microplate reader, where available.

Comments
— The assay may be performed as a tube technique using polystyrene tubes for the reaction, in a 37°C water-bath and 4 times the reagent/plasma dilution volumes. Results are read in a spectrophotometer using semi-microcuvettes.
— If test samples are lipaemic or have high bilirubin levels, the absorbance of the test plasma blank should be subtracted. The latter can be performed by adding the equivalent volume of distilled water instead of plasmin and substrate.

Interpretation
Congenital deficiency of alpha-2-antiplasmin is associated with a marked haemorrhagic diathesis. Levels are reduced in liver disease and DIC, and are temporarily exhausted during streptokinase therapy.

Alpha-2-antiplasmin increases with age and is higher in Caucasians than Africans.

Alpha-2-antiplasmin immunological assay
Most of the regular immunological assays may be used to measure alpha-2-antiplasmin antigen, and antisera are commercially available. These assays may be of some value in investigating functional deficiencies. Assays of plasmin/alpha-2-antiplasmin complexes have also been described, and may be of use in monitoring in vivo fibrinolysis in certain clinical conditions.

Fibrin degradation product (FDP) assays
These are described in a previous section on investigation of prolonged thrombin times (p. 281).

THE FIBRINOLYTIC RESPONSE TO VENOUS OCCLUSION

Subjects are allowed to rest for 20 minutes, and venous blood is collected from the antecubital fossa without using a tourniquet, or with minimal stasis. A sphygmomanometer cuff is applied to the opposite arm, and inflated to midway between systolic and diastolic pressure. The cuff is kept inflated at this pressure for 15 minutes, and blood is drawn from the antecubital fossa of the occluded arm before deflating the cuff. Euglobin lysis times, or fibrin plate assays are performed on the pre- and post-venous occlusion samples, and the difference in lysis time or zone size gives a measure of the response.

Each laboratory must establish its own normal range. Patients should be carefully selected for this test, since it at best causes some discomfort, and in some cases could increase the risk of thrombosis. An alternative approach is to compare samples taken before and after infusion of DDAVP, but again there are some limitations to the use of this test.

LABORATORY CONTROL OF THROMBOLYTIC THERAPY

The main current indication for thrombolytic therapy seems to be in the treatment of massive pulmonary embolus, extensive deep vein thrombosis, or to restore blood flow through occluded coronary arteries, either by local perfusion or systemic treatment. The main agents used are urokinase, which activates plasminogen directly by cleavage to yield plasmin; or streptokinase, which forms a 1:1 stoichiometric complex with plasminogen, resulting in exposure of the active site of plasmin and cleavage of a second non-complexed plasminogen molecule, resulting in free plasmin generation (Chesterman 1981).

There is no standard, well-recognised procedure for monitoring thrombolytic therapy. Thrombolysis is dependent on an adequate plasminogen concentration, and the major side effect is haemorrhage due to fibrinogen depletion. If some measure of fibrinogen concentration is used, information is obtained about the effectiveness of treatment in promoting fibrinolysis as well as the likelihood of haemorrhage due to a low fibrinogen level. The thrombin time reflects both reduction in fibrinogen level and the presence of increased FDP levels. Streptokinase should be given initially as a sufficiently large priming dose to neutralise naturally occurring antibodies that have resulted from previous streptococcal infections. An intravenous loading dose of 250 000–600 000 units over 30 minutes should suffice. Treatment should then be continued by an infusion rate of 100 000–150 000 units per hour. After 2–4 hours of treatment the thrombin time, fibrinogen concentration and plasminogen level should be assessed. The thrombin time should be prolonged by 3–5 times the control value. A lesser degree of prolongation with a fibrinogen concentration above 1 g/l suggests that streptococcal streptokinase antibodies have not been adequately neutralised and the dose should be increased. A thrombin time greater than 5 times the control value suggests excess free plasmin generation. In this situation the streptokinase dose should be increased to 150 000–200 000 units per hour so that more plasminogen becomes complexed to streptokinase and then less free plasminogen is available to be converted to plasmin, thereby reducing the overall fibrinolytic state. The alternative approach is to stop the infusion for 1–2 hours and restart at a lower dose when the thrombin time has returned to the therapeutic range and the fibrinogen concentration recovered to greater than 0.5 g/l. Once therapy has been stabilised monitoring should continue at 12-hourly intervals or be repeated if excessive clinical bleeding episodes develop. Streptokinase therapy should continue for 24–72 hours and, 2–4 hours after the infusion has been terminated, intravenous heparin therapy started and continued for 5–7 days to prevent re-thrombosis.

Urokinase therapy is much easier to monitor. A primary dose of 4000 units/kg is given over 30 minutes and the fibrinolytic effect maintained by an infusion rate of 4000 units per kg per hour. The thrombin time should be maintained at 3–5 times the control value and if the thrombin time exceeds this level the infusion dose of urokinase should be appropriately reduced.

Both agents are also useful to unblock obstructed arteriovenous shunts or in-dwelling Hickman catheters. A local infusion of 25 000 units of streptokinase is usually effective and no laboratory monitoring is required.

The clinical use of tissue-type plasminogen activator produced by tissue culture fluids or recombinant DNA technology has recently been reported and will become widely available in the near future. The theoretical advantage of such activators is that thrombolysis will only occur at the site of thrombus formation, and systemic activation of the fibrinolytic system will not occur. Therefore no changes in fibrinogen, plasminogen or alpha-2-antiplasmin will occur, and laboratory monitoring of dosage to prevent excessive bleeding episodes will not be required. At the present time there is limited experience to confirm these claims, and monitoring of fibrinogen levels may be necessary.

REFERENCES

Chesterman C N 1981 Thrombolytic therapy. In: Bloom A L, Thomas D P (eds) Haemostasis and Thrombosis. Churchill Livingstone, p 693–711

Collen D 1985 Fibrinolysis: mechanism and clinical aspects. In: Walter Bowie E J, Sharp A A (eds) Butterworths, Hemostasis and Thrombosis, p 237–258

Edy J, de Cock F, Collen D 1976 Inhibition of plasmin by normal and antiplasmin depleted plasma. Thrombosis Research 8:513

Friberger P, Knos M 1979 Plasminogen determination in human plasma. In: Scully M F, Kakkar M V (eds) Chromogenic Peptide Substrates. Churchill Livingstone, Edinburgh

Hessel L W, Kluft C 1986 Advances in clinical fibrinolysis.

In: Chesterman CN (ed) Thrombosis and the vessel wall, Clinics in Haematology 15: 443–463

Holvoet P, Cleemput H, Collen D 1985 Assay of human tissue-type plasminogen activator (t-PA) with an enzyme-linked immunosorbent assay (ELISA) based on three murine monoclonal antibodies. Thrombosis and Haemostasis 54: 684–687

Mahmoud M, Gaffney P J 1985 Bioimmunoassay (BIA) of tissue plasminogen activator (t-PA) and its specific inhibitor (t-PA/INH). Thrombosis and Haemostasis 53: 356–359

Ogston D 1976 Assays of the factor XII dependent pathway.

In: Davidson J F, Samama M M, Desnoyers P C (eds) Progress in chemical fibrinolysis and thrombolysis vol II. Raven Press, New York, p 37

Teger-Nilsson A C, Friberger P, Gyzander E 1977 Determination of a new rapid plasmin inhibitor in human blood by means of a plasmin specific tripeptide substrate. Scandinavian Journal of Clinical and Laboratory Investigation 37:403

Walker I D, Davidson J F 1985 Fibrinolysis. In: Thomson J M (ed) Blood coagulation and haemostasis a practical guide. Churchill Livingstone, p 208–263

30

Platelet function tests

The normal physiology of platelet activation and involvement in the haemostatic process has been outlined in the introduction (Chapter 18). It is essential to have a working knowledge of these events so that the relevant platelet-function tests can be performed in an orderly sequence and interpreted correctly (Yardumian et al 1986).

The platelet count, inspection of the blood film and the skin bleeding time are the first-line basic laboratory tests of platelet function used to investigate a bleeding diathesis. If these are normal it is unlikely that a significant platelet defect is responsible for excessive clinical bleeding. The Hess test, a rather outdated test of capillary fragility and platelet reactivity, should not be included as a screening test due to its lack of specificity. If the bleeding time suggests a platelet functional disorder or when there is a high degree of clinical suspicion despite a normal bleeding time, further tests should be planned in a systematic way. Drugs and certain dietary practices are the commonest cause of platelet dysfunction, and ideally patients should refrain from taking drugs with known anti-platelet effects for 7–10 days before blood sampling for more specific function investigation. Clinically the most important of these drugs and dietary food stuffs are listed in Table 30.1. If there is any doubt about a particular drug, the bleeding time and further investigations should be repeated, if possible, two weeks after stopping that drug.

Minimal criteria for diagnosis of the congenital disorders of platelet function are shown in Table 30.2 (Preston et al 1987).

A screening procedure to investigate platelet involvement in a pre-thrombotic or hypercoagulable state is not as straight forward to prepare and follow. However, the platelet aggregate ratio, turbidometric aggregation studies to threshold doses of ADP and arachidonate, spontaneous aggregation, β-thromboglobulin level, platelet factor 4 level, and TXB_2 generation from maximally stimulated platelets are all useful indicators of hyper-reactive circulating platelets.

Table 30.1 Drugs which affect platelet function.

1. Membrane-stabilising agents
   α-antagonists
   β-blockers
   Local anaesthetics, (procaine)
   Antihistamines
   Tricyclic antidepressants
   Frusemide

2. Agents which affect prostanoid synthesis
   Aspirin and proprietary preparations containing ASA
   Non-steroid anti-inflammatory
   Corticosteroids

3. Antibiotics
   Penicillins
   Cephalosporins
   β-lactam derivatives

4. Agents which increase cyclic AMP levels
   Dipyridamole
   Aminophylline
   Prostanoids

5. Others
   Heparin
   Dextrans
   Ethanol
   Phenothiazine
   Clofibrate
   Papaverine

6. Food stuffs
   Alcohol
   Garlic
   Certain Chinese foods

BLEEDING TIME

Principle

A sphygmomanometer cuff is applied to an arm to stress the capillaries; a small incision is made in an area of skin with no major blood vessels. Haemostasis thus depends on extravascular tissues, normal platelet adhesion and function, as well as the presence of certain plasma proteins. A defect in any of these factors will cause a prolongation of the bleeding time (Mielke et al 1969, Ivy et al 1935).

Table 30.2 Congenital platelet disorders: minimal diagnostic criteria.

A. *Glanzmann's disease*
   (i) Absent aggregation responses to ADP *with*:
   (ii) Agglutination response to ristocetin

B. *Bernard-Soulier syndrome*
   (i) Large platelets on peripheral blood film *and*:
   (ii) Absent ristocetin-induced platelet agglutination not corrected by normal plasma (or cryoprecipitate)

C. *Platelet release defects*
   Impaired secondary aggregatory response to ADP. This group can be further categorised by the demonstration of additional features, viz:
   (i) Storage pool disorders
       a. Reduced platelet ADP concentration with increased platelet ATP/ADP ratio
   (ii) Defect of arachidonic acid peroxidation, e.g. cyclo-oxygenase deficiency, thromboxane synthetase deficiency
       a. Impaired arachidonate-induced platelet aggregation with normal primary aggregatory response to ADP
       b. Reduced arachidonate-induced platelet thromboxane production
   (iii) Presumed abnormalities of Ca^{++} mobilisation
       a. Impaired aggregation responses to calcium ionophore (A23187)

D. *Gray platelet syndrome*
   (i) Morphological abnormalities on peripheral blood film (typically, absence of azurophilic granules) *and*:
   (ii) Evidence of reduced intraplatelet levels alpha-granule platelet specific peptides (PF_4 & BTG)

E. *Congenital thrombocytopaenia*
   (i) Giant platelet syndromes (excluding B. Soulier)
       a. Large platelets on blood film *and*:
       b. Exclusion of Bernard-Soulier syndrome
   (ii) Hereditary thrombocytopenia with normal platelet morphology

F. *Platelet-type ('pseudo') von Willebrand's disease*
   (i) Features suggesting Type IIB von Willebrand's disease *and*:
   (ii) Enhanced platelet agglutination with ristocetin or agglutination by cryoprecipitate in the absence of ristocetin

G. It is not currently considered possible to define minimal diagnostic criteria for some other uncommon disorders such as isolated platelet factor 3 deficiency and 'Bolin's disease' in view of the paucity of detailed descriptions to date.

Equipment
○ Sphygmomanometer.
○ Disposable bleeding time templates — Simplate II (Organon Teknika).
○ Stopwatch.
○ Filter papers.
○ Sterile butterfly bandages.

Method
1. A sphygmomanometer cuff is placed on the upper arm and inflated to 40 mmHg.

2. The skin of the forearm distal to the antecubital fossa is cleaned and the disposable template placed over an area where there are no superficial veins.

3. Two horizontal cuts (1 mm × 6 mm), parallel to the antecubital crease, are made.

4. A stopwatch is started and the blood removed at 15 second intervals with a filter paper.

5. The time taken for blood to stop flowing is recorded and the mean time determined.

6. Remove the cuff and place a butterfly bandage over the wound to draw the edges together and reduce scarring.

Comments
— Care must be taken to avoid small veins as these will falsely prolong the test.
— Touching the edges of the wound may disturb haemostatic plug formation and prolong the bleeding time.
— If the bleeding time has not finished at 20 minutes it should be considered whether there is any clinical need to continue with the test (since by that time it is definitely abnormal).
— Individual laboratories and even each qualified operator should determine their own normal range, due to the great reported variability in results (Poller et al 1984).

Interpretation
Normal range — 2–10 minutes.
   Conditions associated with a prolonged bleeding time:
   a. Thrombocytopenia.
   b. Inherited platelet function defects (e.g. Glanzman's thrombasthenia, storage pool defect, Bernard Soulier syndrome).
   c. Inherited plasma defects (e.g. von Willebrand's Disease, afibrinogenaemia, factor V deficiency).
   d. Acquired platelet function defects (e.g. uraemia, paraproteinaemia).
   e. Platelet antibodies.
   f. Platelet inhibitory drugs (see Table 30.1).
   g. Vascular abnormalities (e.g. Ehlers-Danlos syndrome).
   h. Severe anaemia; haematocrit below 20%.

PROTHROMBIN CONSUMPTION INDEX

Principle
When whole blood clots, about 95% of prothrombin is consumed by activation to thrombin and then inhibition by antithrombins. If citrated plasma is clotted, in the absence of platelets, much less prothrombin is consumed. The amount of residual prothrombin in the two sera can be compared by adding brain thrombo-

plastin and calcium ions to serum and citrated plasma, and then adding fibrinogen and measuring the clotting time. By comparing the two times, an estimate of the contribution of platelets to coagulation can be made.

Biochemical basis
Platelets possess coagulant activities of their own, having the ability to activate factor XI and to release a variety of clotting factors e.g. factor V and fibrinogen. After activation they express coagulant active phospholipid (platelet factor III) and have specific receptors for certain coagulation proteins such as factor Xa and factor V. Thus they play an important role in thrombin formation.

Test samples
Citrated plasma. Clotted blood — blood taken into a plain glass tube and left at 37°C for 1 hour before centrifugation for serum.

Reagents
- Brain thromboplastin — Manchester reagent or Diagen phenolysed suspension.
- Calcium chloride 0.025 M.
- Fibrinogen — Diagen bovine fibrinogen.

Equipment
Applicator sticks.

Method
1. Add 0.1 ml serum to duplicate glass tubes at 37°C.
2. Add 0.1 ml brain thromboplastin, and start clock.
3. After 1 minute add 0.1 ml calcium chloride and mix.
4. At 2 minutes add 0.2 ml fibrinogen and time clot formation.
5. Repeat steps 1–4 using citrated plasma. It is necessary to remove any fibrin formed after the addition of calcium ions by winding it onto a pair of applicator sticks.

Calculation
Divide plasma time by serum time and multiply by one hundred.

Prothrombin Consumption Index (PCI)
$$= 100 \times \frac{\text{plasma time}}{\text{serum time}}$$

Interpretation
Normal value — $< 30\%$.
The PCI may be prolonged due to:
a. Thrombocytopenia.
b. Platelet aggregation defects.

c. Platelet coagulant defects. A bleeding diathesis has been described where an abnormal PCI is the only laboratory abnormality (Parry et al 1980).
d. Plasma defects.
e. Drug-induced defects.

PLATELET FACTOR 3 — SCREENING TEST

Principle
Varying mixtures of normal and patient platelet-rich and platelet-poor plasmas are made. The system is activated by adding kaolin and calcium ions, and the platelets accelerate the clotting time by exposing coagulant active phospholipids and receptors for components of the tenase and prothrombinase complexes to the plasma. Individuals lacking in these phospholipids and receptors, or having a platelet defect such that they cannot be made available to the haemostatic process yield prolonged clotting times when their platelets are used (Hardisty & Hutton 1966).

Biochemical basis
The vitamin K-dependent coagulation factors, II, VII, IX, and X bind to negatively charged phospholipids such as phosphatidyl serine in the presence of calcium ions. This interaction is dependent on their gamma carboxy glutamic acid residues, and normally occurs at the surface of ruptured or activated cell surfaces such as platelets. There are also specific platelet membrane receptors for certain coagulation factors, and activated platelets significantly accelerate thrombin generation when added to purified systems or plasma in place of phospholipid micelles.

Test samples
Blood is collected into tri-sodium citrate in the normal way from both patient and a healthy, normal subject of the same blood group. Blood is centrifuged at 170 g for 10 minutes and the platelet-rich plasma (PRP) separated. The blood is then further centrifuged at 2700 g for 15 minutes for platelet-poor plasma (PPP), which is also separated into a plastic tube.

Reagents
- Kaolin (BDH light kaolin) — 0.5% in Tris buffer 0.2 M pH 7.4.
- Calcium chloride 0.035 M.

Preparation of test samples
The following mixtures are prepared in duplicate in glass clotting tubes:

	PPP	PRP
a	100 μl Patient	100 μl Normal
b	100 μl Normal	100 μl Patient
c	100 μl Patient	100 μl Patient
d	100 μl Normal	100 μl Normal
e	200 μl Patient	Nil
f	200 μl Normal	Nil

Method

1. Warm the mixtures of normal and patient plasmas at 37°C.
2. Add 0.2 ml kaolin and mix well.
3. Incubate for 20 minutes at 37°C.
4. Add 0.2 ml calcium chloride and record clotting time.

Comments

— Stagger the kaolin activation of each pair of tubes by 1-minute intervals.
— Remix the kaolin at regular intervals through the incubation period.
— The clotting times of tubes e and f must be greater than 60 seconds to indicate adequate removal of platelets in PPP.

Interpretation

Mixtures a and b compare the activity of normal and patient platelets while the plasma coagulation factors are kept constant. Mixtures c and d test the efficiency of the platelets in their own plasma. Tubes e and f provide controls. If there is a clotting factor deficiency, tube c may give a long time even if the platelets are normal.

PLATELET FACTOR 3 — QUANTITATIVE ASSAY

Principle

Russell's viper venom (RVV) directly activates factors V and X leading to thrombin generation in the presence of calcium ions and phospholipids. If the platelet factor 3 activity of normal and patient platelets is exposed by repeatedly freezing and thawing them, or by activation with ADP, its potency can be tested in an RVV test system in the absence of any other phospholipid source (Sixma & Nijessen 1970).

Test samples

Citrated blood is collected in the normal way, and platelet-rich plasma (PRP) and platelet-poor plasma (PPP) are prepared from both patient and healthy normal donor blood.

Reagents

● Russell viper venom (Diagnostic Reagents Ltd.) — 0.1 mg/ml in Michaelis buffer; store frozen below −20°C.
● Michaelis buffer
   1.943 g sodium acetate trihydrate
   2.943 g sodium barbitone
   3.4 g sodium chloride.
   1 M HCl and distilled water to pH 7.4 and 540 ml volume.
● Calcium chloride 0.05 M.
● ADP (Sigma Chem. Co.) — 100 μM solution in isotonic saline, store below −20°C.

Preparation of working reagent

Dilute RVV to 5 μg/ml in Michaelis buffer immediately before use.

Separate the PRP into two aliquots, and lyse one by freezing and thawing 5 times. Construct calibration curve by mixing frozen/thawed PRP with increasing volumes of PPP from the same donor, i.e. undiluted, 1/2, 1/4, 1/8, 1/16, 1/32.

1. 0.1 ml of each PRP/PPP mixture is added to 0.1 ml normal PPP in a glass tube at 37°C.
2. 0.1 ml RVV is added and the mixture incubated for 30 seconds.
3. 0.1 ml calcium chloride is added, and the clotting time recorded.

Method

1. 270 μl of PRP is stirred in an aggregometer cuvette at 37°C.
2. 30 μl of 100 μM ADP is added, and the cuvette incubated for 30 minutes.
3. 100 μl of the aggregated PRP is diluted with 300 μl PPP from the same donor.
4. 100 μl of this mixture is incubated with 100 μl normal PPP and 100 μl RVV in a glass tube at 37°C.
5. After 30 seconds, 100 μl of calcium chloride is added and the clotting time recorded.

Calculation

A double logarithmic graph of clotting time against dilution is plotted for the calibration curve. 100% platelet factor 3 is the clotting time of the undiluted PRP following the freeze-thaw cycle. The clotting time of the ADP-activated PRP is used to obtain the percentage platelet factor 3 from this graph.

Comments

— If the platelet counts of normal PRP and test sample PRP are brought to the same, the calibration curve may be constructed using normal PRP, and the test result expressed as a percentage of normal rather than a percentage of maximum possible release.

Interpretation

Normal platelets release about 40% of their total platelet factor 3 after ADP activation. A rare platelet disorder associated with a bleeding tendency has been described in which the only laboratory abnormality was decreased platelet factor 3 availability.

CLOT RETRACTION

Principle

Clotted blood incubated at 37°C retracts, expressing serum, and by measuring the ratio of clot volume to total blood volume in a test tube after a fixed incubation time, the degree of clot retraction can be measured.

Test samples

Approximately 1 ml blood is collected into a 75 × 10 mm glass tube at 37°C.

Method

1. The tube of blood is left to clot, and incubated for a further 1 hour at 37°C.
2. The distance from the end of the tube to the meniscus is measured, and the clot is removed carefully with an applicator stick.
3. The distance from the end of the tube to the serum meniscus is measured.

Calculation

The serum distance is divided by the total distance, and multiplied by 100. The result is expressed as the percentage serum expressed.

Comments

— The result may be influenced by anti-platelet drugs and by thrombopenia.
— Careful removal of the clot is essential to avoid fragmentation or squeezing and expression of extra serum.

Interpretation

Normal value — > 40% serum expressed.

Decreased clot retraction may be seen in a number of platelet defects including Glanzman's thrombasthenia.

PLATELET ADHESION

The most widely used test for platelet adhesion measures platelet retention after a single passage through a glass bead column. This test requires strict standardisation, using glass beads of a constant size, packed into a plastic tube of fixed diameter and length (commercially available), with a steady infusion rate, either using a syringe pump and EDTA anticoagulated blood, or non-anticoagulated blood directly from an arm vein, using an evacuated system. The percentage platelet retention is calculated from a pre-column and post-column infusion platelet count. Despite these efforts at standardisation, results are still extremely variable, and decreased glass bead retention of platelets is not only found in platelet adhesion defects. It has been shown that platelet retention also depends on von Willebrand factor activity, fibrinogen binding to the glass bead surface, and on platelet aggregation promoted by locally released ADP from haemolysed red cells in the column. These tests rarely yield any useful information that cannot be obtained from other methods.

Better methods of measuring platelet adhesion are based on the technique developed by Baumgartner and colleagues (Turitto & Baumgartner 1983). These rely on whole blood passing over an everted segment of rabbit aorta with a denuded endothelial surface, in a continuous flow circuit at 37°C. The extent of platelet adhesion is then assessed by light microscopy of the aortic surface, and quantitation of adhesion can be measured if indium-radiolabelled platelets are used in the flow circuit. The shear rate over the vessel surface can be changed by using different diameter chambers, to mimic the in vivo conditions in different sized blood vessels. However, this technique is expensive, time-consuming, and technically difficult, and therefore unsuited to routine diagnostic use.

PLATELET AGGREGATION — TURBIDOMETRIC METHOD

Principle

Blood is centrifuged gently to obtain platelet-rich plasma, which is stirred in a cuvette at 37°C between a light source and a photocell. When an agonist is added (Table 30.3), the platelets aggregate and absorb less light, so that transmission increases and is detected by movement of a pen on the chart recorder. The addition of different agonists, at a range of concentrations, allows the detection of certain aggregation defects.

Biochemical basis

Reagents such as collagen, thrombin, and ADP bind to specific platelet membrane receptors, activating platelets, and triggering a series of reactions which can culminate in shape change, granule release, and aggregation. Whether any or all of these responses occur depends on the normal function of the platelet, the levels of certain inhibitory substances, and the concentration of the agonist used.

There are thought to be three basic pathways of

Table 30.3 Agonists for platelet aggregation studies.

A. Agents routinely used in screening tests	Final concentrations usually employed
ADP	0.5–10.0 μM
Collagen	1.0–4.0 μg/ml**
*Ristocetin	0.5–1.2 mg/ml

B. Other agents in routine use	
Adrenaline	1.0–10.0 μM
Thrombin	0.1–0.5 u/ml
Arachidonic acid	1.0–2.0 mM
Endoperoxide analogues U44069 & U46619	2.5 μg/ml
Calcium ionophores A23187	1.25–10.0 μM
*Porcine factor VIII	2 u/ml

C. Agents used chiefly for research purposes
PAF
Serotonin
Antigen-antibody
complexes Platelet antibodies
Viruses, bacterial products
Particles, e.g. latex &
absorbed C_3 & fibrinogen.
*Concanavalin A
*Phytohaemagglutinins

* Agents causing platelet agglutination, rather than true aggregation.
** This varies according to species and tissue source of collagen. The manufacturer's instructions should be followed.

platelet aggregation: ADP causes a chain of events involving phosphatidyl inositol metabolism leading to the exposure of fibrinogen binding sites on the membrane and aggregation. Low dose collagen causes arachidonic acid mobilisation from the membrane, and this is converted to thromboxane A_2 which is a potent stimulator of aggregation, causing ADP release and calcium flux; higher doses of collagen will also cause release of ADP directly. Low concentrations of thrombin cause aggregation through ADP and arachidonate release, but high doses of thrombin, can induce aggregation through a mechanism independent of thromboxane A_2 and ADP, which may be due to PAF. Serotonin and adrenaline act synergistically with other reagents. The relation of in vitro platelet aggregation in plasma to physiological responses must be considered carefully, since the low extracellular calcium ion concentrations generate artefacts such as the release reactions to ADP and adrenaline, which do not occur if blood is collected into the thrombin inhibitor hirudin, instead of citrate.

Test samples

Citrated blood is centrifuged at 170 g (800–1000 rpm in a 'bench centrifuge) for 10 minutes to prepare platelet-rich plasma (PRP). This must be removed and stored at room temperature in a capped tube. All hand-ling should be kept to a minimum and be performed with plastic pipettes and tubes.

The residual blood must then be centrifuged at 2700 g (approx. 3500 rpm) for 15 minutes and the resulting platelet-poor plasma (PPP) collected.

Equipment

○ Optical aggregometer — e.g. Payton, Biodata or Chronolog. The method described is for a Payton 300BD aggregometer, which does not have an auto-baseline facility, fitted with cuvettes for 250–500 μl.
○ Chart recorder (Rikadenki-Mitsui).
○ Glass cuvettes.
○ Stir bars.
○ Equipment for platelet counting.

Reagents

● ADP (Grade III, Sigma Chemical Co. Ltd.) — 10 mM solution in saline, stored in aliquots at −20°C.
● Collagen (Hormon-Chemie) — 1 mg/ml stored at 4°C.
● Adrenaline (Sigma) — 1 mg/ml (5.5 mM) store at −20°C.
● Sodium arachidonate (Sigma) — 20 mM solution in distilled water, store at −20°C.
● Thrombin (Parke-Davis, bovine) — 50 u/ml solution in saline, at −20°C.
● Endoperoxide analogue U46619 (Upjohn Ltd.). Dissolve vial in a small quantity of ethanol, and dilute to 25 μg/ml (0.071 mM) with saline, store at −20°C in aliquots.
● Calcium ionophore A23187, Ca^{++} + Mg^{++} salt (Sigma) — 500 μg/ml (1 mM) in Dimethyl Sulphoxide at −20°C.
● Ristocetin (Lundbeck) — 12.5 mg/ml in saline, store at −20°C
● Porcine FVIII complex or bovine fibrinogen (Diagnostic Reagents Ltd.), reconstitute according to manufacturer.

Preparation of samples and reagents

– PRP is diluted with autologous PPP to give a final platelet count of 200 × 10⁹/l.
– ADP — prepare 100, 50, 25, 10, and 5 μM solutions in saline on ice.
– Collagen — prepare 40 and 10 μg/ml solutions in SKF buffer (Hormon-Chemie) on ice.
– Ristocetin — thaw stock and keep on ice. Dilute as necessary in saline.
– Adrenaline — prepare 100, 50, and 10 μM solutions in saline on ice.
– Arachidonate — dilute stock solution with an equal volume of distilled water on ice (10 mM).
– Thrombin — dilute in saline to 1 and 5 u/ml, on ice.

– Calcium ionophore A23,187 — dilute in saline to give 5 and 10 μg/ml solutions, store on ice.
– Porcine factor VIII — dilute to 20 u/ml at room temperature.

Method

1. Allow aggregometer to warm to 37°C and set stirrer speed to 900 rpm.

2. Set chart recorder to 10 mv and 3 cm/minute.

3. 300 μl PPP is placed in one cuvette and 270 μl PRP with a stir bar in another; these are used to calibrate the aggregometer signal on the chart recorder to 10% and 95% settings, using the output and zero controls respectively (see manufacturer's instructions).

4. 270 μl of undiluted PRP is placed in a cuvette in the aggregometer, and stirred for 15 minutes to check for spontaneous aggregation (pen deflection >20% of chart).

5. If spontaneity is present, dilute the PRP in PPP and repeat the test, until a dilution is found where spontaneous aggregation disappears. If this point is found at or above a platelet count of 200×10^9/l, aggregation tests may proceed.

6. Place 270 μl dilute PRP in a cuvette and warm until a steady baseline is obtained.

7. Add 30 μl of aggregating reagent (Table 30.3) and record response.

8. Continue with other doses of agonists or other reagents as indicated.

Calculation

The length of the lag phase, aggregation rate, and amplitude of the aggregation wave may be measured (Fig. 30.1). Alternatively, threshold concentrations may be determined by starting with a very low dose of an aggregating agent and progressively adding higher concentrations of the agonist until a response is obtained. Similarly an EC_{50} (50% of effective concentration) value can be obtained by finding the dose of aggregating reagent which causes 50% of the maximum response; this is usually found by drawing a dose/response curve for a number of concentrations of agonist.

Comments

— The volumes of PRP used will depend on the aggregometer and cuvettes used. The smaller the cuvette, the more responses that can be obtained with a given volume of PRP, but the poorer the optical quality (due to a shorter light path) and the more likely the influence of factors such as debris or air bubbles.
— Care should be taken to exclude red cells and granulocytes from PRP, as these will interfere with the light transmittance and cause reduced response

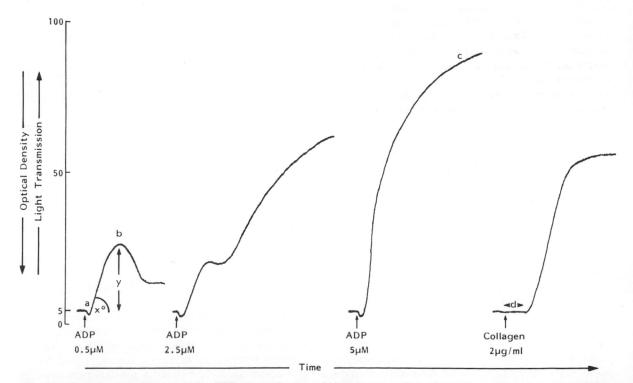

Fig. 30.1 Typical traces obtained during PRP aggregation by turbidometry. a. = shape change; b = primary wave aggregation; c = secondary wave aggregation; x° = angle of ascent of aggregation trace; y = height of aggregation trace; d = lag phase.

heights which can be mistaken for abnormal aggregation. In diseases such as thalassaemia, where there may be red cell fragments and membranes, these may be removed by further centrifugation of PRP at 1500 g for 2 minutes, or after settling has occurred.

— If cryoglobulins are present, they may cause transmission changes similar to spontaneous aggregation. Warming the PRP and PPP to 37°C for 5 minutes allows aggregation to be performed in the normal way.

— Lipaemic plasma may cause problems in adjusting the aggregometer, and the responses may be compressed owing to the small difference in transmitted light between PRP and PPP. Care should be taken in the interpretation of results from such samples.

— The aggregometer calibration must be adjusted if the platelet count of PRP is altered, as this will affect optical density (e.g. when changing from spontaneous aggregation to responses with agonists).

— Aggregation should be performed within 2 hours; if longer delays cannot be avoided, it is best to store the PRP under 5% CO_2, or if this is not available, to leave the smallest possible air gap over the PRP, and cap the tube.

— Lumi-aggregometers are also available; these measure ATP release simultaneously with aggregation. This is possible using a firefly extract containing luciferin and luciferase, which emits energy in the form of luminescence when ATP is available; luminescence can be detected at a specific wavelength in the aggregometer.

— Ristocetin concentrations above 1.4 mg/ml may cause non-specific protein precipitation which can be mistaken for agglutination.

— Thrombin aggregation must be carried out using washed platelets (see later section on platelet washing), to avoid clot formation.

— Cuvettes may be washed by soaking overnight in 2% Decon, rinsing in tap water, soaking in dilute bleach for 30 minutes, rinsing extensively with tap water, and finally rinsing in distilled water and drying in an oven.

— Stir bars may be washed by soaking in 2% Decon for 10 minutes, dilute bleach for 10 minutes, extensive, but rapid washes in tap water followed by rinsing in distilled water and drying in a hot oven on filter paper.

Interpretation

Subjective assessment of aggregation responses by a trained eye is usually sufficient for clinical interpretations, but normal ranges of the lag phase, rate and amplitude of response may be established locally. ADP normally gives a secondary wave at 2.5 μM or above, with no disaggregation, but only a primary wave should be obtained below 1 μM. Both 1 and 4 μg/ml collagen should give a lag phase of 1 minute or less followed by a steep response, spanning the chart paper width. Arachidonate should give a response similar to the secondary wave of ADP. Ristocetin gives a strong response with a steep slope at 1.25 mg/ml, a more protracted response at 1.00 mg/ml, and may give no response at 0.75 mg/ml. Decreased responses at these doses suggest von Willebrand's disease or Bernard Soulier syndrome. This may be differentiated with porcine factor VIII or bovine fibrinogen, or by the addition of normal plasma or cryoprecipitate before the ristocetin. Positive ristocetin responses at 0.5 mg/ml or less may suggest Type IIB von Willebrand's disease. Normal healthy Afro-Caribbean subjects have been shown to have absent ristocetin agglutination, despite having normal levels and function of von Willebrand factor, apparently normal platelets, and no bleeding diathesis. The latter appears to be due to physiological variation and increased levels of a substance which interferes with ristocetin-induced agglutination in PRP. Similar false negatives have been reported after viral illness, in myeloproliferative disorders, and myeloma. Patterns of abnormal aggregation in congenital defects are shown in Table 30.4. The interpretation of aggregation defects is further discussed in the introduction to this section.

PLATELET AGGREGATION IN WHOLE BLOOD — IMPEDANCE METHOD

Principle

Turbidometric methods of platelet aggregation are limited by the need for centrifugation, which is time-consuming, so that labile substances such as cyclic AMP and prostacyclin decay, while red cells, white cells, cell fragments, and some of the larger platelets are removed from the final platelet suspension to be tested. These other blood elements may be important modulators of platelet function in vivo, since they take up adenine nucleotides, synthesise and release regulatory prostaglandins, and bind prostacyclin. Biochemical changes in platelets may also be induced, resulting in prostaglandin synthesis and alteration of cAMP levels, as well as release of ADP from red cells.

The measurement of platelet aggregation by electrical impedance (Cardinal & Flower 1980; Mackie et al 1984) overcomes some of these problems, blood may be analysed immediately after sampling and aggregation is investigated in the presence of all blood elements. A cuvette of blood is placed in the heating block of the impedance aggregometer, where it is stirred at 37°C,

Table 30.4 Platelet aggregation defects.

	ADP	COLL	RIS(H)	RIS(L)	SA	U19	CaI	PVIII	[NUC]
VWD	N	N	O/A	O	N	N	N	N	N
VWD*	N	N	N/H	H	N	N	N	N	N
BSS	N	N	O	O	N	N	N	O	N
GLANZS	O	O	P	O	O	O	?	P	N
SPD	P	A	N/P	O	A	A	A	N/P	A
COX	A/N	A	N	O	A	N	N	N	N
TXSYN	A/N	A	N	O	A	N	N	N	N
TXREC	A/N	A	N	O	A	N	N	N	N
CAL	A	A	N	O	A	A	A	N	N
MEMB	N/A	A	N/A	O	N	N	N	N/A	N
EHLDAN	N	A	N	O	N	N	N	N	N

Key: VWD = von Willebrand's disease; (* = subtype IIB); BSS = Bernard-Soulier syndrome; GLANZS = Glanzman's thrombasthenia; SPD = storage pool defect; COX = cyclo-oxygenase defect; TXSYN = thromboxane A_2 synthetase defect; TXREC = thromboxane A^2 receptor defect; CAL = calcium binding/contractile protein abnormality; MEMB = other membrane receptor defect; EHLDAN = Ehler's Danlos defect.

COLL = collagen; RIS = ristocetin (H = 1–1.25 mg/ml, L = <0.75 mg/ml); SA = sodium arachidonate; U19 = endoperoxide analogue U46619; CaI = calcium ionophore A23187; PVIII = porcine factor VIII; [NUC] = platelet nucleotide concentrations.

N = normal; H = increased; P = primary wave only; A = abnormal/reduced; O = absent.

N.B. Thromboxane A_2 synthetase defect and thromboxane A^2 receptor defects can be differentiated by measuring serum thromboxane B^2 levels.

and an electrode consisting of 2 fine platinum wires set a fixed distance apart is inserted. The electrode immediately becomes covered with a monolayer of platelets and after the addition of a suitable agonist, formed aggregates adhere to the monolayer. The mass of platelets on the electrode influences the electrical impedance between the two wires, and this can be visualised using a chart recorder. A standard resistance of 5 ohms may be applied to the system to enable calibration of the chart recording.

Test samples
Citrated blood.

Preparation of test samples
The haematocrit is determined and the citrated blood diluted to a haematocrit of .300 (PCV 30%) with isotonic saline. The diluted blood is warmed to 37°C in a polystyrene cuvette in the aggregometer heating block. If the haematocrit is unknown at the time of testing, it is suggested that 722 μl of citrated blood is diluted in 253 μl of saline, since this dilution usually reduces the haematocrit to below .300 in most non-anaemic blood samples.

Reagents
- Isotonic saline.
- Collagen (Hormon-Chemie) — for use, dilute in SKF buffer provided by manufacturer to give 200, 100, and 40 μg/ml solutions.
- ADP (Grade III, Sigma Chemical Co. Ltd.). Dissolve in saline to give 10 mM stock solution and store at

−20°C. Before use dilute to 1 mM and make further doubling dilutions in saline.
- Arachidonic acid (Sigma) — dissolve 10 mg in 200 μl absolute ethanol, which has been bubbled with nitrogen. Store under nitrogen at −70°C. Just before use add 20 μl of the stock solution to 80 μl of patient's platelet-poor plasma to obtain working reagent (40 mM).

Equipment
- Model 540 whole blood impedance aggregometer (Chronolog Inc.).
- R302 chart recorder (Rikadenki-Mitsui).
- Cuvettes — polystyrene tubes 9 × 44 mm (Teklab).
- Teflon-coated stir bars (supplied with aggregometer).

Method
1. Switch on aggregometer 30 minutes before required, to warm up.
2. Place 975 μl of diluted citrated blood in a 9 × 44 mm cuvette and allow to warm to 37°C in the machine heating block.
3. Add a Teflon-coated stir bar and place the cuvette in the hole marked 'PRP or Whole Blood' in the aggregometer, carefully position the electrode in the blood; set stirrer speed to 600 rpm.
4. Press the 'Set Aggregation Baseline' button and hold, while the chart recorder zero control is adjusted to give a pen reading of 20% chart width.
5. Adjust the aggregometer 'zero' control to give a pen reading of 20% chart width.
6. Press the 'Calibrate' button and hold, while the

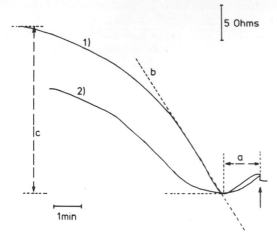

Fig. 30.2 Whole blood impedance aggregation to: 1) 5 μg/ml collagen; 2) 25 μM ADP; A = lag phase; b = rate of aggregation; c = extent of aggregation.

gain control is adjusted to calibrate 10 small divisions of the chart scale to equal 5 ohms; repeat procedure several times to check calibration.

7. Obtain a steady baseline and add 25 μl of aggregating reagent directly into the blood; record impedance change at a chart speed of 2 cm/minute.

Calculation

Three measurements are useful:

The lag period between addition of reagent and beginning of aggregation wave.

The slope, which is measured by drawing a tangent to the initial exponential part of the response, and measuring the angle between this line and the horizontal (Fig. 30.2, a). Alternatively, the rate of aggregation may be assessed by drawing a perpendicular line from the horizontal to the tangent, and dividing the length of the vertical by the length of the base (Fig. 30.2, b).

The extent of response is determined by measuring the vertical height between the minimum point of the trace after addition of reagent and the maximum height, in chart paper units. The extent can then be converted into a resistance (ohms) by referring to the calibration response (Fig. 30.2, c).

Comments

— To check for spontaneous aggregation, blood is stirred at 37°C for 15 minutes without the addition of any reagents; a response is deemed positive if the pen deflects by 10 ohms or more.

— If the baseline decreases before addition of aggregating reagent, it is likely that the blood has not warmed to 37°C, the zero control should be re-

adjusted until the baseline steadies, whereupon the aggregating reagent may be added.

— Changes in haematocrit cause dramatic effects on impedance; high haematocrits cause erratic tracings and poor aggregation with poor precision. Large dilutions with saline also cause a reduction in platelet count, which decreases the aggregation response. Dilution to a haematocrit of less than .350 gives a better wave of aggregation and a less erratic trace.

— Reducing the platelet count causes no significant changes in aggregation down to platelet counts of about $50 \times 10^9/l$.

— The instrument should be recalibrated for each new patient sample or if there is any change in the dilution of blood used. For weak responses the gain may be increased prior to the aggregation response, for greater accuracy.

— High concentrations of ADP are necessary for reasonable levels of aggregation; these are above the physiological range and presumably relate to the uptake of ADP by red and white cell nucleotide salvage pathways, preventing their use by platelets. The type of aggregate formed in whole blood, as well as the way in which that aggregate is detected by the impedance electrode may also contribute, since lower levels of ADP have been used in whole blood counting methods of aggregation.

— Sodium arachidonate frequently causes red cell lysis (certain batches are free of this effect and may be used), and it is therefore preferable to use arachidonic acid.

— After completion of aggregation, scrupulously clean the electrode using isotonic saline and a camel hair brush, to remove all aggregated cells.

— The plastic cuvettes are disposable, but the electrodes and camel hair brush should be soaked for 20 minutes in dilute bleach at the end of a day's use.

— Some whole blood aggregometers have a luminescence facility which enables simultaneous measurement of ATP release from platelets.

— Plastic cuvettes are preferable to glass ones as the latter may cause activation of the sample, and enhanced responses.

Interpretation

Normal ranges should be established for the various agonists under local conditions.

Whole blood impedance aggregation appears to be more suitable than conventional PRP aggregation for samples with low platelet counts, giving good responses at counts as low as $50 \times 10^9/l$. The optical technique is not very effective for diagnostic purposes below $100 \times 10^9/l$. The method may therefore have important applications in the study of patients with mild thrombopenia who are bleeding. It is also useful in assessing prothrombotic patients with hyperaggregability, and for testing compliance during anti-platelet drug treatment, since the action of some drugs such as dipyridamole appears to be influenced by red cells. Patients with certain red and white cell defects may be difficult to investigate in PRP owing to contamination of PRP by the atypical cells, and optical interference. It may be important to be able to measure platelet aggregation in their presence, as they may also be important in modulating platelet function.

An additional method in whole blood has been described (Lumley & Humphrey 1981), which involves incubating whole blood and aggregating reagent in a shaking water-bath at 37°C and removing sequential aliquots for platelet counting. However, this method is tedious, requires a high level of technical presence and training, and is not suited to busy clinical laboratories as a general method.

ADENINE NUCLEOTIDES

Principle
Measurement of platelet ATP/ADP content and release provides a valuable tool for the diagnosis of storage pool and other defects (Summerfield et al 1981). ATP/ADP are released either in response to an aggregating reagent or by in vitro chemical cell lysis. ATP is measured using firefly lantern preparations which produce luminescence in proportion to the ATP concentration. This luminescence can be measured in a luminometer and related to that produced by a standard ATP solution.

Biochemical basis
Platelets contain two separate pools of adenine nucleotides, a metabolic pool and a discrete storage pool which is kept in the dense granules in a complex with calcium ions and pyrophosphate. This latter source is not interchangeable with the metabolic ATP and ADP, and is only liberated after platelet activation, when the granules release their contents to the platelet exterior. Approximately 70% of platelet ADP is contained in the storage pool, whereas most ATP is metabolic.

These nucleotides can be measured by a luminescence method based on the following reactions:

$$\text{ATP} + \text{luciferin} + O_2 \xrightarrow{\text{luciferase}} \text{oxyluciferin} + \text{AMP} + \text{PPi} + CO_2 + \text{luminescence}$$

$$\text{ADP} + \text{PEP} \xrightarrow{\text{PK}} \text{pyruvate} + \text{ATP}$$

An extract of firefly tails contains an enzyme, luciferase and a substance called luciferin. When ATP is provided, a high energy product, oxyluciferin, is formed, and this breaks down, liberating energy as luminescence. ADP can be measured by first converting it to ATP using phosphoenolpyruvate (PEP) and pyruvate kinase (PK).

Test samples
Citrated blood, centrifuged for PRP.

Reagents
- Collagen — 200 μg/ml collagen (Hormon-Chemie).
- 100 mM EDTA 3.71 g Na_2EDTA dissolved in 100 ml distilled water.
- TCA/EDTA solution — equal volumes of: 20% w/v trichloroacetic acid in distilled water and 8 mM Na_2EDTA.
- Absolute alcohol.
- Sample buffer
  12.1 g TRIS
  0.744 g Na_2EDTA
  1 litre distilled water. Adjust pH to 7.75 with acetic acid.
- Assay buffer — prepare as for sample buffer but omit Na_2EDTA.
- BSA buffer — 10 mg bovine serum albumin (Sigma, Fraction V) in 10 ml assay, buffer.
- 0.4 M $MgSO_4$/1.3M KCl 9.86 g $MgSO_4$.7 H_2O 9.69 g KCl 100 ml distilled water.
- 100 mM PEP — 0.234 g phosphoenolpyruvate (Sigma) in 10 ml distilled water — store frozen in aliquots.
- PK — Pyruvate kinase (Sigma Type II ($NH_4)_2$ SO_4 suspension).
- Luciferase — add 10 ml sterile water to a vial of LKB monitoring reagent and freeze in 1 ml aliquots. Thaw when required and keep on ice.

Equipment
Luminescence photometer — e.g. LKB luminometer.

Standard
ATP standard (LKB Ltd.) — Reconstitute with 10 ml sterile water to give a 10 μM stock solution and store frozen in aliquots. Dilute in saline to give working solutions of: 1.0, 0.5, 0.25, 0.125 and 0.063 μM.
ADP standard (Sigma) — Prepare 100 μM stock solution in saline and freeze in aliquots. Prepare 0.5 μM working solution.

Preparation of test samples and reagents

Total platelet ATP/ADP samples
1. Place 0.2 ml undiluted PRP in a 63 × 8 mm plastic tube and add 0.2 ml TCA/EDTA. Mix well, and leave for 10 minutes on ice.

2. Centrifuge for 10 minutes at 2000 g (3500 rpm).

3. Add 10 μl of supernatant to 490 μl sample buffer.

4. Label tube with Name, Date, sample type, and platelet count; store frozen at $-20°C$.

Granule released ATP/ADP

1. Aggregate 270 μl diluted platelets in aggregometer for 4 minutes with 30 μl of 200 μg/ml collagen.

2. Add 30 μl 100 mM EDTA to stop the reaction.

3. Remove stir bar and centrifuge for 5 minutes at 2000 g (3500 rpm).

4. Place 100 μl of supernatant in a polystyrene 63×8 mm tube and add 100 μl absolute alcohol, mix on a vortex mixer.

5. Centrifuge for 10 minutes at 2000 g (3500 rpm).

6. Dilute 10 μl in 490 μl sample buffer.

7. Label tube with Name, Date, sample type and platelet count; freeze at $-20°C$.

Active Buffer:-

Mix 90 μl BSA buffer with 10 μl PK, 84 μl MgSO$_4$/KCl solution and 16 μl PEP in a plastic tube on ice. Add 20 μl to 330 μl of assay buffer in a cuvette.

Inactive Buffer:-

Mix 20.34 ml assay buffer, 504 μl MgSO$_4$/KCl solution, 60 μl PK, and 96 μl PEP in a loosely capped glass universal tube and place in a boiling water bath for 30 minutes. Cool to room temperature and place 350 μl in a cuvette.

Method

1. Turn on luminometer and leave for 20 minutes to warm up.

2. Prepare up to 6 pairs of active and inactive buffer cuvettes as above, add 100 μl luciferase.

3. Place cuvette in holder and measure background luminescence.

4. Add 50 μl of test or ATP standard to each pair of cuvettes, mix and obtain a reading of inactive cuvette.

5. After measuring luminescence of the 6 inactive cuvettes, measure the active cuvettes in the same order.

Calculation

Inactive cuvettes measure ATP levels, active cuvettes measure ATP plus ADP levels. Plot a graph of luminescence response (minus background) against ATP standard concentration. The ATP and ATP plus ADP concentrations of test samples may be abstracted from this graph (after subtracting background from the luminescence values). The concentrations in nMol/10^9 platelets are obtained after the following corrections for dilution and platelet count:-

$$\text{Released ATP} = \text{ATP 1} \times \frac{1000}{P} \times \frac{27\,500}{225}$$

$$\text{Total ATP} = \text{ATP 1} \times \frac{100\,000}{P}$$

Where: ATP 1 = μMol ATP from standard curve
P = platelet count $\times 10^9$/l

Released and total ADP are calculated in the same but the ATP concentration must be subtracted from the ADP plus ATP concentration to give the ADP level.

Comments

— The ADP standard should give a similar response to the equivalent ATP concentration if complete conversion of ADP to ATP occurs.

— If a very low luminescence response is obtained, 5 μl of 10 μM ATP should be added to the cuvette as an internal standard.

— Not more than 6 cuvettes containing luciferase should be prepared at any one time, as the reagent may decay.

Interpretation

Normal ranges for platelet ATP and ADP content and release should be established locally but in our laboratory are as follows:-

	Total	Release	
ATP	41–61	8–20	nMol/10^9 Platelets
ADP	19–38	18–28	nMol/10^9 Platelets

35–55% of total nucleotides are released.

Decreased levels of total ATP/ADP accompanied by decreased release to collagen suggest storage pool defect or in vivo platelet release due to damage or activation (or in vitro mishandling). Decreased release with normal total levels of ATP and ADP suggests a platelet enzyme or membrane defect, or drug-induced defect. Very high levels of nucleotides are sometimes seen if the platelet volume is increased, i.e. if giant platelets are present.

Nucleotides may also be measured by HPLC (Greaves & Preston 1985) in a more sensitive assay, but if not already available, equipment is more expensive than for luminescence assay, and a high degree of technical skill is required.

PLATELET WASHING METHODS

A number of methods such as thrombin aggregation, prostaglandin studies, and platelet coagulant activity require platelets which are not contaminated with plasma proteins or other substances. Since platelets are very sensitive cells, this separation is difficult to achieve without activation and/or loss of function. Various methods have been developed, and the one to be used depends on the application for the washed platelets, and personal experience with each method. Platelets washed in EDTA or gel-filtered platelets are suitable for prostaglandin work, whereas for non-fixed platelets for ristocetin cofactor assay, EDTA/prostacyclin washing is useful; the albumin wash technique for platelet coagulant studies and gel filtration for calcium flux studies. These methods have been discussed by Akkerman et al 1978 and Gerrard 1982.

CENTRIFUGATION WITH INHIBITORS

Principle

This method uses inhibitors to help prevent activation and release. Platelets are diluted in buffer containing prostacyclin analogue and EDTA and sedimented by gentle centrifugation. The supernatant is discarded and the pellet resuspended in buffer with inhibitors; centrifugation is repeated a further two times. Either the EDTA or prostacyclin analogue may be omitted throughout or at final resuspension, depending on the final application of the platelets, but use of both reagents together produces the least activated platelets.

Reagents

- Tyrode's buffer pH 6.5
    - 8.0 g NaCl
    - 0.2 g KCl
    - 0.065 g $NaH_2.PO_4.2H_2O$
    - 0.415 g $MgCl_2.6H_2O$
    - 1.0 g $NaHCO_3$

    Dissolve in 900 ml distilled water and adjust pH to 6.5.
    Make to 1 litre with distilled water.
- Disodium EDTA: 100 mM in Tyrode's buffer.
- Prostacyclin analogue — 100 ng/ml ZK36,374 (Schering Chemicals) in saline.

Method

1. Prepare platelet-rich plasma (PRP) from fresh citrated blood by centrifugation at 170 g for 10 minutes at room temperature.

2. Dilute PRP 1/2 with Tyrode's buffer containing 10 ng/ml ZK36,374 and 10 mM EDTA at room temperature.

3. The diluted platelets are placed in a plastic conical-bottomed centrifuge tube and centrifuged at 850 g for 10 minutes.

4. The supernatant is discarded using a plastic Pasteur pipette and the pellet is slowly and gently resuspended in buffer containing inhibitors (using a plastic pipette to carefully draw solution up and down). When the platelets are completely resuspended, they are again centrifuged. This process is repeated a further two times.

5. The supernatant is discarded, and the platelets resuspended in suitable buffer depending on use.

Comment

— For some methods it may be desirable to make the final resuspension in a solution free of inhibitors; 5.6 mM D-glucose should be added to prevent loss of metabolic activity, apyrase may be added to degrade released ADP; bovine albumin (e.g. 0.2% w/v) can be used to prevent lysis by arachidonic acid, but it can alter the responsiveness to arachidonic acid, A23,187, and endoperoxide analogues. Fibrinogen is required in the resuspending buffer for ADP and adrenaline aggregation, and calcium ions are required for many studies.

— Over-centrifugation or rough resuspension may lead to disruption of platelets.

— Contact with glass or cold solutions should be avoided to prevent gross morphological and functional changes.

GEL FILTRATION

Platelets are applied to the top of a column of agarose gel beads, and are washed downwards by the eluting buffer (calcium-free Tyrode's containing 5.6 mM D-glucose and 0.2% bovine albumin). As the platelets and plasma pass down the column, proteins enter the beads of agarose via pores, and their progress is delayed; platelets are too large to enter the pores and pass on rapidly through the column. Platelets therefore emerge first (in the void volume) at the bottom of the column, and proteins are eluted later. Sepharose 2B (Pharmacia Ltd.) agarose beads are washed with acetone and 0.9% saline, then degassed and packed into a chromatography column or plastic syringe. The size of the column depends on the amount of PRP to be applied and degree of separation of platelets from plasma proteins. The gel volume should be 5–10 times the plasma volume in a long narrow column for good separation. The gel is equilibrated in elution buffer and the PRP applied; the platelets are collected by visual observation of the change in opacity of the column effluent.

TESTS FOR PLATELET HYPERACTIVITY OR ACTIVATION

Numerous tests have been developed to demonstrate hyperactivity of circulating platelets, or to show that platelets have been activated in vivo by some prothrombotic process. These tests require careful interpretation and are unreliable in inexperienced hands.

A method for detecting circulating platelet aggregates

was reported by Wu & Hoak in 1974, and has been modified by others (Bowry et al 1985). Platelet hyperactivity in vitro may be assessed by looking for spontaneous platelet aggregation or a decreased threshold for aggregation to ADP or arachidonate in PRP or whole blood. Assays for various platelet release products have been tried with varying success, since many are already present in plasma from various other sources. The most useful of these assays are perhaps those for β-TG and PF4.

β-TG and PF4 are released from the platelet alpha granules on activation or aggregation, and can therefore provide a means of monitoring platelet activation in vivo due to pathological processes. They have been suggested as indicators of procoagulant states and thromboembolic events. PF4 is readily taken up and stored by the vessel wall, so that low circulating levels are found, whereas β-TG remains in plasma until filtered out by the kidneys. It is therefore useful to measure these two parameters together, as raised B-TG with a low or slightly raised PF4 level suggests in vivo platelet release, while high levels of both suggests in vitro artefactual release. In renal disease, β-TG may be raised due to lack of removal by the kidney, while heparin causes PF4 release from storage sites, giving increased plasma levels.

PLATELET AGGREGATE RATIO

Principle
Small aggregates of platelets may circulate in the blood of patients with thrombotic and hypercoagulable states. A method has been described which allows the quantification of these aggregates (Bowry et al 1985, modified from Wu & Hoak 1974). Blood is collected into buffered EDTA with and without formalin. The formalin fixes any platelet aggregates so that they sediment out with red cells on gentle centrifugation. The platelet count of the formalinised blood will therefore be lower than that of the blood without formalin if circulating aggregates are present, giving a reduced ratio.

Reagents
- 0.017 M EDTA — 0.636 g disodium EDTA in 100 ml distilled water.
- 0.9% w/v saline.
- 40% formalin.
- Sorensen's phosphate buffer
  soln A = 1.03 g KH_2PO_4 in 100 ml distilled water (0.066 M).
  soln B = 0.898 g $Na_2HPO_4.2H_2O$ in 100 ml distilled water (0.066 M).
  Mix 19.2 ml A and 80.8 ml B to obtain pH 7.4.

- PBS — 10 ml Sorensen's buffer plus 90 ml 0.9% w/v saline.
- PBS with formalin — 1 ml 40% formalin plus 19 ml PBS.

Equipment
○ Polypropylene tubes (Sarstedt, Sterilin, Elkay).
○ Coulter S+IV or similar platelet counting instrument.

Preparation of collection tubes
Tube A: buffered EDTA — 0.2 ml EDTA + 0.2 ml PBS
Tube B: buffered EDTA/formalin — 0.2 ml EDTA + 0.2 ml PBS with formalin.

Method
1. Blood is placed in a polypropylene tube and 0.5 ml of blood is pipetted into each of the collection tubes within 1 minute of venepuncture.
2. The tubes are left to stand at room temperature, with regular gentle mixing for 15 minutes.
3. Both tubes are centrifuged at 170 g for 6 minutes.
4. The top 0.4 ml of platelet-rich plasma is removed from each tube to separate clean tubes, and platelet counts are performed using a Coulter S+IV or similar instrument.

Calculation
The platelet count of the buffered EDTA/formalin tube is divided by the count of the buffered EDTA tube, giving a platelet aggregate ratio.

Comments
— Rapid handling of the blood after venepuncture is essential.
— The type of tube used for blood handling and collection should be standardised.
— The platelet counting method should be standardised, and must give reproducible results.
— Patients with thrombocytopenia may give erroneous results in this test.
— Platelet aggregate ratio is influenced by anti-platelet drugs, exercise, and stress.

Interpretation
Normal range — 0.82–1.1.
    Increased platelet aggregates (decreased platelet aggregate ratio) have been found in:
    a. Patients with transient ischaemic attacks.
    b. Ischaemic heart disease.
    c. Acute myocardial infarction.
The platelet aggregate ratio has also been correlated with serum cholesterol concentration, age and smoking.

ADP AGGREGATION THRESHOLD

Platelets are aggregated to various doses of ADP as described in the section on aggregation. The ADP dose which just gives a secondary wave of aggregation is found, and known as the threshold dose; this should be around 2.5 μM. Thresholds of less than 1 μM ADP suggest hyperaggregability. A similar threshold may be determined for arachidonate.

SPONTANEOUS AGGREGATION

Undiluted PRP is stirred in a cuvette in an aggregometer at 37°C for 15 minutes, and the transmission is recorded on a chart recorder. If the platelets aggregate spontaneously to a significant degree, the pen recorder will show a sharp deflection similar to that seen for collagen aggregation, with an amplitude greater than 20% of the chart width. Where positive responses are obtained, PPP should be monitored at 37°C as spontaneity can be mimicked by the warming of cryoglobulins and cold agglutinins which results in a decrease in the optical density of plasma. When spontaneous aggregation is present, the PRP should be diluted 1/2 in autologous PPP, and the test repeated. If it is still present at a count of 200×10^9/l, or occurs in unstirred PRP at room temperature, platelet aggregation to ADP etc. can not be tested. Spontaneity is commonly found in patients with myeloproliferative defects, and in this situation it may well be beneficial to give prophylactic aspirin and persantin, if there is no bleeding diathesis. Spontaneity in other patients, especially at low platelet counts, is even more cause for concern.

Spontaneous aggregation may also be tested for by whole blood impedance aggregation, in a similar fashion. Not all patients with spontaneous PRP aggregation will have a response in whole blood.

BETA-THROMBOGLOBULIN (β-TG)

Principle
This radioimmunoassay technique is based on the competition between unlabelled β-TG and known amounts of ^{125}I-labelled β-TG for binding sites on β-TG specific antibody. The amount of bound ^{125}I-labelled β-TG is inversely proportional to the amount of β-TG in the plasma samples.

Biochemical basis
β-TG is synthesised by the megakaryocyte and stored in the platelet alpha granule; it is not usually present in significant amounts in normal plasma. Various activating stimuli such as exposure to collagen fibrils,

thrombin or ADP can induce its secretion into plasma. The presence of raised levels of plasma β-TG can therefore suggest in vivo platelet activation.

Test samples
Blood is collected by venepuncture with minimal stasis, and the first 5 ml are discarded, or used for other test samples. 2.5 ml blood is rapidly added to a chilled sample collection tube in crushed ice, and gently mixed by inverting 2–3 times, and replaced in crushed ice.

Reagents

Sample collection tubes. In a 75 $\times$ 12 mm polystyrene tube place:
- 140 μl 0.336 M dipotassium EDTA (135 mg/ml in sterile water)
- 36 μl theophylline (12.5 mg/ml in absolute ethanol)
- 10 μl prostaglandin E_1 (25 μg/ml).

Sample collection tubes provided with the Amersham kit are not used.

Amersham β-TG radioimmunoassay kit Sufficient for the determination of β-TG in 19 test samples in duplicate. The following reagents are reconstituted just before use:
- ^{125}I-labelled β-TG.
- anti-β-TG serum.
- Ammonium sulphate solution.
- Reference standards: 10, 20, 50, 100, and 225 ng/ml.

Preparation of reagents
1. Reconstitute each standard with 500 μl distilled water.
2. Reconstitute the antiserum and labelled β-TG with 10 ml distilled water.

Equipment
○ Refrigerated centrifuge.
○ Microcentrifuge.
○ Polypropylene microcentrifuge tubes.
○ Vortex mixer.
○ Gamma counter.

Preparation of test plasmas
1. Keep blood sample on ice for at least 15 minutes and up to 2 hours, before centrifuging at 2000 g at 4°C for 30 minutes.
2. Remove the top third of plasma and collect the next third into a clean polypropylene microfuge tube; freeze at -20°C until assayed.

Method
1. Starting with the lowest concentration, 50 μl of each standard in duplicate is pipetted into the first 10 microfuge tubes.

2. 50 μl of each test sample in duplicate is pipetted into subsequent microfuge tubes.

3. Add 200 μl ^{125}I-labelled β-TG to each tube.

4. Add 200 μl anti-β-TG serum to each tube.

5. Vortex mix all tubes and incubate at room temperature for 1 hour.

6. Add 500 μl ammonium sulphate solution to each tube.

7. Vortex mix all tubes and centrifuge at 1500 g in a microcentrifuge for 15 minutes.

8. Invert each tube and tap gently to remove any fluid. Keeping the tubes inverted, allow them to drain onto tissue paper for 5 minutes.

9. Remove any remaining fluid from the rim of the tube, and place all tubes in a gamma counter and count for 60 seconds, or until 10 000 counts are achieved.

Calculation

A graph of gamma count against the β-TG concentration of the standards is plotted and a smooth curve is drawn. Test sample values are abstracted from the curve using their count values.

Comments

— The theophylline used in the preparation of the sample collection tubes will crystallise at 4°C, and must be warmed to 37°C and vortexed before pipetting the suspension into a tube.

— 'Home-made' tubes are preferred to those provided with the kit, since they may also be used for PF4 assays, there are not always sufficient tubes in the kit, and the assay performs better.

— Careful sample collection and handling is essential to get reproducible results and prevent in vitro release of platelet granular contents.

— Precision pipetting is essential for reconstitution of standards and delivery of reagents to test tubes.

— The tubes should be mixed within 8 minutes of ammonium sulphate addition and centrifuged within 10 minutes of mixing.

— The usual safety regulations and precautions for dealing with radiochemicals should be observed.

Interpretation

Normal values — < 50 ng/ml.

β-TG levels may be raised in venous and arterial thrombosis, pre-eclampsia of pregnancy, and other states where there is platelet activation. Increased levels may occur in renal failure (creatinine × 2 normal) due to decreased catabolism of β-TG by the kidney.

False elevations may be found after poor sample collection or difficult venepunctures — comparison of results with platelet factor 4 levels may help in this situation. Interference with the assay may occur where isotopes are being injected. This most commonly occurs

where a patient is given ^{125}I-labelled fibrinogen for leg scanning. Samples for β-TG measurement should be taken before, or 24 hours after, fibrinogen administration.

The measurement of in vitro β-TG release from platelets in response to various aggregating reagents may be helpful in the investigation of certain platelet dysfunctions.

PLATELET FACTOR 4 (PF4)

Principle

This radio-immunoassay technique is based on the competition between unlabelled PF4 and known amounts of ^{125}I-labelled PF4 for binding sites on PF4 specific antibody. The amount of bound ^{125}I-labelled PF4 is inversely proportional to the amount of PF4 in the plasma samples.

Biochemical basis

PF4 is synthesised by the megakaryocyte and stored in the platelet alpha granule; it is not usually present in significant amounts in normal plasma. Various activating stimuli such as exposure to collagen fibrils, thrombin or ADP can induce its secretion into plasma. Platelet released PF4 is rapidly cleared from plasma by binding to the vascular endothelium. The presence of moderately raised levels of plasma PF4 may therefore suggest in vivo platelet activation.

Test samples

Blood is collected by venepuncture with minimal stasis, and the first 5 ml are discarded, or used for other test samples. 2.5 ml blood is rapidly added to a chilled sample collection tube in crushed ice, and gently mixed by inverting 2–3 times, and replaced in crushed ice.

Reagents

Sample collection tubes. In a 75 × 12 mm polystyrene tube place:
- 140 μl 0.336 M dipotassium EDTA (135 mg/ml in sterile water)
- 36 μl theophylline (12.5 mg/ml in absolute ethanol)
- 10 μl prostaglandin E$_1$ (25 μg/ml).

Platelet factor 4 radioimmunoassay kit (Abbot Laboratories Ltd). The kit is sufficient for 50 test samples in duplicate. The following reagents are included in the kit:
- ^{125}I-labelled PF4.
- PF4 antiserum.
- PF4 standards: 10, 30, 50, and 100 ng/ml.
- Dilution buffer.
- 73% saturated ammonium sulphate.

Preparation of reagents
Bring all reagents to room temperature.

Equipment
○ Refrigerated centrifuge
○ Gamma counter.
○ Vortex mixer.

Preparation of test plasmas
1. Keep blood sample on ice for at least 15 minutes and up to 2 hours, before centrifuging at 2000 g at 4°C for 30 minutes.
2. Remove the top third of plasma and collect the next third into a clean polypropylene microfuge tube; freeze at −20°C until assayed.

Method
1. Label the tubes provided in the kit 1–n, where tubes 1–3 are used for total counts (TC), 4–5 for non-specific binding (NSB), 6–15 for standards in duplicate, and 16–n for test samples.
2. Add 50 μl dilution buffer to tubes 4 and 5.
3. Add 50 μl of each standard in duplicate to tubes 6–15, using dilution buffer as the 0 ng/ml standard.
4. Add 50 μl of each test sample in duplicate to the appropriate tubes.
5. Add 250 μl ^{125}I-labelled PF4 to every tube. Cap tubes 1–3 and place to one side.
6. Add 250 μl dilution buffer to tubes 4 and 5.
7. Add 250 μl anti-PF4 serum to tubes 6–n.
8. Vortex mix all tubes except those for TC.
9. Incubate all tubes at room temperature for 2 hours.
10. Add 1 ml ammonium sulphate solution to each tube except the TC tubes. Mix and allow to stand for at least 10 minutes (but not longer than 60 minutes).
11. Centrifuge all tubes except those for TC at 1500 g for 20 minutes.
12. Carefully decant supernatant from each tube and blot the rim of each tube with a tissue.
13. Obtain gamma counts on all tubes; count for 60 seconds or 10 000 counts.

Calculation
Calculate percentage binding for each tube as follows:

$$\% \text{ Binding} = \frac{\text{cpm test or standard}}{\text{cpm of TC tube}} \times 100$$

Plot the percentage binding for each standard against its concentration to give a smooth curve. Abstract the PF4 values for the test samples from this curve using their percentage binding values.

Comments
— The theophylline used in the preparation of the sample collection tubes will crystallise at 4°C, and must be warmed to 37°C and vortexed before pipetting the suspension into a tube.
— 'Home-made' tubes are preferred to those provided with the kit, since they may also be used for β-TG assays; there are not always sufficient tubes in the kit, and the assay performs better.
— Careful sample collection and handling is essential to get reproducible results and prevent in vitro release of platelet granular contents.
— Precision pipetting is essential for reconstitution of standards and delivery of reagents to test tubes.
— The usual safety regulations and precautions for dealing with radiochemicals should be observed.

Interpretation
Normal values — < 10 ng/ml.

PF4 is rapidly removed from the circulation after platelet release, probably by binding to the vascular endothelium. Smaller increases in PF4 are therefore seen than for β-TG in venous and arterial thrombosis. PF4 is not affected by renal failure, but increased levels may be found after heparin infusion due to displacement of PF4 from the vessel wall. A ratio of β-TG to PF4 less than 2.0 suggests in vitro activation of the sample during collection or handling, causing platelet release. Where the β-TG level is increased to a greater extent than the PF4, ratio >4.0 (in the absence of renal failure), there may be in vivo platelet activation. The concurrent administration of radiolabelled fibrinogen for leg scanning may interfere with PF4 assays.

THROMBOXANE B$_2$ ASSAY

Principle
The assay of thromboxane B$_2$ (TXB$_2$) is performed by a radio-immunoassay technique. The method depends on competition between TXB$_2$ (from the sample) and a ^{3}H-labelled TXB$_2$ reagent for a limited number of binding sites on a TXB$_2$ specific antibody. The TXB$_2$:antibody complexes are separated, and the radioactivity in the supernatant measured. The amount of radioactivity remaining in the supernatant is dependent on the amount of [^{3}H]TXB$_2$ displaced from the antibody by unlabelled TXB$_2$ in the test sample. The measurement of free, unbound [^{3}H]TXB$_2$ in the presence of a series of TXB$_2$ standards allows the concentration of TXB$_2$ in test samples to be interpolated from a standard curve.

Biochemical basis
Certain platelet activators such as collagen cause the

release of arachidonic acid from the platelet membrane phospholipids by phospholipase enzymes. This arachidonate can be rapidly converted to prostaglandin endoperoxides and thromboxane A_2 by cyclo-oxygenase and thromboxane synthetase enzymes. Thromboxane A_2 causes platelet aggregation and smooth muscle contraction, but has a short half-life, rapidly degrading to the stable, but inactive, thromboxane B_2. The measurement of thromboxane B_2 levels therefore reflects the production of thromboxane A_2, and the ability to produce these substances may be used to assess hyperactivity of the platelet cyclo-oxygenase pathway or platelet dysfunctions associated with abnormal thromboxane A_2 generation.

Test samples

Serum thromboxane B_2 — collect 1 ml fresh blood into a plain glass tube and incubate at 37°C for 1 hour. Centrifuge for serum and store this at −20°C until required.

Thromboxane B_2 release — stir 270 μl platelet-rich plasma (platelets $200 \times 10^9/l$) in an aggregometer at 37°C and add 30 μl of either 200 μg/ml collagen or 15 mM sodium arachidonate. Aggregate for 4 minutes and add 30μl 100 mM EDTA. Centrifuge at 1500 g for 10 minutes and store the supernatant at −20°C until assayed.

Plasma thromboxane B_2 — collect blood into β-TG sample tubes and store the plasma at −20°C.

Reagents

- PBS pH 7.3
    0.42 g $NaH_2PO_4.2H_2O$
    1.75 g Na_2HPO_4 (anhydrous)
    0.9 g NaCl
    200 ml distilled water.
- TXB_2 antisera (Universal Biologicals Ltd.).
- $[^3H]TXB_2$ tracer 1 μCi vials (New England Nuclear.).
- TXB_2 standard (Universal Biologicals Ltd., or New England Nuclear).
    Alternatively, kits may be obtained from New England Nuclear or Amersham Ltd.
- Optiphase 'safe' scintillant (LKB Ltd.).
- Dextran T2000 (Pharmacia Ltd.).
- Activated charcoal (BDH Ltd.).
- Bovine serum albumin (Sigma Chem. Co.).

Preparation of reagents and samples
The samples are normally diluted 1/4 and 1/8 in PBS; standards are diluted to give 10, 5, 2.5, 1.25, 0.625, 0.313, 0.156, 0.078, and 0.039 ng/ml solutions.
Charcoal mix. Mix the following reagents immediately before use:
    120 mg activated charcoal
    10 mg dextran T2000

10 mg bovine serum albumin
Add 20 ml of PBS and keep on ice.

Equipment
○ Refrigerated centrifuge.
○ Beta counter.
○ Polystyrene tubes 75 × 12 mm.
○ Vortex mixer.

Method

1. Label a series of polystyrene tubes 1–n, and add 250 μl PBS to tubes 1, 2 for the top count (TC), 100 μl PBS to tubes 3, 4 for non-specific binding (NSB), and 50 μl PBS to tubes 5, 6 for blank (BL). Add 50 μl amounts of each standard concentration in duplicate to further numbered pairs of tubes, and 50 μl of each test dilution in duplicate to subsequent pairs of tubes.
2. Add 50 μl ^3H-labelled TXB_2 tracer to each tube.
3. Add 50 μl TXB_2 antibody to all tubes except tubes 1–4.
4. Mix the contents of each tube and incubate overnight at 4°C.
5. Add 150 μl charcoal mix to all tubes, excluding tubes 1 and 2 (TC). Mix well and centrifuge at 2000 g at 4°C for 15 minutes.
6. Remove 200 μl of supernatant from each tube and add to 5 ml of Optiphase scintillation fluid.
7. The samples are then counted for 2 minutes or 10 000 counts on a beta counter, and cpm obtained.

Calculation
Percentage binding is calculated from the following equation:

$$\% \text{ Binding} = \frac{(\text{sample cpm} \times \text{TC cpm})}{\text{NSB}}$$

A graph of percentage binding against dilution of standard can then be plotted and the test sample values obtained.

Comments
— The top count indicates the amount of tracer added to each tube.
— The non-specific binding tubes give an indication of tracer binding to anything other than the antibody.
— The blank count is a measure of maximum binding of the antibody to the tracer in the absence of any other antigen, and this should be between 35% and 45% to confirm sensitivity.
— There should be a minimum of delay between the addition of charcoal mix and centrifugation. Depending on the capacity of the centrifuge, it may be convenient to precipitate and spin the tubes in

small groups rather than all at the same time.

— Test samples giving values outside the linear portion of the standard curve must be repeated after appropriate adjustment of the sample dilution.

— Careful sample collection and handling is essential to get reproducible results and prevent in vitro release of platelet granular contents.

— Precision pipetting is essential for reconstitution of standards and delivery of reagents to test tubes.

— The usual safety regulations and precautions for dealing with radiochemicals should be observed.

Interpretation

The usual way of estimating the ability of platelets to form thromboxane is to assay serum thromboxane B_2 levels, this gives a maximal challenge to the platelets in a standardised fashion. This measurement may be useful in the investigation of platelet dysfunctions and prothrombotic states, normal range 215–544 ng/ml $(0.89–1.87$ ng/10^6 platelets). Thromboxane B_2 release to collagen in platelet-rich plasma gives a more platelet specific estimation to a standard agonist; normal range 362–722 ng/ml $(1.60–2.68$ ng/10^6/l). Plasma thromboxane B_2 may also be measured to reflect abnormal platelet hyperaggregability in the circulation.

Serum thromboxane B_2 may be reduced if there are platelet membrane abnormalities, deficiency of cyclo-oxygenase or thromboxane synthetase enzymes, or after the ingestion of drugs which inhibit these enzymes, e.g. acetyl salicylic acid, indomethacin, dazoxiben.

PLATELET LABELLING AND KINETIC STUDIES

PLATELET LABELLING

Platelet labelling is best achieved with indium-111 (^{111}In), which has now almost replaced chromium-51 (^{51}Cr) for this purpose (Peters et al 1986). Radiolabelled platelets are used for measurement of mean platelet lifespan (MPLS), quantification of splenic platelet pooling, identification of sites of platelet destruction and thrombus imaging.

Principle

When complexed with certain lipophilic chelating agents, ^{111}In readily enters and stably labels all blood cells to which it is exposed.

[^{111}In] hydroxyquinoline (oxine) is one such complex available commercially. Other chelaters are tropolone and acetylacetone, which, unlike oxine, readily complex with ^{111}In in buffer. Using oxine or acetylacetone, the cells have to be separated from plasma, which otherwise binds the ^{111}In. [^{111}In]tropolonate, on the other hand,

is able to label cells efficiently in plasma if the cell concentration is high. With respect to granulocytes, maintenance in plasma promotes ultimate functional integrity, and this is probably also true for platelets. [^{111}In]tropolonate is therefore preferred, and the technique with this agent will be described. Techniques based on commercially available [^{111}In]oxine are described elsewhere (Hawker et al 1980) and available from the manufacturers (e.g. Amersham International).

Reagents

All materials must be filter sterilised with a 0.22 micron Millipore and checked for sterility and pyrogenicity before in vivo use.

- Anticoagulant
  Acid-citrate-dextrose (ACD) NIH Formula A made up as:

Tri-sodium citrate, $2H_2O$	2.2 g
Citric acid (anyhydrous)	0.8 g
Dextrose	2.5 g
Water for injection	100 ml

- 20 mM HEPES-saline buffer, pH 7.6 made up as:

Sodium chloride	0.804 g
HEPES (acid form)	0.478 g
Sodium hydroxide 1 M	1–2 ml to adjust pH to 7.6
Water for injection	100 ml

  After sterilisation, this buffer may be stored at room temperature.

- Tropolone, 4.4×10^{-3} M $(0.54$ mg/ml). Dissolve 5.4 mg tropolone (Fluka AG) in 10 ml 20 mM.

- Hepes saline buffer pH 7.6. Sterilise the solution using 0.22 μ Millipore filter. Dispense the solution into 1 ml aliquots. It can be stored at 4°C in the dark for several months.

- [^{111}In]chloride in 0.04 M HCl at 370 MBq/ml (Amersham International).

Method

1. Dispense 9 ml ACD into a 60 ml polythene syringe.

2. Collect 51 ml venous blood using a 19 g butterfly needle (or 21 g for children) avoiding undue negative pressure and frothing; this gives a final volume of 60 ml. These volumes can be scaled down for children or patients with normal to high platelet counts $(\geqslant 200 \times 10^9$ per l).

3. Platelet preparation. Transfer 20 ml aliquots of the anticoagulated blood into sterile Sterilin universal containers.

    a. Centrifuge each container at 100 g for 15 minutes.

    b. Collect the platelet-rich plasma (PRP) using a sterile 10 ml syringe without needle, making sure that the buffy coat is not removed.

c. Transfer PRP to new Universal containers, and add 1 ml ACD to each 10 ml PRP in order to lower the pH to 6.5. This inhibits platelet aggregation.

d. Centrifuge at 640 g for 10 minutes.

e. Remove as much of the supernatant (platelet-poor plasma; PPP) as possible from the platelet pellet.

f. Dislodge the platelet pellets by gently tapping the containers and to each add 0.1–0.2 ml of PPP.

g. Pool the platelet pellets and if necessary add more PPP to give a final volume of approx 1 ml.

4. Platelet labelling with $[^{111}In]$tropolonate.

a. Dispense 300 μCi (11 MBq) $[^{111}In]Cl_3$ in 0.04 M HCl (not more than 50 μl), using an automatic micro-litre pipette dispenser with sterile plastic tip, into a 10 ml Universal container.

b. To this $[^{111}In]Cl_3$ add 100 μl tropolone at 4.4 $\times$ 10^{-3} M in 20 mM Hepes-saline buffer, pH 7.6. $[^{111}In]$tropolanate forms immediately. The complex must be pre-formed immediately before use.

c. Add the platelet suspension to the pre-formed $[^{111}In]$tropolonate; this gives a final tropolone concentration of 4 $\times$ 10^{-4} M.

d. Incubate the platelets for 5 minutes at room temperature.

e. Add 5 ml of PPP, retained following step 3e, to the labelled cells.

f. Centrifuge at 640 g for 10 minutes.

g. Withdraw the supernatant PPP containing non-cell bound ^{111}In.

h. Resuspend the labelled platelets in 3–5 ml PPP.

i. Transfer the platelets to a 5 or 10 ml plastic syringe without using a needle and measure the radioactivity in a dose calibrator.

Suggested modifications for patients with severe thrombocytopenia ($<75 \times 10^9/l$)

1. Take more blood, 100–150 ml.

2. Add a red cell sedimenting agent such as Plasmasteril, or Hespan to the whole blood (1 vol to 10 vols blood) prior to the first slow centrifugation (step 3a). This improves the yield of PRP.

3. Resuspend the platelet pellets at step 3g in a 50:50 or 75:25 mixture of plasma:saline for labelling. This improves labelling efficiency. If the patient's platelet count is less than 20 $\times$ $10^9/l$ it is likely that homologous ABO/Rhesus matched platelets will be necessary.

IN VIVO USE OF LABELLED PLATELETS

The in vivo parameters measurable with ^{111}In-labelled platelets are: platelet recovery, distribution, destruction and MPLS.

RECOVERY OF INJECTED PLATELETS

Principle

This is the circulating platelet-bound activity, as a percentage of the injected activity, at 30 minutes after injection. The 'un-recovered' activity is represented by

1. platelets that have entered the splenic platelet pool,

2. damaged platelets rapidly and irreversibly removed by the reticulo-endothelial system, and

3. 'activated' platelets temporarily trapped in the liver and occasionally also in the lung. In the present context, there is not a clear distinction between activated and damaged platelets, and data on the separate kinetics of these cells is limited. There are essentially two causes of reduced recovery. Firstly, splenomegaly, in which the splenic platelet pool is expanded and, secondly, excessive platelet activation and/or damage. The latter may be due to poor technique or, possibly, platelet 'fragility' encountered as part of the disorder under investigation.

Method

1. Prepare a 1 ml standard, containing a known amount of ^{111}In, as follows. Draw up 3–5 ml of unbound ^{111}In (from step 4g, platelet labelling) into a 5 or 10 ml syringe and measure the activity in the same dose calibrator and at the same time as the dose syringe. The syringes containing the standard and dose should be the same size and type, and the standard and dose volumes should be similar. Wash the contents of the syringe in 1 litre of water and then take 1 ml and transfer to tube for well counting.

2. Take a 5 ml i.v. blood sample at 30 minutes and transfer to EDTA tube. Place 1 ml whole blood in well counting tube and centrifuge remainder at 2000 g for 5 minutes. Place 1 ml of cell-free plasma in a well counting tube. Measure haematocrit.

3. Estimate total blood volume from height and weight using tables (Hurley 1975).

Calculation

1. Calculate cell-bound activity in whole blood by subtracting activity in cell-free plasma from the total whole blood activity: $C = W - (1 - H)P$ where C is cell-bound activity in 1 ml whole blood, W is whole blood activity per ml, P is plasma activity in 1 ml plasma and H is haematocrit.

2. $\text{Recovery} = \dfrac{C}{W \text{ std.}} \times \dfrac{TBV}{1000} \times \dfrac{\text{dose std.}}{\text{dose ing.}}$

Where W std. is the counts in the 1 ml well standard, TBV is total blood volume, dose std. is the activity in the standard syringe before dilution and dose ing. is the injected dose. Note that recovery can be expressed for any time after injection and many workers use 1 hour. To have any useful meaning, the time should be long enough to have allowed complete equilibration in the splenic pool, but short enough to be an insignificant fraction of MPLS.

DISTRIBUTION OF INJECTED PLATELETS

Principle

The immediate platelet distribution reflects firstly the integrity of the platelets and secondly the size of the splenic platelet pool. Damaged and/or activated platelets are rapidly taken up by the liver and may also undergo temporary hold-up in the lungs. This liver uptake is partly reversible. For the correct interpretation of liver activity, account must be taken of the platelet disorder; e.g. in severe idiopathic thrombocytopenic purpura (ITP), platelets are destroyed in the liver as part of the disorder.

Method

1. Place the patient supine with the gamma camera underneath viewing the chest and upper abdomen.

2. Inject the labelled platelets and image dynamically, at a frame time of 1 minute, for 30 minutes.

3. Draw regions of interest over the cardiac blood pool, liver and spleen and generate the corresponding time activity curves (Fig. 30.3).

Interpretation and calculation

1. The splenic time activity curve increases monoexponentially to reach a plateau at about 20 minutes. The blood activity decreases with the same time constant and reaches an asymptote which represents the recovery. These two curves are inversely symmetrical because dynamic equilibrium is achieved between platelet flow into, and clearance from, the spleen.

2. Identify the peak of the liver time activity curve. Normally, a liver image is just faintly visible with a peak at 2 to 3 minutes. Because equilibration is established rapidly between blood and the small hepatic platelet

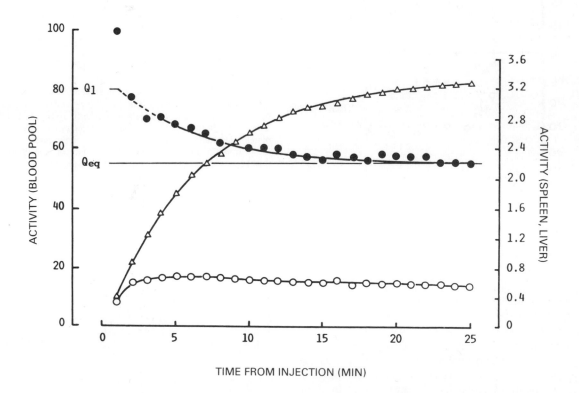

Fig. 30.3 Time activity curves recorded from a gamma camera positioned posteriorly over the chest and upper abdomen following injection of ^{111}In-labelled platelets in a patient with normal platelet kinetics. Regions of interest were drawn over the spleen (triangles), liver (open circles), and cardiac blood pool (closed circles). The blood pool curve has been extrapolated from 4 minutes (the peak of the liver activity) to 1 minute (Q1) and has asymptote Qeq. Ordinate left: percent of maximum (blood); right: counts per second per computer pixel point (liver and spleen). (Reprinted from Thrombosis and Haemostasis)

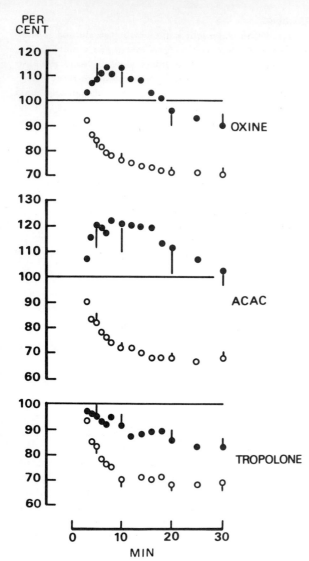

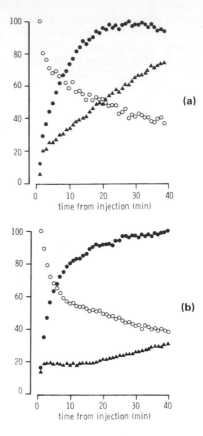

Fig. 30.4 Composite time activity curves generated from regions drawn over liver (closed circles) and cardiac blood pool (open circles) following injection in normal subjects of platelets labelled in saline with [^{111}In] oxine (n = 5; top) or [^{111}In] acetylacetonate (middle; n = 3) and platelets labelled in plasma with [^{111}In] troplonate (n = 10; bottom). Standard errors of the mean are shown at 5, 10, 20, and 30 minutes. Ordinate: per cent of initial activity. Platelets labelled in saline show evidence of activation. (Reprinted from Thrombosis and Haemostasis)

Fig. 30.5 Time activity curves from spleen (closed circles), liver (triangles) and cardiac blood pool (open circles) in patients with severe thrombocytopenia and markedly reduced MPLS. The patient in (**a**) had ITP and shows accelerated hepatic platelet destruction. Having entered the splenic pool, platelets are beginning to show net egress in the face of continuing intrahepatic destruction. The patient in (**b**) had transfusion-induced platelet antibodies and shows abnormal accelerated intrasplenic and intrahepatic destruction. Homologous platelets were labelled and it appears that there is a short latent period before intrahepatic destruction commences. Ordinate: blood-pool-percent of initial value; liver and spleen-count rate per computer pixel point, normalised to maximum splenic value.

pool, the hepatic time activity curve then declines in parallel with blood pool activity (Fig. 30.4). Damaged and/or activated platelets give a curve that peaks at 5 to 10 minutes, maintains a plateau for 10 to 15 minutes and falls at a time when blood pool activity is approaching a steady value (Fig. 30.4). Pathological platelet destruction, as in ITP, gives a liver curve that rises progressively for as long as any platelet-bound activity remains in blood (Fig. 30.5a).

3. Extrapolate the blood pool time activity curve from the time of the liver peak, backwards to 1 minute (Q_1) (Fig. 30.3). Determine the asymptote of the blood pool curve (Qeq). Q_1 and Qeq are best obtained from a computer fit based on the equation $y = A + Be^{-kx}$. A is Qeq and B (at t = 1 min) is Q_1 − Qeq. Then:

$$SPP = \frac{Q_1 - Qeq}{Q_1}$$

where SPP is the fraction of the total circulating platelet population pooled in the spleen, normally about one-third.

DESTRUCTION OF INJECTED PLATELETS

Principle

As circulating platelets are destroyed, ^{111}In is transferred from the blood and SPP to the reticulo-endothelial system. The liver, spleen and bone marrow are periodically imaged to identify the distribution of destruction. Normally, the splenic activity remains essentially constant because the spleen pools almost the same fraction of the platelet population as it destroys (Fig. 30.6). Abnormally increased splenic destruction is recognised, therefore, as an increasing splenic activity signal. In ITP or transfusion-induced platelet immunity with markedly accelerated splenic platelet destruction, this may be evident in the 40-minute dynamic sequence. Thus the splenic curve, after approaching a plateau, continues to increase as the blood level progressively falls (Fig. 30.5b). Pathological hepatic platelet destruction is usually associated with severe thrombocytopenia and very shortened MPLS. It is recognised as a progressive rapid increase in hepatic activity (Fig. 30.5a). Whether the bone marrow ever exclusively causes thrombocytopenia by excessive platelet destruction is not known.

Method

1. Position the gamma camera posteriorly and centre it over the liver and spleen 30 minutes to 1 hour following injection of labelled platelets. Record the activity, centred on both ^{111}In energy peaks, for 2 minutes and store in the computer. Repeat for the anterior view at the same level.

2. Repeat periodically at a rate depending on the MPLS until the blood level of labelled platelets is approaching about 10% of the 30 minute to 1 hour value.

3. Draw regions of interest over the spleen (posterior) and liver (anterior) ensuring that on each occasion they are identically positioned in relation to the respective organs. Record the counts within the regions.

4. Correct the counts for ^{111}In decay, zero time being the time of the first image. The decay constant for ^{111}In is 0.0103 hours[-1] (corresponding to a decay half-time of 67 hours).

5. Plot the time courses of activity within the spleen and liver.

6. Divide the final splenic counts by the initial (t = 0) value. This is the ratio of destruction to pooling within the spleen (D:P).

Interpretation

The normal D:P ratio is slightly heigher than unity. It remains as such in a wide range of spleen sizes and MPLS values (Fig. 30.6). The hepatic activity in the normal rises so that at the completion of radiolabelled platelet clearance from the blood it is about twice the value at t = 0. An increase above 1.5 in the splenic D:P ratio suggests abnormally increased splenic destruction and is commonly seen in ITP (Fig. 30.7). A decrease below unity suggests abnormal platelet destruction elsewhere, either

a. increased peripheral consumption, such as in thrombotic thrombocytopenic purpura, or

b. abnormally increased hepatic destruction, such as in severe ITP.

In the latter, hepatic activity increases progressively in association with a peripheral platelet count of less than $20 \times 10^9/l$ and an MPLS of less than a few hours. In peripheral consumption, hepatic activity would not be expected to show any significant increase, although data on this is limited. The gradual appearance of activity in bone marrow is normal; very little data exists on abnormal marrow uptake.

To summarise: in a patient with thrombocytopenia, a high splenic D:P ratio suggests abnormal splenic destruction, a low D:P ratio suggests abnormal extra-splenic destruction and a normal D:P ratio suggests, especially if there is also splenomegaly, increased splenic pooling.

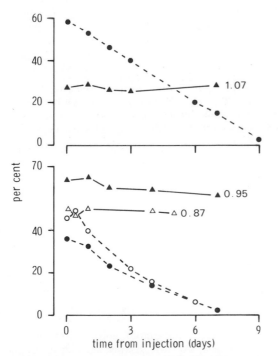

Fig. 30.6 Time courses of blood (circles) and splenic (triangles) activities, corrected for isotope decay, in a normal subject (upper panel) and 2 patients with reduced MPLS and increased splenic platelet pooling (lower panel). The numbers are ratios (DP ratios) of final to initial splenic activities. Ordinate: percent of injected dose. (Reprinted from the British Journal of Haematology)

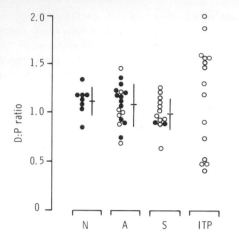

Fig. 30.7 Ratios of platelet destruction to pooling in the spleen (DP ratios) in normal subjects (N), patients with normal sized spleens (A), patients with splenomegaly (S) and patients with ITP. Closed circles: normal MPLS; open circles: reduced MPLS. Mean ± SD is shown for each group (except ITP). (Reprinted from the British Journal of Haematology)

MEAN PLATELET LIFESPAN (MPLS)

Principle

Normally, platelets are destroyed as a result of senescence with a probable small superimposed component of random destruction. The platelet survival curve is therefore almost linear with an MPLS of 8 to 10 days. When MPLS is moderately reduced, the survival becomes curvilinear as the result of an increasing element of random destruction, defined by the proportionality constant K. Increasing K results in a survival curve which approaches a mono-exponential function.

When survival is linear, MPLS is the time at which the plot cuts the time axis. When survival is exponential, the MPLS is the reciprocal of its rate constant K. A linear fit to a platelet survival is appropriate if the plot is perfectly linear, but otherwise overestimates MPLS. On the other hand, an exponential fit to a linear or curvilinear plot, i.e. when the curve is not dominated by K, underestimates MPLS. A relatively simple method of obtaining MPLS when the survival is intermediate between linear and exponential is the weighted mean of linear and exponential fits, the weighting being towards the function which the survival curve most closely approaches. Another simple method is to forward extrapolate the initial, steepest part of the curve (following equilibration in the splenic pool) to the time axis, which is cut at the MPLS.

There are two, more elaborate, techniques in common use for the calculation of MPLS; the Mills-Dornhorst equation and the 'multiple-hit' model. The former is based on the concept of two superimposed destruction processes, one random and the other based on senescence. MPLS is a function of the potential lifespan, T, assumed to be the same for all platelets, and the rate constant of random destruction, K In the multiple-hit model, platelets are conceived to undergo destruction when they have sustained a certain number of insults or 'hits'. The MPLS is a function of the required number of hits, N, and the time interval, a, between hits. Destruction after one hit would give an exponential clearance, whereas the need for an infinite number would give a linear survival. Neither technique has clear merit over the other.

Method

1. Take a 5 ml i.v. blood sample 30 minutes after labelled platelet injection. From this, recovery (R) is calculated and this is the first point on the survival curve.

2. Take further samples at intervals appropriate for the anticipated MPLS. For example, if the patient has a platelet count of $20 \times 10^9/l$ and a clinical diagnosis of ITP, the next sample should be taken no later than 2 hours. Count the early samples in a well-type scintillation counter and estimate the approximate likely MPLS. Take further samples accordingly. The survival curve should ideally be based upon at least 5 points.

3. Separate, from each sample, 1 ml whole blood, and a 1 ml cell-free plasma within 1 hour of collection.

4. When all the samples have been obtained, count them in the well counter. Sample counting time should be such that at least 5000 counts are accumulated from the initial whole blood sample.

5. Subtract background from all samples and then calculate the cell-bound activity present in whole blood as for recovery.

6. Plot cell-bound activity versus time on linear graph paper. If survival is very short, plot it also on semi-logarithmic paper.

7. Calculate MPLS.

a. If survival is clearly linear, perform a least squares linear fit and read MPLS where the fit cuts the time axis.

b. If survival is not linear, perform any of the following:

(i) Weighted mean (see ICSH report on platelet survival, 1977)

(ii) Visualise the maximum slope and extrapolate it to the time axis. For this to work adequately, frequent sampling at the start of the study is necessary.

(iii) Mills-Dornhorst equation. Calculate, using a computer, the parameters MPLS, K and T. Then,

$$MPLS = \frac{1 - e^{-KT}}{K}$$

(iv) Multiple-hit model. Calculate, using a computer, MPLS, N and a.

These last two methods are not necessary for routine use and the reader is referred to the ICSH report (1977). Furthermore, although the parameters K, T, and N have a research importance, they have little practical clinical significance.

c. When it is very short, confirm that the survival is exponential from the semi-logarithmic plot. Perform a least squares fit to this plot and then,

$$MPLS = \frac{t1/2}{0.693}$$

General interpretation of thrombocytopenia

Thrombocytopenia may be the result of

a. decreased platelet production,
b. increased splenic pooling, or
c. decreased MPLS.

The splenic platelet pool (SPP) as a fraction of the total circulating platelet population is approximately equal to $1 - R$ and is normally one-third. It is better obtained from the gamma camera time activity curves, since the component of $1 - R$ that is due to hepatic uptake can be accounted for. The effective platelet production rate (PP) can then be calculated:

$$PP = \frac{\text{peripheral platelet count}}{(1 - SPP) \times MPLS}$$

Splenomegaly causes thrombocytopenia by a dilutional effect. This tendency towards thrombocytopenia can be quantified as an equivalent tendency caused by reduced MPLS. For example, normally the blood platelet space is twice the capacity of the splenic platelet space. A four-fold increase in the latter would, in the absence of any thrombopoietic response, reverse this ratio, give an SPP of two-thirds of the total circulating platelet population, an R of approximately 30%, and halve the peripheral platelet count. This would be the thrombocytopenic equivalent of a reduction in MPLS to half normal. If thrombopoiesis is sensitive to the total platelet mass rather than the peripheral platelet count (P) then the latter can be predicted from the size of the splenic platelet pool from

$$P = \frac{(1 - SPP) \times P\ (norm)}{1 - SPP\ (norm)}$$

(In the presence of reduced MPLS, P(norm) is the platelet count that would result from the MPLS without

splenomegaly). However, if platelet production is regulated by the peripheral count, then increased thrombopoiesis would tend to reverse thrombocytopenia due to splenomegaly. It is not clear which regulatory mechanism predominates and the reader is referred to longer texts for experimental data and discussion (Peters 1985).

PLATELET ANTIBODIES

The detection of platelet antibodies may be useful in the following clinical situations:

1. Unexplained thrombocytopenia due to peripheral destruction of platelets (platelet auto-antibodies).
2. Allo-immune neonatal thrombocytopenia, post-transfusion purpura, and poor survival of transfused platelets (platelet allo-antibodies).
3. Suspected drug-induced immune thrombocytopenia (drug-induced platelet antibodies).

The platelet immunofluorescence test (PIFT), although only semi-quantitative, is suitable for demonstrating platelet antibodies in all of the above conditions and is simple and reliable.

Principle

The PIFT is a fluorescent-labelled anti-human globulin (AHG) technique (von dem Borne et al 1978). It may be used to detect either cell-bound antibody or free antibody in the serum. Fixation of platelets with paraformaldehyde (PFA) largely prevents non-specific adsorption of immunoglobulins and other plasma proteins without affecting cell surface antigens.

Test samples

Clotted blood. 10 ml from patient. Serum can be used fresh or after storage at $-20°C$.

Anticoagulated blood. Platelets from normal Group O donors should be used for the detection of allo-antibodies, and if possible the patient's own platelets should be used when testing for auto-antibodies or drug-dependent antibodies. The usual amount of blood required is 20 ml taken into 5% w/v solution of Na_2 EDTA in distilled water (9 volumes blood to 1 volume EDTA), but larger amounts of anticoagulated blood will be needed from patients with thrombocytopenia.

Platelets should be harvested within 24 hours of collection. They may be used fresh or stored for up to 48 hours suspended in PBS/EDTA at 4°C after fixation in 1% PFA. Alternatively, platelet-rich plasma (PRP) may be stored at $-20°C$ for up to 6 months (Helmerhorst et al 1984).

Reagents

● PBS buffer.

- PBS/EDTA buffer.
- 1% paraformaldehyde (PFA (PFA) solution.
- Glycerol/PBS.
- FITC-labelled anti-human immunoglobulins.
- Chloroquine diphosphate solution.

Equipment
○ Glass or plastic Pasteur pipettes.
○ Glass microscope slides 76 × 26 mm.
○ Glass coverslips 22 × 32 mm.
○ Plastic tubes 7 × 50 mm (precipitin tubes), or U-well microtitre plates.
○ Plastic conical base centrifuge tubes 16 × 10 mm (with caps).
○ Centrifuge(s) capable of holding precipitin and centrifuge tubes.
○ Epifluorescent microscope.
○ 37°C water-bath.

Controls
Positive. Serum containing a platelet-specific antibody.

Negative.   Serum from a pool of non-transfused male group AB donors.

Platelet preparation

Standard technique
1. Centrifuge anticoagulated blood for 10 minutes at 200 g to prepare PRP. Transfer the PRP to a separate tube.
2. Wash the platelets 3 times in PBS/EDTA and resuspend thoroughly each time (centrifuge 5 min at 2500 g).
3. Fix the platelets in 3 ml of 1% PFA for 5 minutes at 22°C.
4. Wash twice PBS/EDTA (centrifuge 5 min at 2500 g).
5. Suspend at a concentration of 250–400 × 10^9/l.

Chloroquine modification (Nordhagen & Flaathen 1985)
The chloroquine modification of the PIFT allows the detection of platelet-specific antibodies in the presence of HLA antibodies. Chloroquine-treated platelets do not react with HLA antibodies, whereas reactions with platelet-specific antibodies are unchanged.

Procedure: as for preparation of normal platelets as far as end of step 2. Add 5 ml of chloroquine diphosphate (200 mg/ml, pH 5.0) to platelet button, mix and leave at 22°C for 2 hours, mixing at frequent intervals. Wash 3 times in PBS/EDTA (centrifuge 5 min at 2500 g) and proceed as for preparation of normal platelets from beginning of step 3.

An additional negative control containing multi-specific HLA antibodies only should be used.

Preparation of FITC-labelled antiglobulin reagents
F $(ab')_2$ fragments of FITC-labelled AHG reagents are used to minimise background fluorescence.

The optimal dilution of each AHG must be established by testing in a chequerboard titration; 10-fold dilutions of the AHG are made in PBS from 1:10 to 1:70. Two-fold dilutions of well-defined platelet and multispecific HLA sera are made in PBS and tested against platelets positive for the antigen against which the antibodies are directed, using each dilution of the AHG. The optimal dilution of each AHG will be the highest dilution which gives a clear negative control and good positivity with the various antisera.

Each diluted AHG should be centrifuged at 2500 g for 10 minutes before use to sediment any particulate fluorescent debris. They should be kept at 4°C and may be used for up to one week.

Method
Each batch of tests should include a positive and negative control, as described in 'Controls' above, and a direct test.

Indirect test
1. Mix 100 μl of serum and 100 μl of platelet suspension (or 50 μl of each using microtitre plates).
2. Incubate 45 minutes at 37°C (anti-IgG, C_3) or 22°C (anti-IgM).
3. Anti-C_3 test only: centrifuge at 1200 g for 3 minutes, remove the supernatant and add 100 μl of fresh AB serum (as a source of complement) mix, incubate for 30 minutes at 37°C.
4. Wash cells 3 times in PBS/EDTA (1200 g for 3 min).
5. Add 100 μl of appropriate fluorescein-conjugated anti-human globulin (anti-IgG, anti-IgM, anti-C_3) and mix.
6. Incubate for 30 minutes at 22°C in the dark.
7. Wash twice in PBS/EDTA (1200 g for 3 minutes and resuspend cells).
8. Add 50 μl of PBS/glycerol and mix.
9. Transfer 1 drop of mixture to a glass microscope slide and a coverslip.
10. Allow cells to settle for 30 minutes in the dark.
11. Examine microscopically using a × 40 objective and epifluorescent UV illuminator. Positive reactions are scored from weak to + + + +.

Direct test
100 μl of appropriate cells are placed in a precipitin-tube. Proceed as for the indirect test from beginning of step 2.

Elution technique (von dem Borne et al 1983)

1. Suspend washed packed platelets, from 50 ml EDTA-anticoagulated blood in PBS at a concentration of $500 \times 10^9/l$.

2. In a glass tube, mix one part of the suspension with two parts of ether and shake vigorously for 2 minutes.

3. Incubate for 30 minutes at 37°C in a water-bath with frequent shaking.

4. Centrifuge for 10 minutes at 1200 g.

5. Remove the eluate (lowest layer).

6. Test the eluate against normal donor platelets.

Drug-dependent antibody testing (Murphy et al 1983, 1984)

Tests should be carried out in three ways:

1. Test the patient's platelets against the patient's serum in the absence of the drug.

2. Incubate PFA-fixed cells, serum and drug together for 45 minutes at 37°C. Proceed from beginning of step 4 of the indirect test.

3. Incubate PFA-fixed cells and drug together for 30 minutes at 37°C, wash twice in EDTA, and continue the test with the addition of serum as from step 1 of the indirect test.

Description of positive reactions in the PIFT.

Anti-IgG — overall increase in cell fluorescence with bright, well-defined points of fluorescent beading on the surface and periphery of the cell. With strong antibodies the beading may coalesce to form an unbroken ring of fluorescence (see Plate 1.6A).

Anti-IgM — large well-defined points of fluorescence over the whole cell.

Anti-C_3 — a bright unbroken ring of fluorescence around the cell, and increased cell fluorescence.

Comments

— Positive reactions should always be assessed against the negative control, even though high background fluorescence is very rarely a problem.

— Group O normal platelet donors are used when testing for platelet allo-antibodies to exclude false positive reactions due to anti-A or anti-B.

— Approximately one-third of chloroquine diphosphate-treated cells show homogenous fluorescence (see Plate 1.6B). These should be ignored and the assessment of positivity should be made on the undamaged cells.

— Frozen and thawed cells show similar damage to chloroquine-treated cells. They are not suitable for chloroquine treatment.

Interpretation

Auto-antibodies

A positive reaction in the direct PIFT may be due to the in vivo attachment of either platelet auto-antibodies or immune complexes. The presence of auto-antibodies may be confirmed by the finding of a positive reaction of the eluate against normal donor platelets. A negative reaction in the direct test but a positive reaction in the indirect auto test is considered to indicate the presence of platelet auto-antibodies as PFA-fixation prevents the in vivo attachment of immune complexes. Positive reactions in the PIFT are found in 65–70% of patients with a clinical diagnosis of idiopathic thrombocytopenia. (Waters & Minchinton 1985).

Allo-antibodies

Positive reactions of patient's sera with PFA-fixed normal donor cells may be either due to HLA antibodies or platelet-specific antibodies, as platelets have both HLA and platelet-specific antigens. Therefore, all sera tested for platelet allo-antibodies should also be tested for HLA antibodies using the lymphocytotoxicity test (LCT). A negative reaction in the LCT and a positive reaction in the PIFT indicate the presence of platelet-specific antibodies. Positive reactions in both LCT and PIFT could either indicate the presence of HLA antibodies alone or both HLA and platelet-specific antibodies; these may be distinguished by testing the patient's sera against chloroquine-treated platelets. Positive reactions with chloroquine-treated platelets indicate the presence of platelet-specific antibodies.

Identification of the specificity of a platelet-specific antibody is carried out by testing against a panel of typed platelets.

Drug-dependent antibodies

By analogy with drug-induced immune haemolytic anaemia, the pattern of serological reactions may illustrate the mechanism of action of drug-dependent platelet antibodies:

Positive reactions only with drug-coated platelets. The drug is adsorbed on to the cell surface, and if anti-drug antibody is formed it will react with the cell-bound drug. Examples — penicillin, Septrin.

Positive reactions only in the presence of the drug. The drug and antibody form circulating immune complexes which attach to platelets. Examples — quinine, quinidine.

Positive reactions even in the absence of the drug. Platelet auto-antibodies are present, possibly due to an alteration in immune regulation caused by the drug. This is similar to methyldopa-induced haemolytic anaemia. Examples — methyldopa, gold. The association of drug and auto-immune thrombocytopenia may only be assumed if there is recovery of the platelet count after withdrawal of the drug, and disappearance of the platelet auto-antibody.

Laboratory confirmation of drug-induced immune thrombocytopenia is often difficult. In the acute phase, if enough platelets can be harvested, the direct PIFT should be performed, and if positive it confirms that there is an immune basis for the thrombocytopenia. Later tests to demonstrate the essential role of the drug should be done after the drug has been eliminated and the direct test is negative. A variety of drug concentrations should be used and if possible testing should be carried out using the patient's own cells collected in recovery with both acute and recovery sera. Tests should be as comprehensive as possible, allowing for all mechanisms of drug action.

Composition of reagents

Phosphate-buffered saline (PBS). Dilute 130 ml concentrated phosphate-buffered saline (Mercia-Brocades Ltd) to 2.5 litres with distilled water (pH 7.2).

PBS/EDTA buffer: dissolve 8.37 g Na_2 EDTA in 2.5 litres PBS.

4% stock paraformaldehyde (PFA) solution. Add 4 g paraformaldehyde to 100 ml PBS. Heat to 70°C with occasional mixing. When the temperature of the mixture reaches 70°C, stop heating and add 1 M NaOH drop-wise, mixing continuously until the solution clears (about 15 drops). This stock solution should be stored at 4°C, and protected from light; it should be used within a few months.

1% working paraformaldehyde solution. Add one part stock 4% PFA solution to three parts PBS and correct pH if necessary to 7.2–7.4 with 1 M HCl. This solution may be used for up to 2 weeks when stored at 4°C protected from light.

Glycerol/PBS. Mix 60 ml glycerol and 20 ml PBS. This may be stored at 4°C for several months.

FITC-labelled anti-human immunoglobulins. FITC-labelled anti-IgG, anti-IgM and anti-C_3 can be obtained from Janssen Pharmaceutical Ltd, or from Dakopatts. The optimal dilution of these reagents may be determined as described under preparation of FITC-labelled antiglobulin reagents.

Chloroquine diphosphate solution. Dissolve 2 g chloroquine diphosphate in 10 ml PBS/EDTA buffer. Adjust pH to 5.0 using 1 M NaOH.

REFERENCES

Akkerman J W N, Doucet-de Bruine M H M, Gorter G et al 1978 Evaluation of platelet tests for measurement of cell integrity. Thrombosis and Haemostasis 39: 146–157.

Bowry S K, Prentice C R M, Courtney J M 1985 A modification of the Wu and Hoak method for the determination of platelet aggregates and platelet adhesion. Thrombosis and Haemostasis 53: 381–385

Cardinal D C, Flower R J 1980 The electronic aggregometer: a novel device for assessing platelet behaviour in blood. Journal of Pharmacological Methods 3: 135–158

Gerrard J M 1982 Platelet aggregation and the influence of prostaglandins. In: Methods in Enzymology, Volume 86. Academic Press p. 642–654

Greaves M, Preston F E 1985 The laboratory investigation of acquired and congential platelet disorders. In: Thomson J M (ed) Blood Coagulation and Haemostasis A Practical Guide. Churchill Livingstone, Edinburgh, p 56–134

Hardisty R M, Hutton R A 1966 Platelet aggregation and the availability of platelet factor 3. British Journal of Haematology 12: 764

Hawker R J, Hawker L M, Wilkinson A R 1980 Indium labelled human platelets. Optimal method. Clinical Science 58: 243–248

Helmerhorst F M, ten Berge M L, van der Plas-van Dalen C M, Engelfriet C P 1984 Platelet freezing for serological purposes with and without a cryopreservative Vax Sanguinis 46: 318–322

Hurley P J 1975 Red cell and plasma volumes in normal adults. Journal of Nuclear Medicine 16: 46–52

International Committee for Standardisation in Haematology 1977 Recommended methods for radioisotope platelet survival studies. Blood 50: 1137–1144

Ivy A C, Shapiro P F, Melnick P 1935 The bleeding tendency in jaundice. Surgery, Gynaecology and Obstetrics 60: 781

Lumley P, Humphrey P P A 1981 A method for quantifying platelet aggregation and analyzing drug-receptor interactions on platelets in whole blood in vitro. Journal of Pharmacological Methods 6: 153–166

Mackie I J, Jones R, Machin S J 1984 Platelet impedance aggregation in whole blood and its inhibition by antiplatelet drugs. Journal of Clinical Pathology 37: 874–878

Mielke Jr C H, Kaneshiro M M, Maher I A, Weiner J M, Rapaport S I 1969 The standardised normal Ivy bleeding time and its prolongation by aspirin. Blood 34: 204

Murphy M F, Riordan T, Minchinton R M, Chapman J F, Amess J A L, Shaw E J, Waters A H 1983 Demonstration of an immune-mediated mechanism of penicillin-induced neutropenia and thrombocytopenia. British Journal of Haematology 55: 155–160.

Murphy M F, Metcalfe P, Grint P C A, Green A R, Knowles S, Amess J A L, Waters A H 1984 Cephalosporin-induced immune neutropenia. British Journal of Haematology 59: 9–14

Nordhagen R, Flaathen S T 1985 Choroquine removal of HLA antigens from platelets for the platelet immunofluorescence test. Vox Sanguinis 48: 156–159

Parry D H, Giddings J C, Bloom A L 1980 Familial haemostatic defect associated with reduced prothrombin consumption. British Journal of Haematology 44: 323–334

Peters A M 1985 Platelet kinetics and imaging in the spleen and hypersplenism. In : Heyns A du P, Badenhorst P N, Lotter M G (eds) Platelet Kinetics and Imaging. II,

Clinical Applications. CRC Press, Florida, p 71–96

Peters A M, Saverymuttu S H, Danpure H J, Osman S 1986 Cell labelling. In : Lewis S M, Bayley R J (eds) Methods in Haematology 14. Radionuclides in Haematology. Churchill-Livingstone, Edinburgh, p 79–109

Poller L, Thomson J M, Tanenson J A 1984 The bleeding time: current practice in the UK. Clinical and Laboratory Haematology 6: 369–373

Preston F E, Hutton R, Ludlam C, Greaves M, Machin S J 1987 personal communication

Sixma J J, Nijessen J G 1970 Characteristics of platelet factor 3 release during ADP-induced aggregation. Thrombosis et Diathesis Haemorrhagica 24: 206

Summerfield G P, Keenan J P, Brodie N J, Bellingham A J 1981 Bioluminescent assay of adenine nucleotides: rapid analysis of ATP and ADP in red cells and platelets using the LKB luminometer. Clinical and Laboratory Haematology 3: 257–271

Turitto V T, Baumgartner H R 1983 Platelet adhesion. In: Harker L A, Zimmerman T S (eds) Measurements of platelet function. Churchill Livingstone, Edinburgh,

pp 46–63 (Methods in Hematology, Vol. 8)

Von dem Borne A E G Kr, Verhengt F W A Oosterhof F, von Riesz E, Brutel de la Riviere A, Enyelfriet C P 1978 A simple immunofluorescence test for the detection of platelet antibodies. British Journal of Haematology 39, 195–207.

Von dem Borne A E G Kr, van der Plas-van Dalen C, Engelfriet C P 1983 Immunofluorescence antiglobulin test. In: McMillan R (ed). Immune Cytopenias. Methods in Haematology, 9. Churchill Livingstone, Edinburgh, p 106–127

Waters A H, Minchinton R M 1985 Immune thrombocytopenia and neutropenia. In: Hoffbrand A V (ed) Recent Advances in Haematology, No. 4 Churchill Livingstone, Edinburgh p 309–332

Wu K, Hoak J C 1974 A new method for the quantitative detection of platelet aggregates in patients with arterial insufficiency. Lancet 2: 924–926.

Yardumian D A, Mackie I J, Machin S J 1986 Laboratory investigation of platelet function: a review of methodology. Journal of Clinical Pathology 39: 701–712

Immunohaematology

31

General approach to blood transfusion and immuno-haematology

This section deals with techniques used in the blood bank and with immuno-haematological techniques for red cells, platelets and white cells. Many of the basic techniques in this section can be applied in several procedures, e.g. the indirect antiglobulin technique can be used for red cell typing with a known antiserum, in antibody screening and identification and in compatibility testing. Such procedures are described in detail. A section on quality control is also included, as well as appendices with formulae for the preparation of reagents.

APPARATUS

- Bench-top centrifuge with a centrifugal force of 100–300 g.
- Automated cell washing centrifuge.
- Small serological centrifuge (to take 75 × 12 mm and/or 75 × 10 mm tubes) with a centrifugal force of 1000 g.
- Refrigerator for storing reagents, cell panels, screening cells, blood samples.
- Deep freezer (-20 to $-30°C$) to store serum samples and complement.
- Microscope with low power objective (an inverted microscope is very useful).
- Illuminated viewing box.
- Water-bath at 37°C (or heated block or incubator).
- Water-bath or heated block with adjustable temperature, 30–60°C.
- Deionised or distilled water.
- Large containers for saline.
- Plastic wash bottles.
- Thermometers.
- Stopwatches (minimum one per member of staff).
- Pasteur pipettes (to deliver 25–30 μl per drop).
- 1 ml graduated pipettes.
- 10 ml graduated pipettes.
- Variable volume pipettes (range 0.1–1 ml and 1–5 ml).

- 75 × 12 mm glass tubes.
- 50 × 7 mm precipitin tubes (glass or plastic).
- Racks for the above tubes.
- Microplates: optional.
- Centrifuge with holder for microplates: optional.
- Glass microscope slides.
- Opal glass tiles.
- Wooden applicator sticks.
- Waterproof markers for glass and plastic tubes.

RED CELL SEROLOGY

Detection of reactions between antigens and antibodies in vitro

The vast majority of techniques used routinely in the blood bank to detect reactions between antibodies and antigens on red cells (RBCs) are based on haemagglutination. Occasionally techniques based on haemolysis or on inhibition of haemagglutination are used and very rarely, for specialised serological work, radio-immunoassay, ELISA or immunofluorescence techniques may be used.

Haemagglutination is the clumping of red cells with a specific antigen on their surface by specific antibody. There are two stages in agglutination:

1. the binding of antigen and antibody (sensitisation) and

2. the formation of the lattice which constitutes the visual stage; not all antigen-antibody reactions involving red cells result in direct agglutination or visible reactions.

Several factors affect the first stage of agglutination such as the equilibrium constant of the antibody which in turn is affected by the ratio of antibody to antigen, the ionic strength of the medium, incubation time, temperature and pH.

The factors that affect the second stage of agglutination are not that clear, but the distance between red cells, the surface charge of the cells, the characteristics of the antigen (density, projection from the membrane),

403

characteristics and immunoglobulin class of the antibody, the size of the hydration layer around the cell, all seem to play a role.

IgM antibody molecules have a span between antigen combining sites of 30 nm and are thus capable of binding to antigen sites on adjacent RBCs forming an intercellular lattice thus causing, in most cases, direct agglutination of red cells. The uptake of antibody by RBC antigens occurs within seconds but the crosslinking to form agglutination requires close proximity between the cells; this can be achieved by allowing the red cells to settle on a tile, in a tube or a well, or it can be speeded by centrifugation of the serum/cell mixture. On the other hand, IgG antibody molecules, with a span between antigen-combining sites of 15 nm, do not usually directly agglutinate RBCs in a saline medium. They do, however, bind to the appropriate antigens, 'sensitising' the RBCs. For IgG antibodies to cause agglutination, indirect techniques with polymers (e.g. albumin, PVP), enzymes or anti-human globulin reagents are necessary.

Some red cell allo-antibodies (e.g. anti-A,-B) activate the full complement cascade up to C9 both in vivo and in vitro leading to lysis of rbcs. On the other hand, a large number of red cell allo-antibodies do not activate the complement cascade or activate complement partially and the classical pathway is halted at the C3 stage by natural inhibitors or regulators in plasma. In vivo, RBCs coated with clinically significant IgG antibodies with or without C3 will be removed from the circulation by phagocytic cells in the reticulo-endothelial system carrying Fc and C3b receptors.

Scoring of haemagglutination. In general the strength of the agglutination reaction (i.e. the size of the clumps) is recorded to reflect the potency of a given antibody. Numerical scores are used when titrating an antibody as a guide to its relative strength since titres alone (i.e. end points of agglutination) may be meaningless. The sum of the scores given to each reaction in a titration is the total score. When titrating test samples in parallel, a difference in total score of 10 or more is considered significant. The following system can be used as a guideline:

C or $++++$ = complete agglutination; one clump of agglutinated cells. Score: 12.

V or $+++$ = visual agglutination; several large clumps of cells. Score: 10.

$++$ = a few large clumps seen with the naked eye. Score: 8.

$+$ = small evenly distributed clumps seen more easily under the microscope. Score: 5.

$(+)$ or $\pm$ = microscopic clumps of 5–10 cells and mainly unagglutinated cells. Score: 3.

w = weak; 3–5 cells per clump. Score 2.

0, neg or $-$ve = negative; no agglutination observed. It is preferable not to use the minus sign '$-$' to record a negative result but 0 or neg.

L = haemolysis; means a POSITIVE reaction. Total haemolysis should be scored as 12 and partial haemolysis as 10.

MF = mixed field reaction; a mixture of agglutinated and unagglutinated cells.

Some general considerations

Blood samples

Samples from patients must be properly identified with the patient's full name, date of birth, hospital number and date of collection. It is mandatory for pre-transfusion testing that the details on the patient's blood samples are identical with the information on the signed request form, which should also be completed fully, including details of previous transfusion and/or pregnancies. Information only on the tubes or on the request forms should not be accepted. Any disagreement between the two should lead to the request of new samples. Remember that the majority of transfusion fatalities are due to **identification mistakes.**

Donor blood should be identified by the unique donation number, ABO and Rh group, date of collection and name or code of the Transfusion Centre.

EDTA and, to a lesser extent, sodium citrate inactivate complement components. Anticoagulated blood samples are used preferably as a source of RBCs for typing but serum, from a clotted sample, is required for antibody screening and identification tests, as complement is required for the detection of some antigen/antibody reactions. Fresh serum or serum stored at $-20°C$ or below should be used wherever possible in pre-transfusion tests.

Centrifuges

Bench-top centrifuges with centrifugal forces of 100–300 g can be used for large numbers of tubes or for microplates. To avoid undue handling of tubes, it is advisable to centrifuge precipitin tubes in the same racks used for setting up and incubation of the tests. Small serological centrifuges can be used for $75×12$ mm tubes and can achieve 900–1000 g. A spin-time of 30 seconds in a serological centrifuge is equivalent to about 2 minutes at 200 g in a larger machine. The centrifugal forces given in this chapter are for the centrifuge we find most appropriate for that technique. However, each machine must be calibrated by the user.

Worksheets

In blood group serology it is important to have standard protocols for the different tests used. The worksheets should be completed before the tests are started, with the date, time, name or number of the patient or donor and reagent/s identified by batch number. The order and position in which the reagents are dispensed should be standard throughout the laboratory. It is important that worksheets are completed clearly and properly so that, in the event of emergency, a different member of staff can take over. When completed, the worksheet should be signed by the person recording the results.

Positive and negative controls

In general, cells used as positive controls in red cell typing should carry a single dose of the relevant antigen to ensure that the reagents are detecting weak expression of the antigen on the cell surface. For example, the positive control cells for D typing should be R_1r (*CDe/cde*).

Cells used as negative controls should lack the relevant antigen but carry the antigen to the most likely contaminating antibody in that serum, e.g. anti-C is often found with anti-D, therefore the negative control in D-typing should be r′r (*Cde/cde*).

Autologous and reagent controls

Whenever red cell typing is performed, the correct autologous or reagent controls must be used.

1. For saline, albumin, enzyme or Polybrene techniques use AB serum. With each cell tested set up an additional tube containing AB serum in place of the antiserum or reagent and adopt the same procedure with both test and control tubes.

2. For the indirect antiglobulin test (IAT), use AB serum in parallel or perform a DAT.

3. For commercial antisera prepared for rapid tests, or for antisera diluted in a low-ionic strength medium, ensure that a reagent control is supplied. This control must be used by the same technique as the antiserum with every cell tested.

If the autologous or reagent control is positive the test is invalidated. If the red cells have a positive DAT, typing by an indirect antiglobulin test is not reliable. In such cases it is recommended to use an IgM saline-agglutinating antibody with AB serum as the reagent control or a reduced-alkylated IgG antibody with the reagent control supplied by the manufacturer.

PRETRANSFUSION TESTING OF RECIPIENTS

The transfusion of blood of the same ABO and Rh(D) group as the recipient is 98–99% safe. This means that,

other than the naturally occurring ABO agglutinins and immune anti-D, clinically significant red cell allo-antibodies are found only in 1–2% of the recipient population. Most transfusion fatalities are due to ABO incompatible transfusions and extreme care should be taken to transfuse ABO compatible blood and to avoid identification mistakes of the donor or the recipient which will lead, in the UK, to a one in three chance of ABO incompatibility. Since, after A and B, the Rh antigen D is the most immunogenic red cell antigen and since anti-D is still the clinically significant immune antibody found most frequently in the recipient population, care should be taken to type properly donors' and recipients' red cells for Rh(D).

An antibody screen, using a combination of two to three sensitive techniques (e.g. saline antiglobulin technique or LISS-antiglobulin technique and two-stage enzyme) needs to be performed on the sera of all prospective recipients of blood. If the antibody screen is negative, in patients who need blood and have not been transfused or been pregnant, ABO and Rh compatible blood can be crossmatched by an immediate spin technique. For those patients who have been transfused or pregnant, a crossmatch by IAT is also recommended. On the other hand, if the screen is positive, the antibody/ies should be identified and, if of clinical significance, (e.g. anti-c; -Fyᵃ), antigen-negative blood (e.g. CDe/CDe; Fyᵃ negative) should be chosen for crossmatching by both an immediate spin and by an indirect antiglobulin technique.

Co-operation between clinicians using blood and the blood transfusion department is needed so that:

1. all patients requiring elective surgery have blood samples taken for grouping, antibody screening and storage of serum in advance of admission to hospital.

2. a surgical blood ordering strategy is devised.

The crossmatch/transfused ratio for units of blood transfused during elective surgery for each specific hospital has to be determined before establishing a maximum surgical blood order schedule. Those surgical procedures with a very high crossmatch/transfused ratio seldom require blood and a 'type and screen' without crossmatching blood pre-operatively is usually sufficient. However, if blood is required unexpectedly, a 'type and screen' programme should be able to supply compatible units within a maximum of 30 minutes of a request for blood.

In summary, pre-transfusion testing consists of ABO and Rh(D) grouping of the patient's red cells followed by antibody screening. If the antibody screening shows positive reactions at 37°C, the presence of a clinically significant antibody should be investigated and identified. A compatibility test or crossmatch should be performed on samples from all patients with a high probability of requiring blood transfusion.

ABO TYPING

ABO typing is usually performed by saline techniques in tubes (T.4) or microplates (T.21) by testing the patient's or donor's rbcs with anti-A, -B and -A,B and the serum or plasma with A_1, A_2, B and O cells.

It is not necessary to perform a serum group on infants under 12 months of age, as they do not start producing antibodies until they are about 6 months old. In old age, and in some haematological diseases, anti-A and anti-B become weaker and may not be detectable; this is often seen in group B individuals where weak reactions are obtained with A_2 cells. In some leukaemias red cell antigens may also become weaker but return to normal during remission.

Control cells for ABO grouping:

	Positive	*Negative*
Anti-A	A_2 (A_2B)	B
Anti-A_1	A_1	A_2
Anti-B	B (A_1B)	A_2
Anti-A,B	A_2B (A_x)	O

Rh(D) TYPING

Typing for D is performed using two different potent anti-D reagents by the manufacturer's recommended technique. The albumin addition technique in tubes (T.6) or microplates (T.21) is inexpensive and easy to perform. AB serum or the manufacturer's reagent control must be used to ensure that the cells are not agglutinated in the test system in the absence of anti-D. A test for D^u (weak expression of D) is not recommended as long as the two anti-D reagents used are potent, specific and free of contaminating allo-antibodies.

Control cells for Rh typing

	Positive	Negative
Anti-D	R_1r (CDe/cde)	r'r (Cde/cde)
-E	r''r (cdE/cde)	R_1r (CDe/cde)
-C	r'r (Cde/cde)	R_2R_2 (cDE/cDE)
-e	R_2r (cDE/cde) or r''r (cdE/cde)	R_2R_2 (cDE/cDE)
-c	R_1r (CDe/cde) or r'r (Cde/cde)	R_1R_1 (CDe/CDe)
Anti-D for D^u tests*	known $R_1^u r$ (CD^{u}e/cde)	r'r (Cde/cde)

*The D^u test is used only rarely. With modern potent anti-D reagents, D^u testing has become obsolete.

ANTIBODY SCREENING AT 37°C

Antibody screening is performed using two or three appropriately selected 'screening cells' **separately, not pooled**, by techniques capable of detecting between them the vast majority of clinically significant antibodies. A two-stage papain technique (T.7) and an indirect antiglobulin technique (T.8 or 9) using LISS or a high ratio of serum to cells (at least 3 volumes of serum to 1 volume of the appropriate cell suspension in saline) are recommended.

The screening cells, in toto, should contain all the antigens necessary for the detection of the most common clinically significant antibodies, particularly C, c, D, E, e, Le^a, M, S, s, K, k, Fy^a, Fy^b, Jk^a, Jk^b, ideally in double dose. It is virtually impossible to have all antigens implicated in in vivo red cell destruction present on the screening cells; the antigens C^w, V, Kp^a, Js^a, and Lu^a are usually absent from screening cells. If antibodies are detected with the screening cells, they should be identified.

Table 31.1 Results of ABO grouping.

Blood group	Cell grouping; reactions of red cells with:				Serum grouping or reverse grouping with:				
	anti-A	-B	-A,B	-A_1	Cells	A_1	A_2	B	O
A_1	C	–	C	C		–	–	C	–
A_2	C	–	C	–		(+)	–	C	–
A_3	++MF	–	+++	–		(+)	–	C	–
A_x	–	–	+++	–		(+)	–	C	–
A_1B	C	C	C	C		–	–	–	–
A_2B	+++	C	C	–		(+)	–	–	–
B	–	C	C	–		C	C	–	–
O	–	–	–	–		C	C	C	–

(+) = anti-A_1 may be present; MF = mixed field agglutination.
Note: identifying other subgroups of A and subgroups of B is of no practical value in a routine blood transfusion laboratory.

ANTIBODY IDENTIFICATION

When an antibody has been detected during antibody screening or crossmatching, the specificity/ies should be determined by testing the serum against a panel of fully phenotyped RBCs by indirect antiglobulin and enzyme techniques. Auto-controls (i.e. the patient's own cells tested against own serum) must be included by the techniques used.

Interpretation of the results must be done with care; it is not sufficient just to try to match the positive and negative results obtained with the positive and negative symbols shown on the panel's antigen profile The following questions must be answered:

1. Is it an auto-antibody or an allo-antibody?

2. Does the antibody react by one technique only, better by one or the same by both?

3. Is there variation in the strength of the reactions with different panel cells?

1. If an auto-antibody is present it may be necessary to perform those tests described in the section on auto-immune haemolytic anaemias.

2. Enzyme-treatment of RBCs destroys some antigens (e.g. M,N, Fy^a, Fy^b); some antibodies react better by IAT than with enzyme-treated RBCs (Table 31.2).

3. Some antibody specificities are commonly associated with the presence of other allo-antibodies e.g. anti-C+D, anti-D+E, anti-c+E, anti-Le^{a+b}. Other

specificities show 'dosage', reacting more strongly with homozygous than heterozygous RBCs, e.g. anti-M and anti-Fy^a react better with MM and Fy(a+b−) cells than with MN and Fy(a+b+) cells respectively.

At least three positive and three negative reactions are required to validate the specificity of an antibody. In addition, the individual's RBCs must be shown to lack the antigen to which the antibody specificity is directed.

COMPATIBILITY TEST OR CROSSMATCH

The crossmatch of the recipient's serum versus donor rbcs of the same ABO and Rh(D) groups must be simple, rapid and safe; for patients whose serum contains antibodies or contained antibodies in the past, it should include an indirect antiglobulin test (T.8 or 9) and be performed with red cells from pre-selected antigen-negative units. Compatibility tests in saline at room temperature are NOT required and are not recommended even for patients undergoing prolonged hypothermia. In the case of cold-reacting antibodies (anti-Le^b, -P$_1$ etc.) crossmatching using a technique performed strictly at 37°C against units unselected for the specific antigen is recommended.

Except for rare emergencies, when there is no time to group the cells of the patient, the indiscriminate use

Table 31.2 Antibodies encountered most commonly in blood group serology.

Specificity	Ig class	Reacts best by	Ag. frequency in Cauc. (%)	HDN	HTR
D	G,(M)	Enzyme, IAT	85	+	+
C	G	Enzyme, IAT	70	rare	rare
c	G	Enzyme, IAT	80	+	+
E	G,M	Enzyme, IAT	28	+	+
e	G	Enzyme, IAT	98	+	+
Le^a	M,(G)	Enzyme,IAT,Saline	22	×	+
Le^b	M,(G)	Enzyme,IAT,Saline	72	×	?
Le^{a+b}	M,(G)	Enzyme,IAT,Saline	94	×	+
P$_1$	M	Saline	79	×	?
I	M	Saline	100	×	rare
M	M(G)	Saline, (LISS)	78	rare	(+)
N	M	Saline, (LISS)	72	rare	rare
S	G	IAT, Saline	55	rare	+
s	G	IAT,	89	rare	+
Fy^a	G	IAT	66	+	+
Fy^b	G	IAT	83	NR	+
Jk^a	G	IAT	77	+	+
Jk^b	G	IAT	72	+	+
K	G	IAT	9	+	+
k	G	IAT	99.8	(+)	+
Lu^a	M?G?A	Saline, IAT	8	NR	×
Lu^b	G	IAT	99.8	(+)	+

Key: Ag — antigen; HDN — haemolytic disease of the newborn; HTR — haemolytic transfusion reaction; + — occurs; × — does not occur; ? — sometimes; (+) — mild; NR — not reported.

of group O blood for non-O patients should be actively discouraged.

INVESTIGATION OF A SUSPECTED HAEMOLYTIC TRANSFUSION REACTION

As soon as a haemolytic transfusion reaction is suspected, the transfusion should be stopped, keeping the i.v. line open with saline. The investigation and treatment should be started immediately.

The following are required:

Recipient's pre-transfusion sample.

Post-transfusion samples (clotted for serology, EDTA for direct inspection and blood culture by the microbiology laboratory).

Any units of blood, blood derivatives or i.v. solutions infused during or immediately prior to the onset of the reaction plus the infusion set.

Post-transfusion urine sample and 24 hour urine collected from the start of the transfusion.

The following procedure should be followed:

1. Check the patient's details, units transfused and any documentation for clerical and/or labelling errors. If a clerical error is found, ensure that other clerical errors endangering other patients have not been made (i.e. errors due to transposition of tubes).

2. Centrifuge and examine the post-transfusion sample for obvious haemolysis. Pink or red serum is a sign of recent haemolysis. Yellow-brown or brown serum indicates that the haemolysis occurred a few hours ago.

3. Check the ABO and Rh(D) groups of both the patient's samples and of the units transfused. These groups should be identical in the pre- and post-transfusion samples. The ABO and Rh groups of the donor units should correspond with the labels. Mixed-field agglutination in the post-transfusion ABO and/or D typing is an indication of an incompatible transfusion.

4. Perform a direct antiglobulin test (T.11) on all samples but especially on the patient's post-transfusion sample. The DAT may be negative in cases of severe intravascular haemolytic transfusion reactions or when the incompatible cells coated with IgG and/or complement have been removed from the circulation by the reticulo-endothelial system. A positive DAT with a mixed-field pattern of agglutination in the post-transfusion sample will support a diagnosis of haemolytic transfusion reaction.

5. Repeat the crossmatch with both pre- and post-transfusion samples on all units transfused.

6. Screen the pre- and post-transfusion serum for atypical antibodies. If any positive results are obtained, the antibody should be identified using a red cell panel.

Any anomalous or unexpected results must be investigated further.

7. Urine samples should be tested on the ward.

8. If no RBC incompatibility is detected and the microbiology results are negative but there are signs of haemolysis, non-immune mechanisms of red cell destruction should be investigated such as mechanical trauma (pumps), thermal damage, etc. . . .

Comment. It is good blood transfusion practice to keep pre-transfusion samples for at least one week in the blood bank in case the patient develops a delayed haemolytic transfusion reaction.

Investigation of non-haemolytic transfusion reactions

a. *Urticarial reactions* are usually due to hypersensitivity to plasma proteins, but so far there are no satisfactory techniques for these investigations.

b. *Febrile reactions* when severe and repeated should be investigated for HLA-, granulocyte- and platelet-antibodies.

SEROLOGICAL TESTS IN PREGNANCY
Antenatal

Red cells from all antenatal patients should be typed for ABO and Rh(D) and their serum screened for atypical antibodies at the first antenatal clinic attendance. If no antibodies are detected, the antibody screen should be repeated at 30–36 weeks of pregnancy. If antibodies are detected at any time, the specificity and titre must be determined; anti-D can be quantitated in the Auto-Analyzer by some reference laboratories to give a value in international units (IU) or μg per ml of serum. Anti-D with a titre by antiglobulin technique of > 32 or a level greater than 4 IU/ml are an indication that the fetus, if Rh-positive, might be affected. Whenever IgG antibodies are detected in a pregnant woman, they should be followed up monthly up to 6–7 months gestation and fortnightly thereafter. If possible, red cells from the husband/partner should be grouped for the relevant antigen and efforts made to determine whether the antigen is present in single or double dose (e.g. DD or Dd), i.e. whether the partner is homo- or heterozygous for the relevant gene.

Post-delivery testing

Cord blood

At delivery of a patient with red-cell allo-antibodies, a cord blood sample (clotted and EDTA) should be collected, for ABO and Rh(D) typing plus a direct antiglobulin test (T.11). If the DAT is positive, a saline-reacting anti-D reagent must be used for reliable typing and an eluate should also be made and tested against a panel of group O cells by an indirect antiglobulin technique.

If haemolytic disease of the newborn (HDN) is suspected after delivery and no allo-antibody is detected in the maternal serum, perform an ABO, Rh type, DAT and prepare and test an eluate from a sample of the infant's blood. If possible, also test the maternal serum against the father's rbcs. Remember that neonatal jaundice can be due to glucose-6-phosphate dehydrogenase deficiency.

If ABO HDN is suspected, a heat (T.15A) or a Lui (T.15B) eluate should be tested by indirect antiglobulin technique against A_1 or B cells, depending on the ABO group of the infant, and also against the group O 'screening cells'. The mother's serum should also be tested for the presence of atypical antibodies using standard antibody screening techniques, and the level of maternal IgG anti-A/B should be determined. (T.18B)

Maternal blood

Ideally, at delivery, the serum from all mothers, and especially from those who are Rh-negative, should be screened for atypical antibodies. Rh(D) negative mothers who have not made anti-D must be given prophylactic anti-D immunoglobulin after delivery of an Rh(D) positive infant or after miscarriage, abortion or termination of pregnancy. Whenever there is doubt about the Rh(D) status of a mother of an Rh-positive infant, anti-D immunoglobulin should be given without delay.

SEROLOGICAL INVESTIGATION OF SUSPECTED IMMUNE HAEMOLYTIC ANAEMIA

When a case of immune haemolytic anaemia is suspected from the clinical and haematological findings, a positive DAT will indicate that more detailed serological investigations are required. Immune haemolytic anaemias may be allo-immune (HDN or haemolytic transfusion reactions), auto-immune (warm-antibody, WAIHA or cold-antibody, CAIHA), or drug-induced.

Auto-immune haemolytic anaemias

The following tests are recommended:

a. ABO and Rh(D) type. A saline anti-D reagent must be used if the autologous control or the DAT is positive.

b. DAT, (T.11) with polyspecific AHGS; if positive, monospecific anti-IgG and anti-C3, should be used. If negative, and there is still a strong suspicion of auto-immune haemolytic anaemia, blood samples should be tested with anti-IgM, -IgA etc, possibly in a reference centre.

An eluate (T.15C or 15D) should be made from the

red cells if any patient is suspected of having WAIHA, and tested in parallel with the last wash and with the patient's serum against a selected panel of group O cells by IAT and enzyme techniques.

If the serum contains an antibody reacting with all panel cells, an auto-absorption using the patient's own ZZAP-(T.16) or enzyme-treated (T.17A) cells, should be performed. The auto-absorbed serum should be retested against the same panel of cells to disclose any allo-antibody that may be present after the removal of auto-antibodies. If the patient requires blood transfusion, blood compatible with the auto-absorbed serum must be found.

If the patient's RBCs are coated with complement alone and if cold haemagglutinin disease (CHAD) is suspected, a cold antibody titre (T.26) should be performed by testing doubling dilutions of serum with group O adult and O cord RBCs at 4°C and at room temperature. The sera from normal individuals have titres below 64 against group O adult cells at 4°C (i.e. anti-I) while the sera from patients with CHAD usually have cold agglutinin titres above 256, and often greater than 1000. For the DAT, RBCs from an EDTA sample should be washed in warm saline to remove any agglutinating antibody.

The rare condition paroxysmal cold haemoglobinuria (PCH) is typified by a positive Donath-Landsteiner (DL) test (T.25), the causative antibody being a biphasic haemolysin, usually an IgG anti-P. The anti-P specificity can only be determined in reference laboratories with the use of the rare P^k and p cells.

Drug-induced haemolytic anaemias (see T.24)

Alpha-methyldopa (Aldomet®) is the drug that most commonly causes immune haemolytic anaemia, but since it causes a classical warm antibody auto-immune haemolytic anaemia, the serological tests will not require the presence of the drug. If a patient who has been on alpha-methyldopa for more than three months presents with warm auto-immune haemolytic anaemia with IgG coating of the rbcs, the drug is likely to be the cause of the anaemia. On the other hand, if the patient has a positive DAT due to IgG coating of the rbcs and is on very high doses of penicillin or if the positive DAT is due to C3 coating and the patient is on any other particular drug or combination of drugs, further tests for drug-dependent antibodies will often be decisive for the correct diagnosis. Except for cases induced by alpha-methyldopa, the eluates prepared from the patient's red cells will be non-reactive against panel cells.

Penicillin (only in large doses) is the second most common drug to cause immune haemolytic anaemia; the drug binds to the red cells and IgG penicillin antibodies will combine with the drug on the cell surface (drug-adsorption mechanism). Very rarely many other drugs can cause immune haemolytic anaemia and they need not be given in large doses. The drug combines with its antibody in the plasma and the immune complexes bind non-specifically to red cells, leading to complement fixation and haemolysis of a proportion of cells (immune-complex mechanism). The unlysed cells have C3 on their surface which is detected in the DAT.

32

Red blood cell serology

TECHNIQUE 1. WASHING CELLS AND MAKING RED CELL SUSPENSIONS

Suspensions of washed red cells are needed for all haemagglutination tests and also for tests based on haemolysis. The cells must be washed at least once in order to remove plasma, which may lead to the formation of small clots which can be confused with agglutinates, leading to false positive results. In addition, blood group substances in plasma may lead to false negative reactions due to neutralisation of the antibody. Weak cell suspensions are used in haemagglutination tests since the ratio of serum to cells affects the sensitivity of most tests; a minimum number of antibody molecules must bind to the RBCs in order to bring about haemagglutination or to be detected in the antiglobulin test.

Materials
○ Sample of blood or RBCs.
○ Saline.
○ Labelled 75 × 12 mm tubes.

Method
1. Place 0.2–0.5 ml of blood into each tube.
2. Fill the tube to within 1 cm of the top with saline.
3. Centrifuge at 200 g for 1–2 minutes, until the RBCs are packed.
4. Decent the supernatant.
5. Tap the tube to resuspend the RBCs in the residual fluid. This constitutes one wash. Repeat steps 2–5 at least twice. The last wash should always have a clear supernant with no signs of haemolysis.
6. To make a 5% cell suspension, add 1 volume of the packed RBCs to 19 volumes of saline.
7. To make a 3% suspension, add 1 volume packed RBCs to 32 volumes of saline.

Comment
— The word SALINE refers to 0.15 mol/l sodium chloride solution, with its pH adjusted to 7 (see reagents). RBCs are suspended in this saline unless otherwise stated.

TECHNIQUE 2. SLIDE (TILE) TECHNIQUE

This is a rapid technique for use with known agglutinating sera. Some potent IgM ABO antibodies, IgG anti-D reagents that are chemically modified or potentiated and some IgM anti-D reagents will agglutinate RBCs directly without the need for sedimentation or centrifugation. The 'strong' cell suspension brings the RBCs into close contact and agglutination quickly develops. However, weakly acting antibodies will not agglutinate red cells directly by this method.

Materials
○ Opal glass tile, or microscope slides.
○ Test serum.
○ Test RBCs: 10–20% suspension.
○ Wooden applicator sticks (may be cut in 2 or 4).

Method
1. Use a single slide for each test or a ruled 3 cm square on an opal glass tile.
2. Label each section of the tile to identify the reagent and cells used.
3. To 1 drop of serum add 1 drop of a 10–20% cell suspension.
4. Mix reactants with a separate, clean applicator stick to an area with a diameter of 2 cm.
5. Rock the tile (slide) gently and look for agglutination.
6. Record the results immediately.

Comments
— Weak reactions may be missed with this method.
— Reactions should be read within 3 minutes; otherwise drying of reagents will give a false positive appearance.
— For ABO grouping the tile must be kept at room temperature. For D-typing, place the tile/slide over a warmed viewing box.
— The tile should be placed in a moist chamber if a longer incubation time is required.

TECHNIQUE 3. IMMEDIATE SPIN (IS) TECHNIQUE

This technique is suitable for use with direct or saline-agglutinating reagents or with enzyme pre-modified rbcs (T.7A). This is a good method for rapid ABO grouping and Rh(D) typing using adequately standardised antisera. It is also suitable for reverse ABO grouping.

Materials
☐ 75 × 12 mm tubes.
☐ Test serum.
☐ 2–5% suspension of test RBCs.

Method
1. In a tube add 2 drops of serum and 1 drop of the cell suspension. Mix by shaking or tapping gently.
2. Centrifuge at 1000 g for 15–20 seconds.
3. Examine macroscopically, over a light source, for evidence of haemolysis in the supernatant and then for agglutination by gently tapping or shaking and rolling the tube to remove the cell button from the bottom.
4. Record the score for lysis and/or agglutination.

Comment
Reagents prepared for use by an IS technique need to be warmed to ambient temperature before use if stored in refrigerator. With some reagents a short incubation period, after step 1, may be required.

TECHNIQUE 4. AGGLUTINATION OF SALINE SUSPENDED CELLS AT 20°C.

This technique is suitable for routine ABO grouping.

Cells and serum are incubated to allow antigen-antibody binding. Agglutination is speeded up by centrifugation or the tubes can be left for the RBCs to sediment.

Materials
☐ 3% cell suspension.
☐ Serum.
☐ 50 × 7 mm precipitin tubes.

Method
1. Place two volumes (drops) of serum into the tube and add one volume (drop) of 3% cell suspension. Mix gently.
2. Incubate in a 20°C water-bath for 30 minutes.
3. Centrifuge for 1 minute at 200 g at room temperature.
4. Alternatively incubate for 60 minutes, and then centrifugation is not required.
5. Read the reaction over a light source; first examine the supernatant for haemolysis and then look for

agglutination by gently tapping or shaking and rolling the tube to remove the cells from the bottom. In case of doubt, some of the cells can be removed and streaked onto a glass slide and then viewed under the low-power objective of the microscope.
6. Record the score for agglutination and/or haemolysis.

Comment
Suitable for use with IgM (saline agglutinating) antisera; i.e. anti-A and anti-B grouping reagents; and for ABO reverse grouping. One drop of antiserum can be used if stated in the manufacturer's instructions but when dealing with patient's sera, two drops are recommended.

TECHNIQUE 5. AGGLUTINATION OF SALINE SUSPENDED CELLS AT 30 OR 37°C

Materials and method are identical to those described for Technique 4, but incubate at 30 or 37°C. RBCs pre-modified with proteolytic enzymes can also be used by this technique (see T.7A)

TECHNIQUE 6. ALBUMIN ADDITION TECHNIQUE USED FOR Rh(D) TYPING.

This test is accomplished in two stages: first the cells and serum are incubated so that antibody binds to the appropriate antigen (first stage of agglutination); then bovine albumin is added and this draws the rbcs closer together so that the IgG antibodies sensitising the RBCs can bind to adjacent cells forming agglutinates. RBCs uncoated with antibody remain unclumped with the concentration of bovine albumin used.

Materials
☐ 3% red cell suspension.
☐ Serum.
☐ 20% bovine albumin (22% or 30% albumin can be used).
☐ 50 × 7 mm precipitin tubes.

Method
1. Place two volumes of serum and one volume of 3% cells into the tube.
2. Incubate for 30 minutes at 37°C.
3. Centrifuge for one minute (200 g) at room temperature. Alternatively incubate for 60 minutes and then centrifugation is not required.
4. Add one drop of albumin so that it slides down the inside of the tube. Do not mix.
5. Incubate for a further 15 minutes at 37°C.
6. Read and record agglutination as in Technique 3.

Comments

— Not all IgG antibodies will agglutinate red cells by this technique; the antiglobulin technique (see T.9) is more sensitive.

— This is a simple technique for use with selected reagents, especially in routine Rh(D) typing. In these circumstances reagent controls are also necessary. An autologous or reagent control must be used with any albumin addition grouping technique.

— Some commercial reagents have albumin and other polymers added at the manufacturing stage so that they react by a saline, direct agglutination technique. A reagent control must also be used with these 'potentiated' reagents.

ENZYME TECHNIQUES

Used for antibody screening, antibody detection and cell typing with certain antisera.

Some antibodies, especially those with Rh, Kidd and Lewis specificities, will agglutinate or even lyse rbcs that have been treated with a proteolytic enzyme such as papain, ficin, trypsin or bromelin. These enzymes remove some of the negatively charged molecules (mainly sialoglyproteins) from the cell surface, allowing the RBCs to come close enough for IgG molecules to agglutinate them when suspended in saline. On the other hand, a different theory suggests that proteolytic enzymes enhance agglutination by removing part of the hydration layer surrounding the red cells.

Enzyme techniques are not suitable for all blood group systems. The following antigens are destroyed or weakened by enzyme treatment of RBCs: Fy^a, Fy^b, M,N,S,s, En^a, Yt^a, Xg^a, Ge, Ch, Rg, JMH, In^b, Yk^a, Tn, Pr. Some proteolytic enzymes affect certain red cell antigens more than others and some have no effect on some of the above antigens, e.g. chymotrypsin destroys the reactivity of Fy^a, S and s whereas purified trypsin has no effect on these antigens.

The reactions of some cold-reacting antibodies, i.e. anti-P_1, -I, -HI, -A, -B are enhanced using enzyme premodified cells.

As discussed above, an immediate spin technique (T.3) can be used with enzyme-treated cells but is less sensitive than incubating the serum and cells prior to centrifugation.

TECHNIQUE 7A. TWO-STAGE PAPAIN TECHNIQUE OR USE OF PAPAIN PREMODIFIED CELLS.

Materials
□ Packed RBCs.

□ Serum.
□ Stock Löws papain diluted 1 in 10 in saline.
□ 50 × 7 mm precipitin tubes.
□ 75 × 12 mm tubes.

Method

a. Papain premodification

1. In a 75 × 12 mm tube add 4 drops of 0.1% papain to 1 drop of packed cells.

2. Incubate at 37°C for 12 minutes, in a water-bath. The time may vary with the batch of papain and needs to be standardised for each new batch.

3. Wash the treated cells twice in saline.

4. Make up a 3% cell suspension in saline. These cells can be stored at 4°C for up to 48 hours.

b. Use of premodified cells

1. In a precipitin tube mix 1 drop of the papain-treated 3% cell suspension and 1 drop of serum.

2. Incubate at 37°C for 20 minutes.

3. Centrifuge at 200 g for 1 minute at room temperature.

4. Alternatively incubate for 60 minutes and then centrifugation is not required.

5. Read as described in Technique 3, but do *not* read microscopically.

Comment

A similar technique can be used with ficin premodified cells.

TECHNIQUE 7B. BROMELIN SUSPENSION TECHNIQUE

Materials
□ Fresh 0.1% bromelin solution.
□ Packed rbcs.
□ Serum.
□ 50 × 7 mm precipitin tubes.

Method

1. Suspend RBCs to 3% in the 0.1% bromelin solution and leave at room temperature for 5 minutes before use.

2. 1 drop of the cell suspension is added to 1 drop of serum and incubated at 37°C for 20 minutes prior to centrifugation and reading as described in Technique 3. Do *not* read microscopically.

Comment

A fresh cell suspension should be made if the RBCs have been suspended in bromelin for more than 1 hour, but after 5 minutes at room temperature they can be washed, suspended in saline and used as bromelin premodified cells. The main application of this technique is in microplate methods when weaker suspensions of RBCs in bromelin are required (i.e. 1%). This technique, though simpler, is not as sensitive and reliable as techniques with enzyme premodified cells.

Each new batch must be standardised and the concentration of enzyme may have to be varied; see Quality Control section, page 430.

ANTIGLOBULIN TECHNIQUES

Used for antibody screening, antibody detection, cell typing with certain antisera and for compatibility testing. The indirect antiglobulin test (IAT) is performed in four stages:

1. The incubation of test RBCs and test serum at 37°C (sensitisation phase).

2. Washing of RBCs to remove excess protein and free IgG in the suspension medium.

3. The addition of anti-human globulin serum (AHGS).

4. The checking of negative results with IgG-coated control RBCs.

In the first stage, antibody in the serum will bind to the corresponding antigen sites on the RBCs, leading to sensitisation or antibody-coating of the red cells. Some antibodies also partially activate the classical pathway of the complement cascade, thus C4 and C3 may also be present on the RBC membrane if the serum is fresh enough to contain active complement components or if fresh serum is added as a source of complement. The cells are washed thoroughly to remove any protein not attached to the RBCs, thus allowing the AHGS to agglutinate antibody- and/or complement-coated RBCs. A polyspecific ('broad spectrum') AHGS, containing optimum dilutions of anti-IgG and anti-C3d is used for most routine IATs. The polyspecific reagent may also contain anti-C3b, -C4b, -C4d, -IgA and/or anti-IgM.

Control (D-positive) cells coated with IgG anti-D are added to any negative test to ensure that the AHGS is active and that it has not been neutralised by any residual proteins present in the system. These control cells should become agglutinated; failure to do so invalidates the test and the whole procedure should be repeated.

Causes of false positive results in the IAT
— Presence of particulate matter, dust, plastic particles in the tubes.
— Presence of substances in saline which lead to non-specific agglutination of the red cells (colloidal silica from glass containers, metallic ions from metal containers or metal connectors).
— Poorly absorbed AHGS (anti-species) will react with uncoated cells.
— Cross-contamination from one tube to the other or from poorly cleaned cell washers.
— Red cells with a positive direct antiglobulin test.
— Over-centrifugation.
— Failure to detect agglutination before washing the cells.

Causes of false negative results in the IAT
— Inadequate washing of the cells. As little as 1 in 4000 serum in saline will neutralise an equal volume of AHGS.
— Failure to add AHGS (this happens sometimes in machines which add the AHGS automatically or when too many tests are carried out simultaneously).
— Inactive antiglobulin reagent due to inadequate storage conditions, contamination with bacteria or serum, use after expiry date, etc.
— Loss of antigens from the red cell surface due to prolonged or inadequate storage.
— Inactive serum due to inadequate storage conditions e.g. repeated freezing and thawing of reagents.
— Inadequate incubation time or temperature.
— Presence of fibrin clots; these will exude serum even after washing and will neutralise the AHGS.
— Cross-contamination with other tubes (e.g. as when a tube is inverted against the finger which may be contaminated with serum or blood).
— Saline at too low a pH (antibodies elute from RBCs at low pH).
— Excess antigen, i.e. too many red cells in the reaction mixture.
— Over-centrifugation or under-centrifugation.
— Leaving cells for too long before adding AHGS (weakly bound antibodies may elute from the RBCs) and after adding AHGS (positive IATs due to IgG-coating become weaker after incubation).
— In addition, some complement-binding antibodies such as examples of anti-Jk^a and Jk^b can only be detected by IAT in the presence of fresh serum as a source of complement; anticoagulants inhibit complement binding (but see T.10).

TECHNIQUE 8. IAT USING SALINE-SUSPENDED RBCs

The ratio of serum to cells is important, and the larger the volume of serum, the more sensitive the IAT. In general it is recommended that for the detection of antibody in patients' sera and for crossmatching, 3–4 volumes of serum to 1 volume of cell suspension should be used. However, for red cell typing with standardised blood grouping reagents, the manufacturer's instructions should be followed since it may be sufficient to add 1–2 volumes of serum to 1 volume of cell suspension.

Materials
○ 5% cell suspension in saline.
○ Serum or grouping reagent.
○ 75 × 12 mm glass tubes.
○ Anti-human globulin serum (polyspecific or 'broad spectrum' AHGS).
○ Control cells: IgG-coated cells washed 4 times (see T.12A).

Method
1. In a tube, mix 3–4 volumes of serum with 1 volume of cells.

2. Incubate at 37°C for 45–60 minutes.

3. Examine for haemolysis and agglutination. If agglutination is observed, record as positive and do not proceed to 4. A positive result in such circumstances should not be interpreted as being due to IgG or C3 coating. Haemolysis should also be recorded; if partial, proceed to 4.

4. Wash at least three times, automatically in a cell washer or manually. If washing manually, ensure that as much supernatant as possible is removed after each wash and that the cell button is totally resuspended in saline before proceeding to the next wash; this is achieved by tapping or shaking the cell button and then adding saline, with force, from a plastic wash bottle.

5. To the washed, packed cell button which has been shaken from the bottom of the tube, add 2 drops of AHGS and mix.

6. Centrifuge the tubes at 1000 g for 15–20 seconds (the speed and time for each centrifuge varies).

7. Remove the tubes and read visually over a light source as described in Technique 3 or by placing the tube on the stage of an inverted microscope. Alternatively, if no inverted microscope is available, some of the cells can be removed using a clean (new) Pasteur pipette and streaked onto a microscope slide. Read using the low power objective of a microscope.

8. Record results.

9. If the test is negative leave the tube at room temperature for 5 minutes, re-centrifuge and read macro- and microscopically.

10. If the test is still negative, add 1 drop of IgG-coated RBCs.

11. Repeat steps 6 and 7.
A positive reaction indicates that the negative result in step 7 is valid, but if the control IgG-coated cells fail to agglutinate, then the test must be repeated.

TECHNIQUE 9. LOW IONIC STRENGTH INDIRECT ANTIGLOBULIN TECHNIQUE (LISS/IAT)

In LISS techniques, lowering the ionic strength of the reaction medium increases the rate of uptake of most antibodies by antigen; hence incubation times can be reduced. However, if the volume of serum is increased from that recommended in a given LISS technique, the ionic strength of the mixture will increase and the benefits of the technique will be lost. It is therefore important not to deviate from the recommended procedure. Some Kell allo-antibodies react more weakly under low-ionic strength conditions while antibodies of most specificities are enhanced. The first stage of agglutination, i.e. sensitisation, can be modified to make use of this enhancement in two different ways: by suspending the test rbcs in a low-ionic salt solution (LISS) or by using a low-ionic salt addition solution.

9A. LISS-SUSPENSION METHOD

Material
○ Glass tubes 75 × 12 mm.
○ LISS.
○ Test RBCs.
○ Serum.
○ AHGS.
○ Control Rh-positive cells pre-coated with anti-D and washed four times.

Method
1. Wash test RBCs twice in saline and then once in LISS.

2. Resuspend test RBCs in LISS to a 3% suspension.

3. In a tube, mix an equal volume of test serum and LISS-suspended cells. (i.e. 2 or 3 drops from a Pasteur pipette or 100 μl measured volume).

4. Incubate tubes at 37°C for 15 minutes (a water-bath is preferable).

5. Remove tubes, examine for haemolysis and/or agglutination.

6. Wash RBCs at least three times manually or in a cell washer and continue as in Technique 8.

Comment
LISS, LISS-suspended cells and serum should be brought to ambient temperature or above, before use. As the rate of antibody uptake onto RBCs is increased using LISS, cold antibodies that are of no clinical significance may bind to the red cells and activate complement before the reactants reach 37°C, and hence an unwanted positive reaction is obtained. If cold-reacting antibodies are suspected to be present, allow the serum and cell suspension to warm to 37°C before mixing the two.

9B. LISS-ADDITION METHOD

Materials
○ LISS-addition solution.
○ AHGS.
○ 75 × 12 mm glass tubes.
○ Test RBCs and serum.

Method
1. In a tube place 3 drops of serum and one drop of a 5% saline suspension of rbcs.
2. Add 3 drops of LISS-addition solution and mix contents (this volume may vary with different makes of reagent).
3. Proceed as from 4 in Technique 9A.

Comments
— If an immediate spin test at room temperature is required, for the detection of ABO incompatibility for example, centrifuge the tubes after step 1 for 15–20 seconds at 1000 g, examine for agglutination and record. Then mix well, add the LISS-addition reagent and proceed as above. If this technique is used, fewer problems are encountered with cold-reacting antibodies.
— The LISS-addition reagent should be allowed to warm to ambient temperature or above before use to avoid positive reactions due to cold-reacting antibodies.

Albumin IAT
The use of bovine albumin to enhance reactions in the IAT is expensive and unnecessary. Some bovine albumin preparations may inhibit antigen-antibody reactions, whilst those made in a low-ionic strength medium may enhance reactions, but this is an expensive method of reducing ionic strength.

Enzyme IAT
Enzyme premodified rbcs can substitute the untreated red cells in the indirect antiglobulin technique (T.8) but with little advantage except for the detection of Kidd antibodies — the reactions of which are enhanced. This technique is not suitable for routine antibody screening or crossmatching as some antigens are denatured by proteolytic enzymes. Moreover, certain AHGS may give false positive results since enzyme-treated cells have enhanced reactivity with anti-species contaminants.

See also microplate techniques (T.21C).

TECHNIQUE 10. TWO-STAGE ANTIGLOBULIN TECHNIQUE

This technique is used in antibody screening if only a stored serum sample is available or in those cases when the presence of complement-binding antibodies is suspected and cannot be detected by conventional IAT. By using a polyspecific AHGS, both antibody and complement can be detected on the surface of RBCs. In the presence of fresh serum, some antibodies (anti-Fy[a], anti-Jk[a]) activate complement to the C3 stage, and in some cases it is C3 rather than IgG that is detectable in the IAT. On storage, some sera become anticomplementary and, although antibody binds to the RBCs, complement activation, even in the presence of fresh serum, is blocked. The addition of EDTA allows antigen-antibody binding but inhibits complement activation. However, in the second stage of this test, fresh serum is added as a source of complement which can then be activated by the cell-bound antibody in the absence of free anticomplementary serum.

Materials
○ Glass tubes 75 × 12 mm.
○ 4.4% K_2 EDTA solution (pH 7.2).
○ Test serum or grouping reagent.
○ Test RBC suspension in saline.
○ Fresh AB serum devoid of atypical antibodies.
○ Polyspecific AHGS.

Method
1. To 1 ml of test serum add 0.1 ml EDTA solution.
2. Proceed as with steps 1–4 in Technique 8.
3. Add 2 volumes of fresh AB serum to each test tube containing washed packed RBCs.
4. In another set of tubes, as controls, add 2 volumes of the fresh AB serum to 1 volume of each of the washed RBC suspension used in the test.
5. Incubate all tubes at 37°C for 15 minutes.
6. Wash three times in saline.
7. Proceed as with steps 5–10 in Technique 8.

Comment
Step 4 is to ensure that the fresh AB serum does not contain antibodies active against the test RBCs.

TECHNIQUE 11. DIRECT ANTIGLOBULIN TEST (DAT)

Anti-human globulin serum is used to detect the presence of antibody and/or complement directly on an individual's RBCs due to in vivo sensitisation. Unlike the indirect test, no incubation of serum and cells is required.

Red cells may be sensitised in vivo by auto-antibodies, as in auto-immune haemolytic anaemias or by allo-antibodies, as in haemolytic transfusion reactions or in haemolytic disease of the newborn.

Materials
○ Glass tubes 75 × 12 mm.
○ 5% cell suspension in saline.
○ Polyspecific AHGS and/or monospecific reagents

Method
1. Wash 1 volume of cell suspension at least three times, automatically in a cell washer, or manually as in step 4 of Technique 8.
2. Add 2 volumes of AHGS and proceed as in steps 5–10 of the IAT (T.8).

Comments
— Polyspecific or monospecific AHGS (anti-IgG, -IgA, -C3d, -C3c, etc.) can be used. For routine testing a polyspecific reagent will suffice, and it is only for the detailed investigation of warm auto-immune haemolytic anaemias that monospecific reagents may be required.
— For reliable results, blood should be collected into an EDTA anticoagulant and the test performed as soon as possible since stored samples tend to bind complement components non-specifically, leading to false positive results.

TECHNIQUE 12. PREPARATION OF CONTROL CELLS FOR THE ANTIGLOBULIN TEST

12A. IgG-COATED RED CELLS.

Group O Rh-positive RBCs are coated with IgG anti-D to give a ++ to +++ reaction when added to the mixture of AHGs and cells of a negative DAT or IAT. These control are added to show that the AHGS is still active.

Materials
○ Group O Rh-positive rbcs.
○ Anti-D (1 IU/ml).

Method
1. Wash the RBCs three times in saline.
2. Add an equal volume of anti-D to the packed RBCs.
3. Incubate at 37°C for 30 minutes.
4. Wash the rbcs four times.
5. Suspend in saline to a 5% suspension.
6. Take 1 volume of the 5% suspension, add 2 volumes of the routine broad spectrum AHGS and test by the antiglobulin technique, which should give a ++++ reaction.
7. These sensitised RBCs can be stored at 4°C for 48 hours.

12B. C3-COATED RED CELLS

As anti-C3d is the most important anti-complement component to be included in a broad spectrum AHGS, it is advisable to have C3-coated cells in the laboratory for use as controls with polyspecific AHGS and monospecific anti-C3 reagents. C3 coated cells are added to all tubes showing negative antiglobulin tests with anti-C3. After re-centrifugation all tubes should give positive reactions for the tests to be considered valid. The cells can also be used to control the presence of anti-C3 activity in polyspecific AHGS.

In very low ionic-strength conditions, complement components present in a fresh blood sample are taken up onto RBCs non-specifically. If these conditions are met in the presence of EDTA and at low temperatures, C3 will preferentially bind to RBCs.

Materials
○ LIS-sucrose solution.
○ Calcium chloride solution.
○ Fresh group O blood (collected into ACD or CPD; not EDTA).
○ Ice-bath.

Method
1. To 10 ml LIS-sucrose solution add 0.05 ml calcium chloride solution. Mix and place the tube into a beaker containing ice.
2. Add 0.5 ml fresh blood, mix contents immediately.
3. Incubate the tube in the melting ice for 15 minutes, mixing occasionally.
4. Wash the RBCs three to four times in ice-cold saline. Usually less washing is required for C-coated than for IgG-coated cells due to the lower concentration of complement components in serum.
5. Make a 5% suspension of the cells in saline.
6. Test by the antiglobulin technique with broad spectrum AHGS or with anti-C3; complete (++++) agglutination should be observed.

TECHNIQUE 13. TITRATION

The titre of an antibody is a semi-quantitative reflection of its concentration in a given serum. Titres can also help to determine the relative strength of a given antigen in different cell samples (e.g. MM cells usually give a higher titre with a given anti-M than MN cells). One of the most useful applications of titrations is in the follow-up of samples from antenatal patients with antibodies that may cause haemolytic disease of the newborn. For results to be meaningful it is important to test samples taken at different stages of gestation in parallel, under the same test conditions.

Occasionally titrations will help to determine the specificity of antibodies in a mixture when the serum is titrated against panel cells of different phenotypes. Titrations may also disclose 'high-titre, low-avidity' (HTLA) antibodies which react only weakly with neat serum but to a high titre.

Materials

○ Glass tubes 75 × 12 mm.
○ Test serum.
○ Cell suspensions of appropriate phenotypes.
○ Hand-held dispenser (pipette) with disposable tips.

Method

Two-fold master dilutions are prepared in 75 × 12 mm tubes as follows:

1. Into 9 tubes, labelled 2 to 10, deliver a constant volume (e.g. 0.5 ml) of isotonic saline or AB serum.

2. Tube no. 1 will contain a fixed volume of neat test serum (e.g. 0.5 ml). Into tube no. 2 add the same volume of test serum as in 1 (i.e. the same as the volume of saline or AB serum). This is mixed several times, using a clean pipette tip, to give a 1 in 2 dilution.

3. Remove a fixed volume from tube 2 and add to tube no. 3, mix to give a 1 in 4 dilution.

4. The process is repeated, with a clean pipette tip for each dilution, to the end of the row of tubes.

5. An aliquot of each dilution is then used and tested against the appropriate cells, depending upon which technique has been selected for the titration (e.g. saline, IAT). The same pipette tip may be used if the highest dilution, i.e. from tube no. 10, is dispensed first.

Techniques are performed, read and scored as described previously (e.g. saline, IAT). The titre is the reciprocal of the highest dilution that shows a positive reaction, (i.e. if the 1 in 64 dilution gives a positive reaction but the 1 in 128 dilution does not, the titre is 64). However, a score provides a better idea of the strength of an antibody than a titre. For example, when comparing two sera containing antibodies of the same specificity and using the scoring system on page 404:

Test serum	Dilutions									Score
	1	2	4	8	16	32	64	128	256	
X	C	C	+++	++	+	+	(+)−	−		55
Y	C	C	C	+++	+++	++	+	−	−	71

Although both test sera have a titre of 64, serum Y contains the stronger antibody with a score of 71, compared with serum X, with a score of 55. As stated previously, a difference in score greater than 10 is significant.

TECHNIQUE 14. MANUAL POLYBRENE TECHNIQUE (MPT)

Can be used as a rapid technique for antibody detection or for red cell typing.

The technique is performed in three stages. The cells and serum are incubated in a low-ionic strength medium to enhance antibody uptake. Polybrene, a polycation, is then added to 'aggregate' the rbcs, this enables IgG antibodies present to form intercellular bridges. The non-specific aggregation is reversed by the addition of sodium citrate, leaving only the specific antibody-mediated haemagglutination.

Materials

○ Glass tubes, 75 × 12 mm.
○ Serum.
○ 3% red cell suspension in saline.
○ LIM (low-ionic strength medium).
○ Polybrene solution (0.05%).
○ Resuspending solution (sodium citrate).

Method

1. To each tube add:
   2 volumes of serum (60 μl approx.)
   1 volumes of RBC suspension
   0.6 ml LIM.
   Mix and incubate at room temperature for 1 minute.

2. Add 2 volumes of Polybrene solution and mix. Incubate for 15 seconds at room temperature.

3. Centrifuge at 1000 g for 10 seconds.

4. Decant supernatant.

5. Add 2 volumes of resuspending solution and mix gently by rolling the tubes over the bench top or light source.

6. Within 10 seconds, the aggregates dissociate leaving behind the true agglutinates, if present.

7. The test can be taken to the antiglobulin phase, without further incubation, by washing three times in saline and adding AHGS in the usual way (see T.8).

Comment

Some antibodies, particularly examples of anti-K and some examples of anti-Fy^a, do **NOT** react by the Polybrene technique even when this is taken to the antiglobulin phase. For this reason, if used in antibody screening, in pre-transfusion testing, the MPT must be used in combination with other techniques. On the other hand, due to its very short incubation time, the technique can be used for rapid RBC typing using standardised antisera or for the rapid detection or identification of antibodies.

TECHNIQUE 15. ANTIBODY ELUTION

Elution techniques are used to remove antibody which has coated the red cells in vivo from patients with auto-immune haemolytic anaemia, haemolytic transfusion reactions or in haemolytic disease of the newborn. The procedure is also useful in specialised antibody identification tests involving in vitro absorption/elution techniques. Antigen-antibody binding is a reversible reaction which depends on weak physico-chemical forces holding the molecules together. To remove or elute antibodies from antigens these forces can be broken by altering the ionic strength or pH of the system, or by using organic solvents or extreme temperature changes. No one red cell elution technique has proved better than the others but some are technically simpler or more efficient at removing particular antibody specificities and are therefore used more often.

General note. With all elution techniques the saline from the last wash must be saved and tested in parallel with the eluate. The last wash must be non-reactive for eluate results to be considered valid.

15A. HEAT ELUTION

Materials
○ 75 × 12 mm tubes.
○ Test RBCs.
○ Water-bath or heating block at 56°C.
○ 3% bovine serum albumin (optional)

Method
1. Wash 0.5–1 ml RBCs six times, packing them firmly during the last wash by centrifugation for 5 minutes at 200 g.
2. To the packed RBCs add an equal volume of saline or 3% bovine albumin.
3. Incubate at 56°C, mixing occasionally, for 10 minutes.
4. Centrifuge immediately for 3 minutes at 200 g (use a centrifuge warmed to 40°C if available).
5. Separate the eluate, i.e. the top layer, from the sedimented stroma and transfer it to a clean tube.

Comments
— Heat elution is efficient for ABO antibodies; it is suitable in those cases where ABO haemolytic disease of the newborn is suspected.
— When it is necessary to dissociate IgG from red cells with a positive DAT, leaving the cells intact for cell typing or for enzyme-treatment, use a mild heat elution at 45–48°C for 3–5 minutes, following the above procedure.

15B. FREEZE-THAW (LUI) ELUTION

Materials
○ 75 × 12 mm tubes.
○ Test RBCs.
○ 20–22% bovine serum albumin.
○ Deep-freezer.

Method
1. Wash 0.5–1 ml RBCs six times and pack them firmly as in 15A.
2. To 10 volumes of packed RBCs add 2 volumes of 20–22% bovine albumin.
3. Cap the tube and roll it on its side so that the cells form a film on the wall.
4. Lay the tube on its side in a deep-freezer at −20°C to −30°C until frozen, (a minimum of 10 min).
5. Thaw the cells at 37°C.
6. Centrifuge at 200 g for 3 minutes.
7. Separate the eluate, which is the top layer, from the RBC stroma.

Comments
— The cells can be left overnight or for longer in the deep-freezer (step 4) if necessary.
— This technique is also suitable for ABO antibodies.

15C. ETHER/HEAT ELUTION

Materials
○ Test RBCs.
○ 56°C water-bath.
○ Large glass tube.
○ Ether.

Method
1. As in Technique 15A, steps 1 and 2.
2. Add 1 volume of ether to 10 volumes of rbc suspension (take care when pipetting ether as heat from the hand on the bulb of the pipette causes rapid expansion of the ether).
3. Mix well by tapping the tube. Do *not* cap the tube.
4. Place in the 56°C water-bath.
5. Mix carefully by agitating the tube whilst the ether boils off.
6. Leave at 56°C for a total of 10 minutes.
7. Centrifuge the tube and remove the eluate, which is the cherry-red top layer. Do not use the eluate until the smell of ether has disappeared completely.

Comment
Ether is highly inflammable and must be stored in a spark-proof refrigerator.

15D. CHLOROFORM ELUTION TECHNIQUE

Materials
○ Chloroform.
○ Test RBCs.
○ 56°C water-bath.
○ Glass tubes 75 × 12 mm.

Method
1. Wash the 0.5–1 ml red cells six times, packing them firmly as in 15A. Transfer the cells to a clean glass tube.
2. Add 1 volume of cells to 1 volume of saline plus 2 volumes of chloroform.
3. Shake hard for 10 seconds, mix several times by inversion for 1 minute.
4. Leave at 56°C for 5 minutes. Stir occasionally with an applicator stick. Do *not* leave tube capped whilst it is at 56°C.
5. Centrifuge at 200 g for 5 minutes; the top layer is the eluate.

Comment
A suitable technique for investigating a suspected case of warm auto-immune haemolytic anaemia or a haemolytic transfusion reaction involving Rh antibodies.

TECHNIQUE 4. AGGLUTINATION OF SALINE RBCs WITH A POSITIVE DAT USING ZZAP

It is sometimes necessary to strip the IgG molecules from cells with a positive DAT (see section on warm auto-immune haemolytic anaemias).

Materials
□ Fresh ZZAP solution (mixture of DTT and a proteolytic enzyme).
□ Test RBCs with a positive DAT.

Method
1. Add 2 volumes of ZZAP to 1 volume of packed RBCs (need not be washed) in duplicate tubes.
2. Mix periodically during incubation at 37°C for 30 minutes.
3. Wash three times in excess saline and pack the cells firmly after the last wash by centrifuging for 5 minutes at 200 g.
4. The DAT should be negative or considerably weaker.

Comments
— The ZZAP-treated cells can be used for typing for most blood group systems, *except* for MNSs, Duffy

or Kell since the antigens in such systems are inactivated by ZZAP.
— If the cells are to be used for auto-absorption, a large volume should be treated with ZZAP and the packed cells should be divided into three tubes. The procedure is the same as in Technique 17A, steps 5–9.

TECHNIQUE 17A. AUTO-ABSORPTION USING PAPAIN-TREATED CELLS

When a papain-reacting, pan-agglutinating auto-antibody is detected in a patient's serum, an auto-absorption is advisable to determine whether an underlying allo-antibody is present. If the DAT is positive, a mild heat elution (see comment in T.15A) should be performed before enzyme treatment.

Materials
○ Glass tubes, 75 × 12 mm.
○ 0.1% papain.
○ Test RBCs.
○ Test serum.

Method

a. Treatment of RBCs
1. Thoroughly wash about 1 ml of patient's cells (obtained from an EDTA sample) with 0.9% saline (minimum of 4 washes).
2. Add 1 volume of packed washed cells (e.g. 1 ml) to 4 volumes of 0.1% papain. Mix and incubate in a water-bath at 37°C for 12 minutes (the incubation time may vary with each papain batch).
3. Wash three times in 0.9% saline. Finally pack the cells by centrifugation.
4. Divide the papain-treated packed cells into three equal parts and dispense into 75 × 12 mm tubes.

b. Auto-absorption
5. To one tube, add an equal volume of patient's serum, mix and incubate at 37°C for 30 minutes. Mix occasionally.
6. Centrifuge and carefully remove the supernatant serum, placing it into the second tube containing papain-treated packed cells.
7. Mix and incubate at 37°C for a further 30 minutes, and repeat the absorption with tube 3.
8. Centrifuge, then carefully remove the auto-absorbed serum into a clean test tube.
9. Test the auto-absorbed serum against a panel of cells by two-stage papain technique. Include the auto control.

Comment

ZZAP-treated cells can be used instead of papain-treated cells from steps 5 to 8.

17B. AUTO-ABSORPTION OF COLD-REACTING ANTIBODIES

If a serum sample contains a cold-reacting auto-antibody that is masking possible reactions in grouping or is interfering with antibody detection techniques, it can be removed by auto-absorption.

Method

If the antibody is weak, place a clotted sample of blood into the refrigerator at 4°C for 30 minutes. Centrifuge the sample and immediately remove the supernatant serum into a clean tube. Warm the serum to the temperature of the test before use, i.e. room temperature or 37°C.

If more potent antibodies are present, adopt the following procedures:

1. Wash three times a large aliquot of RBCs in saline warmed to 37°C. This should remove any antibody bound to the RBCs which can then be used for typing or for the auto-absorption procedures.

2. Add 1 volume of serum to 1 volume of well-packed warm-washed RBCs and incubate at 4°C for 30 minutes.

3. Centrifuge the sample and immediately remove the supernatant serum into a clean tube. Pre-warm the serum to the temperature of the test being used.

If there are still traces of cold auto-antibody after one auto-absorption, the procedure should be repeated until the auto-antibodies fail to interfere with routine tests at room temperature (ABO reverse grouping) or 37°C (antibody screening).

TECHNIQUE 18. INACTIVATION OF THE AGGLUTINATING ACTIVITY OF IgM ANTIBODIES USING DITHIOTHREITOL (DTT)

This technique is used to detect the presence of IgG antibodies when IgM antibodies are also present.

Principle

DTT is a reducing agent which inactivates the agglutinating capacity of IgM antibodies by breaking the inter subunit disulphide bonds and the J chain that hold the 5 subunits of the molecules together. Thus the J chain and the IgM subunits are released. In most cases the subunits will be able to bind to the specific antigen without bringing about agglutination.

18A. STANDARD TECHNIQUE FOR IgM INACTIVATION

Materials

○ Freshly thawed or freshly prepared 0.01 mol/l DTT solution.
○ Test serum.
○ Test RBCs.

Method

1. Incubate 1 volume of test serum with 1 volume DTT at 37°C for 30 minutes.

2. Control: 1 volume serum with 1 volume PBS is incubated simultaneously.

3. The serum is then ready for use, or may be frozen at −20°C or below. Use freshly thawed.

4. Titrate both treated and control sera with saline-suspended cells at 20°C and by IAT with anti-IgG against suitable cells.

18B. RAPID TECHNIQUE FOR IgM INACTIVATION USED IN DETECTING MATERNAL IgG ANTI-A/B

Materials

○ 75 × 12 mm tubes.
○ 0.01 mol/l DTT.
○ Test (maternal) serum.
○ A₁ or B cells.
○ Anti-IgG.

Method

1. In a tube labelled no. 1, place 1 volume of maternal serum and 7 volumes of DTT, mix.

2. Into 9 labelled tubes place 4 volumes of saline.

3. Into tube 2 add 4 volumes of serum/DTT mixture from tube 1 and mix.

4. Continue with the doubling-dilution (see T.11) discarding 4 volumes from tube 10.

5. Add 1 volume of 5% A₁ or B cell suspension to each tube.

6. Mix and incubate at 37°C for 30 minutes.

7. Centrifuge the tubes at 1000 g for 15–20 seconds.

8. Examine visually and record any agglutination seen.

9. Perform an antiglobulin test using anti-IgG, on those tubes not showing agglutination (Technique 8, steps 4–11).

10. The IgG titre of the anti-A or anti-B is the highest dilution giving a positive result with the anti-IgG reagent.

Comment

This is a rapid technique in which maternal serum is

diluted 1 in 8 in the DTT reagent and doubling dilutions are made and tested against suitable cell suspensions without the need for pre-incubation of the serum and DTT. The titre of any IgM antibody present will not be determined but only that of IgG antibodies. An IgG anti-A or anti-B titre greater than 64 can be considered as an indication of an 'immune' maternal anti-A and/or -B. In the vast majority of cases, group O maternal serum is titrated since ABO hdn occurs mainly in A or B infants born to group O mothers.

TECHNIQUE 19. ROSETTE TECHNIQUE FOR THE DETECTION OF A MINOR RED CELL POPULATION

Principle
This technique can be used to demonstrate any minor cell population that has one RBC antigen different to that of the major population and for which a potent specific antibody is available.

If a small proportion of the red cells in a population are coated with IgG it will be difficult to detect them by an IAT. However, indicator red cells, carrying the antigen reactive with the potent IgG antibody used, will adhere specifically to the antibody coating the cells in the minor population, forming clusters or rosettes, easily visible using a microscope. This technique is useful in determining the extent of transplacental haemorrhage of a Rh(D) positive infant into the circulation of its Rh(D) negative mother or the percentage of Rh-positive RBCs in an Rh-negative recipient of a transfusion of Rh-positive blood. An organ transplant contains a small volume of donor blood and if an Rh-negative recipient receives an Rh-positive transplant the volume of Rh-positive blood in the recipient's circulation can be estimated by this technique.

This account describes the detection of Rh(D) positive cells in an Rh(D) negative individual

Materials
- 75 × 12 mm glass tubes.
- Potent anti-D grouping reagent.
- Unknown: 3% washed saline suspension of patient's RBCs.
- Negative control: 3% washed, saline-suspended group O rr (cde/cde) RBCs.
- Positive controls: a) 5% Rh-positive: 1 vol. of 3% O R_2R_2 (cDE/cDE) cells plus 19 vol. of 3% O rr cells; mix well. b) 0.5% Rh-positive: add 1 vol. of the 5% control to 9 vol. 3% group O rr cells; mix well.
- Indicator cells: 0.2% suspension of papain-treated R_2R_2 cells.

Method
1. Add 2 volumes of patient's RBCs to a tube. Do same with each control (i.e. 4 tubes are required altogether).
2. To each tube add 3 volumes of the potent anti-D and mix well.
3. Incubate at 37°C for 30 minutes.
4. Wash tubes five times in saline.
5. Gently resuspend the RBCs and to each tube add 3 volumes of the suspension of papain-treated indicator cells.
6. Incubate at 37°C for a further 30 minutes.
7. Centrifuge for 15 seconds at 1000 g.
8. Examine the test and control tubes microscopically using a low-powered objective.
9. Compare the number of rosettes in the test tube (patient's cells) with the 5% and 0.5% controls and estimate, by approximation, the percentage of Rh-positive cells present in the patient's blood.

TECHNIQUE 20. NEUTRALISATION/INHIBITION TECHNIQUE

Principle
Neutralisation techniques can be used to determine the presence of antigens in body fluids (e.g. ABH in saliva to determine secretor status), fetal ABO type, (from amniotic fluid), or used to confirm the specificity of an antibody using a known 'substance'. Antigens such as A, B, H, Le^a, Le^b, Ch^a, Rg^a and I are found not only on rbcs but also in body fluids: plasma, amniotic fluid, saliva, urine, semen etc. In fact some of these antigens are primarily in plasma and are adsorbed onto red cells. Also, a structure sharing the terminal disaccharide with P and P_1 antigens is present in hydatid cyst fluid (with scolices). If the appropriate fluid is incubated with a serum suspected of having the corresponding antibody, the soluble antigens will readily bind to their specific antibody so that there may not be any antibody remaining to bind to RBC antigens when cells are added to the test system. Thus the soluble antigen has 'neutralised' the antibody or 'inhibited' its activity.

Materials
- Antigen-containing substance or fluid (saliva should be boiled and diluted 1 in 2 in saline).
- Test serum.
- Test RBCs.

(Either the serum or the RBCs are of known specificity.)

Method

1. Mix equal volumes of substance and serum.

2. As a control, mix equal volumes of saline and serum.

3. Incubate for 10–15 minutes at room temperature.

4. Appropriate volumes of the test and control can then be tested by the technique most appropriate for the system, i.e. if an anti-A serum is incubated with saliva, the aliquot of the mixture is tested with group A RBCs by saline room temperature technique.

TECHNIQUE 21. THE USE OF MICROPLATES

Microplates, i.e. plastic plates with 96 U- or V-shaped wells, can be used in any of the preceding techniques in place of 50×7 mm precipitin tubes and also for antiglobulin tests.

Haemagglutination can be read by tilting the plates at an angle of 70° to the horizontal and allowing the cells to 'trail'; with positive reactions the cell button remains in the bottom of the well, negative reactions run or trail. More conventionally, reactions can be read by looking for agglutination after resuspending the cell button. Resuspension can be achieved by tapping the plates or, more conveniently, using a mechanical plate-shaker. The ease of handling microplates makes them efficient to use when testing large numbers of samples, but a centrifuge that can carry these plates is necessary. Many bench-top centrifuges can be adapted to take microplate carriers. Automated and semi-automated pipetting systems that will dispense reagents or cells to several wells simultaneously are available.

In general, the sensitivity of tests in microplates is equal to, or even greater than that of conventional tube techniques. The smaller volumes used mean, generally, that microplate techniques are more economical; but reagents manufactured for tube techniques must be standardised before they are used in microplates.

21A. ABO AND Rh(D) TYPING USING U-WELL MICROPLATES

Materials

○ Test cells and serum.

○ Standard ABO grouping reagents.

○ ABO panel cells.

○ Albumin addition (IgG) anti-D reagent or other IgG anti-D reagent.

○ U-well microplates.

○ 0.1% bromelin.

○ Centrifuge capable of taking microplate carriers.

ABO Typing

Preparation of test red cells

Wash RBCs once in saline and suspend to 1% in either saline or 0.1% bromelin-saline (leave the latter at room temperature for at least 5 minutes before use — if not used within 1 hour, wash, resuspend in saline and use as bromelin-treated cells).

1. Into 3 U-wells place 1 volume ($25 \mu l$) of anti-A, -B and -A,B. Then add 1 volume of patient's cells to each well.

2. As an auto control, in a fourth well, add 1 volume of patient's RBCs to 1 volume of patient's serum.

3. Into the next 4 wells add 1 volume of patient's serum to 1 volume of each of A_1, A_2, B and O panel cells.

4. Mix on a plate-shaker for 5 seconds.

5. Incubate at room temperature for at least 15 minutes; then lightly centrifuge (100 g for 30–60 s).

6. Mix on a plate-shaker for approximately 5 seconds or until the negative controls are resuspended.

7. Read macroscopically with the aid of a plate-reading mirror, looking for agglutination as in tube techniques.

Rh (D) Typing

1. Use either saline- or bromelin-suspended RBCs (see above).

2. Add 1 volume of patient's cells to each of 3 wells containing 1 volume of 2 different anti-D reagents and a control AB serum.

3. Mix on a plate-shaker.

4. Cover the plate with a lid and incubate at 37°C (in an incubator) for at least 15 minutes and centrifuge as 6 above.

5. If saline-suspended cells are used add 1 drop of 20% bovine albumin to each well, and re-incubate at 37°C for 10 minutes before centrifugation. If bromelin-suspended cells are used *do not add albumin*.

6. Mix plate on plate-shaker for approximately 5 seconds.

7. Read macroscopically with aid of a plate-reading mirror.

Comments

— Adequate controls must be set up with each batch tested, i.e. A_2 and B cells as a minimum for ABO grouping and Rh(D) positive and negative cells (preferably r′r Cde/cde), for Rh typing.

— To prevent lysis of reagent red cells in the serum or reverse group, suspend the A_1, A_2, B and O RBCs in EDTA-saline: 4.4 g K_2EDTA added to 100 ml 1 mol/l NaOH and made up to 1000 ml with normal saline pH 7.0.

— If a 'saline-reactive' anti-D is used the rbcs should not be suspended in bromelin nor albumin added.

21B. USE OF ENZYME PREMODIFIED CELLS IN MICROPLATES

Cells pre-treated with proteolytic enzymes can be used in U-well microplates using a 1–2% cell suspension and read as above, (T.21A, step 7). V-well plates have also been used, with reactions read by tilting the plate after centrifugation as in Technique 21C, steps 7 and 8.

21C. INDIRECT ANTIGLOBULIN TESTS (IAT) USING MICROPLATES

The same principles as for the IAT in tubes apply.

Materials
○ V-well microplates.
○ A stand to hold plates at 70° to the horizontal.
○ Test RBCs: 3% suspension in LISS.
○ Sera or IgG reagent.
○ Polyspecific anti-human globulin serum (AHGS).

Method
1. In a well, add 25 μl of serum to 25 μl of test RBCs; mix the contents either on a plate-mixer or by tapping the plate.
2. Cover the plate and incubate in a warm air (37°C) incubator for 20 minutes.
3. Centrifuge the plate (100–200 g for 30–60 s) to pack the RBCs, decant the supernatant.
4. Resuspend the cell button by mixing as in 1, and add 200 μl of saline.
5. Centrifuge the plate again, decant the supernatant (see comments) and repeat this washing process 3 or 4 times.
6. After the last wash, decant the supernatant, resuspend the packed cells in the saline which has remained in the well (*do not add* more saline) and add 1 volume of AHGS.
7. Mix, and centrifuge the plate to lightly pack the RBCs (75–100 g 20–40 s).
8. Tilt the plate at 70° and allow the RBCs to 'trail' for about 5 minutes.
Positive reaction: a monolayer of RBCs or a button of RBCs that stays in the bottom of the well.
Negative reaction: a streak or trail of RBCs.
9. To all negative tests add 1 volume of IgG-sensitised RBCs, mix well, re-centrifuge and read as in 7. The test must now be positive for a valid negative result to be recorded.

Comments
— Centrifugation times and speeds are given as guidelines, but each machine must be calibrated to obtain optimal results. Variations to this technique include the use of saline containing 0.1% bovine albumin and 0.02% Tween 20 for washing the cells. Some workers do not mix after adding the AHGS and the plates are incubated for a further 2–5 minutes before centrifugation.
— During washing, the supernatant can be removed either by 'flicking-off' (a potentially hazardous procedure) or aspirated using a pipette, a multi-channel pipette or a semi-automated system.

TECHNIQUE 22. SOLID-PHASE BLOOD GROUPING

Despite several different approaches, the successful automation of all pre-transfusion tests has not been satisfactorily achieved. The major obstacle, inherent to liquid-phase haemagglutination techniques, is the lack of an objective end point.

We have developed a series of solid-phase assays which utilise red cell adherence as the end point. The sensitivity and specificity of these solid-phase adherence assays compare favourably with conventional haemagglutination methods.

Principle
Solid-phase blood grouping assays depend on the immobilisation of either antigen or antibody on microplate wells. Subsequent capture of analyte, usually red cell-bound antibody or antigen, is recognised by formation of a monolayer of red cells over the entire microplate well. A negative reaction is characterised by a central pellet of red cells. This common objective end point of adherence or non-adherence of indicator red cells permits easy interpretation of results either visually or spectrophotometrically.

Test samples
☐ Venous or capillary blood diluted in bromelin solution for ABO and Rh blood group determination.
☐ Serum for reverse ABO grouping.

Reagents
● Bromelin, (see T.7B).
● Normal saline.
● Monoclonal anti-A.
● Monoclonal anti-B.
● Rabbit anti-human red cell antibody.
● Anti-D.
● Goat anti-human-IgG (affinity purified).
● Group A and B human RBCs.

Equipment

○ Polystyrene U-bottom microplates.
○ Microplate centrifuge.
○ Reagent dispenser.

Methods

A. ABO cell grouping

Preparation of plate

1. Add 100 μl anti-A and anti-B to separate micro-wells.
2. Stand plate overnight at 4°C.
3. Wash 4 times with saline.
4. Store moist at 4°C until use.

Performance of test

1. Add 30 μl of 0.5% saline-suspended bromelin-treated test red cells to each microwell.
2. Centrifuge at 190 g for 1 minute.

B. Rh (D) grouping

Preparation of plate

1. Add 100 μl of goat anti-human IgG to microwells.
2. Stand plate overnight at 4°C.
3. Wash 4 times with saline.
4. Add 100 μl anti-D (eluate or monoclonal).
5. Store moist until use at 4°C.

Performance of test

1. Add 30 μl of 0.5% saline-suspended bromelin-treated test red cells.
2. Centrifuge at 190 g for 1 minute.

C. ABO serum grouping

Preparation of plate

1. Add 100 μl of a 10 μg/μl solution of rabbit anti-human red cell antibody to microplate wells.
2. Stand plate overnight at 4°C.
3. Wash 4 times with saline.
4. Add 100 μl of 0.5% bromelin-treated A_1 or B red cells.
5. Centrifuge to immobilise the cells on wells.
6. Add 100 μl distilled water to haemolyse immobilised red cells.
7. Wash 4 times with saline.
8. Store moist at 4°C until use.

Performance of test

1. Add 30 μl of test serum to wells containing A_1 membranes.
2. Add 30 μl of test serum to wells containing B membranes.
3. Stand 5 minutes at room temperature.
4. Invert plate and blot dry on paper towel.
5. Add 30 μl of 0.5% bromelin-treated A_1 or B indicator red cells (e.g. add A_1 indicator cells to wells coated with A_1 membranes).
6. Centrifuge at 190 g for 1 minute.

Results

Positive reactions are characterised by effacement of the indicator test red cells. Negative reactions result in a central pellet of indicator or test red cells. Results are easily distinguished visually or may be read spectrophotometrically at 405 nm. Using the MR-580 Microelisa Auto Reader (Dynatech Labs. Inc.), modified to offset the light beam 1.5 mm from the centre, an absorbance value of 0.253 was selected as the cut-off to differentiate between positive and negative results.

Comment

Monoclonal sources of anti-A and anti-B have proved superior to eluates. We expect this to hold for anti-D, in which case the initial coat of anti-human IgG would not be required. Solid-phase Rh(D) typing appears to detect D^u samples.

TECHNIQUE 23. PREPARATION AND USE OF LECTINS: APPLICATIONS TO BLOOD GROUP SEROLOGY

The most useful red blood cell antigen- or cryptantigen-specific lectins are obtained from seeds of plants of the Natural Orders *Leguminosae* or *Labiatae*.

Preparation of seed extracts

1. Leguminous seeds are put into a beaker and an excess of water is added.
2. The seeds should be left to soak overnight.
3. Next morning the water is discarded and the now swollen seeds placed in a mortar.
4. About 3 volumes of 0.9% sodium chloride solution are added to 1 volume of swollen seeds and then macerated with a pestle until they are reduced to pulp.
5. Some fluid is lost by evaporation and by continued absorption: the loss should be adjusted by eye by topping up with the saline solution.
6. The mixture is centrifuged and the supernatant crude lectin taken off.

Labiate seeds do not need to be soaked. They should be placed straight into a mortar and treated as described above.

Use of lectins in blood group serology

Lectins act best on white ceramic tiles. The specificity and avidity of a lectin is readily demonstrated by this method. Lectins are also suitable for use in tube techniques, both by gravity sedimentation and 'immediate spin'. A 10% suspension of red cells should be used for tile tests, a 2% suspension for tube tests. The tests are read by the naked eye: tube tests should also be read under the low power of the microscope after carefully pipetting the red cell deposit on to a slide.

ABO grouping

The distinction of A_1 or A_1B red cells from those of weaker forms of A or AB is made by use of the *Dolichos biflorus* lectin.

1. 1 drop of the test red cell suspension and 1 drop each of known A_1, A_2, A_1B and A_2B cells (controls) are placed on the tile and to each is added 1 drop of lectin preparation.

2. The red cells and lectin are mixed thoroughly, preferably with a plastic stirring rod which should be wiped clean with a cloth or tissue after each use.

3. The tile is gently rocked.

The A_1/A_2 or A_1B/A_2B distinction is easily made. A_1 and A_1B cells are strongly agglutinated in a matter of seconds: A_2 and A_2B cells are weakly agglutinated after several minutes. In standard tube tests A_1 and A_1B cells show large agglutinates, A_2 and A_2B cells small agglutinates among unagglutinated cells.

Lectins in the detection of red cell cryptantigens or of polyagglutinable red cells

The panel of lectins shown in Table 32.1 should be used by both tile and tube techniques. The reactions given by various red cell cryptantigens or polyagglutinable erythrocytes are given in Table 32.1. T-cells may be prepared in the laboratory. The other red cells on the panel should be obtained from various donors or patients and stored in the frozen state.

Table 32.1 Lectins in the elucidation of red cell polyagglutinability or detection of red cell cryptantigens

Lectin	Natural Order	Red cells (group O)					
		T	Tk	Th	Tx	Tn	Cad
Arachis hypogaea	Leg	+	+	+	+	−	−
Griffonia simplicifolia II	Leg	−	+	−	−	−	−
Vicia cretica	Leg	+	+	−	−	−	−
Glycine soja	Leg	+	−	−	−	+	+
Salvia sclarea	Lab	−	−	−	−	+	−
Leonurus cardiaca	Lab	w	−	−	−	−	+

Leg = *Leguminosae*; Lab = *Labiatae*

Preparation of T cells

1. Dissolve the contents of one vial (500 units) of Behringwerke Receptor Destroying Enzyme (RDE)® in 2.5 ml distilled water.

2. To 1 volume of washed packed group 0 cells add 1 volume of the enzyme (neuraminidase) solution.

3. Incubate the mixture for 1 hour at 37°C.

4. Wash the cells and resuspend them in 0.9% solution of sodium chloride in distilled water.

TECHNIQUE 24. METHODS FOR THE INVESTIGATION OF A SUSPECTED DRUG-INDUCED IMMUNE HAEMOLYTIC ANAEMIA

Principle

Other, than alpha-methyldopa (Aldomet®) -induced auto-antibodies, some antibodies to drugs, such as penicillin, will react with red cells coated with that drug (drug adsorption mechanism) whilst others will react in the presence of the drug and complement (immune complex mechanism). However, the demonstration in vitro of a drug-dependent antibody does not prove that it is causing the anaemia. In fact, many individuals possess penicillin antibodies without any signs of haemolysis during or after a course of the drug. Clinical evidence that the haemolysis may be due to the drug therapy is required and is of greater importance than the serological tests.

Materials

○ The daily dose of the implicated drug or 1 million units penicillin.
○ Phosphate-buffered saline pH 7.
○ 0.1 mol/l barbital buffer pH 9.6.
○ 1 mol/l NaOH.
○ 1 mol/l HCl.
○ Patient's serum and washed RBCs.
○ 2 or 3 group 0 screening cells containing, between them, the major RBC antigens i.e. routine screening cells.
○ Fresh AB serum.
○ pH meter or suitable indicators.
○ Polyspecific AHGS, anti-IgG and anti-C3d.

24A. DRUG-ADSORPTION MECHANISM

Method

a. Preparation of drug (penicillin)-coated cells

1. Dissolve 1 million units of penicillin in 15 ml 0.1 mol/l sodium barbital solution.

2. Wash the group 0 screening cells three times in saline and pack them firmly.

3. To 1 volume of each of the packed RBCs add approximately 15 volumes of penicillin solution (i.e. to 0.5 ml RBCs add 7.5 ml penicillin solution).

4. Mix and incubate at room temperature for 1 hour with continuous stirring.

5. Wash the cells three times in saline (the first washes may show signs of haemolysis but the last wash should be clear).

6. The penicillin-coated RBCs can be kept in CPD or a preservative solution at 4°C for up to one week but must be washed before use.

Comment. This technique can be used for other drugs suspected to react by the same mechanism as penicillin. In the absence of a barbital buffer, penicillin-coated rbcs can be prepared in saline, but adsorption is more efficient at an alkaline pH.

b. The test

1. Perform a DAT (T.II) on the drug-coated RBCs; this should be negative.

2. Perform standard IATs (T.8) using the patient's serum with the 2–3 drug-coated RBCs and with autologous RBCs.

3. Test the patient's serum against the 2–3 untreated antibody-screening cells by IAT; these should be negative.

Comment. If the patient's DAT is positive the test with autologous RBCs is not required.

24B. IMMUNE COMPLEX MECHANISM

This method is used as a first choice when there is a suspicion of a drug-induced immune haemolytic anaemia not involving alpha-methyldopa or penicillin, and especially when the DAT is positive due to C3 coating the patient's cells.

Method

a. Preparation of the drug

1. If the implicated drug is in tablet form, crush the daily dose and dissolve it/suspend it in 10 ml PBS.

2. Mix overnight at 4°C on a rotating mixer or at 37°C for 1 hour.

3. Centrifuge the suspension and remove the supernatant into a clean tube.

4. Adjust the pH of the supernatant to between 6.5 and 7.5 using either 0.1 mol/l NaOH or 0.1 mol/l HCl (diluting the 1 mol/l stock solutions 1 in 10).

5. Make doubling dilutions of the drug supernatant in PBS and mix 1 volume of each dilution with 1 volume drop of a 5% saline suspension of one of the group 0 screening cells. Incubate at room temperature for 15 minutes, centrifuge the tubes and select, as the working dilution, the highest concentration of drug solution that does not haemolyse the RBCs.

b. The test

1. In a 75 × 12 mm tube add: 1 volume of a 5% suspension of group O screening cells,
   2 volumes of the working dilution of drug solution,
   2 volumes of AB serum and

3 volumes of patient's serum.
Repeat same procedure for each screening RBC sample.

2. Include the following as negative controls for each RBC sample used:

   a. 1 volume of RBC plus 2 volumes of AB serum and 3 volumes of patient's serum.

   b. 1 volume of RBC plus 2 volumes of AB serum and 2 volumes of drug solution.

3. Mix, incubate at 37°C for 60 minutes.

4. Wash the RBCs and perform an antiglobulin test using a polyspecific AHGS. If a positive result is found in the test tubes i.e. the tubes in 1 above, repeat using anti-C3d to confirm that the haemolysis is due to the immune complex mechanism.

Comments

— If there is a positive reaction with only one of the screening cells it may be an indication that the drug may have a 'preference' for a particular RBC antigen, and a whole panel of cells will have to be tested by the relevant technique.

— If a drug-induced haemolytic anaemia is suspected with a drug not known to have been implicated in the past, it is better to start with a test for the immune complex mechanism (T.24B) since, although Aldomet and penicillin-induced haemolytic anaemias are the most common, the majority of cases implicating other drugs are due to the immune complex mechanism.

— Patients treated with alpha-methyldopa may develop true warm auto-antibodies and in such cases the serological tests do not require the presence of the drug in the system. The same procedure as for the investigation of warm auto-immune haemolytic anaemias should be followed.

TECHNIQUE 25. DONATH-LANDSTEINER (D-L) ANTIBODY TEST

Principle

Paroxysmal cold haemoglobinuria, (PCH), is caused by an IgG auto-antibody, usually with anti-P specificity, that binds to the RBCs in the cold but activates complement and causes lysis at or near 37°C. This 'biphasic' antibody can be demonstrated by the direct or indirect Donath-Landsteiner test. Whenever fresh blood samples are available it is better to perform the direct test.

Materials

☐ Ice-bath (0–1°C).
☐ 37°C water-bath or incubator.
☐ Fresh normal serum.
☐ Group O RBCs: 40–50% saline } for the indirect
   suspension } test

Methods

25A. Direct D-L test

1. Collect a sample of blood from the patient, placing 5 ml into each of two plain tubes and take them to the laboratory in a container at 37°C

2. Place one tube in the ice-bath for 30 minutes and leave the other at 37°C for 1 hour.

3. Remove the tube from the ice-bath and incubate it at 37°C for 30 minutes.

4. Centrifuge both tubes for 1 minute at 200 g at room temperature and compare both supernatant sera.

5. The test is positive if there is haemolysis in the tube that has been incubated both in the cold and at 37°C but not in the tube kept at 37°C throughout i.e., the negative control.

25B. Indirect D-L test

1. Use patient's serum that has been separated from a clotted specimen kept at 37°C.

2. Into each of two tubes place:
5 volumes of patient's serum.
5 volumes of fresh normal, ABO-compatible serum.
Place one at 37°C and the other in the ice-bath.

3. As controls, set up two tubes each containing 5 drops of fresh normal serum, place one at 37°C and the other in the ice-bath.

4. Place an aliquot of the 40–50% suspension of group O cells in a tube at 37°C and another aliquot in the ice-bath. After 10 minutes add 1 volume of these RBCs to the corresponding serum at each temperature; mix the contents.

5. The tubes at 37°C are incubated for 1 hour and the tubes in the ice-bath are incubated at this temperature for 30 minutes and then placed at 37°C for 30 minutes.

6. Centrifuge all the tubes at room temperature for 1 minute at 200 g.

7. Read as in the direct test. The test is positive if only the tube containing the patient's serum and incubated sequentially at both temperatures, shows haemolysis. The other 3 tubes are all negative controls.

TECHNIQUE 26. COLD AGGLUTININ TITRE

In cold haemagglutinin disease (CHAD) an antibody, usually with anti-I or, rarely, anti-i specificity, is present to a high titre and reacts optimally at about 4°C and in general at temperatures below 30°C. Depending on the thermal range of the antibody, following exposure to the cold, the patient may suffer from some intravascular haemolysis but those RBCs not destroyed become coated with C3d and, as there are no receptors on macrophages for C3d, these RBCs survive almost normally. In CHAD, therefore, a high titre cold-reacting auto-antibody and RBCs with a positive DAT due to C3d coating are found. Following some acute infections (e.g. mycoplasma) the cold agglutinin titre may also be raised, but rarely is a positive DAT found.

Method

1. Collect a sample of blood from the patient and take it to the laboratory in a container (i.e. a vacuum flask) at 37°C.

2. Place the sample at 37°C to clot, then centrifuge it and immediately remove the supernatant, transferring it to a clean tube.

3. Make doubling dilutions of the serum from a dilution of 1 in 2 to 1 in 32 000 (15 tubes) — see Technique 13. The starting dilution can be 1 in 20 or 1 in 50 and then only 10 tubes are needed.

4. Prepare two sets of precipitin tubes containing 1 volume of each dilution and 1 volume of a 3% suspension of group O adult (I) cells; two sets with serum dilutions and group O cord (i) cells and, another (optional) two sets with group O adult i cells, if available.

5. Incubate one of each sets of tubes at 4°C and the other at room temperature for 1 hour.

6. Score the agglutination as in previous techniques.

Comments

— In CHAD the titre with adult O or cord O cells is usually > 128 at room temperature and > 1000 at 4°C.

— Anti-I reacts more strongly with adult cells and anti-i more strongly with cord cells or with the very rare adult i cells.

TECHNIQUE 27. PRESERVATION OF REAGENT RBCs

27A. STORAGE IN THE LIQUID STATE AT 4°C

Principle

RBCs can be stored for reagent use at 4°C for 3–4 weeks in ACD or CPD or in a solution containing sodium chloride and sodium citrate. A modification of this solution containing buffer salts and antibiotics will prolong RBC storage. Screening cells, ABO control cells for reverse grouping and panel cells need to be preserved for several weeks.

Materials

○ Red cell preservative solution.
○ Sterile bijou bottles or similar vials.
○ Packed red cells.

Method

1. Aliquot 2 ml of the sterile preservative solution into the bijou bottles.
2. Add 2 ml of RBCs and mix.
3. Store at 4°C.
4. For use, wash the RBCs in saline until the supernatant is free of haemoglobin.

Comment

Screening and panel cells can be washed in sterile saline and a 5% suspension made in the modified preservative solution. These can be used for up to 6 weeks with no significant loss of reactivity of the clinically important red cell antigens.

27B. STORAGE IN THE FROZEN STATE USING GLYCIGEL

Principle

RBCs can be preserved in the frozen state using glycerol, which, by increasing the tonicity of the cells, protects them against excessive dehydration and against the formation of water crystals during freezing and thawing. Small volumes of cells with rare groups or with a particular combination of antigens, such as those held by reference laboratories undertaking specialised serological investigations, can be stored for years using this technique.

Materials

☐ Glycigel in 0.5 ml aliquots.
☐ Recovery solutions:
  50% dextrose in water
  10% dextrose saline
  saline.
☐ −60 to −80°C deep freezer.

Method

Freezing the RBCs

1. Wash the RBCs four times in saline. The cells can be collected into any anticoagulant but should be as fresh as possible and ideally not older than one week.
2. Warm sufficient tubes containing Glycigel to 37°C for the contents to liquefy.
3. Add an equal volume of RBCs and mix.
4. Store the tubes at − 60°C or below.

Recovery of the RBCs

1. Thaw the contents of the required number of tubes at 37°C and transfer to a large, 100 × 12 mm or 100 × 16 mm tube. If only a small volume of cells is required, only part of the contents of a tube will be needed and the rest can be returned to the freezer.

2. Add an equal volume of 50% dextrose and mix.
3. Fill the tube with 10% dextrose saline. Centrifuge to pack the RBCs and then decant the supernatant.
4. Wash the RBCs twice in 10% dextrose saline.
5. Then wash the RBCs twice in saline.

Comments

— Both the recovery of RBCs and the maintenance of RBC antigens is good with this technique.
— If a tube is thawed, but the contents are not all used, the remainder can be refrozen without significantly affecting the subsequent survival of the RBCs.

TECHNIQUE 28. CONVERSION OF PLASMA TO SERUM

28A. HEAT TREATMENT

It is preferable to use serum rather than plasma in serological tests because the fibrinogen in plasma may form small clots which may be confused with agglutinates.

Heating plasma to 56°C for 60 minutes denatures fibrinogen, which then precipitates, and concurrently inactivates complement and possibly viruses.

Materials

☐ 56°C water-bath.
☐ Bench-top centrifuge.

Method

1. Separate the plasma from the RBCs and buffy coat.
2. Place the plasma in a container (preferably glass) that can be centrifuged.
3. Place the container at 56°C and allow the contents to warm to 56°C.
4. Leave at 56°C for 1 hour.
5. Centrifuge the heat-treated plasma and transfer the supernatant (serum) to a clean tube.
6. The serum may need further centrifugation and/or filtration before use.

28B. NEUTRALISATION OF HEPARIN

The blood from patients on heparin treatment or undergoing extracorporeal circulation may not clot in vitro when taken into tubes unless the heparin is neutralised.

Materials

☐ 1% saline solution of protamine sulphate.
☐ Patient's blood.

Method

1. To 5 ml of whole blood add 1–2 drops of the protamine sulphate solution and mix well.

2. Leave to stand for 2–5 minutes.

3. Centrifuge for 1 minute at 1000 g and transfer the clear supernatant to a clean tube.

QUALITY CONTROL IN BLOOD GROUP SEROLOGY

(Following recommendations of the Council of Europe)

Saline

Criteria for each batch:

NaCl content: 0.85 g/dl (0.15 mol/l) pH 6.5 to 7.5 (add buffer if necessary)

Visual appearance: clear, no particles or microbial
(check daily)   growth

LISS

Criteria for each batch:

Conductivity: 3.4–3.8 m. mho at 23°C
pH: 6.5 to 7.0

Visual appearance: clear, no particles or microbial
(check daily)   growth

ABO reagents

Potency

Undiluted serum should give a +++ to ++++ reaction in saline tests in tubes using a 3% RBC suspension at room temperature. Titres should be at least 128 for anti-A, anti-B and anti-A, B with A_1 and/or B RBCs; 64 with A_2 and/or A_2B RBCs.

Avidity

Using the slide test, macroscopic agglutination appearing with a 40% RBC suspension in homologous serum within 5 seconds for anti-A, anti-B and anti-A,B with A_1 and/or B-cells, 20 seconds with A_2 and A_2B RBCs.

Reactivity and specificity

No immune haemolysis, rouleaux formation or prozone phenomenon. Clear-cut reactions with RBCs bearing the corresponding antigen(s). No false positive or false negative reactions.

Visual appearance (check daily)

Clear, free from precipitates, particles or gel-formation.

Daily quality control

Clear-cut, +++ to ++++ reactions with RBCs bearing the corresponding antigen(s), no false reactions or haemolysis.

Rh reagents

Potency

Undiluted serum to give a +++ to ++++ reaction with the appropriate positive control cells and a titre of 32 for anti-D, anti-C, anti-E, anti-CD, anti-DE and anti-CDE by the described technique.

Reactivity and specificity

As for ABO-antisera. Free from anti-A and anti-B.

Avidity (for rapid slide anti-D reagents)

Visible agglutination appearing within 30 seconds with 40% R_1r (CDe/cde) RBC suspension in homologous serum.

Visual appearance (check daily)

Clear, free from precipitates, particles or gel-formation.

Daily quality control

Clear-cut, +++ to ++++ reactions with RBCs bearing the corresponding antigens(s), no false reactions or haemolysis.

Proteolytic enzyme preparations

Potency

An IgG antibody, preferably anti-D, standardised to give a titre of 64–128 by the protease technique with positive control cells, should show the same titre on repeated testing with different batches of an enzyme preparation against cells of the same Rh phenotype.

Reactivity (check daily)

No agglutination or haemolysis using inert AB-serum. Visual agglutination of Rh-positive cells with a weak IgG anti-D (0.1 IU/ml). *Note.* 1 μg anti-D = 5 IU.

Polyspecific antiglobulin reagents

Reactivity and specificity

a. No haemolytic activity and no agglutination of unsensitised washed RBCs of any ABO group.

b. No agglutination of washed RBCs from donor blood stored at 4°C until expiry date.

c. Agglutination of RBCs sensitised with anti-D containing 0.2 IU/ml antibody activity.

d. Agglutination of RBCs sensitised with a complement-binding allo-antibody (e.g. anti-Le^a) to a higher titre in the presence than in the absence of complement.

e. Agglutination of RBCs coated with C3b and C3d.

Visual appearance (check daily)

Clear, free from precipitate, particles or gel-formation.

Daily quality control

Agglutination of RBCs sensitised with control 0.2 IU/ml

anti-D. No agglutination of the same RBCs incubated at the same time with inert AB serum, or with unsensitised RBCs from units of donor blood stored for their full shelf life.

Bovine serum albumin

Purity
> 98% albumin as determined by electrophoresis.

Reactivity
No agglutination of unsensitised RBCs; no haemolytic activity; no prozone or 'tailing' phenomena; no rouleaux formation. Agglutination of R_1r (CDe/cde) RBCs sensitised with 0.5 IU/ml anti-D.

Visual appearance
Clear, free from precipitates, particles or gel-formation.

Reagent red cells

Reactivity and specificity
Clear-cut reactions with selected antisera against declared RBC antigens.

Visual inspection (check daily)
No haemolysis or turbidity in the supernatant or discolouration of RBCs; free from fibrin clots.

Red cells used for screening for atypical antibodies should be a pair (or a trio) of group O cells containing between them the following antigens;
D, C, c, E, e, K, k, Fy^a, Fy^b,
Jk^a, Jk^b, M, N, S, s, P_1, Le^a, Le^b;
where possible the Rh, Duffy and Kidd antigens should be expressed in double-dose (e.g. Fy (a+b−).

Equipment
The following daily checks are recommended:

Water-baths, heating blocks, incubators
Check that the temperature is within the stated range before and during use.

Refrigerators/freezers
Check that the temperature has not been out of the acceptable range, re-check during the day.

Centrifuges
Check to ensure each machine is clean before and after use, plus a visual inspection of rotors, buckets and liners for corrosion, cracks, etc.

Cell washers
As for centrifuges, but ensure that the inside of the bowl is not wet (this could indicate tubes are being overfilled) and check to ensure there is no saline (or dried salt) on any electrical connection.

Deionisers/stills
Check water quality.

Storage of donor blood
Blood for transfusion should be stored in a cabinet with a circulating fan at a temperature of 4 to 6°C (British Standard Specification). The cabinet should be fitted with a high (8°C), low (2°C) and mains failure audible and visual alarm sited at a station manned 24 hours a day. A thermograph recording the liquid temperature and a dial or digital thermometer showing the air temperature within the cabinet are also mandatory.

COMPOSITION OF SOLUTIONS USED IN RED BLOOD CELL SEROLOGY

Phosphate buffers

Buffer A — acidic buffer
0.15 mol/l Sodium dihydrogen phosphate

Sodium dihydrogen phosphate dihydrate		23.4 g
(anhydrous	18.0 g)	
Deionised water, up to		1000 ml

Buffer B — alkaline buffer
0.15 mol/l Disodium hydrogen phosphate

Disodium hydrogen phosphate dodecahydrate		53.7 g
(dihydrate	26.7 g)	
(anhydrous	21.3 g)	
Deionised water, up to		1000 ml

Comment
Equal volumes of these two buffers, when mixed, should have a pH 6.7. The pH can be varied by altering the volumes of acidic and alkaline buffers; 40 ml buffer A plus 60 ml buffer B gives pH 7.0.

Saline
(0.85% or 0.15 mol/l sodium chloride solution)
8.5 g NaCl dissolved in 1 litre of fresh distilled or deionised water.

Add 10 ml phosphate buffer pH 7.0.

Check the pH, which should be within the range 6.5–7.5. If the pH is out of range, add more buffer.

Phosphate-buffered saline (PBS)
900 ml saline
100 ml of a mixture of 0.15 mol/l phosphate buffers (see above) at the required pH value.

Low ionic strength salt solution (LISS) of Moore and Mollison

Glycine	18 g
NaCl	1.79 g
NaOH	1 mol/l

Phosphate buffer pH 6.7 (see above)

The glycine is dissolved in approximately 500 ml distilled water. NaOH is added drop-wise while stirring, until the pH reaches 6.7 (approximately 0.35 ml of 1 mol/l NaOH is needed). 20 ml phosphate buffer are added, followed by 1.79 g NaCl dissolved in approximately 100 ml distilled water. The mixture is made up to one litre with distilled water, and 0.5 g sodium azide may be added to stop microbial contamination. The conductivity of the final solution should be 3.4 to 3.8 m mho/cm at 23°C.

Cysteine activated Löws papain solution (1%)

Sorensen's buffer pH 5.4

Potassium dihydrogen phosphate	8.83 g
Disodium hydrogen phosphate dodecahydrate	0.72 g
(dihydrate	0.36 g)
(anhydrous	0.29 g)
Deionised water, up to	1000 ml

B. 1% papain solution

a. 10 g papain powder are ground in a mortar with a small volume of Sorensen's phosphate buffer. The suspension is made up to approximately 500 ml with the same buffer and filtered.

b. 4.375 g L-cysteine hydrochloride are added to the filtrate and the volume made up to 1000 ml with more Sorensen's buffer.

c. The solution is incubated in a water-bath at 37°C for one hour starting from the time when the solution reaches 37°C.

d. Centrifuge and discard any undissolved papain.

e. The activated papain solution is stored in 0.5–1.0 ml aliquots at −20°C or below, for up to 6 months. After thawing, any unused enzyme solution should be discarded and not refrozen.

Bromelin solution (0.1% bromelin in saline)

To 0.1 g bromelin powder add 0.5 ml saline and emulsify, add 9.5 ml saline and mix well for 2–3 minutes, centrifuge, transfer supernatant to a volumetric flask and make the volume up to 100 ml with saline. This solution should be made fresh daily.

0.01 mol/l Dithiothreitol (DTT)

0.154 g DTT dissolved in 100 ml PBS pH 7.

Aliquot and store at −20°C or below for up to 6 months.

LIS-sucrose solution

Sucrose	100 g
$Na_2HPO_4.12H_2O$	0.05 g
KH_2PO_4	1.06 g
Na_2EDTA	0.37 g
Distilled water	1000 ml

The pH of this solution should be 5.15.

Reagents for the manual Polybrene technique

Stock solutions

a. 5% dextrose

Dextrose	5.0 g
Distilled water	100 ml

b. 10% Polybrene (hexadimethrine bromide)

Polybrene	10 g
0.9% NaCl	100 ml

Store in a plastic container.

c. 0.2 mol/l trisodium citrate

Trisodium citrate ($Na_3C_6H_5O_7$. $2H_2O$)	5.8 g

Distilled water to 100 ml in a volumetric flask.

Working solutions

a. LIM or low ionic medium

5% dextrose	100 ml
EDTA (disodium salt)	0.2 g

Adjust pH to 6.4 with 3 mol/l NaOH

b. 0.05% Polybrene

10% Polybrene stock solution	0.5 ml
0.9% NaCl	99.5 ml

c. Resuspension solution

0.2 mol/l trisodium citrate	60 ml
5% dextrose	40 ml

ZZAP

0.2 mol/l DTT	2.5 ml
1% cysteine-activated papain	0.5 ml
Saline (ideally PBS pH 7.3)	2.0 ml

The pH of the final solution should be in the 6–7 range.

Neutralised K_2EDTA solution (pH 7.2–7.3)

$K_2EDTA.2 H_2O$	4.4 g
NaOH 1 mol/l	100 ml

Add 0.1 ml of this solution to 1 ml serum to inactivate complement. A 1 in 10 dilution of the above solution (100 ml solution in 900 ml saline) is used to suspend ABO cells to prevent lysis in the ABO reverse group.

1 mol/l NaOH

40 g NaOH in 1000 ml distilled or de-ionised water.

Calcium chloride solution

$CaCl_2.H_2O$	0.6 g
Distilled water to	10 ml

Glycigel reagent for freezing red cells

For Glycigel

Glycerol	62.9 ml
Sodium chloride	0.9 g
Gelatin	2.5 g
Na$_2$EDTA	0.3 g

a. To 62.9 ml glycerol add distilled water to 100 ml.

b. Add NaCl and warm the solution in a beaker.

c. Stir in the gelatin and warm until liquefied.

d. Finally add EDTA.

e. Aliquot 0.5 ml of the solution in 2 ml plastic tubes and store at 4°C (the capacity of the tubes should be at least twice the volume of Glycigel solution added).

Recovery solutions:

1. 50% w/v dextrose in distilled water.
2. 10% w/v dextrose in saline.

Simple red cell preservation solution

Trisodium citrate (dihydrate)	8.0 g
Dextrose	19.0 g
Sodium chloride	4.2 g
Citric acid (monohydrate)	0.5 g
Water to	1000 ml

Red cell preservation solution

Trisodium citrate (dihydrate)	16.0 g
Sodium chloride	8.4 g
Dextrose	41.0 g
Inosine	0.4 g
Disodium ATP	0.4 g
Chloramphenicol	0.4 g
Neomycin sulphate	0.1 g
Dissolve in distilled water	1000 ml

Modified red cell preservation solution

Solution 1

1. Sodium citrate	2.0	g
2. Citric acid (anhydrous)	0.175	g
3. Sodium chloride	0.375	g
4. Dextrose	8.0	g
5. Chloramphenicol	0.250	g
6. Neomycin sulphate	0.070	g
7. NaH$_2$PO$_4$	0.45	g
8. Na$_2$HPO$_4$	1.75	g
9. Adenine	0.035	g
10. Inosine	0.070	g
11. Magnesium chloride	0.0875	g
12. Potassium chloride	0.125	g
13. Sodium bicarbonate	0.875	g

Dissolve in 200 ml distilled water

Solution 2

Hydrocortisone 0.150 g dissolved in 200 ml hot distilled water.

Solutions 1 and 2 are combined and the total volume made up to 500 ml with water and filtered through a Whatman No. 4 filter paper to remove excess hydrocortisone and then finally sterilised using a sterile membrane filter (0.2 micron).

The hydrocortisone can be omitted with a consequent reduction in shelf life of the stored red cells. The total volume without hydrocortisone should still be 500 ml.

Barbital buffer pH 9.6

20.6 g sodium barbital is dissolve in 1 litre of saline. The pH is adjusted to 9.6 with 0.1 mol/l HCl.

33

White blood cell serology

HLA TYPING

Matching for human leucocyte antigens (HLA antigens) plays an important role in the outcome of organ transplants. The HLA antigens are controlled by a group of linked loci which encode two types of product; the HLA-A, -B and -C (Class I) antigens and the HLA-DR and DQ (Class II) antigens. Each of these series of antigens is polymorphic with, for example, over 30 different HLA-B antigens and over 10 HLA-DR antigens. The majority of individuals are heterozygous for each of the HLA series of antigens.

Principle

HLA antigen determination (tissue typing) is carried out on peripheral blood lymphocytes. Both B and T cells express Class I antigens but only the B cells express Class II antigens. HLA antigens are identified by using panels of allo-antisera with specific activity against the different HLA variants in microcytotoxicity tests. The technique described for Class II typing is based on the identification of B cells using fluoresceinated anti-immunoglobulin and does not require that the B cells be physically separated.

Reagents

- 10% calcium gluconate.
- 1% protamine sulphate.
- Thrombin, 50 IU/ml in phosphate-buffered saline (PBS).
- Ficoll/Isopaque.
- Hanks (HBSS).
- RPMI.
- Complement fixation test (CFT) diluent.
- Fluoresceinated sheep anti-human immunoglobulin (FITC SaH-Ig).
- Paraffin oil.
- Panels of allo-antisera to define HLA Class I and II specificities.
- Selected rabbit complement.
- Ethidium bromide solution.

Equipment

A. Class I
- Plastic test tubes with 10 ml capacity.
- Suitable bench-top centrifuge.
- 60-well plastic Terasaki microtest plates (Sterilin, UK).
- Single and multi (6 channels) 1 μl and 5 μl repeat dispensers (e.g. Hamilton syringes).
- Inverted phase-contrast microscope with plate holder and mechanical stage.

B. Class II
- Plastic tubes with 2 ml capacity.
- Suitable bench-top centrifuge.
- 37°C water-bath or incubator.
- Single 0.5 μl and 2 μl repeat dispensers and a multi (6 channels) 0.5 μl dispenser.
- 60-well glass-bottomed microtest plates (Hamax, Norway).
- Inverted UV epifluorescence microscope (excitation filter 485/20, beam splitter 510 and barrier filter 520) with holder and mechanical stage.

Method

Preparation of typing plates and test samples
For both Class I and Class II typing, the typing plates are prepared in advance in batches and stored at −40°C until required. We use three plates (i.e. 180 different sera) for basic Class I typing and one plate (57 sera) for Class II typing. The sera are added to the plates under paraffin oil using multi-dispensers, 1 μl of serum per well for Class I and 0.5 μl of serum per well for Class II typing.

Lymphocytes for HLA typing are obtained from defibrinated venous blood. If the blood is freshly drawn, defibrinate directly by rotating in a conical flask with 3 mm diameter glass beads for about 10 minutes. If the blood is citrated (2 ml 3.8% sodium citrate/10 ml of blood), add calcium gluconate (0.6 ml/10 ml blood) and

435

thrombin (0.2 ml/10 ml blood) to the flask together with the blood. If the blood is drawn into preservative-free heparin, add protamine sulphate (0.3 ml/10 ml blood) and thrombin (0.2 ml/10 ml blood).

Mix defibrinated blood with an equal volume of Hanks medium. Carefully layer the diluted blood on top of 2.5 ml of Ficoll/Isopaque in 10 ml test tubes. Centrifuge the tubes at 1000 g for 20 minutes. Pipette off the mononuclear cells, the majority of which are lymphocytes, from the interface and wash in medium.

A. Class I typing

1. Wash 1–2 million lymphocytes in CFT diluent and resuspend in CFT at a concentration of 1.25 million cells/ml.

2. Add 1 μl of the cell suspension to the serum in each well of the pre-prepared typing plates. Incubate at 20–22°C for 30 minutes.

3. Add 5 μl of rabbit complement to each of the wells. Incubate the plates at 20–22°C for a further 60 minutes. (The complement is diluted 1 in 2 with CFT diluent before use.)

4. Assess and record the percentage of the cells in each well which are dead (see comments). Under phase contrast live cells have a bright appearance while dead cells appear dark and shrivelled (Fig. 33.1).

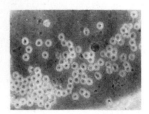 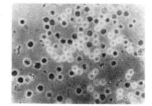

NEGATIVE CONTROL   60% POSITIVE

Fig. 33.1 Complement-mediated lymphocytotoxicity. Lymphocytes treated with antibody and complement. In the negative control, the living cells (light) reflect and do not absorb the light. The 60% positive section shows numerous dead cells visualised as 'flat' dark closed circles. (Phase contrast; Wild-fluotar 20× objective 10× eyepiece)

B. Class II typing

1. Suspend 2 million lymphocytes in RPMI in a 2 ml tube and incubate in a water-bath at 37°C for one hour to reduce non-specific labelling.

2. Centrifuge the cells and resuspend in 0.2 ml of RPMI. Add 10 μl of FITC SaH-Ig diluted 1 in 2 in PBS, mix and incubate at 37°C for 10 minutes.

3. Wash the cells three times to remove excess FITC and resuspend in RPMI at a final concentration of 10–15 million cells/ml (equivalent to 1–1.5 million B cells/ml in normal samples). Check the cell concentration and labelling. For samples with a high proportion of Class II-positive cells (e.g. spleen samples and certain leukaemias) the cell concentration should be reduced accordingly.

4. Dispense 0.5 μl of cell suspension into each well of the prepared typing plate. Incubate at 20–22°C in the dark for 60 minutes.

5. Add 2 μl of rabbit complement to each well and incubate in the dark at 20–22°C for a further 120 minutes.

6. Add 0.5 μl of ethidium bromide solution to each of the wells.

7. Assess and record the percentage of B cells dead in each well. The B cells can be identified by the green label on their surface under epifluorescence, and dead cells take up ethidium bromide, which fluoresces red.

Comments

Class I typing

When using phase-contrast microscopy to determine cell death it is not necessary to add dye (e.g. Eosin or Trypan Blue) to distinguish live and dead cells. However, as the cytotoxic reactions are not halted even by the addition of dye and/or formalin, the plates must be assessed promptly. The plates can also be re-assessed after a further short incubation time, which may clarify previously equivocal reactions with weak antisera.

Class II typing

The main advantages of using the double immunofluorescence technique are that B cell separation can be avoided and fewer lymphocytes are required than when a separation technique is used (2 million vs 5–10 million). However this method does require special equipment (dispensers, plates and microscope) and in the majority of laboratories, B cells are separated using negative (e.g. sheep red blood cell rosetting) or positive (e.g. nylon wool columns or Fab anti-Ig on plates) selection methods. The isolated B cells can then be tested using standard equipment.

For both Class I and Class II

Selection and characterisation of the reagents (human allo-antisera and rabbit complement) are vital factors in obtaining an accurate HLA typing.

In the future, specific monoclonal antibodies may also contribute to HLA typing; at the moment, few are available.

Interpretation

Monospecific Class I antisera are not available for many

specificities and most are defined by panels of sera with different combinations of reactivity. 'Inappropriate' reactions due to cross-reactivity may occur with cells which are not in optimal condition (from patients, for example) and with cells from individuals homozygous for one of the Class I antigens.

Considerable experience and knowledge of the HLA system are required to correctly interpret the results of Class I typing.

Monospecific sera are available for the majority of Class II antigens presently defined, but some definitions do require the use of panels of differently reacting sera, and some assignments of DR specificity are based upon known DQ antigen associations. Factors which can affect the confidence of antigen assignment are the possible presence of Class I antibodies in the sera and (in the case of separation techniques) the purity of the B cell suspension used.

Composition of reagents

RPMI 1640
100 ml of RPMI 1640 (Flow Laboratories UK) is supplemented with 10 ml of L-glutamine (29.23 mg/ml) and 10 ml of cloxacillin-ampicillin-gentamicin (CAG).

CAG
500 mg of Ampiclox and 32 mg of gentamicin are diluted in 20 ml of double-distilled water.

Hanks basal salt solution (HBSS)
50 ml of Hanks (10×), 15 ml of 4.6% $NaHCO_3$, 5 ml of CAG and distilled water up to 500 ml.

Ficoll/Isopaque
72 g of Ficoll (M. Wt. 400 000; Pharmacia Fine Chemicals) and 160 ml of Isopaque (Nyegaard) diluted in 992 ml of distilled water. The density of the solution is adjusted to 1.078 g/ml at room temperature and sterilised in an autoclave.

Ethidium bromide solution
Stock: 100 μg/ml in PBS. Keep in the refrigerator in the dark. Before use, dilute stock 1 in 70 with 5% ethylenediaminetetra-acetic acid, disodium salt (EDTA) in PBS. Can be prepared in advance, aliquoted and kept frozen until required.

Fluoresceinated sheep anti-human immunoglobulin e.g. MFO1: Wellcome
Reconstituted with distilled water, diluted 1:1 with PBS before use.

DETECTION OF NEUTROPHIL-SPECIFIC ANTIBODIES AND ANTIGENS

Antigens on neutrophilic granulocytes may be shared by other cells or may be specific for neutrophils. The shared antigens are HLA Class I antigens and non-HLA antigens, such as antigens from the 5, 9 and Mart systems.

Neutrophil-specific antigens, designated with an N, belong to different systems i.e. the NA, NB, NC, ND and NE systems. Only the NA-system is well characterised; it consists of two antigens, NA1 and NA2, with a frequency of 53.9% and 92.7% respectively in the Northern European population. The frequency of the allelic *NA1* and *NA2* genes is 0.31 and 0.69 respectively. A murine monoclonal antibody against the NA1 antigen has been produced; with this antibody, the NA antigens have been localised on the neutrophilic low-affinity Fc-receptor (50–70 kDa).

Neutrophil-specific antigens may be involved in a number of disease processes. Allo-antibodies against these antigens may give rise to allo-immune neutropenia of the newborn and to transfusion reactions, such as chills and fever and sometimes respiratory distress syndrome. Auto-antibodies against the neutrophil-specific antigens have been found in idiopathic neutropenia, particularly in infants.

For the detection of antibodies against neutrophil antigens two methods have been generally applied, the leucocyte or neutrophil agglutination test (LAT or NAT) and the neutrophil immunofluorescence test (NIFT), also called the granulocyte immunofluorescence test (GIFT).

The NIFT appears to be the most specific and sensitive test available at present. This test can also be used to determine the immunochemical nature of neutrophil antibodies, and their complement-fixing ability. On the other hand, the LAT or NAT is less sensitive and specific, because many neutrophil antibodies are not agglutinins and because of the inherent tendency of leucocytes or neutrophils to adhere to each other. This test is therefore mainly used for typing of neutrophil antigens, with specific antisera, selected for use by this method. But the NIFT is also suitable for this purpose, provided that the typing sera are specific in this assay.

Another test used in neutrophil serology is the neutrophil cytotoxicity test, mostly the double colour fluorescence modification of this method, with fluorescent diacetate and ethidium bromide. However, this test is not suitable for routine investigations because many neutrophil antibodies are non-cytotoxic (non-complement-fixing). Moreover, ill-defined antibodies of unclear nature (such as cold cytotoxins) are often detected in this test.

Principle

Leucocyte- or neutrophil-agglutination test (LAT or NAT)

This test detects the effect of antibody binding indirectly, via the induction of agglutination. Not only IgM but also IgG antibodies may induce agglutination. IgG antibody-mediated agglutination is an active process, which occurs optimally at 37°C; sensitised neutrophils adhere to each other via their Fc receptors (opsonic auto-adherence). The test is done in the presence of EDTA, in order to prevent leucocyte aggregation induced via complement activation by complement-binding leucocyte antibodies or by immune complexes.

Mostly whole leucocyte suspensions are used routinely, but isolated neutrophils may be used as well.

The test detects not only agglutinating neutrophil-specific antibodies but agglutinating HLA-antibodies as well, especially when whole leucocyte suspensions are used. Immune complexes (such as those present in sera from patients with rheumatoid arthritis) and immuno-globulin aggregates (in stored sera) may also be detected in this assay. Bacterial contamination (infected sera) will also lead to agglutination.

Neutrophil- or granulocyte-immunofluorescence test (NIFT or GIFT)

In this test the binding of antibodies to isolated neutrophils is detected directly, with FITC-labelled-antiglobulin reagents. Fluorescence is either read with an UV-microscope or measured in a laser flow-cytofluorometer. Because of the inherent nature of viable neutrophils to actively bind and internalise serum immunoglobulins, the neutrophils must be rendered inactive by fixation in 1% paraformaldehyde. For the same reason pepsin-digested F(ab')2 antiglobulin reagents should be used, in order to avoid binding to the neutrophil Fc-receptors.

For preliminary antibody screening, a FITC-labelled-anti-immunoglobulin reagent is used. For further investigations into the immunochemical characteristics of neutrophil antibodies, antiglobulin sera specific for different immunoglobulin classes, subclasses, light chain types and complement components are used.

The antiglobulin reagents are still mostly polyclonal antisera of rabbit or goat origin, but mouse monoclonal antibodies may prove to be a superior alternative. Not only neutrophil antibodies, but also immune complexes and immunoglobulin-aggregates are detected in the NIFT, especially when incubation is performed at temperatures below 37°C.

Equipment

○ Glass or plastic tubes (45 × 7 mm, 110 × 15 mm, 150 × 15 mm).
○ Pasteur pipettes, Hamilton syringes, jet pipette, automatic pipette (Gilson, Eppendorf).
○ Polystyrene (U-bottom) microplates (Greiner, Dynatech, Falcon).
○ Microplate washer.
○ Glass slides and coverslips.
○ Centrifuges.
○ Incubator.
○ Refrigerator.
○ Freezer.
○ Electronic cell counter.
○ Inverted and fluorescence microscopes (e.g. Leitz or Zeiss).
○ Laser flow cytofluorometer (such as the Epics-C).

Reagents

- EDTA solution (1.5 mol/l; 5% w/v).
- Phosphate-buffered saline (PBS) (NaCl 1.4 mol/l, Na_2HPO_4 + NaH_2PO_4, 0.1 mol/l, pH 7.2–7.4).
- PBS-BSA (PBS with 0.2% w/v bovine serum albumin).
- Dextran solution (Organon Technica) (5% w/v, average M.Wt. 180 000, in PBS) or methyl cellulose solution (Sigma) (1% w/v in PBS, dissolved for 24 h at 4°C).
- Ficoll-Isopaque (s.d. 1.077 g/cm³): Ficoll (Pharmacia). M.Wt. 400 000, 9.556 g in 130.4 ml distilled water. Add 1 ampoule Isopaque (Nyegaard) or Histopaque (Sigma) to 20 ml Ficoll solution.
- NH_4Cl solution (NH_4Cl 1.55 mol/l, $KHCO_3$ 0.1 mol/l, Na_2EDTA 0.1 M mol/l, pH 3 at 0°C).
- Paraformaldehyde stock solution (4% w/v): paraformaldehyde (Merck) dissolved at 70°C, cleared by adding 0.1 mol/l NaOH to pH of 11, millipore-filtered and stored at 4°C in the dark in an aluminium foil-wrapped bottle.
- Paraformaldehyde working solution (1% w/v): stock solution diluted 1:4 in PBS, pH 7.2–7.4 with 0.1 mol/l HCl and stored at 4°C in the dark.
- Mineral oil (Medinol 195).
- Glycerol-PBS: 3 parts of glycerol 85% v/v and 1 part of PBS.
- Normal AB serum: mixture of sera from 10 non-transfused male blood group AB donors, stored at −20°C, in small aliquots.
- Positive control sera: serum with multiple HLA antibodies from a polytransfused patient or serum with anti-NA_1 allo-antibodies with a titre of at least 32, stored at −20°C in small aliquots.
- Antiglobulin sera: FITC-labelled F(ab')$_2$ fragments of rabbit or goat IgG antibodies against Ig, complement, IgG, IgM and IgA (Central Laboratory of the Netherlands Red Cross Blood Transfusion Service).

Method

Serum preparation

The patient's blood is allowed to clot at room temperature and centrifuged. The serum is pipetted off and stored in small aliquots of 0.5–1 ml at −70° to −80°C. Before use the sera are clarified by high-speed centrifugation.

Leucocyte suspension

1. Donor blood anticoagulated with Na_2 EDTA (1 part of EDTA 5% w/v and 9 parts of blood) is used. To sediment the red cells, mix 10 ml of blood with 2.5 ml of dextran (5% w/v) or methyl cellulose solution (1% w/v) and incubate for 20 minutes at room temperature, at a 45° angle, in a test tube (150 × 15 mm). Collect the leucocyte-rich plasma (LRP) into a clean tube.

2. Centrifuge the LRP for 5 minutes at 120 g. Collect the platelet-rich plasma (PRP) into another tube and centrifuge it for 15 minutes at 2000 g. Collect the platelet-poor plasma (PPP) and store it for later use.

3. To lyse the red cells, add 2 ml NH_4Cl solution to the leucocyte-erythrocyte sediment and incubate for 5 minutes on melting ice. Centrifuge for 10 minutes at 500 g. Remove the supernatant, wash the leucocyte sediment twice with PBS-EDTA-BSA (centrifuge each time for 10 min at 500 g).

4. Resuspend the leucocytes in the donor's own PPP. Count the number of leucocytes in an electronic cell counter. Adjust the concentration to 10×10^9 leucocytes/l. Store the leucocyte suspension (LRP) at 4°C until use.

Neutrophil suspension

Distribute the LRP carefully into 2 tubes (110 × 15 mm) on top of 2.5 ml of Ficoll-Isopaque solution. Centrifuge 20 minutes at 500 g. Remove sequentially the plasma layer, the ring fraction (which contains lymphocytes and monocytes) and the Ficoll-Isopaque layer. The bottom layers, i.e. the sediment (containing red cells and neutrophils) of the 2 tubes are then pooled in another tube, the red cells lysed and the neutrophils washed and resuspended as described for the leucocytes. Centrifugation is for 5 minutes at 120 g.

Neutrophil fixation for immunofluorescence

The washed neutrophils are resuspended in 2 ml of 1% paraformaldehyde in PBS and incubated for 5 minutes at room temperature, after which PBS-BSA is added.

The fixed cells are washed once in PBS-BSA (centrifugation 5 min at 200 g) and resuspended in this solution to a concentration of 10×10^9 neutrophils/l. The suspension is stored at 4°C until use.

The tests

Leucocyte agglutination test (micro-method).

1. A microplate is filled with mineral oil (15 μl per well).

2. Under the oil 2 μl of serum are injected in each well, or a 1 in 4 dilution thereof in PBS-EDTA, with a Hamilton syringe, followed by 2 μl of the leucocyte suspension.

3. The trays are covered and incubated for $1\frac{3}{4}$ hours at 37°C. After removal of the cover, agglutination is read under an inverted microscope.

4. A negative and a positive control serum are always tested in parallel.

Neutrophil agglutination test.

This test is performed in exactly the same way, but with a suspension of purified neutrophils.

Neutrophil immunofluorescence test (macro method).

1. 50 μl of serum, or dilutions thereof in PBS-BSA, are mixed with 50 μl of suspension of fixed neutrophils in a tube (45 × 7 mm). The mixture is incubated for 30 minutes at 37°C.

2. For the direct test this first incubation step is not necessary.

3. The cells are washed three times in PBS-BSA (centrifugation 5 min at 300 g) and 50 μl of an optimally diluted FITC-labelled antiglobulin reagent (vide infra) is added to the sediment. The mixture is incubated for 30 minutes at room temperature in the dark.

4. The cells are washed twice in PBS-BSA, the sediment is resuspended in 50 μl of glycerol-PBS, pipetted onto a slide and covered with a coverslip.

5. Immunofluorescence is read under a fluorescence microscope, equipped with water-lenses. It can also be measured in a laser flow fluorocytometer.

6. A negative and a positive control serum are always tested simultaneously.

Neutrophil immunofluorescence (micro-method).

This test is performed in a similar way to the macro-method, except that microplates are used, together with suitably adapted equipment for pipetting, washing and centrifuging.

1. 20 μl of serum, or dilutions thereof, and 20 μl of suspension of fixed neutrophils are pipetted into each well, mixed and incubated for 30 minutes at 37°C.

2. The cells are washed three times with PBS-BSA, using an automatic pipette. Centrifugation is for 1 minute at 200 g, followed by decanting by inversion, shaking and blotting.

3. Incubate the cells with 20 μl of diluted FITC-

labelled antiglobulin reagent for 30 minutes at room temperature in the dark.

4. Wash again three times, resuspend in 20 μl of glycerol-PBS and transfer the cells to a slide, as above.

Determination of the optimal dilution of an FITC-labelled antiglobulin reagent for neutrophil immunofluorescence. This is tested in a chessboard titration.

1. Two-fold dilutions (1 in 2 to 1 in 512) of the antiglobulin reagent are prepared in PBS-BSA.

2. Two-fold dilution (1 in 1 to 1 in 64) of a positive control serum are prepared in PBS-BSA.

3. The serum dilutions, as well as a negative control serum and a PBS control, are incubated with the suspension of fixed neutrophils, washed and incubated with the different antiglobulin reagent dilutions, in amounts and under conditions as described above.

4. The results are read under the fluorescence microscope.

5. The optimal reagent dilution is that which produces the strongest fluorescence with the antiserum and no fluorescence with the negative control serum and the PBS control.

Index